Pathology: A Case-Based Approach

Pathology: A Case-Based Approach

Editor: Hans Affleck

FOSTER ACADEMICS

www.fosteracademics.com

www.fosteracademics.com

FOSTER ACADEMICS

Cataloging-in-Publication Data

Pathology : a case-based approach / edited by Hans Affleck.
p. cm.
Includes bibliographical references and index.
ISBN 978-1-63242-562-1
1. Pathology. 2. Pathology--Case studies. I. Affleck, Hans.
RB112 .P38 2018
616.07--dc23

Foster Academics,
118-35 Queens Blvd., Suite 400,
Forest Hills, NY 11375, USA

ISBN 978-1-63242-562-1 (Hardback)

Printed and bound in China.

Contents

Preface

The main aim of this book is to educate learners and enhance their research focus by presenting diverse topics covering this vast field. This is an advanced book which compiles significant studies by distinguished experts in the area of analysis. This book addresses successive solutions to the challenges arising in the area of application, along with it; the book provides scope for future developments.

Pathology as a branch of medical science refers to the diagnosis and study of diseases and illnesses in general. It uses cells, body fluids and tissues as samples for diagnosing a disease. Pathology has many sub-fields like surgical pathology, clinical pathology, molecular pathology, etc. This book provides comprehensive insights into the field of pathology. It elucidates the various concepts and techniques used in this area. The objective of the book is to give a general view of the different areas of pathology, and its applications. It will prove to be immensely beneficial to students and researchers in this area.

It was a great honour to edit this book, though there were challenges, as it involved a lot of communication and networking between me and the editorial team. However, the end result was this all-inclusive book covering diverse themes in the field.

Finally, it is important to acknowledge the efforts of the contributors for their excellent chapters, through which a wide variety of issues have been addressed. I would also like to thank my colleagues for their valuable feedback during the making of this book.

Editor

1

Correlation of CK5 and EGFR with Clinicopathological Profile of Triple-Negative Breast Cancer

Neelam Sood[1] and Jitendra Singh Nigam[2]

[1] *Department of Pathology, Deen Dayal Upadhyay Hospital, Hari Nagar, New Delhi 110066, India*
[2] *Department of Pathology, Saraswathi Institute of Medical Sciences, Anwarpur, Hapur, Uttar Pradesh 245304, India*

Correspondence should be addressed to Jitendra Singh Nigam; nigamjs@gmail.com

Academic Editor: Luigi M. Terracciano

Purpose. Triple-negative breast cancer (TNBC) is defined by the loss of expression of ER, PR, and Her2*neu* expressions. The aim of this study was to examine the expression of the EGFR, CK5, and Ki-67 among triple-negative breast cancer cases and to correlate the expression of the basal markers with the clinicopathological prognostic parameters. *Materials and Methods.* Thirty-six female patients with TNBC based on ER, PR, and the HER2*neu* negativities were studied by immunohistochemistry for EGFR, CK5, and Ki-67 expression. Statistical analysis was done using the SPSS software version 20. *Results.* The mean and median ages were 45.18 years and 46.70 years, respectively. Infiltrating ductal carcinoma NOS was the predominant histopathological type (29/36 [80.6%]). The commonest histological grade was grade 2 (17/36 [47.2%]). Tumour necrosis was seen in 16/36 (44.4%) patients. Infiltrative margins were shown in 69.44% (25/36) cases. Ki-67 was positive in 80.56% (29/36) cases, 61.11% (22/36) were CK5-positive, and 86.11% (31/36) were EGFR-positive. The only significant positive association observed was between the CK5 and histological grade ($P < 0.05$). *Conclusion.* CK5 shows a statistically significantly correlation with TNBC histological grade. The majority of the specimens show EGFR expression. Therefore TNBCs could potentially benefit from EGFR-targeted therapeutic strategies.

1. Introduction

Triple-negative breast cancer (TNBC) is defined by the loss of expression of estrogen receptor (ER), progesterone receptor (PR), and human epidermal growth factor 2 (Her2*neu*) expressions and associated with biological aggressiveness and poor prognosis and two subtypes, basal and nonbasal, have been described [1]. TNBC and basal type are not synonymous but basal type has similar behavior as TNBC [2]. Basal type was defined as CK5-/6-positive and/or EGFR-positive, and nonbasal type was defined as having no expression of these two markers. Ki-67 is another marker being studied for its implication if any [1]. Bertucci et al. assessed the degrees of correlation and of homogeneity of the TN phenotype (IHC-based definition) and the basal subtype (gene expression-based definition) and observed that tumour classified as TNBC is defined by gene expression profile (GEP) as 71.51% basal (123/172 cases) and 28.49% nonbasal (49/172 cases). Conversely tumors were defined as basal by their gene expression profile and included 76.88% (123/160) TN and 23.12% (37/160) non-TN [3]. Basal type TNBC has high histological grade, p53 mutation, usually expresses basal cytokeratin (CK5/6, CK14, and CK17), epidermal growth factor receptor (EGFR) overexpression, significantly associated with Ki-67 labelling index, p53 expression, and BRCA1 expression, and showed a shorter overall survival than nonbasal type; however, GEP is considered to be the gold standard for basal type TNBC identification [4]. Rao et al. observed that 74% of TNBC showed the expression of the EGFR and/or CK5/6 [5]. CK5/6 and/or EGFR expressing breast tumors showed poorer prognosis in the longer term, and screening for those basal markers is important in determining prognosis and therapeutic strategies in TNBC. Therefore the basal cytokeratins and EGFR in immunohistochemical panel can be used to identify basal-like TNBC [4, 6]. TNBC rates are higher in women of African or Hispanic ancestry, premenopausal and younger age, women with early menarche, higher parity, younger age at full term pregnancy, shorter duration of breast feeding, higher body mass index, and higher waist to hip ratio especially among premenopausal patients [7].

2. Materials and Methods

The present study was done in DDU Hospital, Hari Nagar, New Delhi, during 2010 to 2013 and includes 36 female patients with TNBC based on the ER, PR, and the Her2*neu* negativities. Detailed clinical histories were taken and clinical examinations were done after taking their informed consents. The specimens were processed and fixed in 10% formalin and were examined grossly. Paraffin embedded sections were stained with the haematoxylin and eosin stain. The tumours were classified and graded according to the Nottingham modification of the Scarff-Bloom-Richardson system. The pathological variables were evaluated and pTNM staging was done.

The tissue sections were used for all the immunohistochemical analyses (ER, PR, Her2*neu*, EGFR, CK5, and Ki-67). The antibody clones which were used were for the estrogen receptor (BioGenex: Species mouse, clone 1D5, Isotype IgG1/kappa), the progesterone receptor (BioGenex: Species rabbit, clone SP2, Isotype rabbit IgG1), Her2*neu* (Diagnostic BioSystems: Species rabbit, clone BV5, Isotype IgG), EGFR (Diagnostic BioSystems: Species rabbit, clone SP9, Isotype IgG1/kappa), CK5 (BioGenex: Species rabbit, clone EPR1600Y, Isotype IgG), and Ki-67 (BioGenex: Species mouse, clone Ki-88, Isotype IgG1/kappa). All antibodies are ready to use. After bringing the section to water, antigen retrieval was done by boiling the section in either citrate buffer (pH 6, for CK5/6, Her2*neu*, and Ki-67) or EDTA buffer (pH 9, for ER, PR). For EGFR, antigen retrieval was done by heat induced epitope retrieval. Tissue controls were used for IHC assays. The section was washed with deionized water for 2 to 3 minutes followed by peroxide blocking for 30 minutes using 4% hydrogen peroxide in methanol; then the section was washed by Tris buffer (pH 7.5) for 2 to 3 minutes. Background blocking was done by horseradish peroxidase (HRP) for 10 minutes followed by primary antibody overnight. Next day wash with Tris buffer for 2 to 3 minutes was followed by secondary antibody (Biotin) for 30 minutes; then again wash with Tris buffer and tertiary antibody (Streptavidin) was applied for 30 minutes. Wash with Tris buffer twice and D.A.B. was applied for 10 to 15 minutes and reaction was stopped by using distilled water. Counterstain Hematoxylin was applied for 2 minutes and washed with distilled water.

The ER and PR scores were based on the proportions and the intensities of the stained nuclei, Her2*neu* score was based on the intensities and the proportions of the cells which showed membrane staining, cytokeratin 5 was scored as positive if cells showed any weak or strong cytoplasmic and/or membranous staining, EGFR was scored as positive if more than 1% of the tumour cells showed membrane reactivities, and Ki-67 positivity was quantified as the 10% percent of the positive nuclear staining of the tumour cells [5]. The data were entered and analyzed by using SPSS. The chi-square test was used to compare the association of the expressions of EGFR and CK5 and clinic-pathological characteristics of the tumours. The results were considered as statistically significant if the P value was <0.05.

Table 1: Clinicopathological variables.

Clinicopathological variables	
Age (years)	
Mean	45.18
Tumor size (cm)	
≤2 cm	13
2–5 cm	18
>5 cm	5
Histopathological diagnosis	
IDC, NOS	29
Mucinous carcinoma	2
Metaplastic carcinoma	1
Medullary carcinoma	3
Mixed ductal-lobular carcinoma	1
Tumor necrosis	
Present	16
Absent	20
Margin	
Infiltrative	25
Pushing margin	11
Lymphocytic infiltrate	
Present	23
Absent	13
Tumor grade	
Grade I	5
Grade II	17
Grade III	14
Lymph node metastases	
Absent	12
1 to 3	14
>4	10
Tumour stage	
Stage I	5
Stage II	16
Stage III	13
Stage IV	2
Ki-67	
Positive	29
Negative	7
Immunohistochemical panel	
CK5+ EGFR+	22
CK5+ EGFR−	5
CK5− EGFR+	9
CK5− EGFR−	Nil

3. Results

A total of 36 cases of infiltrating TNBC were included. The age of patients was ranged from 19 to 78 years with

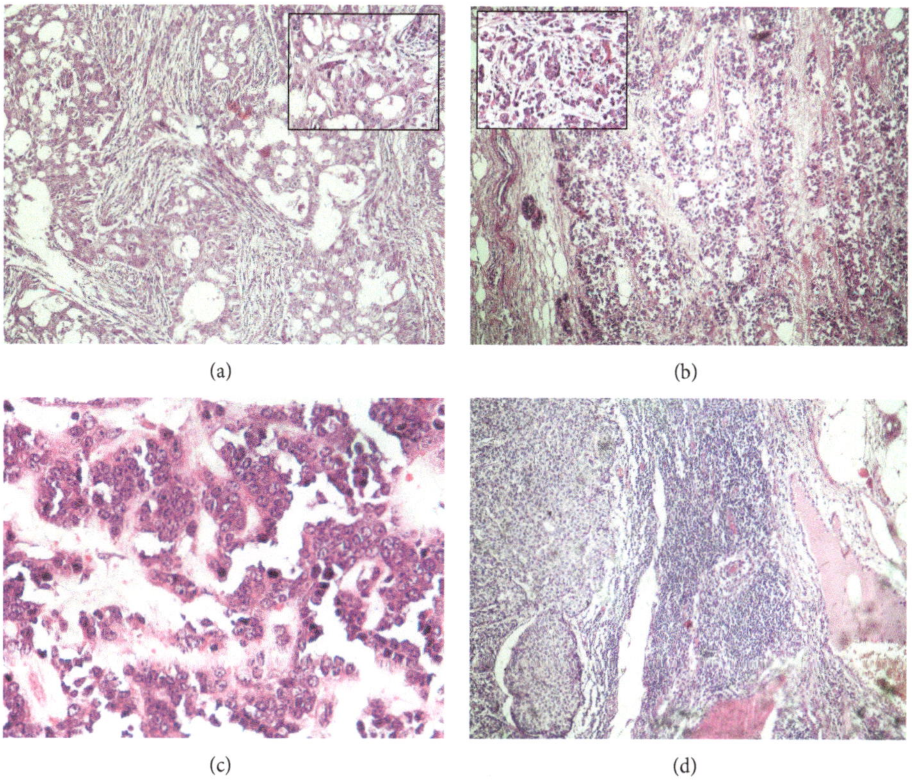

FIGURE 1: (a) Histological grade 1: tumour with tubular differentiation, regular outlines, and uniform nuclear chromatin (H&E ×100, Inset-H&E ×400). (b) Histologic grade II: tumours with cords, islands with tubular differentiation, open vesicular nuclei, and visible nucleoli (H&E ×100, Inset-H&E ×400). (c) Histologic grade III: infiltrative islands, with minimal tubular differentiation, marked variability in size and shape, open vesicular nuclei, and visible nucleoli (H&E ×400). (d) Invasive breast carcinoma involving lymph node (H&E ×400).

mean age of 45.18 years and median age of 46.7 years. Infiltrating ductal carcinoma NOS was the predominant histopathological type (80.56%, 29/36). In a majority of the patients, the tumour size was between 2.1 and 5 cm (50%, 18/36) followed by <2 cm (36.11%, 13/36). The commonest histological grade was grade 2 (47.22%, 17/36) followed by grade 3 (38.89%, 14/36) and grade 1 (13.89%, 5/36) (Figure 1). In grade 1 tumours, 2 cases show adenoid cystic pattern and 3 cases showed ductal carcinoma in situ (DCIS). In grade 2, 14 cases were associated with infiltrative borders, 3 cases were associated with DCIS, and 1 case was associated with intraductal papillomatous. In grade 3, 2 cases were associated with atypical medullary features, 1 case was associated with metaplastic carcinoma with osteoclastic giant cells, 1 case was associated with lobular carcinoma, and 2 cases were associated with DICS. Four cases of grade 3 and two cases of grade 2 tumours showed recurrence or metastasis within 5 years. Three cases of grade 3 and 2 cases of grade 2 died within 5 five years of surgery. Three cases of grade 1, 3 cases of grade 2, and 1 case of grade 3 were survived without any recurrences or metastasis. The rest of the cases were lost for follow-up. The commonest histological pTMN stage was stage II (44.44%, 16/36) followed by stage III (36.11%, 13/36) and stage I (13.89%, 13/36). The tumour necrosis was seen in 44.44% patients. Lymphocytic infiltrates were observed in 63.89% patients. 69.44% (25/36) cases showed infiltrative margins and 30.56% (11/36) cases showed pushing tumour margins. Ki-67 was positive in 80.56% (29/36) (Table 1). Out of the 36 TNBC cases, 61.11% (22/36) were CK5-positive and 86.11% (31/36) were EGFR-positive Figure 2. We studied the association between the CK5 and EGFR expression with the clinicopathological prognostic parameters. A significant positive association was observed between the histological grade and CK5 but not with EGFR (Table 2).

4. Discussion

Breast cancer is a biologically heterogeneous disease and clinical outcomes of patients with the same diagnostic and clinical prognostic profiles are markedly different possibly due to molecularly distinct diseases into group into classes based mainly on morphology [8]. Breast cancers can be divided into five molecular subtypes which are two ER positive types (luminal A and luminal B) and three ER negative types (HER-2 expressing, basal-like, and normal breast-like) and have distinct clinical features, with markedly differing prognosis and clinical outcomes [8]. Nielsen et al. studied the immunohistochemical profile for breast basal-like tumors for the protein patterns that are characteristic of this subtype and examined the significance of these protein patterns using tissue microarrays and evaluated the prognostic

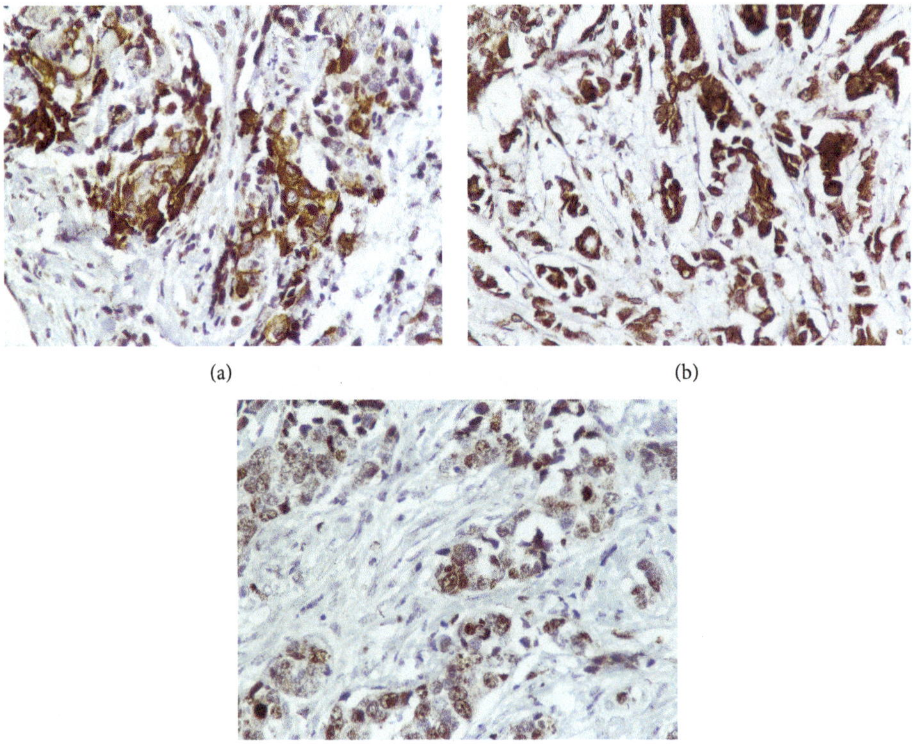

(a) (b) (c)

FIGURE 2: (a) Cytokeratin 5 positivity in tumour cells. (b) EGFR positivity in tumour cells. (c) Ki-67 positivity in tumour cells.

significance of these findings [9]. They concluded that a panel of four antibodies (ER, HER1, HER2, and cytokeratin 5/6) can accurately identify basal-like tumors using standard available clinical tools and shows high specificity [9]. In the present study, the triple-negative breast cancer was correlated with age, tumour size, histolopathological type, tumour necrosis, tumour margin, lymphocytic infiltrate, lymph node status, tumour grades, tumour stages, and Ki-67. The commonest age group in the present study was ≤40 years (14/36) followed by >50 years (12/36); however, Tan et al. observed TNBC common in age >40 years and Rao et al. observed that mean age of TNBC is 46.8 years [5, 10]. In the present study CK5 and EGFR do not show significant correlation with age as observed by other studies [1, 5]. The commonest tumour size was ranged from 2 to 5 cm (18/36) and did not significantly correlate with basal markers as observed by other workers [1, 5, 10]. In the present study, the majority of the TNBCs were grade 2 (17/36) instead of grade 3 (10/36) but significant correlation with CK5 was noted unlike observation by Rao et al. where grade 3 was the commonest grade and was statistically not significantly correlated [5]. This could be possibly due to higher associated DCIS pattern and infiltrative margins in such cases. Low-grade TNBCs have also been observed by other too as observed in the present study [4]. The important histologic basal-like carcinomas are usually high histologic grade, pushing, noninfiltrative borders, and large zones of geographic or comedo-type necrosis; stromal lymphocytic infiltrates; scant stromal content; lack of tubule formations; marked cellular pleomorphism; high nuclear-cytoplasmic ratios; vesicular chromatin; prominent nucleoli; high mitotic indices; and frequent apoptotic cells, presence of metaplastic elements, and glomeruloid microvascular proliferation as also seen in the present study [4]. Infiltrative margins were more commonly observed than pushing margins in the present study; however, margins were statistically not significant which are also corroborated with results of other studies [5, 11]. Lymphocytic infiltrates and necrosis were present in 23 and 16 cases, respectively, and were statistically not significantly correlated with CK5 and EGFR. Other workers also observed lymphoid infiltrate which is statistically not significantly correlated with basal markers as in the present study; however necrosis shows statistically significant correlation [1, 5]. In the present study lymph node involvements were observed in 24 cases and were statistically not significantly correlated with CK5 and EGFR. Lymph node involvement is also observed by other studies [1, 5, 11] and is statistically not significantly correlated with basal markers [5]. In the present study, the commonest histological pTMN stage was stage II followed by stage III and stage I and histological stages were not significantly correlated with CK5 and EGFR. Kutomi et al. also observed that stage II is the commonest pTNM stage followed by stage I and stage III. Ki-67 was positive in 29 cases and was statistically not significantly correlated with basal markers similar to Rao et al. findings [5]. Foulkes et al. observed that TNBC which also expresses CK5/6, EGFR, or

Table 2: Correlation of EGFR and CK5 with clinicopathological variables.

(a)

Prognostic parameters	EGFR Positive	EGFR Negative	*P* value	CK5 Positive	CK5 Negative	*P* value
Age						
≤40	13	1		7	7	
41–50	8	2	>0.05	6	4	>0.05
>50	10	2		9	3	
Tumor size (cm)						
≤2	11	2		9	4	
2.1–5	15	3	>0.05	11	7	>0.05
>5	5	0		2	3	
Histopathological diagnosis						
IDC, NOS	24	5		17	12	
Mucinous carcinoma	2	0		1	1	
Metaplastic carcinoma	1	0	>0.05	1	0	>0.05
Medullary carcinoma	3	0		3	0	
Mixed ductal-lobular carcinoma	1	0		0	1	
Tumour grades						
Grade I	4	1		2	3	
Grade II	17	0	>0.05	8	9	**0.052**
Grade III	10	4		12	2	

(b)

Prognostic parameters	EGFR		*P* value	CK5/6		*P* value
Tumour stage						
Stage I	5	0		2	3	
Stage II	12	4	>0.05	11	5	>0.05
Stage III	12	1		7	6	
Stage IV	2	0		2	0	
Margins						
Infiltrative margin	22	3	>0.05	13	12	>0.05
Pushing margin	9	2		9	2	
Necrosis						
Present	12	4	>0.05	11	5	>0.05
Absent	19	1		11	9	
Infiltrate						
Present	20	3	>0.05	15	8	>0.05
Absent	11	2		7	6	
Lymph node metastases						
Absent	11	1		6	6	
1 to 3	11	3	>0.05	11	3	>0.05
>4	9	1		5	5	
Ki-67						
Positive	25	4	>0.05	16	13	>0.05
Negative	6	1		6	1	

both may have a worse outcome than the TNBCs that are negative for both of these markers and the overexpression of EGFR is more common in the TNBCs than in other subtypes of breast cancer, and cetuximab, which is targeted against EGFR, is being further studied in combination with carboplatin [12]. To conclude, among the clinic-pathological factors in the present study, age, tumour size, histological type, tumour stage, tumour margin, presence of lymphoid infiltrate and necrosis, lymph node metastasis, and Ki-67 positivity did not show statistically significantly correlation with CK5 and EGFR; however tumour grade shows statistically significantly correlation with CK5 only but not with EGFR. TNBCs are heterogeneous group of breast tumours that possess distinctive pathological and clinical features and TNBC and basal-like breast carcinoma should not be used as synonymous. By using CK5 and EGFR, the basal-like breast carcinoma can be identified and the majority of the TNBC patients show EGFR expression; however CK5 shows the statistically significantly correlation with histological grade. Therefore basal-like breast cancers could potentially benefit from EGFR-targeted therapeutic strategies.

Conflict of Interests

The authors declare that there is no conflict of interests regarding the publication of this paper.

References

[1] G. Kutomi, T. Ohmura, Y. Suzukil et al., "Clinicopathological characteristics of basal type breast cancer in triple-negative breast cancer," *Journal of Cancer Therapy*, vol. 3, pp. 836–840, 2012.

[2] R. Rouzier, C. M. Perou, W. F. Symmans et al., "Breast cancer molecular subtypes respond differently to preoperative chemotherapy," *Clinical Cancer Research*, vol. 11, no. 16, pp. 5678–5685, 2005.

[3] F. Bertucci, P. Finetti, N. Cervera et al., "How basal are triple-negative breast cancers?" *International Journal of Cancer*, vol. 123, no. 1, pp. 236–240, 2008.

[4] E. Rakha and J. S. Reis-Filho, "Basal-like breast carcinoma: from expression profiling to routine practice," *Archives of Pathology & Laboratory Medicine*, vol. 133, no. 6, pp. 860–867, 2009.

[5] C. Rao, J. Shetty, and H. L. Kishan Prasad, "Immunohistochemical profile and morphology in triple—negative breast cancers," *Journal of Clinical and Diagnostic Research*, vol. 7, no. 7, pp. 1361–1365, 2013.

[6] L. M. Sutton, J. S. Han, K. H. Molberg et al., "Intratumoral expression level of epidermal growth factor receptor and cytokeratin 5/6 is significantly associated with nodal and distant metastases in patients with basal-like triple-negative breast carcinoma," *American Journal of Clinical Pathology*, vol. 134, no. 5, pp. 782–787, 2010.

[7] K. Aysola, A. Desai, C. Welch et al., "Triple negative breast cancer—an overview," *Hereditary Genetics*, vol. S2, p. 001, 2013.

[8] K. Munjal, A. Ambaye, M. F. Evans, J. Mitchell, S. Nandedkar, and K. Cooper, "Immunohistochemical analysis of ER, PR, Her2 and CK5/6 in infiltrative breast carcinomas in indian patients," *Asian Pacific Journal of Cancer Prevention*, vol. 10, no. 5, pp. 773–778, 2009.

[9] T. O. Nielsen, F. D. Hsu, K. Jensen et al., "Immunohistochemical and clinical characterization of the basal-like subtype of invasive breast carcinoma," *Clinical Cancer Research*, vol. 10, no. 16, pp. 5367–5374, 2004.

[10] G. H. Tan, N. A. Taib, W. Y. Choo, S. H. Teo, and C. H. Yip, "Clinical characteristics of triple-negative breast cancer: experience in an Asian developing country," *Asian Pacific Journal of Cancer Prevention*, vol. 10, no. 3, pp. 395–398, 2009.

[11] A. A. Thike, J. Iqbal, P. Y. Cheok et al., "Triple negative breast cancer: outcome correlation with immunohistochemical detection of basal markers," *American Journal of Surgical Pathology*, vol. 34, no. 7, pp. 956–964, 2010.

[12] W. D. Foulkes, I. E. Smith, and J. S. Reis-Filho, "Triple-negative breast cancer," *The New England Journal of Medicine*, vol. 363, no. 20, pp. 1938–1948, 2010.

2

A Prospective Study of Soft Tissue Tumors Histocytopathology Correlation

Priyanka Bhatia Soni,[1] Anand Kumar Verma,[2] Raj Kumar Chandoke,[2] and Jitendra Singh Nigam[3]

[1] *Department of Pathology, Deen Dayal Upadhyay Hospital, Hari Nagar, New Delhi 110066, India*
[2] *Department of Pathology, Employees' State Insurance Scheme of India (ESI) Hospital, Basaidarapur, New Delhi 110015, India*
[3] *Department of Pathology, Saraswathi Institute of Medical Sciences, Hapur, Uttar Pradesh 245304, India*

Correspondence should be addressed to Raj Kumar Chandoke; drchandoke@gmail.com

Academic Editor: Oscar W. Cummings

Background. Soft tissue tumors are defined as nonepithelial extraskeletal tissue of the body exclusive of the reticuloendothelial system, glia, and supporting tissue of various parenchymal organs. The absence of recognizable tissue architectural patterns in cytological preparation makes diagnosis by FNAC more difficult. *Aims.* To assess the utility of FNAC in diagnosing soft tissue tumors and to determine their patterns compared with with the respective histopathology results. *Materials and Methods.* 150 cases of soft tissue tumors were included in this study for cytologic and histologic correlation. FNAC air dried smears were stained with Giemsa stain and 95% ethanol fixed smears were stained with Papanicolaou stain. The smears were studied for cytological diagnosis and were categorized as benign, suspicious of malignancy, and malignant along with specific subtyping of the lesion. All diagnostic FNAC results were compared for diagnostic concordance using histology results as the "gold standard." *Results.* The sensitivity, specificity, positive predictive value, negative predictive value, and efficiency were 70%, 100%, 97.90%, 100%, and 98%, respectively. P value was <0.0001 which shows statistically extreme significant correlation. *Conclusion.* FNAC is a very important preliminary diagnostic tool in palpable soft tissue lumps with high degree of correlation with the final histopathology report.

1. Introduction

The field of soft tissue tumors (STT) is enormously vast, and yet as cytologically, relatively undiscovered. The rarity of primary tumors of soft tissue and large range of different types of tumors, the diagnosis and classification of soft tissue tumors become most difficult areas in surgical pathology and absence of recognizable tissue architectural patterns in cytological preparation makes diagnosis by fine needle aspiration cytology (FNAC) even more difficult [1]. STT are defined as mesenchymal proliferations that occur in the extraskeletal, nonepithelial tissues of the body, excluding the viscera, coverings of the brain, and lymphoreticular system, and benign tumors are more common than malignant counterparts (sarcomas) with a ratio of at least 100 : 1 [2]. FNAC is almost painless, easy to perform, safe, and cost effective, without any anesthesia, and acts as a useful diagnostic technique in the initial diagnosis of tumors [3]. FNAC is fairly specific and sensitive in the diagnoses of primary, recurrent, and metastatic STT [3]. For distinguishing benign from malignant soft tissue tumors FNAC was very useful except for exact categorization of tumors, where it was not so effective [4]. However FNAC as a preliminary diagnostic tool offers several advantages as it can provide a predictive diagnosis of a benign or malignant neoplasm. In benign neoplasm, surgery can be avoided in the patients who are of poor surgical risk, and in malignant or recurrent cancers, FNAC allows the administration of a palliative treatment [5]. Present study was performed with the aim of assessing the utility of FNAC in diagnosing STT and determining their patterns compared with the respective histopathology results.

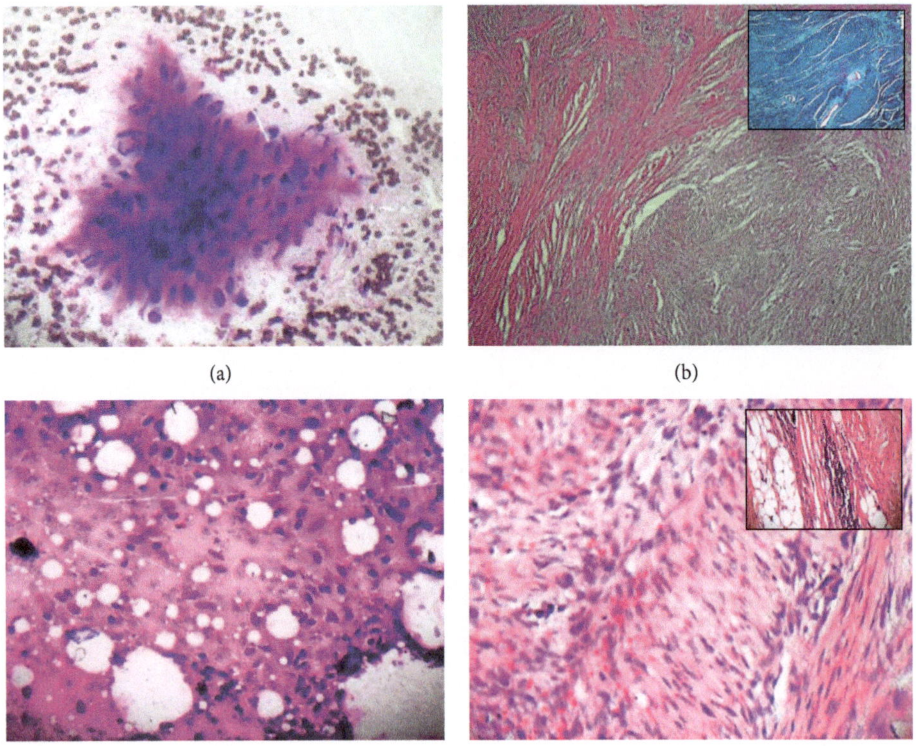

(a) (b) (c) (d)

FIGURE 1: (a) Benign mesenchymal lesion (nodular fasciitis) cytology: myxoid background matrix with dispersed fibroblasts (Giemsa ×100). (b) Nodular fasciitis: plump, randomly oriented spindle shaped cells surrounded by myxoid stroma with dominating fibrous component (inset, Masson Trichrome) (H&E ×200). (c) Benign mesenchymal lesion (extra-abdominal desmoid) cytology: loosely arranged fibroblast-like cells with ovoid nuclei and greyish blue cytoplasm (Giemsa ×100). (d) Extra-abdominal desmoids: cellular proliferation of bland spindle shaped cells arranged into ill-defined long fascicles along with infiltration of spindle cells (inset) between skeletal muscle and fat (H&E ×100).

2. Materials and Methods

The study was undertaken in the Department of Pathology, Employees' State Insurance Scheme of India (ESI) Hospital, Basaidarapur, New Delhi, from February 2009 to February 2011. A total of 150 cases of soft tissue tumors were included in this study for cytologic and histologic correlation. Patients with palpable soft tissue lumps of size more than 1 cm were included in this study. Complete clinical details, examination findings, and radiological investigations of all patients were studied. FNAC was done with 23/24G needle attached to 10 mL disposable plastic syringe and air dried smears were stained with Giemsa stain and 95% ethanol fixed smears were stained with Papanicolaou stain if required. The smears were studied for cytological details/diagnosis and were categorized as benign, suspicious of malignancy, and malignant along with specific subtyping of the lesion. The smears were also assessed for the principle pattern shown by the tumor cells. The excised tissue specimens of all the above cases were processed routinely and stained with hematoxylin and eosin and examined, while special stains/immunohistochemistry was performed as and when required. All diagnostic FNAC results from patients who underwent a subsequent surgical excision were compared for diagnostic concordance using histology results as the "gold standard." In addition FNAC results were analyzed for ability to recognize malignancy using statistical parameters of sensitivity, specificity, positive predictive value, and negative predictive value. Efficacy of FNAC in the diagnosis of soft tissue tumors was determined by calculating efficiency.

3. Results

On FNAC 95.3% (143/150) of patients had benign lesions, 3.34% (5/150) had malignant lesions, and 1.3% (2/150) were suspicious. The commonest age group for benign soft tissue lesions was between 2nd and 4th decades and for malignant lesions was between 4th and 5th decades of life. 54% (81/150) of cases with soft tissue tumors including both benign and malignant were males and 46% (69/150) were females. The commonest site of involvement of the benign tumors was upper extremities 43.5% (61/140) cases, followed by trunk and the head and neck region; however for malignant lesions it was the lower extremities followed by trunk region. On cytology the commonest benign lesion was lipoma in 48.2% (69/143) followed by vasoformative lesion (hemangioma) in 16% (23/143). All the benign lesions which could not be categorized into a particular group were labeled as BML (BML) 27.27% (39/143) (Figures 1 and 2).

The FNA of lipoma in all cases showed a uniform pattern consisting of fragments of adipose tissue composed of clusters

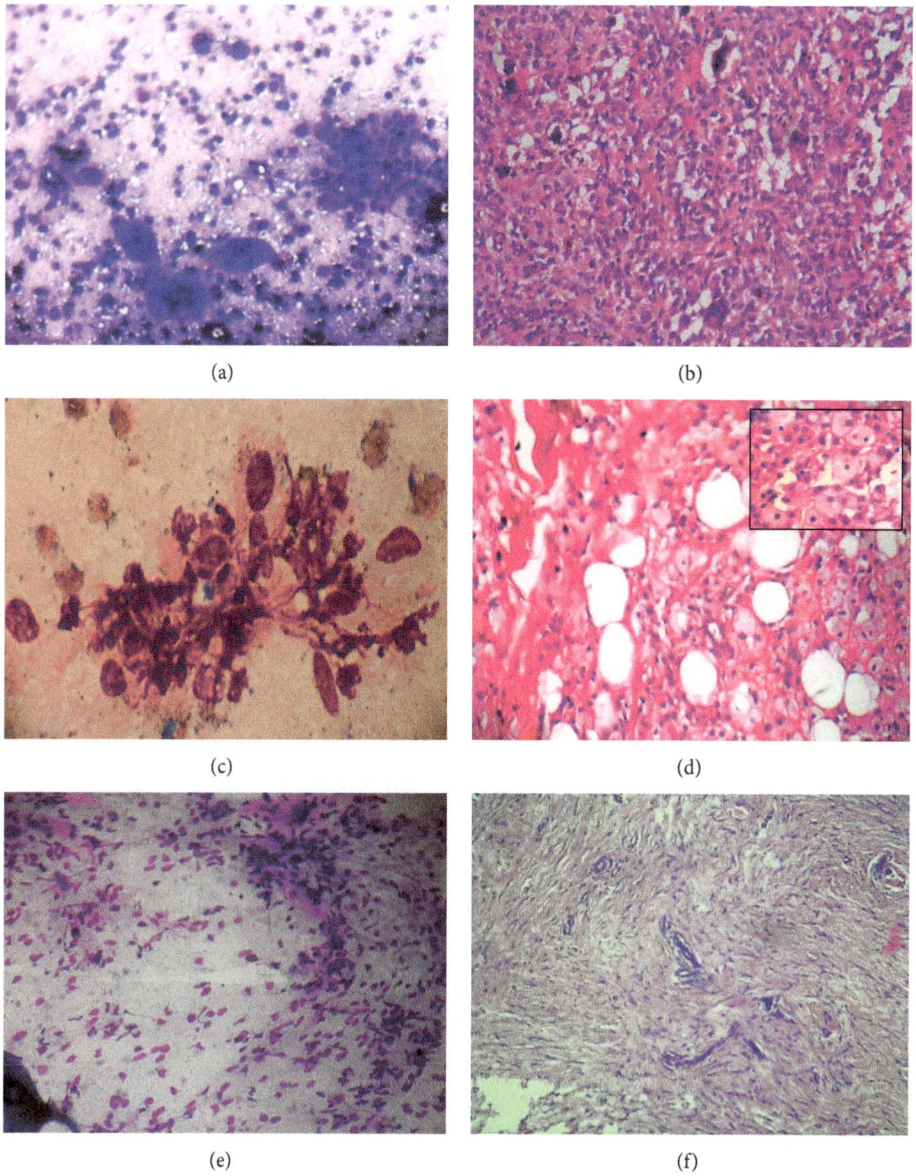

FIGURE 2: (a) Benign mesenchymal lesion (giant cell tumor of tendon sheath) cytology: dispersed rounded cells with rounded nuclei exhibiting moderate cellular pleomorphism and osteoclast like giant cells (Giemsa ×100). (b) Giant cell tumor of tendon sheath: mononuclear histiocytoid cells with variably prominent eosinophilic cytoplasm and scattered osteoclastic giant cells (H&E ×200). (c) Benign mesenchymal lesion (tuberous xanthoma) cytology: ovoid to plump benign spindle cell clusters (Giemsa ×400). (d) Tuberous xanthoma: large and small aggregates of foamy cells admixed with few nonfoamy cells and interspersed collagen bundles (H&E ×100, inset ×400). (e) Benign mesenchymal lesion (neurofibroma) cytology: highly cellular smears consisting of plump to tapered spindle shaped cells (Giemsa ×100). (f) Neurofibroma: arranged tumor cells nuclei which show a typical fascicular pattern of growth and serpentine shape (arrow) (H&E ×200).

of univacuolated fat cells and a small dark peripheral nucleus without evidence of atypia and confirmed on histology with few variants (Table 2). The FNAC of liposarcoma showed lipoblasts with significant mild to moderate pleomorphism, with focal areas showing adipocytic nuclear atypia, and the diagnosis of malignant adipocytic lesion was given.

The FNAC of nodular fasciitis cellular aspirates consisting of dispersed cells mixed with packed clusters of spindle shaped cells showing marked pleomorphism with fusiform nuclei, fine chromatin, and cytoplasmic processes. Few plump cells with ovoid, rounded, and irregular nuclei were also found, lying against myxoid background matrix. Two cases were accurately diagnosed on cytology.

FNAC of calcifying aponeurotic fibroma, collagenous fibroma, and fibroma of tendon sheath showed spindle cells lying dispersed and in packed clusters against clean background, showing predominantly a spindle cell pattern. None of them could be categorized broadly and were labelled as BML cytologically.

FNAC of extra-abdominal desmoids tumor showed good cell yield, with spindle cells lying singly and in loose clusters against a fatty and myxoid background. Few cells showed tapered and wavy nuclei. Cytological diagnosis of BML, probably of neurogenic origin, was given, thus not giving an accurate diagnosis. Diagnosis was given on histology and immunohistochemistry.

Keloid FNAC smears showed very few scattered spindle shaped cells with glassy collagenized material and were not correctly diagnosed and confirmed on histology.

FNAC of low grade fibromyxosarcoma yielded myxoid material and smears showed moderate cellularity of loosely cohesive spindled fibroblast-like cells with moderate atypia arranged in a myxoid background. However already bland looking cells were masked with abundant myxoid material and so the nuclear features were not too prominent to call them malignant and therefore diagnosis given was suspicious for malignancy.

FNAC of giant cell tumor of tendon sheath showed mild to moderate cellularity, composed of numerous dispersed and clustered mononuclear rounded cells showing moderate amount of pleomorphism ranging from plump stellate to round cells. In addition, multinucleated giant cells of histiocytic origin were also seen, the nuclei of which resembled those of stromal cells. In the background brown pigment laden macrophages and few inflammatory cells were observed. Accurate cytological diagnosis was rendered in all the cases and duly confirmed by subsequent histopathological study.

FNAC of benign fibrous histiocytoma showed solid cell clusters and dispersed spindle shaped cells, thereby giving predominantly a spindle cell smear pattern. However, in none of the cases accurate broad categorization could be done and thus a diagnosis of BML was given.

FNAC of dermatofibroma showed low cellularity consisting of scattered spindle shaped cells lying against a fatty background. It was labelled as BML and could not be broadly categorized.

FNAC of tuberous xanthoma yielded scant aspirate, with low cellular smears showing scattered spindle shaped cells. Accurate diagnosis could not be made and so labelled as BML.

FNAC of undifferentiated pleomorphic sarcoma yielded blood admixed aspirate and smears showed high cellularity composed of bizarre tumor cells lying singly and entangled clusters. Individual cells were round to oval with indistinct cytoplasm, high nuclear : cytoplasmic ratio (N : C ratio), and prominent nucleoli and labelled as malignant mesenchymal tumor (MMT).

FNAC of dermatofibrosarcoma protuberans cases showed scanty to moderate cellularity, consisting of small cohesive clusters of short spindle cells and a diagnosis of BML was given.

FNAC of angioleiomyoma showed poor cell yield with predominating dissociated spindle cells lying singly against bloody background in one case and slightly collagenous in another. Exact categorization could not be done and labelled as BML.

The FNAC of pericytic tumor shows uniform pattern consisting of fragments of adipose tissue composed of a single large vacuole of fat and a small dark peripheral nucleus with no evidence of atypia. A cytological diagnosis of lipoma was given, thus not accurately diagnosed.

FNAC of vascular tumors showed yielded copious blood. Majority of the smears were poor in cells and showed blood only. Few cases showed spindle shaped cells with ovoid nuclei and a varying amount of indistinct cytoplasm. All cases were diagnosed as benign vascular lesion except one case showing occasional cohesive epithelioid cells with moderate cytoplasm, ovoid nuclei, and small nucleoli with mildly pleomorphic nuclei and irregular nuclear contours against a largely bloody background and diagnosed as vascular BML.

FNAC of chondroosseous lesion showed spindle cells arranged in packed clusters only. Broad categorization could not be done and diagnosis given was BML.

FNAC of schwannoma showed moderate cellularity with mainly cohesive spindle cell clusters having long-slender nuclei with pointed ends and indistinct cytoplasm with at places the arrangement was suggestive of palisading. A probable diagnosis of neurilemmoma was given in 5 cases only as they experience sharp radiating pain when tumor was aspirated and this would also suggest a neurogenic tumor. The rest of the 10 cases were not broadly categorized and showed mainly spindle cell clusters and cells lying singly and were labelled as BML.

FNAC of four cases of neurofibroma showed good cellularity consisting of clustered and scattered spindle shaped, elongated cells with poorly preserved, pale staining cytoplasm and irregular, elongated nuclei. Scattered naked nuclei were also noted. These cases were accurately diagnosed on FNAC. Two cases of neurofibroma showed moderate to high cellularity consisting of occasional clustered aggregates of plump to tapered spindle cells with irregular, hyperchromatic nuclei. These were diagnosed as BML.

FNAC of traumatic neuroma yielded scant aspirate. Hypocellular smears showed scattered spindle shaped cells lying singly and in small clusters. A diagnosis of BML was given.

FNAC of malignant peripheral nerve sheath tumor with low malignant potential yielded blood admixed aspirate. Smears showed mainly tissue fragments, with few dispersed cells. Individual cells were ovoid to spindle shaped admixed with wavy cells. The case was labelled as BML probably of neurogenic origin.

FNAC of alveolar soft part sarcoma yielded blood admixed aspirate. Smears show clusters of spindle shaped to epithelioid cells (polygonal) entangled in stroma. Numerous scattered plump cells were seen against dense hemorrhagic background. Individual cells show high N : C ratio, with round to oval irregular nucleus, prominent pale blue nucleoli, and scant cytoplasm. A diagnosis of malignant mesenchymal tumor with predominantly epithelioid smear pattern was given.

FNAC of PEComa yielded blood admixed material. Cellular smears show numerous scattered large round to oval spindle shaped cells with high N : C ratio and bizarre looking nuclei with prominent nucleoli. Few cells entangled in stroma were seen as well. Diagnosis made was malignant mesenchymal tumor, as it could not be accurately categorized.

FNAC of clear cell sarcoma showed loosely cohesive atypical spindle to oval cells entangled in stroma. Individual

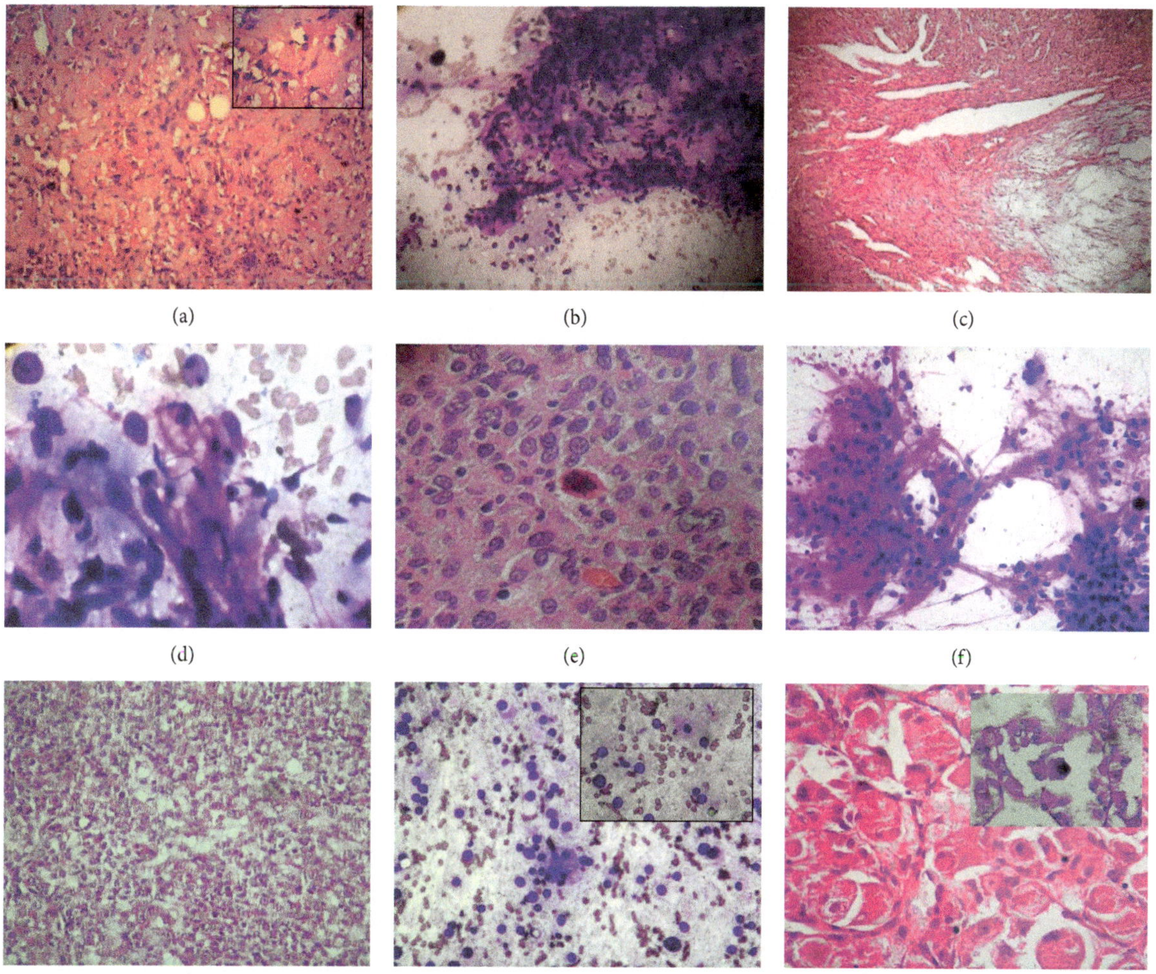

(a) (b) (c) (d) (e) (f) (g) (h) (i)

FIGURE 3: (a) Well differentiated liposarcoma: lipoblasts with atypical hyperchromatic nuclei and multinucleated giant cell (H&E ×100, ×400 inset). (b) Malignant mesenchymal lesion (low grade fibromyxoid sarcoma) cytology: loosely arranged bland spindle cells with slight to moderate atypia arranged in a myxoid background (Giemsa ×100). (c) Low grade fibromyxoid sarcoma: abrupt transition from fibrous areas (composed of bland spindle cells) to myxoid areas (H&E ×100). (d) Malignant mesenchymal lesion (malignant fibrous histiocytoma) cytology: bizarre tumor cells with prominent nucleoli (Giemsa ×400). (e) Malignant fibrous histiocytoma: cells with marked pleomorphism and mitosis (H&E ×400). (f) Malignant mesenchymal lesion (clear cell sarcoma) cytology: atypical spindle to oval cells entangled in stroma. (Giemsa × 400). (g) Clear cell sarcoma: Tumor cells in short fascicles separated by dense fibrous septa exhibiting prominent vesicular nuclei with large single nucleolus (H&E ×400). (h) Malignant mesenchymal lesion (alveolar soft part sarcoma) cytology: spindle to epithelioid cells with prominent nucleoli and high N : C ratio (Giemsa ×100, inset ×400). (i) Alveolar soft part sarcoma: tumor cells in typical organoid/nesting pattern are separated by delicate partitions of connective tissue containing vascular channels (H&E ×100) with chunky crystalline inclusions (inset) (PAS × 400).

cells had high N : C ratio. Diagnosis given was malignant mesenchymal lesion.

All malignant lesions on cytology were labelled as malignant mesenchymal tumor (MMT) (Figure 3). Excluding lipoma, the most common pattern observed was spindle cell pattern in 48% (72/150), followed by myxoid pattern in 4% (6/150) (Table 1). On histopathological examination (Table 2) 93.33% (140/150) of the soft tissue tumors were benign and 6.67% (10/150) malignant. Amongst malignant lesions, two cases of liposarcoma, 2 cases of dermatofibrosarcoma protuberans, and one case of each of malignant peripheral nerve sheath tumor, low grade fibromyxosarcoma, undifferentiated pleomorphic sarcoma, alveolar soft part sarcoma, PEComa, and clear cell sarcoma were seen. Three cases reported as BML on cytology were diagnosed as dermatofibrosarcoma protuberans in two cases and malignant peripheral nerve sheath tumor in one case on histopathology. Three cases reported as MML on cytology were diagnosed as alveolar soft part sarcoma, undifferentiated pleomorphic sarcoma, and clear cell sarcoma on histopathology. Both the cases reported as suspicious for malignancy were malignant on histopathology (low grade fibromyxosarcoma and PEComa). One case of lipoma on FNA turned to be glomus tumor on histopathology.

Correlation of cytodiagnosis and histopathological diagnosis in case of benign soft tissue tumors showed accurate categorization in 77.14% of cases (108/140). (Table 3) Among

Table 1: Cytomorphological pattern and spectrum of soft tissue tumors on FNAC.

(a) Cytomorphological pattern of STT on FNAC.

S. no.	Pattern	Benign	Suspicious	Malignant	Total
1	Spindle cell	45	01	0	72
2	Pleomorphic	0	0	02	02
3	Myxoid	04	01	01	06
4	Small round cell	0	0	0	0
5	Epithelioid	0	01	0	01

(b) Spectrum of soft tissue tumors on FNAC.

S. no.	Category	Benign	Malignant
1	Adipocytic tumor	Lipoma = 69	Atypical lipomatous tumor = 2
2	Fibroblastic tumors	Nodular fasciitis = 2	0
3	Fibrohistiocytic tumors	GCT = 06	0
4	Vascular tumor	23	0
5	Peripheral nerve sheath tumor	Neurofibroma = 04	0
6	Mesenchymal lesion	BML = 39	MML = 03
	Total	143	05

Suspicious cases = 2.

individual tumors entity adipocytic tumor had the best cyto-histological correlation with 100% (68/68) correctly identified on FNAC, followed by 95.84% correlation for vascular tumors (23/24). Least correlation was observed in cases of fibroblastic tumors 20% (2/10) followed by peripheral nerve sheath tumor 39.13% (9/23). 22.86% (32/140) of cases were diagnosed as benign but not accurately categorized. The correlation of cytodiagnosis and histopathological diagnosis in cases of malignant soft tissue tumors showed accurate categorization in only 2 cases (20%) out of 10 cases (Table 4). Three (30%) cases diagnosed as malignant on FNAC could not be accurately categorized. Two cytological suspicious diagnoses were evaluated histologically and both of them confirmed as malignancy whereas three cases diagnosed as benign on FNAC turned out to be malignant. Overall accurate/exact categorizations for both benign and malignant tumors (total STT studied) were seen in 70% (105/150) of cases. Because FNAC is a screening test with relatively high sensitivity for the diagnosis of malignancy, suspicious cases were included in the category of malignant lesions for statistical analysis. The sensitivity, specificity, positive predictive value, negative predictive value, and diagnostic accuracy of FNAC were calculated taking histology as gold standard. The sensitivity, specificity, positive predictive value, negative predictive value, and efficiency were 70%, 100%, 97.90%, 100%, and 98%, respectively. Pearson chi-square test with Yates' corrections was 87.665 with 1 degree of freedom and P value was <0.0001 which shows statistically extreme significant correlation.

4. Discussion

FNAC has numerous advantages over open biopsy, because it is relatively inexpensive and easy to perform and yields clinically useful results with a rapid turnaround time. Despite these benefits the present study depicts the difficulty of categorizing soft tissue lesion cytologically. If FNAC is to be of value the cytologists must be able to differentiate primary malignant soft tissue tumors from benign lesions and from other malignancies, such as metastasis of carcinomas and malignant lymphomas and tumors of dermal appendages. Kilpatrick et al. observed the extent to which cytology can be utilized in effective diagnosis of STT and influence on initial therapy in adults and pediatric sarcoma [6]. Rekhi et al. concluded that FNAC is fairly specific and sensitive in STT diagnoses for primary, recurrent, and metastatic lesions and the cytological types, especially round cell and pleomorphic sarcomas, can be quickly identified [3].

Parajuli and Lakhey also conclude that FNAC is highly sensitive to detect benign soft tissue tumors and highly specific for malignant soft tissue tumors [7]. Kulkarni et al. concluded that FNAC of STT provided acceptable diagnostic accuracy when supported by appropriate clinical and other diagnostic data [8]. The benign tumors are more common than malignant tumors with a ratio of at least 100 : 1 [2], and in the present study, ratio was 14 : 1. Roy et al. observed that benign STT were relatively common above third decade of life, while malignant STT occurred in patients of all ages [5]. Rekhi et al. observed that the commonest age group is 21–30 years for STT [3]. In present study, the commonest age group was 21–30 years and 40–50 years for benign and malignant STT, respectively. In present study, the commonest site for benign and malignant STT was upper extremities followed by trunk and the lower extremities followed by trunk region, respectively. Roy et al. observed that benign tumors are roughly equally distributed across all parts of the body with a slight predilection for the upper parts and the commonest site of involvement of the malignant tumors was trunk [5], in contrast to present study. Roy et al. [5] also observed that the most common benign tumour was lipoma followed by neurofibroma followed by haemangioma,

TABLE 2: Spectrum of soft tissue tumors on histopathology.

Categories	Number of cases	Percentage (%)
Benign		
Adipocytic tumors	**68**	**45.34**
Classic lipoma	54	36
Angiolipoma	6	4
Myxolipoma	1	0.67
Fibrolipoma	6	1
Pleomorphic lipoma	1	0.67
Vascular tumors	**24**	**16**
Hemangioma	23	15.33
Epithelioid hemangioma	1	0.67
Peripheral nerve sheath and related tumors	**23**	**15.33**
Schwannoma	15	10
Neurofibroma	06	4
Traumatic neuroma	02	1.33
Fibrohistiocytic tumors	**11**	**7.34**
Giant cell tumor of tendon sheath	6	4
Benign fibrous histiocytoma	3	2
Dermatofibroma	1	0.67
Tuberous xanthoma	1	0.67
Smooth muscle tumors	2	1.33
Angioleiomyoma		
Pericytic tumors	1	0.67
Glomus tumor		
Fibroblastic tumors	**10**	**6.67**
Nodular fasciitis	3	2
Collagenous fibroma	1	0.67
Fibroma of tendon sheath	2	1.33
Calcifying aponeurotic fibroma	1	0.67
Extra abdominal desmoids	1	0.67
Keloid	2	1.33
Chondroosseous tumor	1	0.67
Soft tissue tumor		
Malignant		
Fibrohistiocytic tumors	3	2
Dermatofibrosarcoma protuberans	2	1.33
Tumors of uncertain differentiation	**3**	**2**
Alveolar soft part sarcoma	1	0.67
PEComa	1	0.67
Clear cell sarcoma	1	0.67
Undifferentiated sarcomas		
Undifferentiated pleomorphic sarcoma	1	0.67
Peripheral nerve sheath and related tumor	1	0.67
Fibroblastic tumors	1	0.67
Low grade fibromyxoid sarcoma		
Adipocytic tumors	2	1.33
Liposarcoma		

TABLE 3: Correlation of cytodiagnosis and histopathological diagnosis in benign tumors.

Histopathology	Total number of cases	Correlation with cytological diagnosis	
		Accurately categorized	Diagnosed as benign but not accurately categorized
Adipocytic tumors	68	68	0
Fibroblastic tumors	10	2	8
Fibrohistiocytic tumors	11	6	5
Smooth muscle tumors	2	0	2
Pericytic tumors	1	0	1
Vascular tumors	24	23	1
Chondroosseous tumors	1	0	1
Peripheral nerve sheath and related tumors	23	4	19
Total	140	108 (77.14%)	32 (22.86%)

TABLE 4: Correlation of cytodiagnosis and histopathological diagnosis in malignant tumors.

Histopathology	Total number of cases	Correlation with cytological diagnosis			
		Accurately categorized	Diagnosed as malignant but not accurately categorized	Diagnosed as benign on FNAC	Suspicious
Adipocytic tumors	2	2	0	0	0
Fibroblastic tumors	1	0	0	0	1
Fibrohistiocytic tumors	2	0	0	2	0
Peripheral nerve sheath and related tumors	1	0	0	1	0
Tumors of uncertain differentiation	3	0	2	0	1
Undifferentiated sarcomas	1	0	1	0	0
Total	10	2 (20%)	3 (30%)	3 (30%)	2 (20%)

and Parajuli and Lakhey [7] observed lipoma followed by benign mesenchymal tumor followed by benign fibrohistiocytic tumor, while in present study adipocytic tumours were commonest followed byvascular tumours followed by peripheral nerve sheath tumors. In malignant cases, Roy et al. observed malignant fibrous histiocytoma followed by rhabdomyosarcoma and liposarcoma [5]. In the present study tumors of uncertain differentiation were the commonest tumors followed by fibrohistiocytic and adipocytic tumors. The sensitivity, specificity, positive predictive value, negative predictive value, and efficiency in the present study were 70%, 100%, 97.90%, 100%, and 98%, respectively. Rekhi et al. observed the diagnostic accuracy of FNAC in STT was 98%, with a positive predictive value of 98% in malignant cases and a negative predictive value of 100% in benign cases [3]. Dey et al. observed the sensitivity, specificity, and positive predictive value of FNAC in diagnosis of STT were 91.5%, 92.5%, and 95.5%, respectively [4]. Roy et al. observed that the diagnostic accuracy of FNAC of STT for benign and malignant tumours was 90.6% and 91.3%, respectively, with overall accuracy rate of 90.8% [5]. In the present study overall accuracy rate was 98%. Parajuli and Lakhey observed that the overall diagnostic accuracy of FNAC in STT was 80% and the sensitivity and specificity of diagnosing benign soft tissue tumors were 97.36% and 66.67%, respectively, and for malignant soft tissue tumors 66.67% and 97.36%, respectively [7]. Kulkarni et al. observed that the overall diagnostic accuracy of FNAC in STT was 93.33% for all lesions, 93.93% for malignant mesenchymal tumour, 93.33% for benign mesenchymal lesion, and 100% for metastasic tumours [8]. Layfield et al. observed that the diagnostic sensitivity of FNAC for detecting malignant neoplasm was 95% and the specificity was 95% [9]. Wakely and Kneisl observed 100% sensitivity and 97% specificity in STT diagnosis with FNAC and concluded that aspiration cytopathology of soft tissue mass lesions using FNA biopsy can be an accurate and minimally invasive method for the initial pathologic diagnosis of primary benign and malignant soft tissue masses, for the pathologic confirmation of metastatic tumors to soft tissue and for the documentation of locally recurrent soft tissue neoplasms [10].

5. Conclusion

FNAC is a very important preliminary diagnostic tool in palpable soft tissue lumps and done by expert hands; the results show a high degree of correlation with the final histopathology report.

Conflict of Interests

The authors declare that there is no conflict of interests regarding the publication of this paper.

References

[1] M. Akerman and H. Domanski, "Soft tissues," in *Orell and Sterrett's Fine Needle Aspiration Cytology*, S. R. Orell and G. F. Sterrett, Eds., pp. 387–400, Churchill Livingstone, Edinburgh, Scotland, 5th edition, 2012.

[2] A. E. Rosenberg, "Bones, joints, and soft-tissue tumorseditors," in *Robbin's and Cotran Pathologic Basis of Disease*, V. Kumar, A. K. Abbas, N. Fausto, and J. C. Aster, Eds., pp. 235–249, Saunders, Philadelphia, Pa, USA, 8th edition, 2010.

[3] B. Rekhi, B. D. Gorad, A. C. Kakade, and R. Chinoy, "Scope of FNAC in the diagnosis of soft tissue tumors—a study from a tertiary cancer referral center in India," *CytoJournal*, vol. 4, article 20, 2007.

[4] P. Dey, M. K. Mallik, S. K. Gupta, and R. K. Vasishta, "Role of fine needle aspiration cytology in the diagnosis of soft tissue tumours and tumour-like lesions," *Cytopathology*, vol. 15, no. 1, pp. 32–37, 2004.

[5] S. Roy, A. K. Manna, S. Pathak, and D. Guha, "Evaluation of fine needle aspiration cytology and its correlation with histopathological findings in soft tissue tumours," *Journal of Cytology*, vol. 24, no. 1, pp. 37–40, 2007.

[6] S. E. Kilpatrick, J. O. Cappellari, G. D. Bos, S. H. Gold, and W. G. Ward, "Is fine-needle aspiration biopsy a practical alternative to open biopsy for the primary diagnosis of sarcoma? experience with 140 patients," *American Journal of Clinical Pathology*, vol. 115, no. 1, pp. 59–68, 2001.

[7] S. Parajuli and M. Lakhey, "Efficacy of fine needle aspiration cytology in diagnosing soft tissue tumors," *Journal of Pathology of Nepal*, vol. 2, pp. 305–308, 2012.

[8] D. R. Kulkarni, H. R. Kokandakar, N. R. Kumbhakarna, and K. S. Bhople, "Fine needle aspiration cytology of soft tissue tumours in correlation with histopathology," *Indian Journal of Pathology & Microbiology*, vol. 45, no. 1, pp. 45–48, 2002.

[9] L. J. Layfield, K. H. Anders, B. J. Glasgow, and J. M. Mirra, "Fine-needle aspiration of primary soft-tissue lesions," *Archives of Pathology and Laboratory Medicine*, vol. 110, no. 5, pp. 420–424, 1986.

[10] P. E. Wakely and J. S. Kneisl, "Soft tissue aspiration cytopathology," *Cancer*, vol. 90, pp. 292–298, 2000.

3

In Vitro Studies on the Antioxidant Property and Inhibition of α-Amylase, α-Glucosidase, and Angiotensin I-Converting Enzyme by Polyphenol-Rich Extracts from Cocoa *(Theobroma cacao)* Bean

Ganiyu Oboh, Ayokunle O. Ademosun, Adedayo O. Ademiluyi, Olasunkanmi S. Omojokun, Esther E. Nwanna, and Kuburat O. Longe

Functional Foods and Nutraceuticals Unit, Biochemistry Department, Federal University of Technology, PMB 704, Akure 340252, Nigeria

Correspondence should be addressed to Olasunkanmi S. Omojokun; sunjoks@live.com

Academic Editor: Shahid Pervez

Background. This study sought to investigate the antidiabetic and antihypertensive mechanisms of cocoa (*Theobroma cacao*) bean through inhibition of α-amylase, α-glucosidase, angiotensin-1 converting enzyme, and oxidative stress. *Methodology.* The total phenol and flavonoid contents of the water extractable phytochemicals from the powdered cocoa bean were determined and the effects of the extract on α-amylase, α-glucosidase, and angiotensin-1 converting enzyme activities were investigated *in vitro*. Furthermore, the radicals [1,1-diphenyl-2 picrylhydrazyl (DPPH), 2,2..-azino-bis(3-ethylbenzthiazoline-6-sulphonic acid) (ABTS), hydroxyl (OH), and nitric oxide (NO)] scavenging ability and ferric reducing antioxidant property of the extract were assessed. *Results.* The results revealed that the extract inhibited α-amylase (1.81 ± 0.22 mg/mL), α-glucosidase (1.84 ± 0.17 mg/mL), and angiotensin-1 converting enzyme (0.674 ± 0.06 mg/mL [lungs], 1.006 ± 0.08 mg/mL [heart]) activities in a dose-dependent manner and also showed dose-dependent radicals [DPPH (16.94 ± 1.34 mg/mL), NO (6.98 ± 0.886 mg/mL), OH (3.72 ± 0.26 mg/mL), and ABTS (15.7 ± 1.06 mmol/TEAC·g] scavenging ability. *Conclusion.* The inhibition of α-amylase, α-glucosidase, and angiotensin-1 converting enzyme activities by the cocoa bean extract could be part of the possible mechanism by which the extract could manage and/or prevent type-2 diabetes and hypertension.

1. Introduction

The studies of cocoa and their related products have become an area of interest owing to their health-promoting properties. In recent years, cocoa and cocoa products, namely, cocoa powder, dark chocolate, and cocoa liquor, have been shown to suppress atherosclerosis and reduce the risk of heart disease [1], increase dermal blood circulation, and decrease platelet activation, adhesion, and function, as well as function as cancer protective agent by inhibiting the proliferation of human cancer cells and also exerted hypoglycemic properties [2] owing to the presence of the phenolic compounds in it. Polyphenols have been researched for decades, mostly because of their antioxidant properties [3].

Dietary antioxidants sourced from the diet such as fruits and vegetables are capable of counteracting the damaging but normal effects of the physiological process of oxidation reactions that occur in animal tissue [4]. These antioxidants are considered beneficial because of their protective role against oxidative stress, which is involved in the pathogenesis of multiple diseases such as cardiovascular and cerebrovascular diseases [5]. Diabetes mellitus is a complex disease that is characterized by chronic hyperglycemia. The peculiar clinical features like excessive urination, thirst, weight loss. and secondary complications observed in diabetes mellitus are primarily an indication of the hyperglycemic state [6]. Type 1 diabetes results from inadequate synthesis of insulin by β-cells of the pancreas, while type II diabetes is characterized primarily by insulin resistance (a condition in which peripheral cells do not respond normally to insulin) or β-cell dysfunction [7].

Alpha-amylase is a prominent enzyme found in the pancreatic juice and saliva which breaks down large insoluble starch molecules into absorbable molecules [8]. On the other hand, mammalian α-glucosidase is an enzyme found in the mucosal brush border of the small intestine which catalyzes the end step of digestion of disaccharides that are abundant in human diet to its corresponding monosaccharide [9]. Effective means of lowering the levels of postprandial hyperglycemia have been offered by α-amylase and α-glucosidase inhibitors by delaying the breakdown of ingested carbohydrates in the small intestine thereby reducing the postprandial blood glucose excursion [10]. Several inhibitors of α-amylase and α-glucosidase have been isolated from medicinal plants to serve as an alternative drug with increased potency and less adverse effects than existing synthetic drugs [11].

Angiotensin-I converting enzyme (ACE) activity has been linked to hypertension. Inhibition of ACE is considered a useful therapeutic approach in the treatment of high blood pressure and dietary phenolic phytochemicals have shown promising potential while previous *in vitro* and *in vivo* animal and clinical studies have also indicated the potential of specific phenolic phytochemicals in hypertension management with absorption into the blood [12]. However, despite the documented antidiabetic [13] and antihypertensive potential of *Theobroma cacao* [14] no previous report has been given on the mechanism by which it exerts this effect.

2. Materials and Methods

2.1. Chemicals. All chemicals used were sourced from Sigma Corporation (St. Louis MO). Except stated otherwise, all the chemicals and reagents used are of analytical grade, while the water used was glass distilled.

2.2. Plant Material Collection and Preparation. Cocoa beans were bought at a local market in Ibule-soro (a suburb of Akure) near Federal University of Technology, Akure, Ondo State, Nigeria. The authentication of the bean was done at the Department of Crop, Soil and Pest Management, Federal University of Technology, Akure, Nigeria. Subsequently, the dried beans were then milled into fine powder. The aqueous extracts of the bean were prepared by soaking 5 g of the grinded samples in 100 mL of distilled water for 24 hrs at 37°C. The mixture was later filtered through Whatmann number 2 filter paper and centrifuged at 4000 rpm to obtain a clear supernatant which was then stored in the refrigerator for subsequent analysis [15].

2.3. Total Phenol Determination. The total phenol content was determined by mixing 0.2 mL of the sample extract with 2.5 mL 10% Folin-Cioalteau reagent (v/v) and 2.0 mL of 7.5% sodium carbonate was subsequently added. The reaction mixture was incubated at 45°C for 40 min, and the absorbance was measured at 765 nm using a spectrophotometer. Gallic acid was used as standard phenol; the total phenol content was subsequently calculated as gallic acid equivalent [16].

2.4. Total Flavonoid Determination. The total flavonoid content was determined by mixing 0.5 mL of appropriately diluted sample with 0.5 mL methanol, 50 μL 10% $AlCl_3$, 50 μL 1 M Potassium acetate, and 1.4 mL distilled water and allowed to incubate at room temperature for 30 min. The absorbance of the reaction mixture was subsequently measured at 415 nm; quercetin is used as standard flavonoid. The total flavonoid content was subsequently calculated as quercetin equivalent. The nonflavonoid polyphenols were taken as the difference between the total phenol and total flavonoid content [17].

2.5. Enzyme Inhibition Assay

2.5.1. Angiotensin I Converting Enzyme (ACE) Inhibition Assay. Appropriate dilution of the aqueous extract (0–500 μL) and ACE solution (50 μL, 4 mU) was incubated at 37°C for 15 min. The enzymatic reaction was initiated by adding 150 μL of 8.33 mM of the substrate Bz - Gly - His - Leu in 125 mM Tris-HCl buffer (pH 8.3) to the mixture. After incubation for 30 min at 37°C, the reaction was arrested by adding 250 μL of 1 M HCl. The Gly-His bond was then cleaved and the Bz-Gly produced by the reaction was extracted with 1.5 mL ethyl acetate. Thereafter the mixture was centrifuged to separate the ethyl acetate layer; then 1 mL of the ethyl acetate layer was transferred to a clean test tube and evaporated. The residue was redissolved in distilled water and its absorbance was measured at 228 nm [18]. The ACE inhibitory activity was expressed as percentage (%) inhibition.

2.5.2. α-Amylase Inhibition Assay. This was measured using the dinitrosalicylic acid method as described by Worthington Biochemical Corporation 1978 [19]. Appropriate dilution of the pastes (500 μL) and 500 μL of 0.02 M sodium phosphate buffer (pH 6.9 with 0.006 M NaCl) containing pancreatic α-amylase (EC 3.2.1.1) (0.5 mg/mL) were incubated at 25°C for 10 min. Then, 500 μL of 1% starch solution in 0.02 M sodium phosphate buffer (pH 6.9 with 0.006 M NaCl) was added to each tube. The reaction mixtures was incubated at 25°C for 10 min and stopped with 1.0 mL of dinitrosalicylic acid colour reagent. Thereafter, the mixture was incubated in a boiling water bath for 5 min and cooled to room temperature. The reaction mixture was then diluted by adding 10 mL of distilled water, and absorbance measured at 540 nm. The EC_{50} (the extract concentration inhibiting 50% of the α-amylase activity) of the pastes was calculated.

2.5.3. α-Glucosidase Inhibition Assay. The extract (50 μL) and 100 μL of α-glucosidase solution (1.0 U/mL) in 0.1 M phosphate buffer (pH 6.9) was incubated at 25°C for 10 min. Then, 50 μL of 5 mM p-nitrophenyl-α-D-glucopyranoside solution in 0.1 M phosphate buffer (pH 6.9) was added. The mixtures were incubated at 25°C for 5 min before reading the absorbance at 405 nm in the spectrophotometer. The α-glucosidase inhibitory activity was expressed as percentage inhibition. The EC_{50} of the pastes was calculated [20].

2.6. In Vitro Antioxidant Studies

2.6.1. Determination of Reducing Property. The reducing property was determined by assessing the ability of the sample extract to reduce $FeCl_3$ solution as described by Pulido et al., 2002 [21]. Briefly, appropriate dilutions (0–1.0 mL) were mixed with 2.5 mL 200 mm sodium phosphate buffer (ph 6.6) and 2.5 mL of 1% potassium ferricyanide. The mixtures were incubated at 50°C for 20 min. Thereafter, 2.5 mL 10% trichloroacetic acid was added and subsequently centrifuged at 650 rpm for 10 min. Then 5 mL of the resulting supernatant was mixed with equal volume of water and 1 mL of 0.1% ferric chloride. The absorbance was taken at 700 nm against a reagent blank.

2.6.2. DPPH Free Radical Scavenging Assay. The free radical scavenging ability of the extract against DPPH (1,1-diphenyl-2picrylhdrazyl) free radical was evaluated as described by Gyamfi et al., 1999 [22]. Briefly, appropriate dilution of the extracts (0–500 μL) was mixed with 1 mL, 0.4 mM methanolic solution containing DPPH radicals; the mixture was left in the dark for 30 min and the absorbance was taken at 516 nm. The DPPH free radical scavenging ability was subsequently calculated.

2.6.3. $ABTS^{\cdot+}$ Radical Scavenging Ability Assay. The $ABTS^{\cdot+}$ (2,2′-azino-bis(3-ethylbenzthiazoline-6-sulphoic acid) scavenging ability of the extract was determined according to the method described by Re et al., 1999 [23]. The $ABTS^{\cdot+}$ was generated by reacting 7 mM ABTS aqueous solution with $K_2S_2O_8$ (2.45 mmol/L, final concentration) in the dark for 16 hrs and adjusting the Abs 734 nm to 0.700 with ethanol. Thereafter, 200 μL of appropriate dilution of the extract was added to 2.0 mL $ABTS^{\cdot+}$ solution and the absorbance was measured at 734 nm after 15 min. The trolox equivalent antioxidant capacity was subsequently calculated using trolox as the standard.

2.6.4. Inhibition of the Fenton Reaction (Degradation of Deoxyribose). The method of Halliwell and Gutteridge 1981 [24] was used to determine the ability of the extract to prevent Fe^{2+}/H_2O_2 induced decomposition of deoxyribose. The extract (0–100 μL) was added to a reaction mixture containing 120 μL of 20 mM deoxyribose, 400 μL of 0.1 M phosphate buffer, 40 μL of 500 μM $FeSO_4$, and the volume were made up to 800 μL with distilled water. The reaction mixture was incubated at 37°C for 30 min and the reaction was then stopped by the addition of 0.5 mL of 2.8% trichloroacetic acid (TCA). This was followed by addition of 0.4 mL of 0.6% thiobarbituric acid (TBA) solution. The tubes were subsequently incubated in boiling water for 20 min and the absorbance was measured at 532 nm in a spectrophotometer.

2.6.5. Nitric Oxide Radical Scavenging Assay. The scavenging effect of the extract on nitric oxide (NO) radical was measured according to the method of Marcocci et al., 1994 [25]. Samples of 100–400 μL of the oil extract were added in the test tubes to 1 mL of Sodium nitroprusside solution (25 mM) and tubes incubated at 37°C for 2 hours. An aliquot (0.5 mL) of the incubation was removed and diluted with 0.3 mL Griess reagent (1% sulphanilamide in 5% H_3PO_4 and 0.1% naphthlethylenediaminedihy drochloride). The absorbance of the chromophore formed was immediately read at 570 nm against distilled water as blank with catechin (50 μg) used as standard. Results were expressed as percentage radical scavenging activity (RSA).

2.7. Lipid Peroxidation Assay

2.7.1. Preparation of Tissue Homogenates. The rats were decapitated under mild diethyl ether anaesthesia; the pancreas was rapidly isolated, placed on ice, and weighed. This tissue was subsequently homogenized in cold saline (1/10, w/v) with about 10-up-and down strokes at approximately 1200 rev/min in a Teflon glass homogenizer. The homogenate was centrifuged for 10 min at 3000 ×g to yield a pellet that was discarded, and a low-speed supernatant (S1) that was kept for lipid peroxidation assay.

2.7.2. Lipid Peroxidation and Thiobarbituric Acid Reactions. The lipid peroxidation assay was carried out using the modified method of Ohkawa et al., 1979 [26]. Briefly 100 μL Sl fraction was mixed with a reaction mixture containing 30 μL of 0.1 M pH 7.4 Tris-HCl buffer, extract (0–100 μL) and 30 μL of 250 μM freshly prepared $FeSO_4$ (the procedure was also carried out using 7 μM sodium nitroprusside). The volume was made up to 300 μL by water before incubation at 37°C for 1 hr. The reaction was developed by adding 300 μL 8.1% Sodium doudecylsulphate (SDS) to the reaction mixture and this was subsequently followed by the addition of 600 μL of acetic acid/HCl (pH 3.4) and 600 μL 0.8% thiobarbituric acid (TBA). This mixture was incubated at 100°C for 1 hr and the thiobarbituric acid reactive species (TBARS) produced were measured at 532 nm. Subsequently, the lipid peroxidation was calculated as MDA produced (percentage of control).

2.8. Data Analysis. The results of three replicates were pooled and expressed as mean ± standard deviation (SD). One-way analysis of variance (ANOVA) and least significance difference (LSD) were carried out [27]. Significance was accepted at $P \leq 0.05$. EC_{50} was determined using linear regression analysis

3. Results

The total phenolic content reported as gallic acid equivalent, total flavonoid content reported as quercetin equivalent, $ABTS^*$ scavenging ability reported as trolox equivalent, and ferric reducing antioxidant property reported as ascorbic acid equivalent as presented in Table 1 were 17.9 mg·GAE/100 g, 6.84 mg·QUE/100 g, 15.7 mmol/TEAC·g, and 14.92 mg/AAE·g, respectively.

As shown in Table 2, the cocoa bean aqueous extract scavenged DPPH, OH, and NO radicals in concentration-dependent manners, with EC_{50} values of 16.94 mg/mL, 3.72 mg/mL, and 6.98 mg/mL, respectively.

TABLE 1: The total phenol content reported as gallic acid equivalent, total flavonoid content reported as quercetin equivalent, ABTS* scavenging ability reported as trolox equivalent antioxidant capacity, and ferric reducing antioxidant property reported as ascorbic acid equivalent of aqueous extract of cocoa bean.

Parameter	Value (unit)
Total phenol	17.9 ± 0.96 (mg·GAE/100 g)
Total flavonoid	6.84 ± 0.10 (mg·QUE/100 g)
ABTS* scavenging ability	15.7 ± 1.06 (mmol/TEAC·g)
Ferric reducing antioxidant property	14.92 ± 0.82 (mg/AAE·g)

Values represent means ± standard deviation of triplicate readings.

TABLE 2: EC_{50} values of DPPH, OH, and NO radical scavenging ability of aqueous extract of cocoa bean.

Parameter	EC_{50} value (mg/mL)
DPPH radical scavenging ability	16.94 ± 1.34
OH radical scavenging ability	3.72 ± 0.26
NO radical scavenging ability	6.98 ± 0.88

Values represent means ± standard deviation of triplicate readings.

The antioxidant effect of the cocoa powder by interacting the aqueous extract with isolated rat pancreas in the presence of sodium nitroprusside (SNP) and Fe^{2+} as prooxidants was investigated. As shown in Table 3, the EC_{50} results show that the extract inhibits SNP (11.47 mg/mL) and Fe^{2+} (2.12 mg/mL) induced lipid peroxidation in rat's pancreas. In assessing the antihypertensive and antidiabetic potentials of the extract, the results revealed that the bean extracts inhibited angiotensin-I converting enzyme, α-amylase, and α-glucosidase activities. The EC_{50} values as presented in Table 3 were found to be 1.81 mg/mL (α-amylase), 1.84 mg/mL (α-glucosidase), 0.674 mg/mL (ACE in the lungs), and 1.01 mg/mL (ACE in the heart).

4. Discussion

Previous studies on the health benefits of cocoa have primarily focused on its effects on the risk of cardiovascular diseases and reduction of blood glucose levels [28], with a dearth of information on the possible mechanisms of action. The inhibition of α-amylase slows down the breakdown of starch to disaccharide, while the inhibition of α-glucosidase slows down the breakdown of the disaccharides to the simple monosaccharide, glucose, thereby reducing the amount of glucose absorbed into the blood stream [10]. Angiotensin-1 converting enzyme (ACE) cleaves angiotensin I which is a decapeptide to produce angiotensin II, an octapeptide and potent vasoconstrictor that has been identified as a major factor in hypertensive conditions [29]. Therefore, ACE inhibitors have been widely considered to prevent angiotensin II production in cardiovascular diseases, and utilized in clinical applications since the discovery of ACE inhibitors in snake venom [29]. The inhibition of α-amylase and α-glucosidase activities by the cocoa powder aqueous extracts could have

TABLE 3: EC_{50} values of SNP and Fe^{2+} induced lipid peroxidation in rat's pancreas, angiotensin-I converting enzyme inhibitory activity in the lungs and heart, and α-amylase and α-glucosidase inhibitory activity of aqueous extract of cocoa bean.

Parameter	EC_{50} value (mg/mL)
SNP induced lipid peroxidation	11.47 ± 1.07
Fe^{2+} induced lipid peroxidation	2.12 ± 0.10
ACE (lungs)	0.674 ± 0.06
ACE (heart)	1.006 ± 0.08
α-amylase	1.81 ± 0.22
α-glucosidase	1.84 ± 0.17

Values represent means ± standard deviation of triplicate readings.

contributed to its use in the management of diabetes, thereby slowing down the breakdown of starch to disaccharide. The extract inhibited both α-glucosidase and α-amylase in a dose-dependent manner; pointing to its potential of being of great pharmaceutical importance, in addressing some of the side effects (like flatulence and abdominal distention) associated with the drugs (Acarbose, Miglitol, and Voglibose) presently used for the management of diabetes. Furthermore, the dose-dependent ACE inhibitory activity of the cocoa powder aqueous extract reveals that this could explain the likely mechanism for its use in the treatment of hypertension and possibly address the side effects of some class of antihypertensive drugs (diuretics, beta blockers, and synthetic ACE inhibitors) used in managing hypertension.

Polyphenols have received wide attention because of their antioxidant properties which refers to their ability to prevent damage from reactive oxygen species through free radical scavenging or prevent the generation of these species by iron chelation as well as bind and inhibit the enzymes α-amylase and α-glucosidase [30]. The antioxidant activity of fruits and vegetables significantly increases with the increase in polyphenol content in it [31]. The total phenol and flavonoid content of this cocoa bean extract was found to be 17.9 mg·GAE/100 g and 6.84 mg·QUE/100 g, respectively. This finding was in agreement with previous study which demonstrated that high flavonoid (a class of polyphenol) content of cocoa extract correlated with its strong antioxidant capacity [28].

The free radical scavenging ability of this extract was also studied making use of moderately stable nitrogen-centred radical species-ABTS radical [32]. The result obtained here agrees with the phenolic content in earlier research articles, where correlations were reported between phenolic content and antioxidant capacity of some plant foods [33]. The extract was found to also demonstrate strong free radical scavenging abilities as exemplified by their scavenging activity of moderately stable $ABTS^{\cdot+}$, NO, OH^{-}, and DPPH radicals *in vitro*. However, there is an agreement between the $ABTS^{\cdot+}$, NO, OH^{-}, and DPPH free radical scavenging ability, which agrees with earlier findings where plant antioxidant properties (free radical scavenging ability) correlates with their phenolic content [34]. A study showed that decrease in antioxidant capacity in cocoa beverages stored at different temperature and time was due to loss of its phenolic content [35].

Antioxidants neutralize the electrical charges on free radicals and prevent them from taking electrons from other molecules [36]. They are needed to prevent the formation and oppose the actions of reactive oxygen and nitrogen species, which are generated *in vivo* and cause damage to DNA, lipids, proteins, and other biomolecules. Antioxidants are naturally powerful substances that help slow the aging process, fight diseases such as diabetes mellitus and hypertension, and prevent some deadly and incurable diseases like cancer [37]. The protective ability of the extract against Sodium nitroprusside and Fe^{2+} induced lipid peroxidation in cultured rats' pancreas assessed revealed that incubation of the pancreas tissues in the presence of Fe^{2+} caused a significant ($P < 0.05$) increase in the MDA content (181%). Likewise, incubation of the pancreas tissue in the presence of sodium nitroprusside caused a significant ($P < 0.05$) increase in the MDA content (249%). These findings agree with earlier reports, where phenolics had been reported to be potent inhibitors of lipid peroxidation in several animal tissues [38]. Sodium nitroprusside; a component of antihypertensive drugs is known to cause cytotoxicity through the release of cyanide and/or nitric oxide (NO). NO is a universal neuronal messenger in the central nervous system and acts independently, it may also cause neuronal damage in cooperation with other reactive oxygen species (ROS) [39]. It could be suggested that the higher ACE inhibitory ability of the aqueous extracts of the cocoa powder aqueous extract is due to its higher NO^* scavenging ability. However, we advise that further work should be done to isolate the phytoconstituents in the cocoa bean which may be responsible for eliciting the biological activities. Also, *in vitro* works do not automatically translate to human body response; hence, we suggest that further *in vivo* work should be carried out.

5. Conclusion

Conclusively, cocoa bean is rich in phenolic compounds and exhibits a high antioxidant activity. Its ingestion as a functional food lowers plasma glucose level by inhibiting α-amylase and α-glucosidase and could be of importance in the management of diabetes mellitus as it also addresses some side effects associated with synthetic antidiabetic drugs. In addition, cocoa seed extract inhibition of ACE also explains the likely mechanism for its use in the treatment of hypertension. Hence, cocoa bean ingestion will improve the quality of life of hypertensive patients and the diabetics.

Conflict of Interests

There is no conflict of interests regarding the publication of this paper.

References

[1] J. W. Erdman Jr., L. Carson, C. Kwik-Uribe, E. M. Evans, and R. R. Allen, "Effects of cocoa flavanols on risk factors for cardiovascular disease," *Asia Pacific Journal of Clinical Nutrition*, vol. 17, no. 1, pp. 284–287, 2008.

[2] D. Ramljak, L. J. Romanczyk, L. J. Metheny-Barlow et al., "Pentameric procyanidin from *Theobroma cacao* selectively inhibits growth of human breast cancer cells," *Molecular Cancer Therapeutics*, vol. 4, no. 4, pp. 537–546, 2005.

[3] M. Netzel, G. Strass, I. Bitsch, R. Könitz, M. Christmann, and R. Bitsch, "Effect of grape processing on selected antioxidant phenolics in red wine," *Journal of Food Engineering*, vol. 56, no. 2-3, pp. 223–228, 2003.

[4] G. Oboh, "Antioxidant properties of some commonly consumed and underutilized tropical legumes," *European Food Research and Technology*, vol. 224, no. 1, pp. 61–65, 2006.

[5] M. Alía, C. Horcajo, L. Bravo, and L. Goya, "Effect of grape antioxidant dietary fiber on the total antioxidant capacity and the activity of liver antioxidant enzymes in rats," *Nutrition Research*, vol. 23, no. 9, pp. 1251–1267, 2003.

[6] O. Klein, J. Lynge, L. Endahl, B. Damholt, L. Nosek, and T. Heise, "Albumin-bound basal insulin analogues (insulin detemir and NN344): comparable time-action profiles but less variability than insulin glargine in type 2 diabetes," *Diabetes, Obesity and Metabolism*, vol. 9, no. 3, pp. 290–299, 2007.

[7] T. Heise, L. Nosek, B. B. Roønn et al., "Lower within-subject variability of insulin detemir in comparison to NPH insulin and insulin glargine in people with type 1 diabetes," *Diabetes*, vol. 53, no. 6, pp. 1614–1620, 2004.

[8] A. F. Afifi, A. E. Kamel, A. A. Khalil, M. A. Foaad, E. M. Fawziand, and M. Houseny, "Purification and characterization of α-amylase from penicillium olsonii under the effect of some antioxidant vitamins," *Global Journal of Biotechnology and Biochemistry*, vol. 3, no. 1, pp. 14–12, 2008.

[9] V. Manohar, N. A. Talpur, B. W. Echard, S. Lieberman, and H. G. Preuss, "Effects of a water-soluble extract of maitake mushroom on circulating glucose/insulin concentrations in KK mice," *Diabetes, Obesity and Metabolism*, vol. 4, no. 1, pp. 43–48, 2002.

[10] Y.-I. Kwon, E. Apostolidis, and K. Shetty, "Evaluation of pepper (*Capsicum annuum*) for management of diabetes and hypertension," *Journal of Food Biochemistry*, vol. 31, no. 3, pp. 370–385, 2007.

[11] T. Matsui, I. A. Ogunwande, K. J. M. Abesundara, and K. Matsumoto, "Anti-hyperglycemic potential of natural products," *Mini-Reviews in Medicinal Chemistry*, vol. 6, no. 3, pp. 349–356, 2006.

[12] Y.-I. I. Kwon, D. A. Vattem, and K. Shetty, "Evaluation of clonal herbs of Lamiaceae species for management of diabetes and hypertension," *Asia Pacific Journal of Clinical Nutrition*, vol. 15, no. 1, pp. 107–118, 2006.

[13] I. Amin, H. A. Faizul, and R. Azli, "Effect of cocoa powder extract on plasma glucose levels in hyperglycaemic rats," *Nutrition and Food Science*, vol. 34, pp. 116–121, 2004.

[14] B. Buijsse, E. J. M. Feskens, F. J. Kok, and D. Kromhout, "Cocoa intake, blood pressure, and cardiovascular mortality: the Zutphen Elderly Study," *Archives of Internal Medicine*, vol. 166, no. 4, pp. 411–417, 2006.

[15] G. Oboh, R. L. Puntel, and J. B. T. Rocha, "Hot pepper (*Capsicum annuum*, Tepin and *Capsicum chinese, Habanero*) prevents Fe^{2+}-induced lipid peroxidation in brain—in vitro," *Food Chemistry*, vol. 102, no. 1, pp. 178–185, 2007.

[16] V. L. Singleton, R. Orthofer, and R. M. Lamuela-Raventós, "Analysis of total phenols and other oxidation substrates and antioxidants by means of folin-ciocalteu reagent," *Methods in Enzymology*, vol. 299, pp. 152–178, 1998.

[17] A. Meda, C. E. Lamien, M. Romito, J. Millogo, and O. G. Nacoulma, "Determination of the total phenolic, flavonoid and proline contents in Burkina Fasan honey, as well as their radical scavenging activity," *Food Chemistry*, vol. 91, no. 3, pp. 571–577, 2005.

[18] D. W. Cushman and H. S. Cheung, "Spectrophotometric assay and properties of the angiotensin-converting enzyme of rabbit lung," *Biochemical Pharmacology*, vol. 20, no. 7, pp. 1637–1648, 1971.

[19] Worthington Biochemical Corporation, *Enzyme and Related Biochemicals*, Worthington Biochemical Corporation, Freehold, NJ, USA, 1978.

[20] E. Apostolidis, Y.-I. Kwon, and K. Shetty, "Inhibitory potential of herb, fruit, and fungal-enriched cheese against key enzymes linked to type 2 diabetes and hypertension," *Innovative Food Science and Emerging Technologies*, vol. 8, no. 1, pp. 46–54, 2007.

[21] R. Pulido, L. Bravo, and F. Saura-Calixto, "Antioxidant activity of dietary polyphenols as determined by a modified ferric reducing/antioxidant power assay," *Journal of Agricultural and Food Chemistry*, vol. 48, no. 8, pp. 3396–3402, 2000.

[22] M. A. Gyamfi, M. Yonamine, and Y. Aniya, "Free-radical scavenging action of medicinal herbs from GhanaThonningia sanguinea on experimentally-induced liver injuries," *General Pharmacology*, vol. 32, no. 6, pp. 661–667, 1999.

[23] R. Re, N. Pellegrini, A. Proteggente, A. Pannala, M. Yang, and C. Rice-Evans, "Antioxidant activity applying an improved ABTS radical cation decolorization assay," *Free Radical Biology and Medicine*, vol. 26, no. 9-10, pp. 1231–1237, 1999.

[24] B. Halliwell and J. M. C. Gutteridge, "Formation of a thiobarbituric-acid-reactive substance from deoxyribose in the presence of iron salts: the role of superoxide and hydroxyl radicals," *FEBS Letters*, vol. 128, no. 2, pp. 347–352, 1981.

[25] L. Marcocci, J. J. Maguire, M. T. Droy-Lefaix, and L. Packer, "The nitric oxide-scavenging properties of Ginkgo biloba extract EGb 761," *Biochemical and Biophysical Research Communications*, vol. 201, no. 2, pp. 748–755, 1994.

[26] H. Ohkawa, N. Ohishi, and K. Yagi, "Assay for lipid peroxides in animal tissues by thiobarbituric acid reaction," *Analytical Biochemistry*, vol. 95, no. 2, pp. 351–358, 1979.

[27] J. H. Zar, *Biostatistical Analysis*, Prentice-Hall, 1984.

[28] K. A. Cooper, J. L. Donovan, A. I. Waterhouse, and G. Williamson, "Cocoa and health: a decade of research," *British Journal of Nutrition*, vol. 99, no. 1, pp. 1–11, 2008.

[29] A. Villar, M. Paya, and M. C. Terencio, "Plants with antihypertensive action," *Fitoterap*, vol. 57, pp. 131–145, 1986.

[30] N. R. Perron and J. L. Brumaghim, "A review of the antioxidant mechanisms of polyphenol compounds related to iron binding," *Cell Biochemistry and Biophysics*, vol. 53, no. 2, pp. 75–100, 2009.

[31] K. Ghasemi, Y. Ghasemi, and M. A. Ebrahimzadeh, "Antioxidant activity, phenol and flavonoid contents of 13 citrus species peels and tissues," *Pakistan Journal of Pharmaceutical Sciences*, vol. 22, no. 3, pp. 277–281, 2009.

[32] M. Benderitter, V. Maupoil, C. Vergely, F. Dalloz, F. Briot, and L. Rochette, "Studies by electron paramagnetic resonance of the importance of iron in the hydroxyl scavenging properties of ascorbic acid in plasma: effects of iron chelators," *Fundamental & Clinical Pharmacology*, vol. 12, no. 5, pp. 510–516, 1998.

[33] J. Sun, Y.-F. Chu, X. Wu, and R. H. Liu, "Antioxidant and antiproliferative activities of common fruits," *Journal of Agricultural and Food Chemistry*, vol. 50, no. 25, pp. 7449–7454, 2002.

[34] A. A. Oluwaseun and O. Ganiyu, "Antioxidant properties of methanolic extracts of mistletoes (Viscum album) from cocoa and cashew trees in Nigeria," *African Journal of Biotechnology*, vol. 7, no. 17, pp. 3138–3142, 2008.

[35] S. Sang, M.-J. Lee, Z. Hou, C.-T. Ho, and C. S. Yang, "Stability of tea polyphenol (-)-epigallocatechin-3-gallate and formation of dimers and epimers under common experimental conditions," *Journal of Agricultural and Food Chemistry*, vol. 53, no. 24, pp. 9478–9484, 2005.

[36] G. Oboh and J. B. T. Rocha, "Antioxidant in foods: a new challenge for food processors," in *Leading Edge Antioxidants Research*, H. V. Panglossi, Ed., pp. 35–64, Nova Science Publishers, New York, NY, USA, 2007.

[37] R. H. Liu, "Health benefits of fruit and vegetables are from additive and synergistic combinations of phytochemicals," *The American Journal of Clinical Nutrition*, vol. 78, no. 3, pp. 517S–520S, 2003.

[38] I. Klimczak, M. Małecka, M. Szlachta, and A. Gliszczyńska-Świgło, "Effect of storage on the content of polyphenols, vitamin C and the antioxidant activity of orange juices," *Journal of Food Composition and Analysis*, vol. 20, no. 3-4, pp. 313–322, 2007.

[39] G. Oboh and J. B. T. Rocha, "Antioxidant and neuroprotective properties of sour tea (*Hibiscus sabdariffa*, calyx) and green tea (*Camellia sinensis*) on some pro-oxidant-induced lipid peroxidation in brain in vitro," *Food Biophysics*, vol. 3, no. 4, pp. 382–389, 2008.

4

Evaluation of Various Nuclear Cytological Changes in Normal Buccal Mucosa and Peritumoural Area in Patients with Oral Squamous Cell Carcinoma Receiving Concomitant Chemoradiotherapy

Sadia Minhas,[1] Muhammad Kashif,[2] and A. H. Nagi[3]

[1]*Department of Oral Pathology, Akhtar Saeed Medical and Dental College, Bahria Town, Lahore 54000, Pakistan*
[2]*Department of Immunology, University of Health Sciences, Lahore, Pakistan*
[3]*Department of Morbid Anatomy and Histopathology, University of Health Sciences, Lahore, Pakistan*

Correspondence should be addressed to Sadia Minhas; sadiawasif81@gmail.com

Academic Editor: Elizabeth Wiley

Objectives. To evaluate the role of serial cytological assay in calculating the nuclear response of contralateral normal buccal mucosa and peritumoural area of squamous cell carcinoma of oral cavity in patients receiving fractionated radiotherapy (RT) and chemotherapy. *Materials and Methods.* This prospective, nonrandomized study was comprised of 76 histologically confirmed cases of oral squamous cell carcinoma on cyclical chemoradiation treatment. Chemoradiosensitivity was evaluated using serial scrape smears taken before and after immediate exposure to CCRT, at 17th day of CCRT (mid of treatment), and at the end of treatment. The nuclear changes, such as multinucleation, micronucleation, karyorrhexis, karyolysis, nuclear budding, prominent nucleoli, and binucleation occurring in both irradiated cancer cells and contralateral normal buccal mucosa, had a statistically significant dose related increase with concomitant chemoradiotherapy ($p < 0.05$). *Conclusion.* We recommend regular use of serial cytological assay during CCRT as it may prove to be a valuable tool for assessment of chemoradiosensitivity and persistence of tumour/dysplastic cells after radiotherapy.

1. Introduction

Globally, oral cancer is the eighth most common cause of cancer-related deaths, although many people are unaware of its presence [1]. Of these oral cancers, more than 90% are oral squamous cell carcinomas (OSCC) arising in the mucous membranes of the oral cavity, floor of the mouth, ventral surface of the tongue, and oropharynx [2]. A study conducted by Bhurgi in Pakistan, reported that it is the most common cancer in Pakistan, whereas Rehman and Jafferi found that oral carcinoma constitutes about 10% of the malignancies in Pakistan [3]. The early oral cancers are usually treated with surgery and radiation therapy, whereas patients with advanced oral tumours may undergo combination of treatments, that is, radiation therapy, chemotherapy, and concomitant chemoradiotherapy. The selection of treatments depends on patient general health, the size of tumour, and metastasis [4]. The radiation which is used for the treatment of cancers is ionizing radiation because it produces ions in the cells of the tissue from where it passes. This can kill cells or alter genes so that the cells cannot grow [5].

The drugs flow all-round the body in the blood and reach cancer cells nearly anywhere in the body. This is called systemic treatment. Chemotherapy drugs deteriorate the genes inside the nucleus of cells. A combination of different chemotherapy drugs are used for the treatment of cancer. The combination of chemotherapy drugs damages cells at different stages in the course of cell division. There is more chance of killing more cells with the use of more than one type of drug [6]. A concurrent chemoradiotherapy (CCRT) regimen represents the most excellent current standard therapy for many patients with regionally advanced solid tumours and improves the likelihood of cure. The clinical goal of administrating chemotherapy and radiation concurrently is to develop both locoregional and systemic tumour control [7].

For oral cancer, cytology has been an option and proved to be a consistent primary diagnostic test. It can also be of value where surgical biopsy is not indicated or in postradiotherapy follow-up cases. The combined histological and cytological assessment of a lesion has been found to give the highest percentage of early diagnosis of oral cancers [8]. Cytological effects of radiation on oral mucosa and in oral cancers were reported in 1957 and 1959, respectively [9]. Numerous reports have described different cytoplasmic and nuclear changes following radiation therapy. These changes consist of cytoplasmic granulation, cellular enlargement, vacuolization, pyknosis, binucleation, karyorrhexis, karyolysis, micronucleation, nuclear budding, nuclear enlargement, and multinucleation [10].

By the 1960s, the nuclear morphological alterations that were calculated by cytology became well established and included karyorrhexis, karyolysis, multinucleation, and crenation of nuclear membrane [11]. Despite a high incidence of oral cancer in Asian region, studies on prediction of effectiveness of various treatment modalities are inadequate and sparse, in this region [12]. The present study was taken forward to see whether serial cytological evaluation from normal buccal mucosa and peritumoural area in oral squamous cell carcinoma patients receiving concomitant chemoradiotherapy at four different stages can predict the chemoradiosensitivity of peritumoural area and response of normal buccal mucosa.

2. Materials and Methods

The study was conducted in Department of Morbid Anatomy and Histopathology, University of Health Sciences Lahore Pakistan, during the period of one year. A total of 76 patients with histologically proven squamous cell carcinoma of oral cavity, on fractionated radiotherapy on a dose of 70–90 Gy in 5 fractions/week for a span of 7 weeks (total 35 fractions), were included in the study. Scrape smears were collected from peritumoural area (the peritumoural area is defined as a 2 mm wide band of host tissue adjacent to the invasive front. The tumour periphery is defined as a 2 mm wide band of tumour immediately adjacent to the invasive front, and tumour center is defined as an inner center area) and contralateral normal buccal mucosa of each patient before the start, after immediate exposure to CCRT, on 17th day, and at the end of treatment. The cytological smears were obtained by scraping the peritumoural area and contralateral normal buccal mucosa using the rounded end of Ayre's spatula and slides were fixed in 95% alcohol for haematoxylin and eosin and Papanicolaou (Pap) stains, while some slides were air dried for May-Grunwald-Giemsa (MGG) stain. Smears were examined at both 20x and 40x with an eyepiece of 10x. Around 500–1000 cells were evaluated from the samples collected on each occasion. The nuclear changes were observed, that is, multinucleation, nuclear budding, karyolysis, karyorrhexis, micronuclei, binucleation, and prominent nucleoli. Data were entered and analyzed using the SPSS 20.0. The variation in the frequency of these changes in relation to cumulative radiation dose was analyzed using Chi-square test/Fisher exact test and a p value < 0.05 was considered as statistically significant. The study was approved and certified by Institutional Ethical Review Committee and Advanced Studies & Research Board, UHS Lahore, Pakistan.

3. Results

In 304 smears from normal buccal mucosa on all respective days of CCRT, karyolysis was seen in $n = 156$ (51.3%) smears and it was absent in $n = 148$ (48.7%) smears. Out of 76 smears from normal buccal mucosa on each day, that is, before and immediately after first dose, at 17th day, and at end of CCRT, karyolysis was seen in $n = 1$ (1.3%), $n = 3$ (3.9%), and $n = 76$ (100%) for 17th day and end of therapy smears, respectively. In overall 304 smears from peritumoural area on all respective days of sampling, karyolysis was seen in $n = 180$ (59.2%) smears and it was absent in $n = 124$ (40.8%) smears.

Considering the karyolysis in peritumoural area before and after immediate exposure to CCRT it was seen in $n = 7$ (9.2%) and $n = 21$ (27.6%) smears, respectively. Smears were taken on each day, that is, at the 17th day and at the end of therapy; all the smears (100%) were positive for karyolysis.

Destructive fragmentation of nucleus (karyorrhexis) in normal buccal mucosal cells on all particular days of treatment from 76 patients was observed in $n = 154$ (50.6%) smears and absent in $n = 150$ (49.3%) smears. Among 76 smears from normal buccal mucosa on all sampling days, that is, before and after immediate exposure, at 17th day, and at end of CCRT, karyorrhexis was observed in 1.3%, 2.6%, 98.7%, and 100% smears, respectively.

While inspecting the 304 smears from peritumoural area on all specific days of CCRT, karyorrhexis was seen in $n = 174$ (57.2%) smears. In $n = 130$ (42.7%) smears no karyorrhexis was seen in peritumoural area. Out of 76 smears from peritumoural area on each day, that is, before CCRT $n = 7$ (9.2%), after immediate exposure $n = 15$ (9.7%), at 17th day, and at end of CCRT, $n = 76$ (100%) of smears were positive for karyorrhexis (Table 1).

Regarding binucleation in contralateral normal buccal mucosal cells, it was present in $n = 190$ (62.5%) out of 304 smears while it was absent in $n = 114$ (37.5%) smears. A total of 76 smears from normal buccal mucosa before CCRT $n = 7$ (9.2%), after immediate exposure to CCRT $n = 32$ (42.1%), at the 17th day of treatment 98.7%, and at the end of treatment $n = 76$ (100%) smears were positive for binucleation (Figure 1).

Among all the 304 smears from peritumoural on all particular days of sampling, binucleation was observed in $n = 263$ (86.5%) and absent in $n = 41$ (13.5%) smears (Figure 1). On each day of sampling, binucleation was observed in $n = 49$ (64.5%) before CCRT, after immediate exposure to CCRT in $n = 63$ (82.9%), at the 17th day of treatment in 98.7% (Figure 1), and at the end of CCRT in 100% of smears (Table 1).

Considering the nuclear budding in normal buccal mucosal cells on all specific days of CCRT, it was present in

Table 1: Frequencies of different variables of nuclear atypia in cells of peritumoural area on different days of CCRT.

Variables/days of CCRT	Before	Immediate	17th day	End
Karyolysis	9.2%	27.6%	100%	100%
Karyorrhexis	9.2%	9.7%	100%	100%
Binucleation	64.5%	82.9%	98.7%	100%
Multinucleation	0%	0%	30.3%	92.1%
Nuclear budding	1.3%	1.3%	36.8%	98.7%
Micronuclei	23.7%	69.7%	98.7%	100%
Prominent nucleoli	82.9%	98.7%	100%	100%

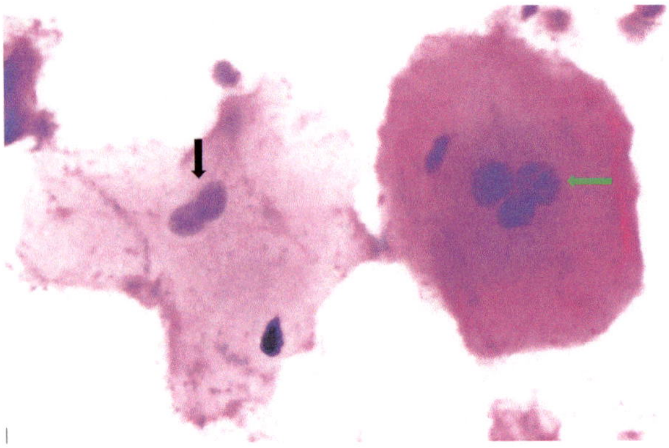

Figure 1: Photomicrograph with H&E stain shows multinucleated cell (green arrow) and binucleated cell (black arrow) in smears from contralateral normal buccal mucosa obtained at end of CCRT.

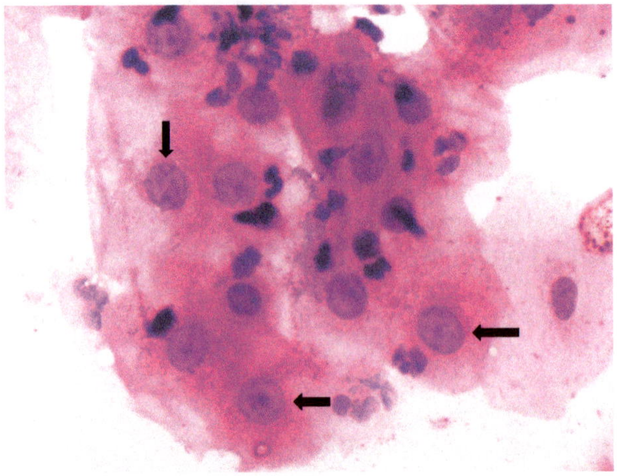

Figure 2: Photomicrograph reveals prominent nucleoli in almost each and every cell in smears obtained from contralateral normal buccal mucosa at 17th day of CCRT.

$n = 90$ (29.6%) smears and was absent in $n = 214$ (70.3%) smears. From normal buccal mucosa on each specific day, that is, before and after immediate exposure to CCRT none of the smears showed nuclear budding. However, at the 17th day and at the end of treatment (Figure 5) nuclear budding was observed in $n = 16$ (21.1%) and $n = 74$ (97.4%) smears, respectively.

In a total of 304 smears from peritumoural area from 76 patients on all respective days of treatment, nuclear budding was observed in $n = 105$ (34.5%) smears and absent in $n = 199$ (65.4%) smears. Before and after immediate exposure to CCRT nuclear budding was observed in $n = 1$ (1.3%) smears for both days of therapy. Whereas $n = 28$ (36.8%) smears were taken at the 17th day of treatment and at the end of treatment $n = 75$ (98.7%) smears were positive for nuclear budding.

Regarding micronucleation in a total of 304 smears from normal buccal mucosa on all specific days of sampling, it was seen in $n = 173$ (56.9%) smears and absent in $n = 131$ (43.1%) smears. Out of 76 smears from normal buccal mucosa, before CCRT $n = 3$ (3.9%) and after immediate exposure to treatment $n = 18$ (23.7%) smears were positive for micronucleation. However, in smears taken on each day, that is, at the 17th day of therapy and at the end of therapy, 100% of smears were positive for micronucleation.

In a total of 304 smears from peritumoural area on all particular days of treatment, micronucleation was observed in $n = 222$ (73.0%) smears. However it was absent in $n = 82$ (26.9%) smears. In a total of 76 smears taken at each specific day of CCRT, that is, before CCRT, after immediate exposure to CCRT, at the 17th day of CCRT (Figure 3), and at end of therapy micronucleation was observed in smears as follows: $n = 18$ (23.7%), $n = 53$ (69.7%), 98.7%, and 100%, respectively (Table 1).

Among 304 smears from normal buccal mucosa on all specific days of CCRT from 76 patients, prominent nucleoli were seen in $n = 225$ (74.0%) smears and were absent in $n = 79$ (25.9%) smears. Among 76 smears from normal buccal mucosa on each specific day of sampling, that is, before CCRT and after immediate exposure to CCRT, prominent nucleoli were seen in $n = 15$ (19.7%) and 76.3% smears, respectively, while smears both at 17th day (Figure 2) and at end of therapy were 100% positive for prominent nucleoli.

On peritumoural area, prominent nucleoli were present in $n = 290$ (95.4%) smears and were absent in $n = 14$ (4.6%) smears. Among 76 smears on each day, that is, before and after immediate exposure to CCRT, prominent nucleoli were seen in $n = 63$ (82.9%) and 98.7% smears, whereas prominent nucleoli were observed in 100% smears taken at each day, that is, at the 17th day and end of therapy, respectively, from peritumoural area.

In normal buccal mucosal cells, multinucleation was observed in $n = 69$ (22.6%) smears on all specific days of sampling from 76 patients. No such changes were seen

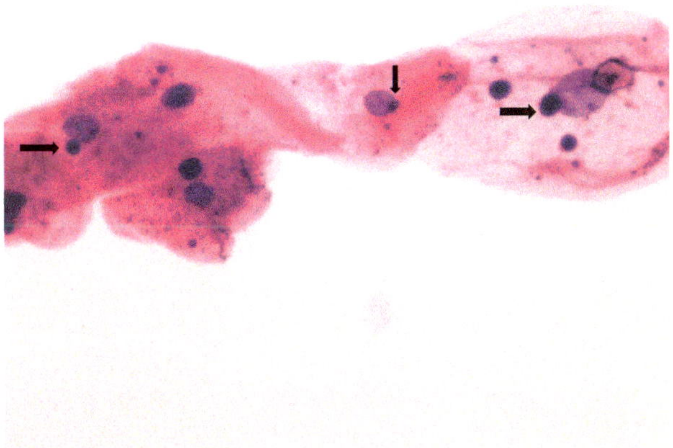

Figure 3: Photomicrograph with H&E stain shows feature of nuclear atypia, that is, micronuclei (arrows) in smears obtained at the 17th day of CCRT from peritumoural area.

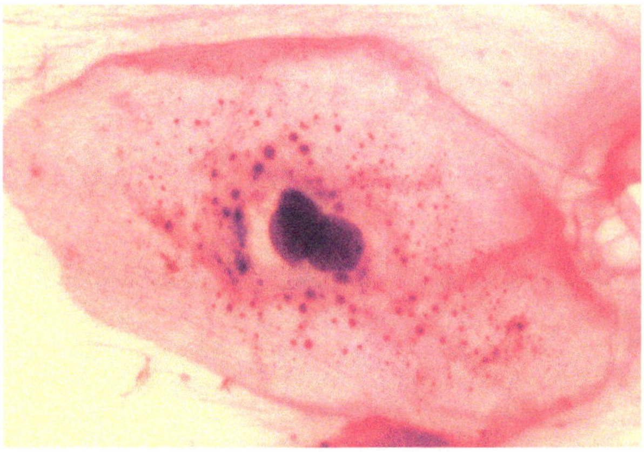

Figure 4: Photomicrograph with H&E stain shows a multinucleated cell in smear obtained from peritumoural area at the 17th day of CCRT.

in $n = 235$ (77.3%) smears (Figure 1). As considering the smears from peritumoural area on all particular days of CCRT, multinucleation was observed in $n = 93$ (30.5%) smears (Figure 4). Detailed distribution of multinucleation both on normal buccal mucosa and on peritumoural area on different days of sampling is given in Table 1.

4. Discussion

Oral squamous cell carcinoma is a serious fatal disease. The outcomes from management of advanced carcinoma of the head and neck are unfortunate. The conventional management procedures for SCC of head and neck are radiotherapy and surgery, which are mostly curative in early stages of disease and are less efficient in more advanced patients. Although squamous cell carcinoma of the head and neck is chemosensitive, it is not treatable by chemotherapy alone [13–15]. One method, in an attempt to improve clinical outcomes, is to give radiotherapy and chemotherapy concomitantly [16].

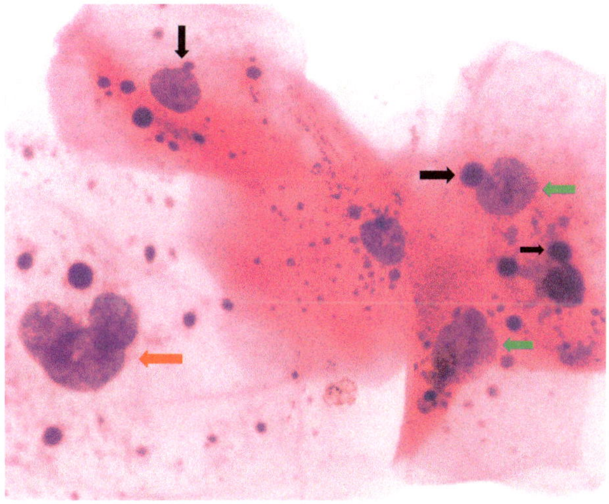

Figure 5: Photomicrograph of smear obtained at the end of CCRT from contralateral normal buccal mucosa shows features of nuclear atypia, micronuclei (black arrow), mild to moderate degree of pleomorphism (green arrow), and nuclear budding (red arrow).

Responses of malignant cells as well as the surrounding normal oral tissues to radiotherapy are based on their radiosensitivity but the inconsistency in host-tumour reaction makes it complicated to evaluate and predict the effect of such treatment in a particular patient. Radiation puts forth its effects on both malignant and normal cells mostly by inducing chromosomal injury, the end result of which can be distinguished by the occurrence of micronuclei in dividing cells [17].

Improvement of the radiation response was usually less marked in the tumour model as compared to normal tissues. The combined drug-radiation effect was actually less time-dependent in the tumour than in the normal tissues [18].

The present study was designed to determine the cytological changes following concomitant chemoradiotherapy (radiochemoreaction) and predict the strength of association among duration and dose of chemoradiation therapy to these changes.

In this study, the changes were evaluated in peritumoural area around the tumour and benign cells collected from contralateral normal buccal mucosa. Our results showed that various quantifiable cellular changes become evident in the initial few days of concomitant chemoradiotherapy but are more prominent at the end of CCRT where they illustrate strong statistical significance (Table 2).

Karyorrhexis is the destructive fragmentation of the nucleus of a dying cell whereby its chromatin is distributed irregularly throughout the cytoplasm. It signifies nuclear breakup into smaller fragments, whereas karyolysis indicates a progressive dissolution of chromatin. Karyolysis and karyorrhexis were reported on both normal and malignant oral cells and also noted a statistically significant increase with radiotherapy dose ($p = 0.01$) [19–21]. Serial cytological

TABLE 2: Association between days of CCRT and various variables of nuclear abnormalities on both sites (contralateral normal buccal mucosa and peritumoural area).

Variables/site	Buccal mucosa	Peritumoural area
Karyolysis	$p = 0.000$	$p = 0.000$
Karyorrhexis	$p = 0.000$	$p = 0.000$
Multinucleation	$p = 0.000$	$p = 0.000$
Nuclear budding	$p = 0.000$	$p = 0.000$
Prominent nucleoli	$p = 0.000$	$p = 0.000$
Binucleation	$p = 0.000$	$p = 0.000$
Micronuclei	$p = 0.000$	$p = 0.000$

smears from OSCC show that both karyorrhexis and karyolysis were more pronounced at the end of therapy [10].

Nuclear budding is defined as production of two daughter nuclei of unequal size by constriction of the parent nucleus. It represents the rounded nuclear material mimicking a micronucleus and can often be found close to the nucleus without any definite separation. Nuclear budding can occur in the nuclear envelope and when it ruptures it leads to transfer of DNA material to cytoplasm. Nuclear budding can be considered to be stimulated by a direct, localized consequence of radiation on nuclear membrane [22, 23]. The frequency of nuclear budding was increased with increased radiotherapy dosages in serial scrape smears from contralateral normal buccal mucosa and malignant tissue, and a statistically significant association has been reported with the radiotherapy dose ($p < 0.001$) on each site (Table 2) [19]. Similarly, serial scrape smears from radiotherapy receiving patients for OSCC reported that statistically significant association was observed between nuclear budding and radiotherapy dosages on tumoural area ($p = 0.034$) (Table 2) [21].

Cell division is accomplished when the splitting up of cell membrane happens subsequent to nuclear division. Incomplete cell division occurs due to cell membrane damage which directs to the development of binucleated and multinucleated cells by recurring nuclear division. Membrane lipids can undergo peroxidation subsequent to irradiation and this injury might be adequate to avoid cell wall division in sensitive cells [24]. Multinucleation (Figure 4) is considered by having more than one nucleus per cell. It is caused by membrane damage related with increased proliferation of the nucleus resulting in lack of ability of the membrane to continue with the nuclear division. Silverman et al. stated that multinucleation is a frequent radiation-induced change in oral cancers and this was accepted by other researchers later on [25, 26]. Radiation stimulated multinucleation has been noted in cell culture and animals experiments. Damage to nuclear membrane has been suggested as a mechanism that directs to cell death; as a result multinucleated cells are considered to be dead cells and unable of giving rise to colonies [27]. Mehrotra and his colleagues observed that in normal mucosa and malignant cells, the frequency of multinucleation was increased with increased radiotherapy dosage in a serial scrape smears from both sites. They also reported a significant association between multinucleation on normal mucosa and malignant cells and radiation dose ($p < 0.001$) [22]. Similarly, the frequency of multinucleated cells in tumoural area in irradiated serial smears was increased with increased radiotherapy dosages [21, 26].

Binucleation is defined as formation of two nuclei within a cell through division of the nucleus without division of the cytoplasm. The study conducted in India on binucleation and radiation response in normal buccal mucosa and malignant cells stated that there was increased incidence of binucleation on both sites as the radiotherapy dose increased. Similarly, a significant association was observed between radiotherapy dose and binucleation on both contralateral normal mucosa and in malignant cells ($p < 0.001$) in present study [22].

Micronucleation is also the name given to the small nucleus that forms whenever a chromosome or a fragment of a chromosome is not incorporated into one of the daughter nuclei during cell division. Micronuclei are intracytoplasmic DNA staining bodies found in the same level as the main nucleus with the equal or a little staining intensity, one-third to one-fifth of the size of the main nucleus placed within two nuclear diameters from the main nucleus but distinctly separated from it. The micronuclei represent the genomic damage of the cell and to calculate the genomic damage as a result of radiotherapy. The micronuclei present in normal buccal mucosa cells are noteworthy, because they are in irradiated field. The existence of micronucleus shows that the cell has undergone through unrepaired DNA damage and the cells containing micronuclei are considered as dead cells that are unable to give rise to progeny [28]. Existence of a micronucleus is a recognized test for observing the toxicity of chemicals in normal tissues and efficiency of chemopreventive agents against cancer [29]. The number of micronucleated cells raises and achieves a plateau with repetitive chemical and radiation injuries [22]. Hintzsche et al. examined normal buccal mucosa cells for genomic damage at four different times during radiation therapy. A clear increase was observed in normal buccal mucosa for every time point [30]. The frequency of MN in oral mucosal cells of patients with OSCC was three- to fourfold higher as compared with the control group [31]. In a study, Dórea and his colleagues stated that incidence of micronuclei was seen considerably more commonly in cells collected from lesions than in cells from normal areas [32]. Similar findings were reflected in our study with the frequency of micronuclei increasing with radiation dose on both sites. Previous multiple studies with multinucleation and micronucleation assays during the first 15–18 days of radiotherapy showed that serial cytology has important and significant correlations with cell proliferation and radiosensitivity [12, 25, 33].

Prominent nucleoli are defined as small, typically round granular bodies composed of protein and RNA in the nucleus of a cell. Nucleoli are usually associated with a specific chromosomal site and involved in ribosomal RNA synthesis and the formation of ribosomes. The study conducted in USA reported that the incidence of prominent nucleoli was raised in smears obtained from benign prostate glands after radiotherapy [34]. A study carried out in Chicago stated that chemotherapy could induce prominent nucleoli [35].

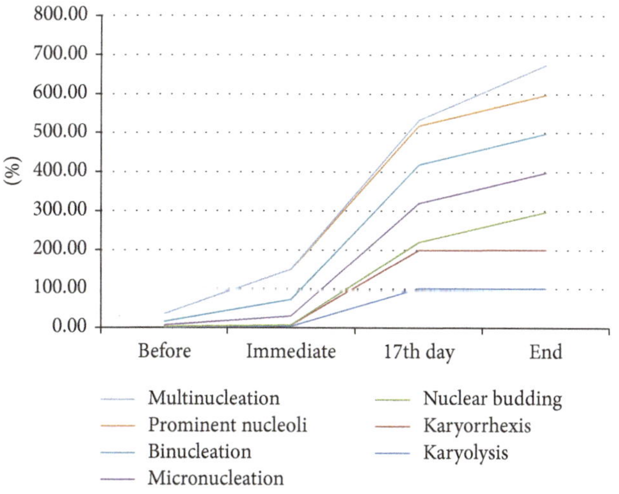

FIGURE 6: Nonlinear increase among the variables of nuclear atypia and different days of CCRT in smears obtained from contralateral normal buccal mucosa.

Significant association was observed among different variables of nuclear atypia (karyolysis, karyorrhexis, nuclear budding, micronucleation, prominent nucleoli, binucleation, and multinucleation) and days of CCRT in present study (Table 2).

Another finding which is apparent in the present study is a nonlinear increase in the numbers of nuclear abnormalities on exposure to increasing doses of concomitant chemoradiotherapy. It can be observed from the graphs (Figure 6) that the rise in the frequencies of the different nuclear abnormalities follows a gentle curve up till after immediate exposure to CCRT but after that the rise is relatively much steeper. A similar "hockey stick" curve for stimulation of micronuclei in lymphocytes exposed to ionizing radiation has been stated earlier and might result from DNA repair processes taking place at low radiation doses promoting reattainment of DNA strand breaks at some stage in the S phase of cell cycle prior to the cell entry in mitotic phase [36]. With a raise in the chemoradiation dose the repair ability of the cell decreases while the amount of chromosomal damage increases accelerating to increase in unrepaired DNA fragments which may lead to development of more number of micronuclei and nuclear buddings. An almost identical accumulation of unrepaired damage to the cell membrane at elevated doses of chemoradiation may cause an increase in the counts of multinucleated and binucleated cells too.

All the nuclear abnormalities that were studied, that is, micronucleation, nuclear budding, binucleation, and multinucleation, showed a dose dependent increase in response to concomitant chemoradiotherapy for both sites (contralateral normal buccal mucosa and peritumoural area) and these changes were more marked in CCRT receiving patients as compared to patients receiving radiotherapy alone.

These all previously described features, that is, karyolysis, karyorrhexis, binucleation, nuclear budding, and multinucleation, are collectively called nuclear atypia (Figure 5). The study conducted by Bhattathiri called the "abnormal nucleated cells" with these features and many other international studies reported that these features are indicators/markers of radiosensitivity of tumour. It is a useful tool in the assessment of biological damage that can help in radiosensitivity of tumour whereas tumours which are radioresistant exhibited lesser degree of change as compared to radiosensitive tumours [10, 26, 37]. We observed that when different parameters (multinucleated cells, nuclear budding, micronucleation, and bizarre cells) were taken together, the increase in dose related response was significantly high. These abnormally nucleated cells had a mean value four times higher than pretreatment count at 38.5 Gy, thus indicating these combined parameters to be a better indicator of radiosensitivity than any single parameter [37, 38].

5. Conclusion

It is concluded from the findings of present study that various nuclear abnormalities reveal a statistically significant increase with increasing chemoradiation doses and time interval. Persistence of dysplastic and malignant cells from peritumoural area during and at end of this treatment can be a sign of resistant or recurrent carcinoma. Similarly, the relationship among different days of CCRT and high frequency of nuclear abnormalities in normal buccal mucosa suggests that the serial smears of these changes have potential use for the early prediction of inflammatory-benign-precancerous and then malignant lesions in patients receiving CCRT. We, therefore, suggest serial cytological assays of peritumoural area and from contralateral normal buccal mucosa till the end of therapy and also on longer term follow-ups.

Competing Interests

All the authors also assure that they have no potential competing interests (financial or nonfinancial interests) in the subject matters or materials discussed in this paper.

Acknowledgments

The authors are grateful to University of Health Sciences Lahore, Mr. Sameer Anjum, Lab Tech, Department of Morbid Anatomy and Histopathology, UHS Lahore, and the staff of Department of Chemoradiotherapy, Institute of Nuclear Medicine Lahore (INMOL), for their technical and logistic support.

References

[1] N. W. Johnson, P. Jayasekara, A. A. Amarasinghe, and K. Hemantha, "Squamous cell carcinoma and precursor lesions of the oral cavity: epidemiology and aetiology," *Periodontology 2000*, vol. 57, no. 1, pp. 19–37, 2011.

[2] M. L. Darby and M. M. Walsh, *Dental Hygiene Theory and Practice*, Saunders Elsevier, St. Louis, Mo, USA, 3rd edition, 2010.

[3] M. A. Musani, I. Jawed, S. Marfani, Y. Khambaty, M. Jalisi, and S. A. Khan, "Carcinoma cheek: regional pattern and

management," *Journal of Ayub Medical College, Abbottabad*, vol. 21, no. 3, pp. 87–91, 2009.

[4] NCI, *What Do You Need to Know about Oral Cancer?* National Cancer Institute at the National Institutes of Health, 2009, http://www.cancer.gov/publications/patient-education/wyntk-oral-cancer.

[5] American Cancer Society, *Types of Radiation Used to Treat Cancer. Radiation Therapy Principles*, American Cancer Society, 2013, http://www.cancer.org/treatment/treatmentsandsideeffects/treatmenttypes/radiation/radiationtherapyprinciples/radiation-therapy-principles-types-of-radiation.

[6] Cancer Research UK, *How Chemotherapy Kills Cancer Cells. How Chemotherapy Works*, Cancer Research UK, 2013, http://www.cancerresearchuk.org/about-cancer/cancers-in-general/treatment/chemotherapy/about/how-chemotherapy-works.

[7] T. Y. Seiwert, J. K. Salama, and E. E. Vokes, "The chemoradiation paradigm in head and neck cancer," *Nature Clinical Practice Oncology*, vol. 4, no. 3, pp. 156–171, 2007.

[8] J. G. Cowpe, R. B. Longmore, and M. W. Green, "Quantitative exfoliative cytology of abnormal oral mucosal smears," *Journal of the Royal Society of Medicine*, vol. 81, no. 9, pp. 509–513, 1988.

[9] K. Rimpu, A. Chaugule, and P. K. Goyal, "Karyoanomalic frequency during radiation therapy," *Journal of Cancer Research and Therapeutics*, vol. 1, no. 3, pp. 187–190, 2005.

[10] L. Bindu, P. Balaram, A. Mathew, P. Remani, V. N. Bhattathiri, and M. K. Nair, "Radiation-induced changes in oral carcinoma cells—a multiparametric evaluation," *Cytopathology*, vol. 14, no. 5, pp. 287–293, 2003.

[11] E. G. Wachtel, "Radiation changes in vaginal smears," in *Exfoliative Cytology in Gynecological Practice*, pp. 175–193, Butterworths, London, UK, 1964.

[12] T. Ramaesh, N. Ratnatunga, B. R. Mendis, and S. Rajapaksa, "Exfoliative cytology in screening for malignant and premalignant lesions in the buccal mucosa," *The Ceylon Medical Journal*, vol. 43, no. 4, pp. 206–209, 1998.

[13] P. M. Stell, J. E. Dalby, P. Strickland, J. G. Fraser, P. J. Bradley, and L. M. Flood, "Sequential chemotherapy and radiotherapy in advanced head and neck cancer," *Clinical Radiology*, vol. 34, no. 4, pp. 463–467, 1983.

[14] I. F. Tannock, "Combined modality treatment with radiotherapy and chemotherapy," *Radiotherapy and Oncology*, vol. 16, no. 2, pp. 83–101, 1989.

[15] P. M. Stell and N. S. B. Rawson, "Adjuvant chemotherapy in head and neck cancer," *British Journal of Cancer*, vol. 61, no. 5, pp. 779–787, 1990.

[16] E. E. Vokes and R. R. Weichselbaum, "Concomitant chemotherapy: rationale and clinical experience in patients with solid tumours," *Journal of Clinical Oncology*, vol. 8, pp. 911–934, 1990.

[17] F. Sarto, R. Tomanin, L. Giacomelli, G. Iannini, and A. R. Cupiraggi, "The micronucleus assay in human exfoliated cells of the nose and mouth: application to occupational exposures to chromic acid and ethylene oxide," *Mutation Research Letters*, vol. 244, no. 4, pp. 345–351, 1990.

[18] H. von der Maase, "Experimental studies on interactions of radiation and cancer chemotherapeutic drugs in normal tissues and a solid tumour," *Radiotherapy and Oncology*, vol. 7, no. 1, pp. 47–68, 1986.

[19] R. Mehrotra, Madhu, and M. Singh, "Serial scrape smear cytology of radiation response in normal and malignant cells of oral cavity," *Indian Journal of Pathology and Microbiology*, vol. 47, no. 4, pp. 497–502, 2004.

[20] R. Mehrotra, A. Gupta, M. Singh, and R. Ibrahim, "Application of cytology and molecular biology in diagnosing premalignant or malignant oral lesions," *Molecular Cancer*, vol. 5, article 11, 2006.

[21] D. Agarwal, N. Khan, S. A. Siddhiqui, and N. Afroz, "Assessment of various cytological changes for predicting radiosensitivity of oral cavity cancer by serial cytology," *JK Science*, vol. 13, no. 4, pp. 171–175, 2011.

[22] R. Mehrotra, N. Goel, M. Singh, and D. Kumar, "Radiation-related cytological changes in oral malignant cells," *Indian Journal of Pathology and Microbiology*, vol. 47, no. 3, pp. 343–347, 2004.

[23] V. Raj and S. Mahajan, "Dose response relationship of nuclear changes with fractionated radiotherapy in assessing radiosensitivity of oral squamous cell carcinoma," *Journal of Clinical and Experimental Dentistry*, vol. 3, no. 3, pp. e193–e200, 2011.

[24] G. R. Ogden, S. McQueen, D. M. Chisholm, and E. B. Lane, "Keratin profiles of normal and malignant oral mucosa using exfoliative cytology," *Journal of Clinical Pathology*, vol. 46, no. 4, pp. 352–356, 1993.

[25] N. V. Bhattathiri, L. Bindu, P. Remani, B. Chandralekha, and K. M. Nair, "Radiation-induced acute immediate nuclear abnormalities in oral cancer cells: serial cytologic evaluation," *Acta Cytologica*, vol. 42, no. 5, pp. 1084–1090, 1998.

[26] R. Kumari, C. Arun, and P. K. Goyal, "Karyoanomalic frequency during radiation therapy," *Journal of Cancer Research and Therapeutics*, vol. 1, no. 3, pp. 187–190, 2005.

[27] Y.-G. Man and H. E. Nieburgs, "A subset of cell clusters with malignant features in morphologically normal-appearing and hyperplastic tissues," *Cancer Detection and Prevention*, vol. 30, no. 3, pp. 239–247, 2006.

[28] G. R. Ogden, J. G. Cowpe, and A. J. Wight, "Oral exfoliative cytology: review of methods of assessment," *Journal of Oral Pathology and Medicine*, vol. 26, no. 5, pp. 201–205, 1997.

[29] H. F. Stich and M. P. Rosin, "Micronuclei in exfoliated human cells as a tool for studies in cancer risk and cancer intervention," *Cancer Letters*, vol. 22, no. 3, pp. 241–253, 1984.

[30] H. Hintzsche, B. Polat, V. Schewe et al., "Micronucleus formation kinetics in buccal mucosa cells of head and neck cancer patients undergoing radiotherapy," *Toxicology Letters*, vol. 212, no. 1, pp. 33–37, 2012.

[31] K. Jadhav, N. Gupta, and B. R. Ahmed Mujib, "Micronuclei: an essential biomarker in oral exfoliated cells for grading of oral squamous cell carcinoma," *Journal of Cytology*, vol. 28, no. 1, pp. 7–12, 2011.

[32] L.-N. T. M. Dórea, J. R. C. Meireles, J. P. R. Lessa et al., "Chromosomal damage and apoptosis in exfoliated buccal cells from individuals with oral cancer," *International Journal of Dentistry*, vol. 2012, Article ID 457054, 6 pages, 2012.

[33] P. Sharma, N. Kumar, A. K. Bahadur, and A. K. Mandal, "Ki-67 expression in cytologic scrapes from oral squamous cell carcinoma before and after 24 gray radiotherapy—a study on 43 patients," *Medicina Oral, Patología Oral y Cirugía Bucal*, vol. 10, pp. E15–E17, 2005.

[34] L. Cheng, J. C. Cheville, and D. G. Bostwick, "Diagnosis of prostate cancer in needle biopsies after radiation therapy," *American Journal of Surgical Pathology*, vol. 23, no. 10, pp. 1173–1183, 1999.

[35] M. I. Doria Jr., L. K. Doria, J. Faintuch, and B. Levin, "Gastric mucosal injury after hepatic arterial infusion chemotherapy with floxuridine: a clinical and pathologic study," *Cancer*, vol. 73, no. 8, pp. 2042–2047, 1994.

[36] J. C. Mitchell and A. Norman, "The induction of micronuclei in human lymphocytes by low doses of radiation," *International Journal of Radiation Biology*, vol. 52, no. 4, pp. 527–535, 1987.

[37] N. V. Bhattathiri, C. Bharathykkutty, R. Prathapan, D. A. Chirayathmanjiyil, and K. M. Nair, "Prediction of radiosensitivity of oral cancers by serial cytological assay of nuclear changes," *Radiotherapy and Oncology*, vol. 49, no. 1, pp. 61–65, 1998.

[38] V. N. Bhattathiri, L. Bindu, P. Remani, B. Chandralekha, C. A. Davis, and M. K. Nair, "Serial cytological assay of micronucleus induction: a new tool to predict human cancer radiosensitivity," *Radiotherapy and Oncology*, vol. 41, no. 2, pp. 139–142, 1996.

5

Diagnostic Modalities of Precancerous and Cancerous Cervical Lesions with Special Emphasis on CD31 Angiogenesis Factor as a Marker

Bandana Sharma, Neetu Singh, Neena Gupta, Pavika Lal, Shefali Pande, and Shashi Chauhan

Department of Obstetrics & Gynaecology, GSVM Medical College, Kanpur 208002, India

Correspondence should be addressed to Bandana Sharma; bandanasharma20@gmail.com

Academic Editor: Piero Tosi

Objectives. To evaluate the role of angiogenesis tumor marker CD31 in the detection of precancerous and cancerous cervical lesions and to compare its efficacy with colposcopy and histopathology. *Materials and Methods.* 230 patients with a suspicious looking cervix and an abnormal Pap smear attending the Outpatient Department of Obstetrics and Gynaecology of GSVM Medical College were subjected to a colposcopic examination. 180 patients with suspected colposcopic findings were subjected to a colposcopic directed biopsy. Biopsy tissues were sent for histopathological examination out of which 50 biopsied samples were sent for immunostaining of CD-31. Statistical analysis was done. *Results.* Comparison of microvessel density (MVD) count by haematoxylin and eosin staining (HE) and immunostaining of CD31 in preinvasive group were 4.012 ± 2.57 and 5.44 ± 2.21, respectively, and in invasive group were 9.18 ± 2.32 and 12.82 ± 4.07, respectively, which showed that MVD was higher by CD31 both in preinvasive and invasive group, and it was statistically significant. *Conclusion.* Angiogenesis is a marker of tumor progression, and CD31 fixes up vessel better as compared to HE, so aggressiveness of the tumor can be better predicted by MVD-CD31 as compared to MVD-HE.

1. Introduction

Worldwide cervical cancer is the most common gynaecological malignancy and the third most common frequently diagnosed cancer in female after breast and colorectal cancer. It is the commonest cause of gynaecological cancer death and responsible for about 190,000 deaths every year [1].

Both the incidence and mortality from cervical cancer have been reduced by various systematic screening methods and treatment of premalignant cervical lesions. The introduction of practical cytology by Papanicolaou and Traut in 1943 and its later widespread use into clinical practice represented the major development in cervical cancer preventions further assisted by the use of colposcopy which allows the clinician to visually identify these preinvasive lesions on the cervix, determine their extent, and select a site for biopsy confirmation.

Angiogenesis is a better correlate of malignancy and a requisite for metastasis. Tumor growth is thus controlled by the balance between angiogenic factors (vascular endothelial growth factor, fibroblast growth factor, and platelet derived growth factor) and antiangiogenic factors (thrombospondin, angiostatin, and endostatin). Intensity of tumor angiogenesis is supposed to be reflected by intratumoral microvessel density (MVD), but it is difficult to assess revascularization by normal microscopy; therefore various antibodies members for endothelial cells have been used to demarcate the area of vascularity within the tumor out of which CD-31 has the best documented specificity for endothelial cells. CD-31 is a cluster of differentiation molecule with molecular weight of 130–140 Kilodaltons belonging to the immunoglobuin supergene family. It plays a major role in tissue regeneration and is normally found on endothelial cells, platelets, and on macrophages along with the expression on vascular tumors.

The importance of screening of carcinoma cervix by CD31 angiogenesis marker is that it may provide a better detection of precancerous and cancerous lesions along with its aggressiveness, therefore, being of great help in prognostication of patients.

TABLE 1: Sociodemographic characteristics of the study population.

Histopathological findings	Age (mean ± SD)	Parity (number)				Socioeconomic status (number)			Age at first coitus (number)		
		P_0	P_1	P_2	$\geq P_3$	Low	Middle	High	10–20 yrs	21–30 yrs	>30 yrs
Normal	27.71 ± 5.44	17	27	23	03	21	36	13	04	64	02
Inflammatory	28.37 ± 5.74	7	28	26	02	27	25	11	03	59	01
CIN-I	36.67 ± 7.20	—	19	21	20	30	21	09	35	25	—
CIN-II	39.33 ± 6.39	—	08	07	15	17	09	04	28	02	—
CIN-III	46.39 ± 5.33	—	03	03	10	11	05	—	16	—	—
Carcinoma		—	—	—	11	09	02	—	11	—	—

TABLE 2: Correlation of cytological findings with histopathological findings in 180 patients.

Cytological finding	Histopathological findings					
	Normal	Inflammatory	CIN-I	CIN-II	CIN-III	Carcinoma
Normal	—	08	05	—	—	—
Inflammatory	—	51	11	02	—	—
Mild dysplasia	—	04	40	04	02	—
Moderate dysplasia	—	—	04	24	03	—
Severe dysplasia	—	—	—	—	11	—
Carcinoma	—	—	—	—	—	11
Total	—	63	60	30	16	11

2. Materials and Methods

This was a prospective study with total number of 250 patients who attended the Outpatient Department of Obstetrics and Gynaecology of GSVM Medical College, Kanpur, from January 2007 to October 2008, out of which 230 patients with suspicious looking cervix and abnormal pap smear were subjected to colposcopy between the 8th and the 12th days of the menstrual cycle. 180 patients with suspected colposcopic findings were subjected to a colposcopy directed biopsy, and tissues were sent for histopathological examination in the Department of Pathology, GSVM Medical College Kanpur. Biopsy tissues of 50 patients were sent for immunostaining of CD-31 angiogenesis tissue marker using streptavidin biotin immunoperoxidase method at a laboratory in Mumbai. A monoclonal antibody against CD-31 was used as a primary antibody.

Patients were studied according to their sociodemographic characteristics and correlation of cytological, colposcopic, and histological findings was done along with comparison of MVD by haematoxylin and eosin staining (HE) and CD-31 immunostaining. Statistical analysis was applied wherever applicable.

3. Observations and Results

Mean age for CIN III and carcinoma was 46.39 ± 5.33 years in our study. 34.42% (21/61) of patients with parity ≥3 had CIN III and carcinoma lesions, whereas in patients with parity ≤2 it was only 3.17% (6/189). 52.2% (94/180) of patients with cervical lesions belonged to a lower socioeconomic status, whereas only 13.3% (24/180) belonged to a higher socioeconomic status. Mean age at first coitus for inflammatory lesion was found to be 24.61 ± 3.37 years and for dysplasia and carcinoma was 17.67 ± 3.86 years (Table 1).

A Pap smear was taken in 250 patients out of which the total number of premalignant and malignant cases (mild to severe dysplasia and carcinoma) detected was 95 (38%). 2.8% was an unsatisfactory cytology due to the presence of a large number of red cells or mucus and drying artifacts. Among 180 patients whose tissues were biopsied, distribution of cases according to histopathological findings was inflammatory (63), CIN-I (60), CIN II (30), CIN III (16), and carcinoma (11). Therefore our study showed that inflammation (35%) followed by CIN-I (33.3%) was the commonest histological finding, when colposcopic directed biopsy was done (Table 2).

Acetowhite epithelium was the most common colposcopic finding in 100% of cases, and also the grade of dysplasia increases as mosaic and punctuation pattern increases. Atypical vessels were the finding which was present in 100% of the cases of carcinoma and in 12.5% cases of CIN III of the whereas no abnormal vessels were seen in inflammatory or CIN-I lesions (Table 3).

Reid's colposcopic index is based on 4 colposcopic signs that is, colour, margin, vascular pattern, and vascular response [2]. Using Reid's colposcopic index in our study, the sensitivity and the specificity were 100% and 87.3%, respectively (Table 4).

Advanced cervical lesions showed higher MVD count both by HE and CD-31 which was statistically significant that is $P < 0.0001$ (Table 5).

Mean MVD in preinvasive as well as in invasive lesions by CD-31 immunostaining was higher when compared with HE staining which was also found to be statistically significant (Table 6, Figures 1, 2, and 3).

TABLE 3: Colposcopic findings of the study population (230).

Histological diagnosis	Normal	Colposcopic findings Acetowhite No. (%)	Mosaic No. (%)	Punctation No. (%)	Atypical vessels No. (%)	Schiller's positive No. (%)	Unsatisfactory No. (%)	Total
Normal (%)	50	—	—	—	—	—	—	50
Inflammatory (%)	—	63 (100)	06 (9.52)	08 (12.69)	—	14 (22.22)	—	63
CIN-I (%)	—	60 (100)	15 (25)	22 (36.6)	—	36 (60)	02 (3.33)	60
CIN-II (%)	—	30 (100)	14 (46.6)	16 (53.3)	02 (6.67)	19 (63.3)	—	30
CIN-III (%)	—	16 (100)	06 (37.5)	04 (25)	02 (12.5)	16 (100)	06 (37.5)	16
Carcinoma (%)	—	11 (100)	11 (100)	11 (100)	11 (100)	11 (100)	—	11

TABLE 4: Correlation of colposcopic findings using colposcopic index with histopathological findings.

Colposcopic index	Histopathological findings Inflammatory (No.)	CIN-I (No.)	CIN-II (No.)	CIN-III (No.)	Carcinoma (No.)
0	—	—	—	—	—
1	32	17	—	—	—
2	23	23	—	—	—
3	06	12	09	—	—
4	02	08	08	05	—
5	—	—	08	07	—
6	—	—	05	04	—
7	—	—	—	—	—
8	—	—	—	—	11
Total	63	60	30	16	11

4. Discussion

The detection rate of Pap smear was 38% [3]. In our study, mean age for inflammatory lesions was found to be 28.37 ± 5.74 years whereas that for CIN-I, CIN II, and CIN III was 36.67 ± 7.2, 39.33 ± 6.39, and 46.39 ± 5.33 years, respectively, which was found to be similar in a study conducted by Rohtagi [4]. Severity of lesions increased with increasing parity indicating that trauma and child birth are predisposed to cervical lesions. The results of our study correlate with that of Rohtagi and Wahi et al. [4, 5]. CIN III and carcinoma were found in 52.2% of patients which belonged to a lower socioeconomic status, whereas only 13.3% belonged to higher socioeconomic status which was in concordance with the study conducted by Sankaranarayanan et al. who found that 8% of their cases was a from higher socioeconomic group [6].

In our study, the mean age at the first coitus for inflammatory lesions was found to be 24.67 ± 3.37 years and that for CIN-I, CIN II, CIN III, and carcinoma was 17.67 ± 3.86 years which was similar to the study conducted by Rotkin who found that among patients who began the coitus between the age group of 15 to 17 years had twice the incidence of cervical cancer than the control group [7].

The sensitivity of colposcopic index in our study was 100% as no patients with cervical dysplasia were missed; however, the specificity was 87.3% with no false negatives. Hordhanger et al. reported the accuracy in detecting preinvasive lesions of cervix by colposcopy to 89% as against 99% by colposcopy and targeted biopsy [8].

Ozalp et al. study showed that CIN II and CIN III show higher MVD count as compared to normal and CIN I lesions [9].

Comparison of mean of MVD in the preinvasive and invasive lesions by HE showed that in preinvasive group mean MVD was 4.01 ± 2.57, and in the invasive group it was 9.18 ± 2.32 which shows that MVD was higher in the invasive group as compared to the preinvasive group, and it was statistically significant $P < 0.0001$. Comparison of mean of MVD in the preinvasive and invasive carcinoma by CD31 showed that in preinvasive group mean MVD was 5.44 ± 2.21, and in the invasive group it was 12.82 ± 4.07 showing that MVD was higher in the invasive group, and it was also statistically significant $P < 0.0001$. Dellas et al. also showed similar results [10].

Silva-Filho et al. to evaluated the association between the expression of CD31 in the tumor and histopathologic finding in patients with cancer cervix of the expression; CD31 was significantly associated with tumor size [11].

Comparison of mean MVD count by HE and CD31 shows that mean MVD in the preinvasive group by HE was 4.01 ± 2.57 and by CD31 was 5.44 ± 2.21. It shows that mean MVD detected by CD31 was higher, and it was also statistically significant. Similarly, mean MVD in invasive lesions by HE was 9.18 ± 2.32 and by CD31 was 12.82 ± 4.07. It shows that mean MVD detected by CD31 was higher, and it was also statistically significant. Angiogenesis is a marker of tumor progression, and CD31 fixes up vessel better as

TABLE 5: Comparison of mean vascular density in different stages of preinvasive and invasive lesions using haematoxylin and eosin staining and CD-31 immunostaining (per high power field).

S. no.	Stage	No. of cases	MVD-HE		MVD-CD31	
			Mean ± SD	S.E. of mean	Mean ± SD	S.E. of mean
1	CIN-I	17	2.53 ± 1.007	0.24	4.06 ± 0.83	0.20
2	CIN-II	05	3.64 ± 1.10	0.29	5.40 ± 1.84	0.48
3	CIN-III	07	8.43 ± 2.64	0.99	8.86 ± 1.46	0.55
4	Carcinoma	11	9.18 ± 2.32	0.69	12.82 ± 4.07	1.23

TABLE 6: Comparison of mean vessel density by HE and CD-31 staining (per high power field).

S. no.	Group	No. of cases	Mean ± SD	*P* value
		Preinvasive		
1	HE	39	4.01 ± 2.57	0.011
2	CD31	39	5.44 ± 2.21	
		Invasive		
3	HE	11	9.18 ± 2.32	0.018
4	CD31	11	12.82 ± 4.07	

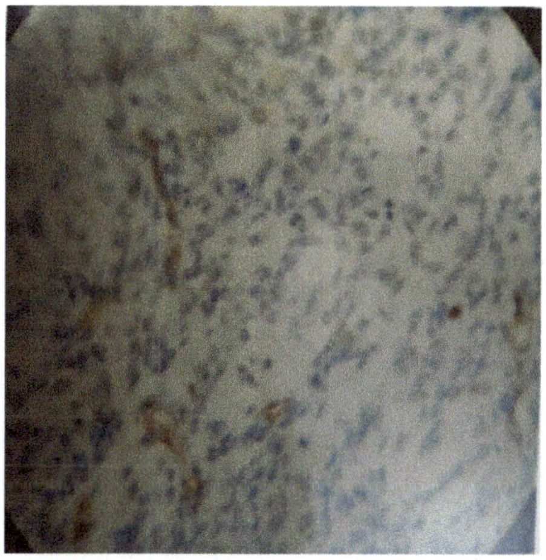

FIGURE 1: CIN 1 showing low CD31 positivity (×400).

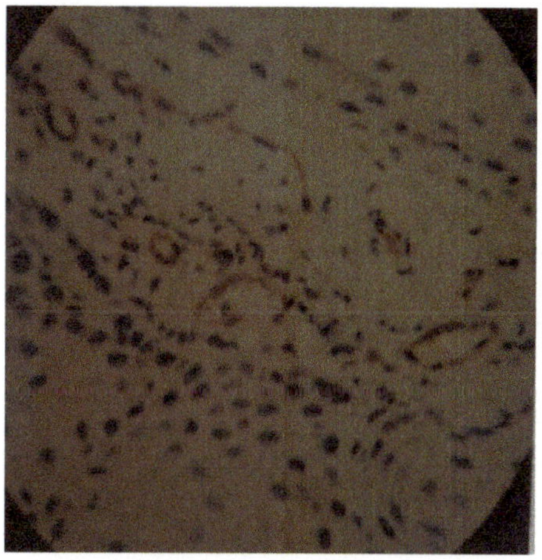

FIGURE 2: CIN II showing moderate CD31 positivity (×400).

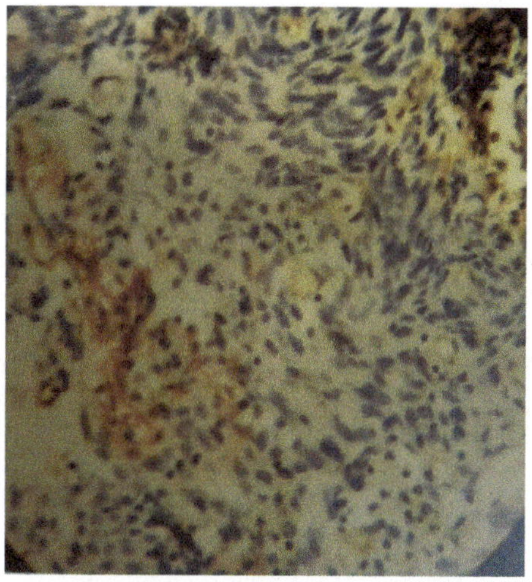

FIGURE 3: CIN III showing high CD31 positivity (×400).

compared to HE, so the aggressiveness of the tumor can be assessed better by CD31 as compared to HE.

Sapino et al. also showed increased expression of CD31 by cell of ductal carcinoma in situ and invasive carcinoma of breast which was associated with more poorer prognosis [12].

Arihiro et al. also concluded increased CD 31 expression with increased incidence of lymph node metastasis in breast cancer [13].

In a study conducted by Alexander-Sefre et al., the detection rate for tumor metastasis in lymphovascular space is three fold greater by CD31 marker as compared to conventional HE staining methods [14].

5. Conclusion

With the introduction of various effective screening programmes, the mortality and morbidity have declined rapidly associated with cervical cancer but, still there is a need for a better screening test because the existing screening test lacks the appropriate sensitivity and specificity.

The Pap test may be unable to achieve concurrently high sensitivity and specificity [3].

The major drawback of primary colposcopy is its low specificity with the consequence of high false positive rates and over treatment in substantial number of cases [15].

MVD was higher both in the invasive and the preinvasive groups by CD31 immunostaining as compared to HE.

We concluded that CD31 immunostaining is a better quantitative prognostic marker, so it should be done in all cases of preinvasive and invasive lesions.

More studies are required for the evaluation of this marker to be incorporated in the existing screening programs because of its limited availability and higher cost.

Conflict of Interests

The authors declared that they have no conflict of interests.

References

[1] S. Dennis, R. Nadeem, and Abu Rustam, "Cancer of the cervix," in *T-Lindes Operative Gynaecology*, Chapter 47, pp. 1227–1290, Wolters Kluver Pvt, 10th India, 2011.

[2] R. I. Reid and M. Coppleson, "The reid colposcopic index for lesion grading," in *Colposcopy: Principles and Practice*, B. Apgar, G. Brotzman, and M. Spitzer, Eds., Elsevier, Amsterdam, The Netherlands, 2nd edition, 2008.

[3] M. T. Fahey, L. Irwig, and P. Macaskill, "Meta-analysis of pap test accuracy," *American Journal of Epidemiology*, vol. 141, no. 7, pp. 680–689, 1995.

[4] A. Rohtagi, "Evaluation of cervix with colposcope, acetowhite patches ic colposcopically screened womens," *The Journal of Obstetrics and Gynaecology of India*, vol. 39, pp. 433–435, 1989.

[5] P. N. Wahi, S. Mali, and U. K. Luthra, "Factors influencing cancer of the uterine cervix in North India," *Cancer*, vol. 23, no. 5, pp. 1221–1226, 1969.

[6] R. Sankaranarayanan, M. Krishnan Nair, P. G. Jayaprakash et al., "Cervical cancer in Kerala: a hospital registry-based study on survival and prognostic factors," *British Journal of Cancer*, vol. 72, no. 4, pp. 1039–1042, 1995.

[7] I. D. Rotkin, "Relation of adolescent coitus to cervical cancer risk," *The Journal of the American Medical Association*, vol. 179, pp. 486–491, 1962.

[8] P. Hordhanger, U. Mehra, and A. Torranga, "Comparison of colposcopy biopsy and cold knife conization in patients with abnormal cytology," *Surgery, Gynecology and Obstetrics*, vol. 142, p. 333, 1976.

[9] S. Ozalp, O. T. Yalcin, U. Oner, H. M. Tanir, M. Acikalin, and I. Sarac, "Microvessel density as a prognostic factor in preinvasive and invasive cervical lesions," *European Journal of Gynaecological Oncology*, vol. 24, no. 5, pp. 425–428, 2003.

[10] A. Dellas, H. Moch, E. Schultheiss et al., "Angiogenesis in cervical neoplasia: microvessel quantitation in precancerous lesions and invasive carcinomas with clinicopathological correlations," *Gynecologic Oncology*, vol. 67, no. 1, pp. 27–33, 1997.

[11] A. L. Silva-Filho, P. Traiman, S. A. Triginelli et al., "Association between CD31 expression and histopathologic features in stage IB squamous cell carcinoma of the cervix," *International Journal of Gynecological Cancer*, vol. 16, no. 2, pp. 757–762, 2006.

[12] A. Sapino, L. Righi, P. Cassoni, M. Papotti, P. Gugliotta, and G. Bussolati, "Expression of apocrine differentiation markers in neuroendocrine breast carcinomas of aged women," *Modern Pathology*, vol. 14, no. 8, pp. 768–776, 2001.

[13] K. Arihiro, M. Kaneko, S. Fujii, and K. Inai, "Loss of CD9 with expression of CD31 and VEGF in breast carcinoma, as predictive factors of lymph node metastasis," *Breast Cancer*, vol. 5, no. 2, pp. 131–138, 1998.

[14] F. Alexander-Sefre, N. Singh, A. Ayhan, H. B. Salveson, G. Wilbanks, and I. J. Jacobs, "Detection of tumour lymphovascular space invasion using dual cytokeratin and CD31 immunohistochemistry," *Journal of Clinical Pathology*, vol. 56, no. 10, pp. 786–788, 2003.

[15] I. Pete, V. Toth, and P. Bosze, "The value of colposcopy in screening cervical carcinoma," *European Journal of Gynaecological Oncology*, vol. 19, no. 2, pp. 120–122, 1998.

6

Diagnosis of B-Cell Non-Hodgkin Lymphomas with Small-/Intermediate-Sized Cells in Cytopathology

Joerg Schwock and William R. Geddie

Division of Anatomical Pathology, Department of Laboratory Medicine and Pathobiology, University of Toronto, Toronto General Hospital, Room E11-219, Toronto, ON, Canada M5G 2C4

Correspondence should be addressed to William R. Geddie, william.geddie@uhn.ca

Academic Editor: Gary Tse

Fine needle sampling is a fast, safe, and potentially cost-effective method of obtaining tissue for cytomorphologic assessment aimed at both initial triage and, in some cases, complete diagnosis of patients that present clinically with lymphadenopathy. The cytologic diagnosis of B-cell non-Hodgkin lymphomas composed of small-/intermediate-sized cells, however, has been seen as an area of great difficulty even for experienced observers due to the morphologic overlap between lymphoma and reactive lymphadenopathies as well as between the lymphoma entities themselves. Although ancillary testing has improved diagnostic accuracy, the results from these tests must be interpreted within the morphological and clinical context to avoid misinterpretation. Importantly, the recognition of specific cytologic features is crucial in guiding the appropriate selection of ancillary tests which will either confirm or refute a tentative diagnosis. For these reasons, we here review the cytologic characteristics particular to five common B-cell non-Hodgkin lymphomas which typically cause the most diagnostic confusion based on cytological assessment alone: marginal zone lymphoma, follicular lymphoma, mantle cell lymphoma, chronic lymphocytic leukemia/small lymphocytic lymphoma, and lymphoplasmacytic lymphoma. We summarize the most pertinent cytomorphologic features for each entity as well as for reactive lymphoid hyperplasia, contrast them with each other to facilitate their recognition, and highlight common diagnostic pitfalls.

1. Introduction

Over the past 25 years, a large number of articles have been published and significant academic discourse has occurred, and continues to occur, around the usefulness and role of cytopathology in the diagnosis of lymphoma [1–3]. Sophisticated ancillary techniques have changed the landscape considerably and now play a major role in the diagnosis of lymphoproliferative disorders. We decided therefore to revisit the cytologic diagnosis of the five most common B-cell non-Hodgkin lymphomas (NHL) with small-/intermediate-sized cells with a renewed focus on morphology itself. In the following article, we will focus on cytologic samples obtained from lymph nodes by the use of small caliber needles, that is, fine-needle sampling/aspiration. We will not discuss the specifics of other specimen types such as samples of body cavity effusions or cerebrospinal fluid.

The primary and most significant role of fine-needle sampling in undiagnosed lymphadenopathy is to triage the patient appropriately for further management which may include subsequent diagnostic procedures such as excisional or core biopsy. Broadly, fine needle specimens can be categorized into neoplastic and nonneoplastic. Among the nonneoplastic specimens, the possible diagnoses include normal lymphoid tissue, nonspecific reactive change, inflammatory changes indicative of a specific process such as suppurative or granulomatous lymphadenitis, or rarely lymphadenopathies of unknown etiology such as Rosai-Dorfman disease. Within the neoplastic category, the most important distinction to be made is between primary lymphoid and secondary metastatic neoplasms. Subsequent considerations include the type and, if possible, the grade of the neoplasm in order to assign the patient to the most appropriate path for further management. In patients with a prior diagnosis of lymphoma additional questions arise such as the potential presence of changes related to therapy, the assessment for transformation/progression from a low-grade lymphoma to a higher grade, the recurrence of previously treated lymphoma, and the exclusion or inclusion of a synchronous or metachronous second malignancy.

The principle advantage of fine-needle sampling, particularly in superficial palpable lymph nodes, is the ease of specimen acquisition, which provides rapid access to diagnostic material not requiring the extensive tissue processing associated with excisional biopsies. Fine needle sampling causes only minimal patient discomfort and has the potential to spare at least a proportion of patients from a surgical procedure if subsequent lymphadenectomy is deemed unnecessary. When small caliber needles are used (25 gauge or 27 gauge), the risk of subsequent histology being compromised in any way by infarction, hematoma, or other artifact is very small. In selected patients with a single accessible enlarged lymph node and with an established diagnosis of lymphoma, the node can be spared from excision for later clinical assessment of a therapeutic response. In patients with multifocal disease multiple fine-needle samples permit the mapping of sites of involvement and planning of the optimal site for excisional biopsy where required. Also, fine-needle sampling maybe the most practical way to assess patients with deep seated lymphadenopathy or those who are too ill to undergo more invasive procedures [4, 5]. Disadvantages of fine-needle sampling of lymph nodes are mainly associated with the nature of the specimen in which architectural features, although not completely absent, are less obvious than in histologic preparations. There is a known potential for sampling error and bias which may be alleviated to some degree by using multiple needle passes into a single lymph node, ultrasound guidance to ensure sampling of different areas of a node, and sampling of multiple lesions in patients that present with more than a single enlarged lymph node. Concurrent core needle biopsy or fine-needle sampling with on-site evaluation and possible conversion to core biopsy have both been advocated to improve specimen adequacy [5–7]. Interestingly, Gong et al. concluded that there was no clear advantage in the diagnosis and classification of small B-cell NHL by adding core needle biopsy to fine-needle sampling [6].

Opponents may argue that fine-needle sampling provides only limited material for ancillary testing. Lymphoid tissues are, however, predisposed to a rich cellular harvest due to a lack in cellular cohesion. Even in the case of a paucicellular specimen, appropriate sample processing will permit subsequent studies with minimal amounts of material. Finally, the technique of fine-needle sampling itself requires a certain amount of training: failure to render a specific cytologic diagnosis is frequently associated with a lack of recognition that the component steps of sample acquisition and handling are simple, but not trivial.

2. Prerequisites and Techniques for Lymph Node Cytology

Difficulties associated with the diagnosis of B-cell NHL with small-/intermediate-sized cells by cytomorphology alone are mostly related to the morphologic overlap between the entities as well as with the changes that occur normally in benign, reactive lymph nodes [8, 9]. Some cases may display partial involvement of a lymph node by a neoplastic process, adding to the diagnostic challenge. Familiarity with the spectrum of "normal" changes in a lymph node, and the morphologic findings associated with them is essential. Lymph node morphology may also vary with respect to the body site as exemplified by an increased number of secondary follicles in cervical lymph nodes, the increased occurrence of plasma cells, monocytes, macrophages and mast cells in deep/mesenteric nodes, and the presence of pigment and/or benign cellular inclusions in lymph nodes from body sites such as the mediastinum or axillary region.

The background of a smear produced from a cytologic specimen of a lymph node usually shows an abundance of Söderstrom bodies, mostly referred to as lymphoglandular bodies (LGB), which measure 2–10 micrometers in size and occur both in benign and malignant lymph node aspirates [10]. These structures may be fragments of fragile lymphoid cell cytoplasm avulsed from cells during sampling. Occasionally though, LGBs are found within the cytoplasm of histiocytes which may indicate their existence *in vivo*. The presence or absence of LGBs is not entirely specific for a lymphoid proliferation since occasional lymph node aspirates may display a paucity of these structures whereas samples from some nonlymphoid tumors can have frequent, easily identifiable cytoplasmic fragments [11]. In general, the presence of LGBs in an aspirate, especially if there are more than 20 per high power field, indicates sampling of a lymphoid organ such as lymph node, spleen, thymus, tonsil, or of an extranodal lymphoid proliferation [12, 13]. The number of LGBs may be conspicuously increased if a lymphoid neoplasm is present.

Fine-needle sampling performed with a needle as thin as 27 gauge leaves components of the lymph node architecture intact and, if conventional smears rather than liquid-based cytology are used, these structures will be present on the slide. The most commonly observed part of the native lymph node architecture present in cytological preparations is the lymphohistiocytic aggregate (LHA) or germinal center fragment. LHAs are characterized by the presence of cells of the mononuclear phagocyte system, especially tingible body macrophages (TBMs), which are frequently observed in benign, reactive, or "follicular" lymphoid hyperplasia. Like the secondary follicles of follicular hyperplasia, LHAs are quite variable in size and may be dominated by activated cells (centroblasts) associated with the germinal center reaction. A follicle center fragment (FCF), on the contrary, is an aggregate of lymphoid cells arranged around a meshwork of follicular dendritic cells ("kissing cells") the interdigitating cytoplasm of which can be highlighted by immunohistochemical staining for CD21 and/or CD23. The latter type of cell aggregate, by some authors referred to as pseudo-LHA [12], may also occur in benign samples, but is seen in increased frequency in smears prepared from lymph nodes involved by follicular lymphoma (FL), constituting an important diagnostic clue in this particular setting. Notably, FCFs in FL are often small and similar in size imparting an "architectural" monomorphism which can be recognized, often grossly, in smear preparations [14]. FCFs may be mimicked in smears occasionally by other cell aggregates such

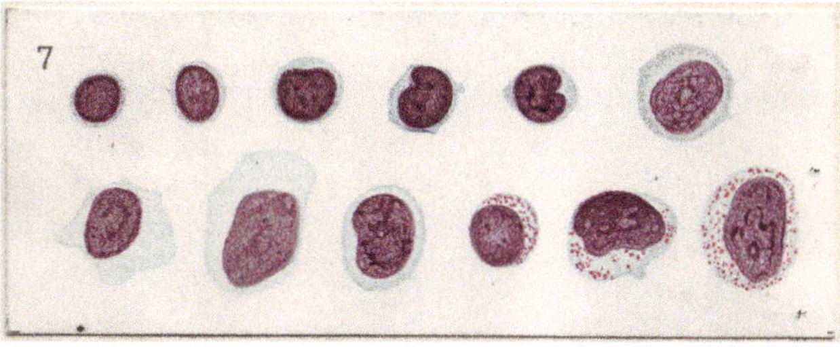

FIGURE 1: Historical depiction of different lymphoid cell types. Schleip examined the heterogeneity of lymphoid cells in peripheral blood films. This image taken from the atlas published based on his observations illustrates the variable nuclear morphology and cytoplasmic content of benign lymphoid cells in different states of activation.

as the densely packed groups of cells associated with proliferation centers, or pseudofollicles, seen in chronic lymphocytic leukemia/small lymphocytic lymphoma (CLL/SLL). In CLL/SLL, no follicular dendritic cells should be visible, but prolymphocytes and paraimmunoblasts will be present. Also, it is important to note that occasional "true" FCFs can be found in mantle cell lymphoma (MCL) and marginal zone lymphoma (MZL), and that LHAs can be seen whenever benign lymphoid tissue is sampled at the same time as lymphoma. Other, less frequently observed cell aggregates in smear preparations may consist of capillary-size vessels with attached lymphoid tissue or occasional aggregates of adipose tissue infiltrated by lymphoid cells.

Readily recognizable normal lymphoid constituents seen in fine-needle samples from benign/reactive lymph nodes include small round lymphocytes (either functionally "naïve" or terminally differentiated memory cells or unstimulated T-cells), centrocytes, centroblasts, immunoblasts, and plasma cells. Common nonlymphoid cell types present in the aspirate are follicular and interdigitating dendritic cells located mainly in germinal centers and paracortex, respectively. Constituents such as histiocytes, macrophages, plasmacytoid monocytes, and epithelioid cells are related to the mononuclear-phagocyte system. Other cell types are mast cells, basophils, neutrophils, eosinophils, endothelial cells, and occasional fat cells. Small lymphocytes have an approximate size of 6–12 micrometers, comparable to a histiocyte nucleus. Practically, erythrocytes and neutrophils are more convenient comparators. The small lymphocyte is usually about twice the size of an erythrocyte and somewhat smaller than the nucleus of a segmented neutrophil. Mature, circulating lymphocytes dominate at the lower end of this size spectrum and activated lymphocytes at the upper end. Large lymphocytes may exceed 20 micrometer size, equivalent to or greater than the diameter of 3 erythrocytes, and larger than a histiocyte or neutrophil nucleus. Lymphocytes that fulfill neither size criterion, usually designated as "intermediate," include many centrocytes and some centroblasts. It is not unusual for a "small" B-cell lymphoma to be composed mainly of cells that fall into this intermediate size range. This broad spectrum of lymphocyte size and morphology has been long recognized and documented (Figure 1) [15].

The character of the nuclear chromatin, the presence or absence and size of nucleoli, and the character of the cytoplasm (including cytoplasmic granulations) provide better clues to the identification of the position of a lymphoid cell within the functional spectrum than size alone. The typical cytologic features of small round lymphocytes are a regular nuclear contour, dense chromatin, invisible nucleoli, and a narrow rim of cytoplasm. Cells with these properties in medullary cords and sinuses are mainly B cells, but in the paracortex of the lymph node will mainly consist of T-cells. Some small round T-lymphocytes are also present within the germinal centers. The naïve cells of the primary follicle and the mantle zone are very similar but display a slightly more irregular nuclear contour and slightly more open chromatin. B-cells of the marginal zone are characterized by slightly irregular nuclear contours and moderate amounts of pale cytoplasm. Cell types of the lymphoid lineage recognizable in fine-needle specimens include centrocytes, centroblasts, prolymphocytes/(para-)immunoblasts, plasmablasts, plasmacytoid lymphocytes, plasma cells, and monocytoid lymphocytes. Overlap between these cell types occurs, so that it may be difficult to definitively classify some individual cells based on cytomorphology alone. Overall, the small round lymphocyte is always the most frequent cell in reactive lymph nodes. However, the predominance or increased occurrence of any of these cell types, including the small round lymphocyte, should lead at least to the consideration of a neoplastic process as part of the differential diagnosis.

The success of fine-needle cytology is dependent on samples of high cellularity and excellent technical preparation. Several articles and textbooks have detailed descriptions of the technique of fine-needle sampling with aspiration [16]. Briefly, fine-needle sampling of superficial nodes with suction is performed using a 23–27 gauge needle fitted to a 10 mL syringe which may be attached to a one hand grip syringe holder for convenience. Larger needles should be avoided since they will cause considerable admixture of the sample with peripheral blood. Local anesthesia is rarely required for the sampling of superficial, palpable lesions which should be almost painless. Local anesthesia, however, is used in cases where penetration of pleura or peritoneum is necessary. The sampling of a superficial lesion is performed with the mass immobilized between two fingers while one or two needle passes consisting of several (5–10) strokes each are performed. At this stage, the sampling is for the most part due to detachment of cells and tissue fragments by the cutting edge of the needle as described in the method published by Zajdela et al. [17] whereas excessive aspiration may increase the blood content of the sample. The material obtained in this way is often sufficient for several smears and a cell suspension for ancillary studies. Nonpalpable lesions are sampled with the aid of imaging modalities such as ultrasonography or computer tomography.

The obtained sample is then placed on a glass slide and a "splitting" or "touch-off technique" can be used to generate several matching smears from the same sample (Figure 2). After the sample is expelled onto the slide, the smear is produced by even and thin spreading of the cells with a second "spreader" slide using the so-called "one-step" technique

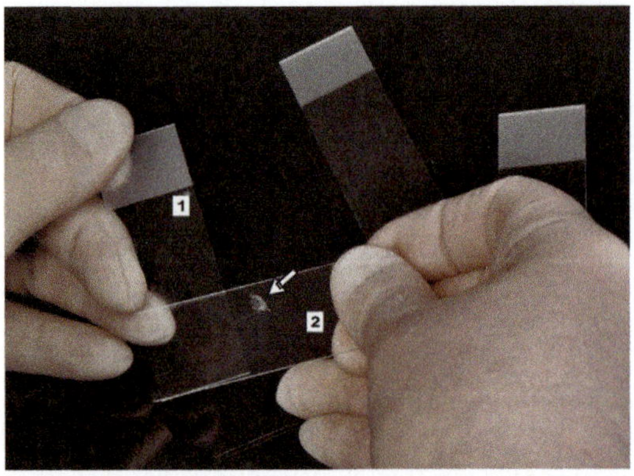

Figure 2: Hand position during the one-step smear with touch-off which allows multiple smears to be produced from a single fine-needle sample. The sample is expelled from the needle and placed near the frosted end of the "receiver" slide (1). The "spreader" slide (2) is then lowered in a hinge-like fashion onto the receiver slide from above, allowing the sample to disperse by capillary action, and then drawn down the length of the receiver slide producing the characteristic "bullet shape with feather edge." If using the touch-off technique, the spreader slide is lowered to pick up a small amount of the specimen and then turned over so that a clean glass surface can be used to spread the remaining sample on the receiver slide. The picked up sample on the reverse of the spreader slide (arrow) is then used to generate a second smear.

[18]. During this step, it is important not to apply too much pressure which will destroy fragile cells. Ideally direct smears are subsequently processed using both Papanicolaou and Romanowsky-type stains on paired slides after alcohol fixation and air-drying, respectively. The two staining methods highlight distinct cellular features thereby producing complimentary diagnostic information. In general, alcohol fixation with Papanicolaou stain emphasizes nuclear detail whereas air-drying with Romanowsky-type stains demonstrates the cytoplasm more effectively. Also, Romanowsky-type stains differentially color DNA a metachromatic purple and RNA blue. Diff-Quik, a proprietary "quick" stain, or other non-proprietary modified staining methods are frequently used and are particularly suitable for immediate specimen assessment in situations where confirmation of specimen adequacy is crucial [19]. It should be noted, though, that the higher concentration of methylene blue present in Diff-Quik and similar rapid stains can sometimes cause fine blastic chromatin to appear darker and more mature than it otherwise would, and produce the appearance of "pseudonucleoli" in cells if staining is performed on an incompletely dried smear. May-Grünwald-Giemsa (MGG) stain provides more subtle coloration of nuclei and is superior for staining of cytoplasmic granulations. MGG is highly pH-dependent and may be difficult to standardize. Finally, cell suspensions are produced by aspiration of sterile physiological saline, phosphate-buffered saline solution, or cell culture medium from a tube through the sampling needle into the syringe. The cell suspension can then be used for ancillary testing purposes and either directly submitted for flow or slide-based cytometry or, after further processing as cytospin preparation or cell block, for immunocytochemistry or fluorescence *in-situ* hybridization (FISH). Cell suspensions are ideal material for more specialized molecular methods that may be required for diagnostic and research purposes including polymerase-chain reaction (PCR) and gene expression profiling. Very small amounts of residual cell suspension can be expelled onto an FTA card or paper for indefinite storage of DNA.

3. Differential Diagnosis of B-Cell NHLs Composed of Small-/Intermediate-Size Cells

A sequential approach to the examination of fine-needle samples from lymph nodes includes the initial assessment of cellularity and adequacy of the sample. As with samples from other sites, an absolute definition of adequacy is difficult. Pambuccian and Bardales propose a minimum number of 40 lymphoid cells per high power field in the area of highest cellularity as criterion to consider an aspirate as adequate in cases not showing granulomas or metastatic malignancy [12]. By this definition, an extensively hemodiluted specimen would be considered inadequate for the purpose of establishing a complete diagnosis, although it still might yield useful information. Other adequacy criteria related to the quality of the cytologic preparation include a uniform, thin smear resulting in a "bullet shape with feather edge" appearance, lack of involvement of the slide margins, and absence of extensive artifacts [12]. The slide should be examined grossly to determine if the cells smeared diffusely or focally form small or large aggregates. Next, there should be an assessment of the slide background which, in the case of reactive lymph nodes or small B-cell NHLs, should contain numerous LGBs without presence of extraneous elements. Depending on the anatomic site sampled, however, a variety of noncellular material may be present such as anthracotic pigment in mediastinal nodes sampled by endobronchial ultrasound with transbronchial needle aspiration or melanin pigment in axillary lymph nodes involved by dermatopathic lymphadenopathy. The subsequent steps include a low power assessment of the lymphoid cell population for its (a) composition (mono-/dimorphic *versus* polymorphic), (b) presence, density, and nature of cell aggregates (FCF *versus* LHA), and (c) any cell predominance or presence of atypical cells (small *versus* intermediate *versus* large cells). The final step is the assessment of the sample at high power during which the specific nature of the lymphoid population is elicited through recording of the cytologic features of any predominant cell population with or without admixed minor cellular component(s).

In the following section, we will review the cytologic features of B-cell lymphomas characterized by a predominance of cells with small to intermediate size and consider possible diagnostic pitfalls. In the context of the most pertinent clinical scenarios, we will discuss areas of morphologic overlap and important differential diagnoses.

3.1. Reactive Lymphoid Hyperplasia. Reactive lymphoid hyperplasia (RLH) is the most common cause for a polymorphic lymphoid cell pattern in a fine-needle sample and

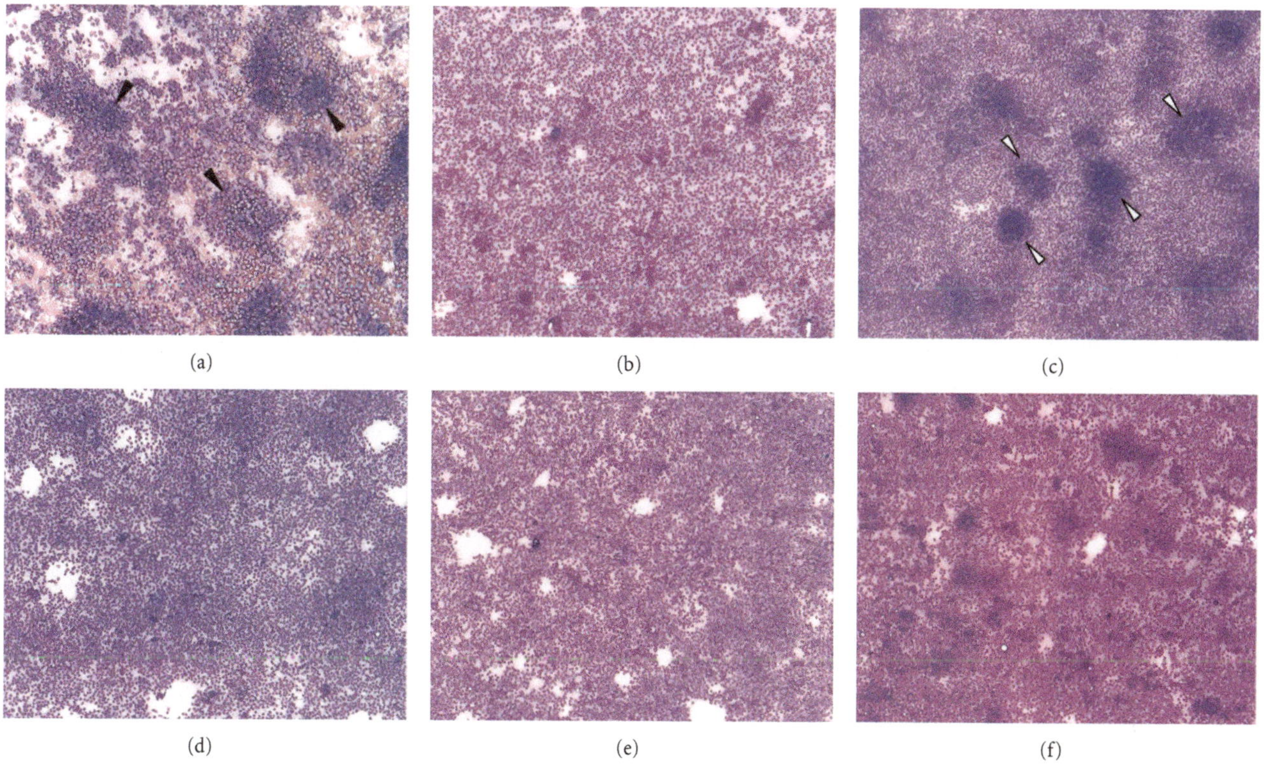

Figure 3: Smears produced from lymph node fine-needle samples and examined at low power. Low power assessment shows the differences in cell composition and the presence or absence of cell aggregates in reactive lymphoid hyperplasia (a), marginal zone lymphoma (b), follicular lymphoma (c), mantle cell lymphoma (d), chronic lymphocytic leukemia/small lymphocytic lymphoma (e), and lymphoplasmacytic lymphoma (f). Note the variable size and frequency of aggregates in reactive lymphoid hyperplasia (black arrowheads). Compare with the monomorphism of the small aggregates in follicular lymphoma (white arrowheads) and the absence or vague delineation of aggregates in the other lymphoma cases. Also, there is a markedly more polymorphic cell composition in reactive lymphoid hyperplasia as compared to the other cases. (d: Diff-Quik, all other: May-Grünwald-Giemsa; 10x).

is mostly associated with benign, reactive and reversible lymphadenopathy. The histologic correlate is an expansion of the sinusoidal, follicular, paracortical, or medullary area of a lymph node leading to corresponding changes in cellular composition. Two distinct patterns of RLH exist with (a) follicular hyperplasia as correlate of a B-cell response and (b) paracortical hyperplasia as correlate of a T-cell response [12]. Both patterns are characterized by a spectrum of differentiation of the lymphoid cells with numerous small mature lymphocytes in the background resulting in a polymorphic impression at low power assessment (Figure 3(a)). In follicular hyperplasia, LHAs of variable size with conspicuous TBMs are often evident at low power, and a mixture of centrocytes, centroblasts, and plasma cells is prominent (Figure 4(a)). Immunoblasts are dominant in paracortical hyperplasia, particularly viral lymphadenopathy. It is important to note, however, that the two reaction patterns, follicular and paracortical hyperplasia, often present together. Also, temporal changes in the cell composition occur until the RLH resolves and are associated with concomitant cytologic variations.

In most cases the etiology of the RLH remains unknown. RLH most frequently affects children and young adults. Bacteria, viruses, chemicals, and drugs are the most common inciting agents [12]. Considering patient age and cytomorphology, the differential diagnosis in most cases will include Hodgkin lymphoma, T-cell lymphoma, and FL. Depending on the degree of cytomorphologic change, ancillary testing may need to be employed to exclude those mimics. After cytologic diagnosis of RLH an attempt should be made to establish the cause by appropriate history, serology, or other investigations, but as mentioned above the etiology may remain undetermined. If resolution of the lymphadenopathy does not occur, excisional biopsy is warranted.

3.2. Marginal Zone B-Cell Lymphoma. Nodal MZL is a rare neoplasm (1.5–1.8% of all lymphoid neoplasms [20]) which, similar to RLH, presents with a distinctly polymorphic cytologic pattern [21, 22]. By definition, nodal MZL presents without evidence of extranodal or splenic disease. However, the similarly rare splenic MZL and the more common extranodal MZL of mucosa-associated lymphoid tissue (MALT) may resemble nodal MZL in cytomorphology. LHAs may be present, and only careful examination at higher power may suggest the presence of monotonous neoplastic cells within a background resembling nonspecific RLH. This may be particularly problematic in partially involved nodes. In contrast, in cases with follicular colonization, the smear may

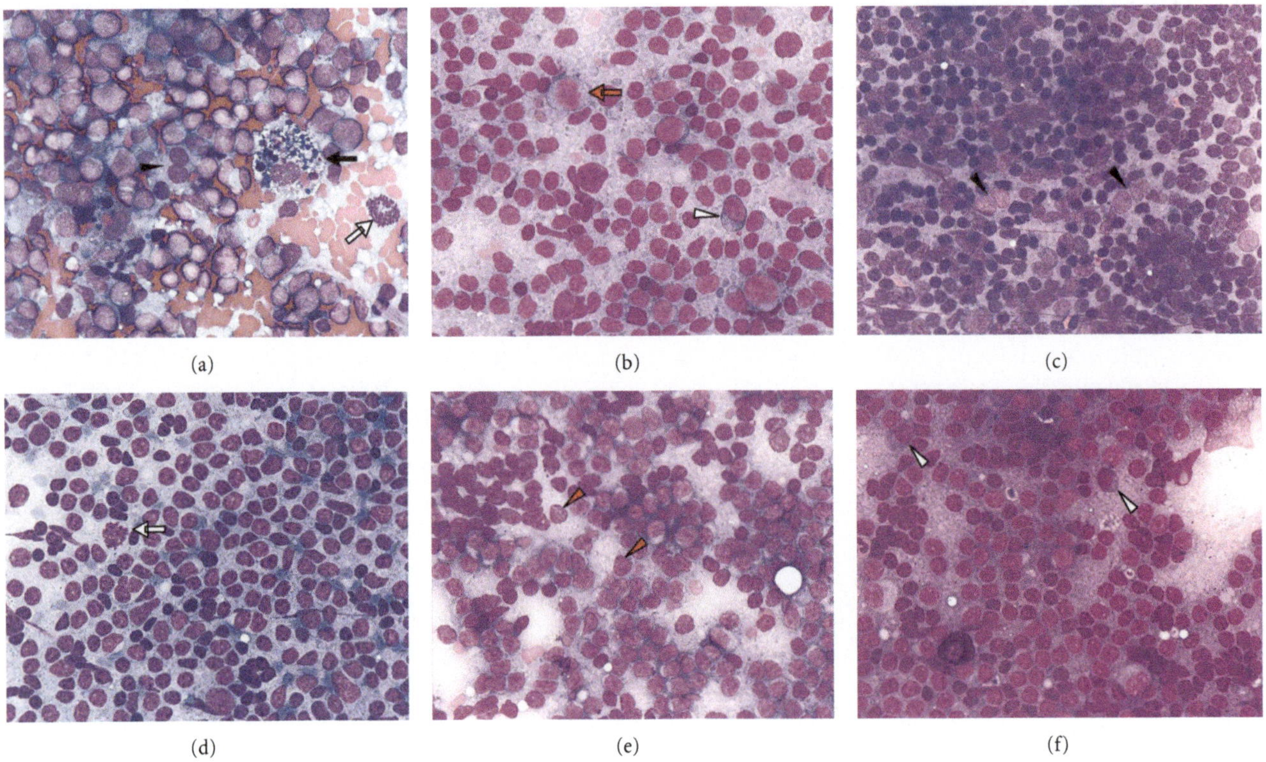

FIGURE 4: Smears produced from lymph node fine-needle samples and examined at high power. High power assessment shows the differences in cell composition between reactive lymphoid hyperplasia (a) and the cytological features of the neoplastic cells in marginal zone lymphoma (b), follicular lymphoma (c), mantle cell lymphoma (d), chronic lymphocytic leukemia/small lymphocytic lymphoma (e), and lymphoplasmacytic lymphoma (f). Follicular dendritic cells (black arrowheads), tingible body macrophages (black arrow) and mitoses (white arrows) are present within a lymphohistiocytic aggregate seen in reactive lymphoid hyperplasia. Monocytoid B-cells (red arrow) and plasmacytoid cells (white arrowheads) are often found in marginal zone lymphoma. Follicular dendritic cells are a prominent feature of follicle center fragments present in samples of follicular lymphoma. These follicle center fragments do not show the other constituents seen in the lymphohistiocytic aggregates of a reactive lymph node. Mitoses are also a frequent finding in mantle cell lymphoma, but are not commonly seen in the other types of B-cell non-Hodgkin lymphoma illustrated here. Prolymphocytes (red arrowheads) are often found in areas of vague nodularity present in smears of chronic lymphocytic leukemia/small lymphocytic lymphoma and identified by a nucleolus which has a tinctorial quality similar to the cytoplasm of the cell. Plasmacytoid cells and mast cells (f: left lower image quadrant) are constituents seen in lymphoplasmacytic lymphoma. (d: Diff-Quik, all other: May-Grünwald-Giemsa; 63x).

contain numerous FCFs. Rare cases show a monotonous intermediate-size cell pattern at low power assessment. The neoplastic cells may be exclusively monocytoid, but more typically are cytologically polymorphic with monocytoid cells occurring alongside small lymphocyte- and centrocyte-like cells [12] as well as with elements showing plasma cell differentiation [20] (Figures 3(b) and 4(b)). The cytomorphology of such samples, therefore, leads frequently to a broad differential diagnosis including RLH as well as the spectrum of lymphomas with small and intermediate-sized cells [23]. Finally, an important potential pitfall is peripheral T-cell lymphoma which can mimic MZL morphologically [24].

MZL usually affects the middle-aged and elderly, although it may occur in children. Clinical history is important with regard to multiple sites of involvement including intra-abdominal lymphadenopathy and presence of constitutional symptoms. Consideration should be given to the possibility of nodal dissemination of extranodal MZL which occurs in approximately one third of the cases [20]. The clinical course is indolent, but transformation to a large B-cell lymphoma may occur. Ancillary studies are particularly important in making the diagnosis of MZL, but cases in which the reactive cells obscure the neoplastic B-cell population even by immunophenotyping may occur [25]. A further complication is the well-documented occurrence of small clonal, but non-neoplastic, B-cell populations in some of the chronic inflammatory conditions, such as Sjögren's syndrome, which may be associated with extranodal marginal zone (MALT) lymphoma.

3.3. Follicular Lymphoma. FL grade 1-2 is characterized by a monotonous to somewhat dimorphic pattern, respectively. FL grade 3A or 3B is characterized by a dominant population of large cells resembling centroblasts and is, therefore, not discussed here. The dimorphic pattern may initially cause the false impression of a polymorphic cell composition at low power. Regardless of grade, smears often give the low-power impression of a nodular pattern which can be an important clue to the diagnosis (Figure 3(c)). At higher power, the nodules correspond to numerous FCFs populated by small to intermediate-sized centrocytic cells with cleaved nuclei and clumped chromatin (Figure 4(c)). Cells with deeply cleaved, apparently bilobed nuclei can be conspicuous [26]. Larger centroblasts characterized by noncleaved nuclei, less dense chromatin, and a narrow rim of dense cytoplasm are rare in grade 1 FL, but occur with increasing frequency in grade 2 where both cell populations may be present in equal numbers. Rarely, LHAs with TBMs may occur which should not distract from the overall impression. LHAs and mitotic activity are both uncommon, and the presence of either should raise suspicion for a reactive process which then needs to be distinguished from partial lymph node involvement by lymphoma. Of note, a rare signet-ring variant of FL exists and is due to immunoglobulin stored within the cytoplasm of the neoplastic cells. A diagnostic challenge can be posed by diffuse FL which is rare and characterized by a lack of follicular architecture in which case FCFs would be absent. The differential diagnosis in this situation would include insufficient sampling of a FL displaying a focal diffuse component.

FL accounts for approximately 20% of all lymphomas, and affects adults and elderly individuals. FL occurring before the age of 20 years is rare. Characteristically there is often widespread nodal involvement at diagnosis. Histologic grading of FL is based on the number of centroblasts per high-power field (HPF, $0.159\,mm^2$) counted in ten HPFs within different representative follicles [20]. Similar grading can be performed on cytological preparations but is not universally accepted [27, 28]. The vast majority of FLs are grade 1 or 2. As distinction between these two is poorly reproducible and not clinically important, the diagnostic terminology usually reported is "follicular lymphoma, grade 1-2/3." Although an indolent lymphoma, transformation to diffuse large B-cell lymphoma (DLBCL) is more frequent than with other low-grade lymphomas [12] and areas of DLBCL are present in a substantial proportion of grade 3 FLs. Fine-needle sampling plays an important role in the initial assessment of FL since it allows sampling of multiple sites of involvement so that the optimal site for excisional biopsy (if required) can be determined. Similarly, in a case of suspected transformation multiple fine-needle samples improve the chances of finding and documenting progression.

3.4. Mantle Cell Lymphoma. MCL is characterized, in contrast to the lymphomas considered previously, by a distinctly monomorphic cell composition [29, 30]. Histologically three patterns of MCL occur: diffuse, vaguely nodular, and mantle zone pattern, the latter with preservation of preexisting follicles. Accordingly, smears may be diffuse, show poorly formed FCFs, or contain intact LHAs. The mantle zone pattern, however, is rarely seen in cytologic material. Most commonly, smears consist of a highly monotonous population of lymphoid cells interrupted only by small round lymphocytes and occasional histiocytes [12] (Figure 3(d)). At higher magnification, the cells have subtly irregular nuclear contours reminiscent of centrocytes, dispersed to clumped chromatin, mostly inconspicuous nucleoli, and moderate amounts of cytoplasm. Mitotic figures may be observed, and this feature can be used together with monomorphism and nuclear contour irregularities in differentiating MCL from other lymphomas [31] (Figure 4(d)). Diagnostic challenges may be posed by any of the variants of MCL. Marginal zone-like MCL and small cell MCL may be confused with MZL or small lymphocytic lymphoma, respectively. The blastoid and pleomorphic variant both display a more aggressive clinical behavior and may enter the differential diagnosis in cases sampled at relapse which can show increased nuclear size, pleomorphism and mitotic activity [20]. The latter two variants, again, can be confused with DLBCL.

MCL comprises 3–10% of lymphomas and predominantly occurs in middle-aged to older males. Lymphadenopathy, hepatosplenomegaly, bone marrow, and peripheral blood involvement are frequent. The median survival is 3–5 years and the majority of patients cannot be cured [20]. Grading of MCL is not performed. However, the estimation of the proliferative fraction either by counting mitotic figures or Ki67 staining has shown prognostic impact [32]. Given the different prognosis of MCL, ancillary testing to discriminate the above-mentioned variants of MCL from their less aggressive counterparts is crucial.

3.5. Small Lymphocytic Lymphoma/Chronic Lymphocytic Leukemia. SLL/CLL is characterized by a monomorphic cellular aspirate often without conspicuous nodularity or presence of aggregates. Thicker areas of a smear occasionally show poorly defined aggregates of cells that may correspond to the proliferation centers associated with SLL/CLL (Figures 3(e) and 5(a)). In Romanowsky-stained smears these are appreciated as darker zones at low power, whereas in H&E-stained histologic sections proliferation centers appear as pale zones. Proliferation centers differ from FCFs in that they do not contain follicular dendritic cells. At higher magnification, small lymphoid cells with smooth-contoured nuclei and minimal cytoplasm predominate (Figure 4(e)). The chromatin frequently has a peculiar coarsely clumped appearance best appreciated on Papanicolaou-stained slides which led to the original designation as "cellules grumelées" [33, 34] (Figure 5(b)), a term which refers to clotted milk or cheese curd. "Soccer balls" might be a better modern appellation. Most cases have interspersed intermediate-sized prolymphocytes with dispersed chromatin and obvious nucleolus as well as paraimmunoblasts with broader, pale cytoplasm, vesicular chromatin, and large central nucleolus (Figures 4(e) and 5(b)). Both cell types are most often seen in those ill-defined aggregates corresponding to the proliferation centers, and their presence provides a clue towards the diagnosis. A common artifact in smears from patients with CLL/SLL is the presence of smudge cells, also referred to as basket cells or shadow cells of Gumprecht, which are lymphoid cells stripped of their cytoplasm with the nuclear material dispersed on the slide. This artifact, however, is not specific to CLL/SLL. In samples with more than a few cells with plasmacytoid features, lymphoplasmacytic lymphoma (LPL) needs to be considered in the differential diagnosis to CLL/SLL. Another important differential diagnosis is the benign, minimal enlarged lymph node with a high proportion of small lymphocytes and few secondary follicles which,

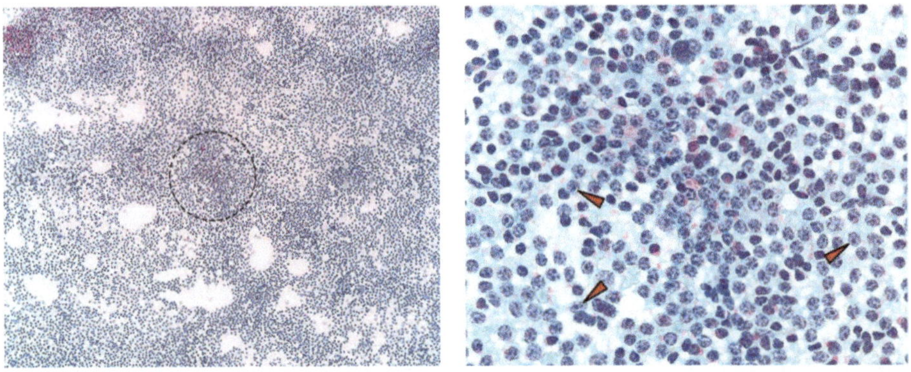

(a) (b)

Figure 5: Fine needle samples of chronic lymphocytic leukemia/small lymphocytic lymphoma examined after Papanicolaou stain. Several ill-defined cellular aggregates (circle) are visible at low power inspection giving the impression of vague nodularity (a). High-power examination reveals the peculiar chromatin distribution and presence of numerous prolymphocytes (red arrowheads) within this area of increased cell density (b). Note the coarse distribution of the chromatin and tinctorial quality of the nucleoli in the prolymphocytes in this stain. ((a) and (b): Papanicolaou; (a): 10x, (b): 63x).

at first glance, may cause a similarly monotonous impression as CLL/SLL [35].

CLL/SLL is, in general, an indolent disease and occurs at a mean age of 65 years. It is the most common lymphoproliferative disorder of adults in Western countries and shows a slight male preponderance. The disease is rarely seen in individuals of Asian descent. Fine-needle sampling is often done to exclude Richter's transformation to DLBCL which occurs in 2–8%. Transformation to Hodgkin lymphoma occurs in less than 1% of the patients. Immunoglobulin gene mutation status and specific cytogenetic abnormalities correlate with disease prognosis [20], and can be examined using cytologic material.

3.6. Lymphoplasmacytic Lymphoma. Fine-needle specimens from patients with LPL show a monomorphic, rarely more polymorphic cell composition without a significant number of cell aggregates. The hint to the diagnosis is an admixture of small lymphocytes and plasmacytoid cells (Figures 3(f) and 4(f)). Mature plasma cells may be present, but if dominant, plasmacytoma should be considered in the differential diagnosis. Intranuclear Dutcher bodies and intracytoplasmic Russell bodies may be seen in the neoplastic cells, and occasional multinucleated cells can be present. Mast cells are often seen and are diagnostically helpful when frequent, but they may also occur in other B-cell lymphomas with small-/intermediate-sized cells [22]. In contrast to CLL/SLL, prolymphocytes and paraimmunoblasts are absent which is useful in excluding this differential diagnosis. Importantly, LPL may be indistinguishable from MZL both histologically or cytologically in which case ancillary testing and correlation with clinical presentation are indispensable.

LPL is a rare lymphoma and most frequently occurs in elderly patients with slight male predominance. The disease is often associated with a paraprotein of IgM type, but this is not required for diagnosis. Bone marrow involvement and IgM monoclonal gammopathy are the diagnostic features of Waldenström macroglobulinemia found in a significant subset of patients with LPL. Autoimmune phenomena, hyperviscosity, cryoglobulinemia, coagulopathies, and/or neuropathy characterize the clinical course in a significant proportion of these patients. The lymphoma is typically indolent, but transformation to DLBCL and, rarely, Hodgkin lymphoma occurs in a small number of cases [20].

4. The Role of Ancillary Testing in Small B-Cell Non-Hodgkin Lymphoma

Due to the morphologic overlap between different B-cell NHLs with small-/intermediate-sized cells as well as with RLH, ancillary testing plays a central role in their workup [34, 36]. This is true regardless of the method with which the specimen was obtained: excisional biopsy or fine-needle sample. Although smears can be used for immunocytochemistry, it is much more practical to use cell suspensions which can be submitted directly for flow- or slide-based cytometry, or for further processing as cytospins or cell blocks [37]. Each of these methods has advantages and disadvantages, and their use is guided by the particular clinical circumstance and, importantly, by the cytomorphology of the sample which is the basis for a tentative diagnosis. Because material for ancillary testing may be limited, the initial morphological assessment becomes a crucial step and determines if a particular investigative pathway will ultimately lead to the correct diagnosis. Flow cytometry has become indispensable in the diagnosis and classification of B-cell NHLs with small-/intermediate-sized cells [38, 39]. Some institutions have developed expertise in slide-based cytometry which can be used with specimens of very low cellularity and yields immunophenotyping results similar to flow cytometry [14, 40, 41]. However, flow cytometry protocols using ten or more colors can be similarly informative with extremely paucicellular specimens.

The selection of the antibodies, again, is guided by cytomorphology, clinical history, and the amount of material available for testing. A stepwise approach may be employed which includes, at a minimum, kappa, lambda, CD19, CD20, CD3, CD5, CD10, and CD23 for the initial assessment. Additional markers such as CD4, CD8, CD7, CD2, CD43, and FMC7 may be included upfront or subsequently. A kappa : lambda ratio exceeding a threshold between 4 : 1 to 6 : 1 or a lambda : kappa ratio exceeding 3 : 1 on flow cytometry are generally sufficient to prove light chain restriction, that is, monoclonality [12, 42]. The exact thresholds depend on the cut-off(s) set by the individual laboratory. However, in most cases of NHL, these ratios will be clearly surpassed. Flow- or slide-based cytometry are ideal for markers with cell surface expression and invaluable for the assessment of antigen coexpression. Also, some intracellular antigens such as Bcl-2 can be assessed by flow cytometry after cell permeabilization. In contrast, the nuclear expression of Cyclin D1 is best examined using standardized immunohistochemical staining protocols on cell block sections. MIB-1 as an indicator of the proliferative activity may aid in the classification of a B-cell lymphoma according to its expected biological behavior and can be evaluated by immunocytochemistry [43].

Since normal lymph nodes show a predominance of T-cells, a large proportion of CD20-positive B-cells in a fine-needle sample will raise the suspicion of lymphoma. Expression of CD5 and CD23 is indicative of CLL/SLL, the presence of Bcl-2 in a population of germinal center cells positive for CD10 or Bcl-6 is seen in FL, and staining for Cyclin D1 is diagnostic for MCL. LPL will usually lack CD5 and CD23 and show expression of CD38 as well as presence of cytoplasmic immunoglobulin which distinguishes this entity from CLL/SLL. Immunophenotyping by flow cytometry may be the most informative test in cases of MZL where it can reveal a population of B-cells with light chain restriction which, by cytomorphology, may be obscured by a reactive background [38]. Variations may occur with any of the mentioned immunophenotypic markers as exemplified by a range of CD23 expression in CLL/SLL [44]. Consequently, a high level of vigilance is required as well as interpretation of the flow cytometric data in the context of morphological and clinical information. Limitations to the use of flow cytometry, which occur particularly with lymphoid neoplasms that have a rich background of benign cells such as in Hodgkin lymphoma or that have particularly fragile cells such as in some large cell lymphomas, are not usually encountered in B-cell NHLs with small-/intermediate-sized cells.

Cytogenetic testing, most commonly FISH, can be used to demonstrate genetic abnormalities which are either (a) recurrent and diagnostic for a specific lymphoma type, (b) occur at an increased frequency, thus supporting a tentative diagnosis, or (c) confer prognostic information [45]. Trisomy of chromosome 12 is most commonly seen in CLL/SLL where it occurs in approximately 25% of the cases [12]. Trisomy 12 and to a greater extent deletions on chromosomes 11, 17, and 6 are associated with a poorer prognosis in CLL/SLL whereas an isolated deletion of 13q14.3 is a positive prognostic marker. MCL is characterized in almost all cases (>95%) by translocation *t*(11;14)(q13;q32) which involves the genes *IGH* and *CCND1*. Although rare cases may have an alternative translocation, the diagnosis of MCL should be made with caution in cases that are *t*(11;14) negative [46]. Slightly less frequent is the translocation *t*(14;18)(q32;q21) which is seen in approximately 80% of FLs and results in rearrangement of *IGH* and *BCL2*. In contrast, translocation *t*(11;18)(q21;q21) which affects the *API2* and *MALT1* genes is only present in MZL of the extranodal sites (MALT), but not in nodal MZL. Trisomies of chromosome 3 and 18 are nonspecific, but may support the diagnosis of MZL in the appropriate context. There are marked variations in the rate with which these genetic alterations can be detected depending on the anatomic site involved by lymphoma with reported frequencies for *t*(11;18), trisomy 3, and trisomy18 ranging between 0–56%, 11–75%, and 0–25%, respectively [20]. No specific cytogenetic abnormalities have so far been found for LPL leaving cytomorphology and immunophenotyping as primary diagnostic tools. Molecular studies, mostly PCR-based assays for clonality and translocation detection with or without sequencing, are, at the present time, rarely used in the diagnostic workup of B-cell NHLs with small-/intermediate-sized cells. Their application will depend on specific situations where an attempt to classify a neoplasm with the aforementioned techniques has left questions unanswered.

5. Summary

The current World Health Organization (WHO) classification of tumors of the hematopoietic and lymphoid tissues emphasizes cellular morphology in addition to immunophenotypic and genotypic characteristics [20]. Since a fine-needle sample, if properly obtained and processed, provides excellent material for both cytomorphologic assessment and ancillary testing, the acceptance of cytology as diagnostic tool in lymphoma diagnosis has increased considerably. Much progress has been made since the publication by Chhieng et al. [9] who, like various other groups, emphasized the difficulty inherent in the cytologic recognition of B-cell NHLs, especially those with predominant small cell component. They reported that these low-grade lymphomas accounted for a significant percentage of false-negative or indeterminate cases. However, they also stated that the diagnosis of malignant lymphoma could be made in 82% of their cases with a significant contribution occurring through the use of immunophenotyping which led to a substantial improvement in diagnostic accuracy. Remarkably, when they compared the results of the histologic assessment based on REAL with their cytologic diagnosis, there was agreement in 85% of the cases. In a similar vein, Wakely Jr [8] reported a sensitivity of >80% and specificity of >90% in the majority of studies focused on the cytologic diagnosis of NHL. However, these results may reflect the best possible scenario which may not be accomplished in each setting [3].

Although much progress has been made over the past decade and despite the development of sophisticated methods for ancillary testing, there is still significant skepticism towards the role of cytology in this setting, and excisional biopsy is frequently regarded as essential for an accurate initial diagnosis and classification of malignant lymphoma [47]. Some of this skepticism is attributed to the overlap

Table 1: Summary of the cytologic features of B-cell non-Hodgkin lymphomas with small-/intermediate-sized cells.

	Gross	Low Power			High Power							
	Smear	Composition	Aggregates	Cell Size	Nuclei	Nucleoli	Chromatin	Cytoplasm	Mitotic activity	Plasma/-cytoid Cells	Mast Cells	Other Cells
RLH	Large and small aggregates	Polymorphic	LHA and FCF are key features	Small to intermediate	N/A	N/A	N/A	N/A	Present	Present	Present	Complete spectrum
MZL	Large and small aggregates	Polymorphic	LHA and FCF possible	Intermediate	Smooth to mildly irregular	Inconspicuous to large	Open to clumped	Conspi-cuous, abundant in mono-cytoid forms	Low	Present	Present	Large activated cells, histiocytes, immunoblasts
FL Grade 1/2	Numerous small aggregates	Monomorphic to dimorphic (grades 1-2)	Repetitive FCF common	Intermediate	Irregular, bilobed or "divided" nuclei common	Inconspicuous	Open to clumped	Scant	Low	Absent	Present	Centroblasts
MCL	Vague aggregates	Markedly monomorphic	Vague aggregates (FCF/LHA possible in mantle zone pattern)	Intermediate (small and large cell variants occur)	Subtly irregular	Inconspicuous to large	Dispersed to clumped	Variable, moderate	Possible	Absent/ Rare	Infrequent	Scattered EH present, PLC and PIB *absent*
SLL/CLL	Vague aggregates	Monomorphic	Vague aggregates (proliferation centers)	Small	Smooth	Absent/In-conspicuous	Coarse -clumped	Scant	Low	Infrequent	Infrequent	PLC, PIB, smudge cells, rarely RS cells
LPL	Vague aggregates	Mono-, rarely polymorphic	Rare/ Absent aggregates	Small	Smooth, possible Dutcher bodies	Absent/In-conspicuous	Coarse–clumped, "cart-wheel"	Scant to plasma-cytoid, Russell bodies	Low	Common	Present, often frequent	PLC and PIB *absent*

CB: centroblasts, EH: epithelioid histiocytes, FCF: follicle center fragments, FDC: follicular dendritic cell, FL: follicular lymphoma, LHA: lymphohistiocytic aggregate, LPL: lymphoplasmacytic lymphoma, MCL: mantle cell lymphoma, MZL: marginal zone lymphoma, PLC: prolymphocytes, PIB: paraimmunoblasts, RLH: reactive lymphoid hyperplasia, RS: Reed-Sternberg, SLL/CLL: small lymphocytic lymphoma/chronic lymphocytic leukemia; N/A: not applicable.

in morphologic features between B-cell NHLs with small-/intermediate-sized cells as well as with benign reactive and inflammatory lymphadenopathies. In fact, the significant impediments to fine-needle sampling as stand-alone approach to NHL diagnosis were discussed in a recent commentary which also stressed the need for interdisciplinary collaboration, multiparametric testing and on-site specimen adequacy assessment as requirements for optimal results [3]. Undoubtedly there are situations where even a tentative diagnosis can only be rendered with great difficulty. Such cases, however, are not unique to cytological specimens, and this morphologic ambiguity is part of the reason why ancillary testing, in particular immunophenotyping studies, are considered mandatory in the diagnosis of lymphoproliferative disorders. It is important to emphasize, though, that ancillary studies are crucially guided by the initial cytologic evaluation of the sample which also provides the framework for the proper interpretation of the immunophenotypic and molecular testing results.

Some of the cytologic features of the B-cell NHLs reviewed here have been recognized for some time, whereas others are less well known or have been applied somewhat more variably depending on the training of the individual cytopathologist. An example is the recognition of FCFs in cases of FL initially reported by Suh et al. [48], and their distinction from LHAs based on the presence of follicular dendritic cells alone in the former versus TBMs, follicular dendritic cells and activated cells in the latter. A stepwise approach as summarized in Table 1, which includes a low power assessment for cellularity, monomorphism, and predominant cell size with an astute examination for residual architectural features, that is, cell aggregates, followed by a detailed interrogation of the cytologic features at high power will yield the largest amount of information on which a tentative diagnosis can be built, and has the least potential to cause diagnostic confusion.

Awareness of the diagnostic limitations and pitfalls is of key importance in advancing the acceptance for a cytologic diagnosis of lymphomas. Other sampling techniques including excisional biopsy should be considered where the cytologic diagnosis is equivocal or lymphadenopathy persists without definitive cause. Situations in which other sampling modalities may be given preference include, but are not limited to, suspected T-cell lymphoma, Hodgkin lymphoma and composite lymphomas [49]. Excisional biopsies may also be necessary to satisfy criteria for participation in a clinical trial or for purposes of tissue banking for potential future diagnostic and therapeutic developments. Finally, histologic examination may also be necessary due to persistent controversies such as those related to the grading of FL. On the other hand, excisional biopsy in SLL/CLL is probably never warranted, unless Richter's transformation is suspected, and it can be argued that in the case of the indolent, but currently incurable, B-cell NHL with small-/intermediate-sized cells under clinical observation alone, excisional biopsy is best left for a point in the illness when therapeutic intervention becomes necessary.

6. Conclusion

With the advent of sophisticated techniques for ancillary testing and with the emphasis on cytomorphologic and immunophenotypic characteristics for the classification of NHLs, there has been a resurgence in interest in cytologic diagnosis of lymphoproliferative disorders. The cytomorphologic features of B-cell NHLs with small-/intermediate-sized cells in many cases are sufficiently characteristic to permit at least some degree of differentiation. The assessment of these features can be applied in a stepwise or algorithmic fashion to discriminate between entities and to arrive at a final differential diagnosis which can be resolved with additional testing. Clinical data, immunophenotyping and cytogenetics provide the context for cytomorphology, and permit accurate diagnoses to be rendered even in this challenging area. Hence, we conclude that the medical community has come closer to realizing the full potential of fine-needle cytopathology.

References

[1] N. A. Young and T. Al-Saleem, "Hematopathologists and cytopathologists: enemies or allies?" *Diagnostic Cytopathology*, vol. 21, no. 5, pp. 305–306, 1999.

[2] L. M. Sandhaus, "Fine-needle aspiration cytology in the diagnosis of lymphoma: the next step," *American Journal of Clinical Pathology*, vol. 113, no. 5, pp. 623–627, 2000.

[3] P. E. Wakely Jr., "The diagnosis of non-Hodgkin lymphoma using fine-needle aspiration cytopathology: a work in progress.," *Cancer Cytopathology*, vol. 118, no. 5, pp. 238–243, 2010.

[4] L. L. Cafferty, R. L. Katz, N. G. Ordonez, C. H. Carrasco, and F. R. Cabanillas, "Fine needle aspiration diagnosis of intraabdominal and retroperitoneal lymphomas by a morphologic and immunocytochemical approach," *Cancer*, vol. 65, no. 1, pp. 72–77, 1990.

[5] E. Ravinsky and C. Morales, "Diagnosis of lymphoma by image-guided needle biopsies: fine needle aspiration biopsy, core biopsy or both?" *Acta Cytologica*, vol. 49, no. 1, pp. 51–57, 2005.

[6] J. Z. Gong, M. J. Snyder, A. S. Lagoo et al., "Diagnostic impact of core-needle biopsy on fine-needle aspiration of non-hodgkin lymphoma," *Diagnostic Cytopathology*, vol. 31, no. 1, pp. 23–30, 2004.

[7] S. Bandyopadhyay, V. Pansare, J. Feng et al., "Frequency and rationale of fine needle aspiration biopsy conversion to core biopsy as a result of onsite evaluation," *Acta Cytologica*, vol. 51, no. 2, pp. 161–167, 2007.

[8] P. E. Wakely Jr., "Fine-needle aspiration cytopathology in diagnosis and classification of malignant lymphoma: accurate and reliable?" *Diagnostic Cytopathology*, vol. 22, no. 2, pp. 120–125, 2000.

[9] D. C. Chhieng, J. M. Cohen, and J. F. Cangiarella, "Cytology and immunophenotyping of low- and intermediate-grade B-cell non-Hodgkin's lymphomas with a predominant small-cell component: a study of 56 cases," *Diagnostic Cytopathology*, vol. 24, no. 2, pp. 90–97, 2001.

[10] N. Söderström, *Fine-Needle Aspiration Biopsy: Used as a Direct Adjunct in Clinical Diagnostic Work*, Almqvist & Wiksell, Stockholm, Sweden, 1966.

[11] E. Flanders, M. J. Kornstein, P. E. Wakely Jr., T. F. Kardos, and W. J. Frable, "Lymphoglandular bodies in fine-needle aspiration cytology smears," *American Journal of Clinical Pathology*, vol. 99, no. 5, pp. 566–569, 1993.

[12] S. E. Pambuccian and R. H. Bardales, *Lymph Node Cytopathology in Essentials in Cytopathology*, Springer, Science, Business Media, New York, NY, USA, 2011.

[13] M. Bangerter, F. Herrmann, M. Griesshammer et al., "The abundant presence of Soderstrom bodies in cytology smears of fine-needle aspirates contributes to distinguishing high-grade non-Hodgkin's lymphoma from carcinoma and sarcoma," *Annals of Hematology*, vol. 74, no. 4, pp. 175–178, 1997.

[14] W. R. Geddie, "Cytology and laser scanning cytometry," in *Wintrobe's Atlas of Clinical Hematology*, chapter 7, Williams & Wilkins, Philadelphia, Pa, USA, 2007.

[15] K. F. W. Schleip, *Hematological Atlas with a Description of The Technic of Blood Examin*, Rebman, New York, NY, USA, 1908.

[16] L. Skoog and E. Tani, "Techniques.," *Monographs in Clinical Cytology*, vol. 18, pp. 5–10, 2009.

[17] A. Zajdela, P. Zillhardt, and N. Voillemot, "Cytological diagnosis by fine needle sampling without aspiration," *Cancer*, vol. 59, no. 6, pp. 1201–1205, 1987.

[18] J. S. Abele, T. R. Miller, E. B. King, and T. Lowhagen, "Smearing techniques for the concentration of particles from fine needle aspiration biopsy.," *Diagnostic Cytopathology*, vol. 1, no. 1, pp. 59–65, 1985.

[19] H. M. Ko, G. D. C. Santos, G. Darling et al., "Diagnosis and subclassification of lymphomas and non-neoplasticlesions involving mediastinal lymph nodes using endobronchial ultrasound-guided transbronchial needle aspiration," *Diagnostic Cytopathology*. In press.

[20] S. H. Swerdlow, E. Campo, N. L. Harris et al., *WHO Classification of Tumours of Haematopoietic and Lymphoid Tissues*, IARC Press, Lyon, France, 2008.

[21] A. Y. Matsushima, D. Hamele-Bena, and B. M. Osborne, "Fine-needle aspiration biopsy findings in marginal zone B cell lymphoma," *Diagnostic Cytopathology*, vol. 20, no. 4, pp. 190–198, 1999.

[22] U. N. Saikia, P. Dey, B. Saikia, and A. Das, "Fine-needle aspiration biopsy in diagnosis of follicular lymphoma: cytomorphologic and immunohistochemical analysis," *Diagnostic Cytopathology*, vol. 26, no. 4, pp. 251–256, 2002.

[23] J. P. Crapanzano and O. Lin, "Cytologic findings of marginal zone lymphoma," *Cancer*, vol. 99, no. 5, pp. 301–309, 2003.

[24] P. Uherova, C. W. Ross, W. G. Finn, T. P. Singleton, R. Kansal, and B. Schnitzer, "Peripheral T-cell lymphoma mimicking marginal zone B-cell lymphoma," *Modern Pathology*, vol. 15, no. 4, pp. 420–425, 2002.

[25] H. Y. Dong, N. L. Harris, F. I. Preffer, and M. B. Pitman, "Fine-needle aspiration biopsy in the diagnosis and classification of primary and recurrent lymphoma: a retrospective analysis of the utility of cytomorphology and flow cytometry," *Modern Pathology*, vol. 14, no. 5, pp. 472–481, 2001.

[26] K. Kishimoto, T. Kitamura, K. Fujita, G. Tate, and T. Mitsuya, "Cytologic differential diagnosis of follicular lymphoma grades 1 and 2 from reactive follicular hyperplasia: cytologic features of fine-needle aspiration smears with Pap stain and fluorescence in situ hybridization analysis to detect t(14;18)(q32;q21) chromosomal translocation," *Diagnostic Cytopathology*, vol. 34, no. 1, pp. 11–17, 2006.

[27] N. A. Young, T. I. Al-Saleem, Z. Al-Saleem, H. Ehya, and M. R. Smith, "The value of transformed lymphocyte count in subclassification of non-hodgkin's lymphoma by fine-needle aspiration," *American Journal of Clinical Pathology*, vol. 108, no. 2, pp. 143–151, 1997.

[28] G. D. Brandao, R. Rose, S. Mckenzie, P. Maslak, and O. Lin, "Grading follicular lymphomas in fine-needle aspiration biopsies: the role of ThinPrep slides and flow cytometry," *Cancer*, vol. 108, no. 5, pp. 319–323, 2006.

[29] G. Z. Rassidakis, E. Tani, E. Svedmyr, A. Porwit, and L. Skoog, "Diagnosis and subclassification of follicle center and mantle cell lymphomas on fine-needle aspirates: a cytologic and immunocytochemical approach based on the Revised European-American Lymphoma (REAL) classification," *Cancer*, vol. 87, no. 4, pp. 216–223, 1999.

[30] D. Gagneten, Y. M. Hijazi, E. S. Jaffe, and D. Solomon, "Mantle cell lymphoma: a cytopathological and immunocytochemical study," *Diagnostic Cytopathology*, vol. 14, no. 1, pp. 32–37, 1996.

[31] B. A. Murphy, B. A. Meda, D. H. Buss, and K. R. Geisinger, "Marginal zone and mantle cell lymphomas: assessment of cytomorphology in subtyping small B-cell lymphomas," *Diagnostic Cytopathology*, vol. 28, no. 3, pp. 126–130, 2003.

[32] R. Schaffel, C. V. Hedvat, J. Teruya-Feldstein et al., "Prognostic impact of proliferative index determined by quantitative image analysis and the international prognostic index in patients with mantle cell lymphoma," *Annals of Oncology*, vol. 21, no. 1, pp. 133–139, 2010.

[33] T. Strunge, *La ponction des ganglions lymphatiques (une description cytologique controlée par la clinique)*, Ph.D.thesis, Munksgaard, Copenhagen, Denmark, 1944.

[34] L. Skoog and E. Tani, "B cell neoplasms," *Monographs in Clinical Cytology*, vol. 18, pp. 19–37, 2009.

[35] P. E. Wakely Jr., "Fine needle aspiration cytopathology of malignant lymphoma," *Clinics in Laboratory Medicine*, vol. 18, no. 3, pp. 541–559, 1998.

[36] N. P. Caraway, "Strategies to diagnose lymphoproliferative disorders by fine-needle aspiration by using ancillary studies," *Cancer*, vol. 105, no. 6, pp. 432–442, 2005.

[37] L. Skoog and E. Tani, "Immunocytochemistry: an indispensable technique in routine cytology," *Cytopathology*, vol. 22, no. 4, pp. 215–229, 2011.

[38] A. Demurtas, G. Accinelli, D. Pacchioni et al., "Utility of flow cytometry immunophenotyping in fine-needle aspirate cytologic diagnosis of non-Hodgkin lymphoma: a series of 252 cases and review of the literature," *Applied Immunohistochemistry and Molecular Morphology*, vol. 18, no. 4, pp. 311–322, 2010.

[39] S. Barrena, J. Almeida, M. D. C. Garcia-Macias et al., "Flow cytometry immunophenotyping of fine-needle aspiration specimens: utility in the diagnosis and classification of non-hodgkin lymphomas," *Histopathology*, vol. 58, no. 6, pp. 906–918, 2011.

[40] R. J. Clatch and J. L. Walloch, "Multiparameter immunophenotypic analysis of fine needle aspiration biopsies and other hematologic specimens by laser scanning cytometry," *Acta Cytologica*, vol. 41, no. 1, pp. 109–122, 1997.

[41] A. M. AlZa'abi, W. B. Geddie, and S. L. Boerner, "Equivalence of laser scanning cytometric and flow cytometric immunophenotyping of lymphoid lesions in cytologic samples," *American Journal of Clinical Pathology*, vol. 129, no. 5, pp. 780–785, 2008.

[42] M. D. Jeffers, J. Milton, R. Herriot, and M. McKean, "Fine needle aspiration cytology in the investigation of non-hodgkin's lymphoma," *Journal of Clinical Pathology*, vol. 51, no. 3, pp. 189–196, 1998.

[43] A. E. Ali, E. K. Morgen, W. R. Geddie et al., "Classifying B-cell non-Hodgkin lymphoma by using MIB-1 proliferative index

in fine-needle aspirates.," *Cancer Cytopathology*, vol. 118, no. 3, pp. 166–172, 2010.

[44] G. Barna, L. Reiniger, P. Tatrai, L. Kopper, and A. Matolcsy, "The cut-off levels of CD23 expression in the differential diagnosis of MCL and CLL," *Hematology & Oncology*, vol. 26, no. 3, pp. 167–170, 2008.

[45] G. D. C. Santos, H. M. Ko, W. R. Geddie et al., "Targeted use of fluorescence in situ hybridization (FISH) in cytospin preparations: results of 298 fine needle aspirates of B-cell non-Hodgkin lymphoma.," *Cancer Cytopathology*, vol. 118, no. 5, pp. 250–258, 2010.

[46] S. Gesk, W. Klapper, J. I. Martín-Subero et al., "A chromosomal translocation in cyclin D1-negative/cyclin D2-positive mantle cell lymphoma fuses the CCND2 gene to the IGK locus," *Blood*, vol. 108, no. 3, pp. 1109–1110, 2006.

[47] S. T. Hehn, T. M. Grogan, and T. P. Miller, "Utility of fine-needle aspiration as a diagnostic technique in lymphoma," *Journal of Clinical Oncology*, vol. 22, no. 15, pp. 3046–3052, 2004.

[48] Y. K. Suh, A. Shabaik, W. T. Meurer, and S. S. Shin, "Lymphoid cell aggregates: a useful clue in the fine-needle aspiration diagnosis of follicular lymphomas," *Diagnostic Cytopathology*, vol. 17, no. 6, pp. 467–471, 1997.

[49] O. Landgren, A. P. MacDonald, E. Tani et al., "A prospective comparison of fine-needle aspiration cytology and histopathology in the diagnosis and classification of lymphomas," *Hematology Journal*, vol. 5, no. 1, pp. 69–76, 2004.

7

Upregulation of Serum Vascular Endothelial Growth Factor in Patients with Salivary Gland Tumor

Azadeh Andisheh Tadbir,[1] Bijan Khademi,[2] Mahyar Malekzadeh,[3] Maryam Mardani,[4] and Bahar Khademi[5]

[1] *Department of Oral and Maxillofacial Pathology, School of Dentistry, Shiraz University of Medical Sciences, Ghom Abad, Ghasrodasht Avenue, Shiraz 71956-15878, Iran*

[2] *Department of Otolaryngology, Khalili Hospital, Shiraz Institute for Cancer Research, Shiraz University of Medical Sciences, Shiraz 71348-45794, Iran*

[3] *Shiraz Institute for Cancer Research, Shiraz University of Medical Sciences, Shiraz 71348-45794, Iran*

[4] *Department of Oral Medicine, School of Dentistry, Shiraz University of Medical Sciences, Ghom Abad, Ghasrodasht Avenue, Shiraz 71956-15878, Iran*

[5] *School of Dentistry, Shiraz University of Medical Sciences (International Branch), Azadi Square, Jahad Sazandegi Street, Shiraz 71447-16699, Iran*

Correspondence should be addressed to Azadeh Andisheh Tadbir; andisheh@sums.ac.ir

Academic Editor: Piero Tosi

Neoangiogenesis is essential for tumor development, invasion, and dissemination. The most potent of the cytokines associated with angiogenesis is vascular endothelial growth factor (VEGF). The aim of the present study was to determine VEGF serum level in patients with salivary gland tumor. Using an ELISA kit, the circulating levels of VEGF in sera from 58 patients with salivary gland tumor and 30 healthy controls were assessed. Mean VEGF levels in sera of patients with salivary gland tumors (574.9 ± 414.3) were significantly higher than those in controls (263.9 ± 310.0) ($P = 0.009$). Within the salivary gland tumor group, mean serum VEGF concentration in malignant tumors ($n = 27$) was 727.3 ± 441.8 pg/mL, and that in benign tumors ($n = 31$) was 442.2 ± 343.3 pg/mL. Mean serum VEGF concentration was significantly higher in malignant tumors than in benign tumors ($P = 0.008$) and was higher in benign tumors than in controls ($P = 0.03$). The data in the present study clearly show that VEGF level was consistently upregulated in benign and malignant tumors in comparison to healthy controls. However, the role of VEGF as a prognostic factor in salivary gland tumor and its application in antiangiogenic therapy require further clinical research.

1. Introduction

Neoangiogenesis, the development of new vessels from pre-existing ones, is necessary for tumor development, invasion, and dissemination. Angiogenic process not only delivers nutrients for tumor growth but also increases the chance for tumor cells to enter the circulation and metastasis [1].

A variety of signals such as diminished nutrition or oxygen in tissue or genetic changes in oncogenes or tumor suppressor genes can start angiogenic process. Different factors produced from stromal and tumor cells such as growth factors, cytokines, enzymes, and adhesion molecules are involved in this process, and the most potent of them is vascular endothelial growth factor (VEGF) [2].

Among the VEGF family, which consists of VEGF-A, VEGF-B, VEGF-C, VEGF-D, and VEGF-F, VEGF-A is a key angiogenic factor and is mostly used to promote angiogenic phenotype by a tumor [3].

VEGF-A is a dimeric glycoprotein with a molecular weight of 34–45 KDa, consisting of two subunits. Increased VEGF expression was seen in different physiologic and pathologic conditions which was associated with hypoxia [4].

VEGF is expressed in several malignant tumors which indicates its importance in angiogenesis process.

TABLE 1: Serum VEGF level in benign, malignant salivary gland tumors and normal controls as measured by Sandwich ELISA.

Groups	Mean serum VEGF (pg/mL)	*P* value
Controls	263.9 ± 310 ± 0.0	Controls versus benign tumors $P = 0.03$
Benign salivary gland tumor	442.2 ± 343.3	Controls versus malignant tumors $P = 0.001$
Malignant salivary gland tumor	727.3 ± 441.8	Benign tumors versus malignant tumors $P = 0.008$

Overexpression of VEGF was found in body fluids and solid tumors such as brain, colon, breast, kidney, bladder, lung, and oral cancer [5].

However, no investigations have been conducted regarding serum VEGF levels in patients with salivary gland tumor, so the aim of the present study was to determine VEGF serum level in patients with salivary gland tumor.

2. Materials & Methods

2.1. Subjects. For the purpose of this case-control study, 58 serum samples from the patients diagnosed with salivary gland tumor (24 males, 34 females, age: 44.8 ± 16.6 years) consisting of 31 pleomorphic adenoma, 17 adenoid cystic carcinoma, and 10 mucoepidermoid carcinoma and 30 serum samples from healthy control subjects (12 males, 18 females, age: 44.6 ± 16.6 years) were collected.

Study subjects were the patients admitted to the Department of Otolaryngology, Khalili Hospital, Shiraz University of Medical Sciences, and diagnosed with salivary gland tumor histopathologically.

Control cases were healthy blood donors, who were matched for age and gender. Exclusion criteria for both groups were based on the presence of any systemic disease, use of corticosteroid or nonsteroid anti-inflammatory medication, or a history of malignancy of any type.

All the participants were informed about the research study and agreed to participate by signing an informed consent form.

2.2. Serum Analysis. Serum samples were obtained from clotted blood following the centrifugation at 4°C and storing at −80°C until analysis. VEGF concentrations were measured by Sandwich ELISA, in accordance with the manufacturer's instructions (BMS, GmbH, Germany).

2.3. Statistical Analysis. Statistical analysis was performed using Mann-Whitney test. A *P* value less than 0.05 was considered significant.

3. Results

Mean serum VEGF levels in malignant tumors, benign tumors, and controls are shown in Table 1. Mean VEGF levels in sera of patients with salivary gland tumors (574.9 ± 414.3) were significantly higher than those in controls (263.9 ± 310.0) ($P = 0.009$). Within the salivary gland tumor group, mean serum VEGF concentration in malignant tumors ($n = 27$) was 727.3 ± 441.8 pg/mL, and that in benign tumors ($n = 31$) was 442.2 ± 343.3 pg/mL. Mean serum VEGF concentration was significantly higher in malignant tumors than in benign tumors ($P = 0.008$) and was higher in benign tumors than in controls ($P = 0.03$).

No relation was found between mean VEGF levels and sex and age of the patients and controls.

4. Discussion

Angiogenesis is necessary for tumor growth. It is a multifaceted process which is regulated by a variety of inducers and inhibitors, which are produced by different cell types like stromal cells, endothelial cells, and tumor cells [6]. Different angiogenic factors have been described. VEGF plays an important role in both pathologic and physiologic conditions [7].

VEGF is one of the most important angiogenic factors involved in tumor angiogenesis. It has been suggested that VEGF is a potent mitogen for endothelial cells and can directly induce new blood vessels formation. Concurrently, increased VEGF will enhance microvascular permeability and will lead to plasma protein extravasation (e.g., fibrinogen) into the extravascular area. Then, extra vascular fibrinogen causes clot formation and other proteins like fibronectin are added to fibrin clot and formed a suitable matrix for growth of endothelial cells [8].

Numerous studies have shown that VEGF is involved in tumor progression. VEGF can increase tumor cell extravasation and metastasis through inducing angiogenesis, enhancing vascular permeability, and stimulating immunosuppression [8–10].

Clearly, identification of different biologic markers and understanding of underlying mechanisms may provide useful markers for determining prognosis and effective treatment.

Recently, different functions such as lymphangiogenesis, enhanced vascular permeability, and antiapoptosis activity have been recognized for VEGF which all have a role in tumor progression [10, 11].

VEGF overexpression has been reported in different tumors. Kulapaditharom et al. (2012) found that the most aggressive head and neck squamous cell carcinoma showed the highest VEGF expression. These findings suggest that VEGF has a role in the progression of head and neck squamous cell carcinoma toward an aggressive and invasive phenotype [12].

Lequerica-Fernández et al. (2007) showed that VEGF can contribute to the progression of salivary gland carcinomas and seems to be associated with lymph node metastasis and worse survival [13].

Recently, Ke-Xiong et al. (2011) suggested that inducible nitric oxide synthase can motivate the expression of VEGF, and its expression status may help evaluate tumor malignancy and prognosis of the patient [14].

A study conducted by Hao et al. (2010) showed that overexpression of VEGF was seen in adenoid cystic carcinoma and its expression was higher in solid form and in advanced-stage group. Also VEGF expression was related to invasion and metastasis and proposed as a prognostic factor [15].

Swelam et al. (2005) suggest that tumor cells of pleomorphic adenoma secrete functional VEGF in different forms that induce their proliferation and differentiation, and VEGF expression is regulated by hypoxic conditions [16].

Recently, circulating VEGF levels have been reported to be a reliable and noninvasive marker of angiogenic activity and were shown to be independent prognostic factors which are correlated with survival in various malignant neoplasms [17], but fewer studies were carried out to evaluate its circulating level.

Shang et al. showed serum VEGF levels to be significantly elevated in oral cancers compared to control group [18].

Dirix et al. (1996) showed that high serum VEGF was associated with the large size of the primary tumor in advanced colorectal cancer [19].

Khademi et al. (2013) reported that increased preoperative or postoperative serum levels of VEGF can predict disease recurrence and are associated with poor disease-free and overall survival of patients with HNSCC [20].

In the present study, ELISA kit was used to measure serum VEGF concentrations in patients with salivary gland tumor. By reviewing the articles, this study was the first report to do so.

Results of this study indicate a significant increase in VEGF level from healthy controls to benign and malignant tumors.

So VEGF levels can significantly discriminate patients from controls and malignant from benign tumors. Also our results suggest that VEGF levels play a role in the progression of salivary gland tumors which was similar to those of Doi et al. (1999) and de Faria et al. (2011) [21, 22].

5. Conclusion

The data in the present study clearly show that VEGF level was consistently upregulated in benign and malignant tumors in comparison to healthy controls. However, the role of VEGF as a prognostic factor in salivary gland tumor and its application in antiangiogenic therapy require further clinical research.

Acknowledgments

This paper has been extracted from Mrs. Bahar Khademi's DDS thesis which was conducted under supervision of Dr. Azadeh Andisheh Tadbir and Dr. Bijan Khademi. This study was approved, registered with ID Grant no. 8591019, and supported by the Vice-Chancellery of International Branch of Shiraz University of Medical Sciences.

References

[1] S. Pourshahidi, A. A. Tadbir, H. Ebrahimi et al., "Serum level of vascular endothelial growth factor-c in patients with head and neck squamous cell carcinoma," *Australian Journal of Basic and Applied Sciences*, vol. 5, no. 9, pp. 426–429, 2011.

[2] D. Hodorowicz-Zaniewska, W. Kibil, A. Małek, J. Szpor, J. Kulig, and K. Sztefko, "Evaluation of serum concentrations of vascular endothelial growth factor (VEGF) in breast cancer patients," *Polish Journal of Pathology*, vol. 63, no. 4, pp. 255–260, 2012.

[3] S. Nayak, M. M. Goel, S. Chandra et al., "VEGF-A immunohistochemical and mRNA expression in tissues and its serum levels in potentially malignant oral lesions and oral squamous cell carcinomas," *Oral Oncology*, vol. 48, no. 3, pp. 233–239, 2012.

[4] M. Farzin, M. Mardani, J. Ghabanchi et al., "Serum level of matrix metalloproteinase-3 in patients with oral Lichen planus," *Iranian Red Crescent Medical Journal*, vol. 14, no. 1, 2012.

[5] C.-J. Liu, K.-W. Chang, S.-C. Lin, and H.-W. Cheng, "Presurgical serum levels of matrix metalloproteinase-9 and vascular endothelial growth factor in oral squamous cell carcinoma," *Oral Oncology*, vol. 45, no. 10, pp. 920–925, 2009.

[6] D. Hanahan and J. Folkman, "Patterns and emerging mechanisms of the angiogenic switch during tumorigenesis," *Cell*, vol. 86, no. 3, pp. 353–364, 1996.

[7] M. Sawatsubashi, T. Yamada, N. Fukushima, H. Mizokami, O. Tokunaga, and T. Shin, "Association of vascular endothelial growth factor and mast cells with angiogenesis in laryngeal squamous cell carcinoma," *Virchows Archiv*, vol. 436, no. 3, pp. 243–248, 2000.

[8] Z.-J. Shang, J.-R. Li, and Z.-B. Li, "Upregulation of serum and tissue vascular endothelial growth factor correlates with angiogenesis and prognosis of oral squamous cell carcinoma," *Journal of Oral and Maxillofacial Surgery*, vol. 65, no. 1, pp. 17–21, 2007.

[9] M. E. Baldwin, S. A. Stacker, and M. G. Achen, "Molecular control of lymphangiogenesis," *BioEssays*, vol. 24, no. 11, pp. 1030–1040, 2002.

[10] J. A. Nagy, E. Vasile, D. Feng et al., "Vascular permeability factor/vascular endothelial growth factor induces lymphangiogenesis as well as angiogenesis," *Journal of Experimental Medicine*, vol. 196, no. 11, pp. 1497–1506, 2002.

[11] J. E. Ohm, D. I. Gabrilovich, G. D. Sempowski et al., "VEGF inhibits T-cell development and may contribute to tumor-induced immune suppression," *Blood*, vol. 101, no. 12, pp. 4878–4886, 2003.

[12] B. Kulapaditharom, V. Boonkitticharoen, and C. Sritara, "Plasma vascular endothelial growth factor dysregulation in defining aggressiveness of head and neck squamous cell carcinoma," *Journal of Oncology*, vol. 2012, Article ID 687934, 7 pages, 2012.

[13] P. Lequerica-Fernández, A. Astudillo, and J. C. De Vicente, "Expression of vascular endothelial growth factor in salivary gland carcinomas correlates with lymph node metastasis," *Anticancer Research*, vol. 27, no. 5 B, pp. 3661–3666, 2007.

[14] O. Y. Ke-Xiong, L. Jun, and H. Zhi-Quan, "Association of clinicopathologic parameters with the expression of inducible nitric oxide synthase and vascular endothelial growth factor in mucoepidermoid carcinoma," *Oral Diseases*, vol. 17, no. 6, pp. 590–596, 2011.

[15] L. Hao, N. Xiao-lin, C. Qi, Y. Yi-ping, L. Jia-quan, and L. Yan-ning, "Nerve growth factor and vascular endothelial growth factor: retrospective analysis of 63 patients with salivary adenoid cystic carcinoma," *International journal of oral science*, vol. 2, no. 1, pp. 35–44, 2010.

[16] W. Swelam, H. Ida-Yonemochi, S. Maruyama, K. Ohshiro, J. Cheng, and T. Saku, "Vascular endothelial growth factor in

salivary pleomorphic adenomas: one of the reasons for their poorly vascularized stroma," *Virchows Archiv*, vol. 446, no. 6, pp. 653–662, 2005.

[17] R. T.-P. Poon, S.-T. Fan, and J. Wong, "Clinical implications of circulating angiogenic factors in cancer patients," *Journal of Clinical Oncology*, vol. 19, no. 4, pp. 1207–1225, 2001.

[18] Z.-J. Shang, J.-R. Li, and Z.-B. Li, "Circulating levels of vascular endothelial growth factor in patients with oral squamous cell carcinoma," *International Journal of Oral and Maxillofacial Surgery*, vol. 31, no. 5, pp. 495–498, 2002.

[19] L. Y. Dirix, P. B. Vermeulen, G. Hubens et al., "Serum basic fibroblst growth factor and vascular endothelial growth factor and tumour growth kinetics in advanced colorectal cancer," *Annals of Oncology*, vol. 7, no. 8, pp. 843–848, 1996.

[20] B. Khademi, M. Soleimanpour, A. Ghaderi, and M. Mohammadianpanah, "Prognostic and predictive value of serum vascular endothelial growth factor (VEGF) in squamous cell carcinoma of the head and neck," *Oral and Maxillofacial Surgery*, 2013.

[21] R. Doi, I. Kuratate, E. Okamoto, K. Ryoke, and H. Ito, "Expression of p53 oncoprotein increases intratumoral microvessel formation in human salivary gland carcinomas," *Journal of Oral Pathology and Medicine*, vol. 28, no. 6, pp. 259–263, 1999.

[22] P. R. de Faria, R. A. Lima, F. L. Dias et al., "Vascular endothelial growth factor and thymidine phosphorylase expression in salivary gland tumors with distinct metastatic behavior," *Journal of Oral Pathology and Medicine*, vol. 40, no. 6, pp. 456–459, 2011.

8

Thyroid Cytopathology Reporting by the Bethesda System: A Two-Year Prospective Study in an Academic Institution

Payal Mehra and Anand Kumar Verma

Department Of Pathology, Employees State Insurance (ESI) Postgraduate Institute of Medical Sciences and Research and ESI Model Hospital, Basai Darapur, New Delhi 110015, India

Correspondence should be addressed to Anand Kumar Verma; anandverma1961@gmail.com

Academic Editor: Marco Volante

Background. The Bethesda System for Reporting Thyroid Cytopathology (TBSRTC) has attempted to standardize reporting and cytological criteria in aspiration smears. *Aims.* The objective of this study was to analyze the thyroid cytology smears by TBSRTC, to determine the distribution of diagnostic categories and subcategories, to analyze cytological features, and to correlate the cytopathology with histopathology, wherever surgery was done. *Materials and Methods.* This was a prospective study of 225 fine needle aspirations (FNA) of thyroid nodules. All fine needle aspiration cytology (FNAC) diagnoses were classified according to the features given in the monograph of TBSRTC into nondiagnostic/unsatisfactory (ND/UNS), benign, atypia of undetermined significance/follicular lesion of undetermined significance (AUS/FLUS), follicular neoplasm/suspicious of a follicular neoplasm (FN/SFN), suspicious for malignancy (SFM), and malignant. Cytohistological correlation was done, when surgical material was available. *Results.* The distribution of various categories from 225 evaluated thyroid nodules was as follows: 7.2% ND/UNS, 80.0% benign, 4.9% AUS/FLUS, 2.2% FN, 3.5% SFM, and 2.2% malignant. Sensitivity, specificity, positive predictive value, and negative predictive value were calculated. *Conclusions.* TBSRTC is an excellent reporting system for thyroid FNA. It also provides clear management guidelines to clinicians to go for follow-up FNA or surgery and also the extent of surgery.

1. Introduction

Fine needle aspiration cytology (FNAC) of thyroid occupies an extremely important role worldwide. This minimally invasive and cost-effective technique is extremely useful in identifying a substantial proportion of thyroid nodules as benign and reducing unnecessary surgery for patients with benign disease.

However, terminology of reporting thyroid FNACs has varied markedly. Various reporting formats of thyroid FNACs have been used varying from two category schemes to six or more category schemes [1]. While some of them tried to diagnose various lesions using histology-equivalent categories, other formats had categories like equivocal, inconclusive, indeterminate, atypical, suspicious, uncertain, malignancy suspicious, possibly neoplastic, possibly malignant, and probably malignant to report thyroid aspirates that fell between benign and malignant diagnostic categories [1]. It made it difficult for clinicians to interpret the reports. To address terminology and other issues related to thyroid FNACs, the National Cancer Institute (NCI) hosted "The NCI Thyroid Fine Needle Aspiration State of the Science Conference" at Bethesda, Maryland. There were six committees which dealt with different areas regarding thyroid cytology. Committee IV dealt with diagnostic terminology and morphologic criteria for cytological diagnosis of thyroid lesions. Its recommendations were widely published [2, 3]. Subsequently a monograph "The Bethesda System for Reporting Thyroid Cytopathology" (TBSRTC) which includes definitions, diagnostic/morphologic criteria, explanatory notes, and a brief management plan for each diagnostic category was published [4]. TBSRTC is a six-category scheme of thyroid cytopathology reporting (Table 1). Each category has an implied cancer risk, which ranges from 0% to 3% for the "benign" category to virtually 100% for the "malignant" category. It uses three categories, AUS/FLUS, SFN/Hürthle cell neoplasm, and SFM, to report thyroid aspirates that fall between benign and malignant. As a function of these risk associations, each

TABLE 1: The Bethesda System for reporting thyroid cytopathology: recommended diagnostic categories, implied risk of malignancy, and recommended clinical management.

Diagnostic category	Risk of malignancy (%)	Usual management[a]
(I) Nondiagnostic or unsatisfactory (ND/UNS)		Repeat FNA with ultrasound guidance
Cyst fluid only		
Virtually acellular specimen		
Other (obscuring blood, clotting artifact, etc.)		
(II) Benign	0–3	Clinical follow-up
Consistent with a benign follicular nodule (includes adenomatoid nodule,colloid nodule etc.)		
Consistent with lymphocytic (Hashimoto) thyroiditis in the proper clinical context		
Consistent with granulomatous (subacute) thyroiditis		
Other		
(III) Atypia of undetermined significance or follicular lesion of undetermined significance (AUS/FLUS)	5–15[b]	Repeat FNA
(IV) Follicular neoplasm or suspicious for follicular neoplasm (FN/SFN)	15–30	Surgical lobectomy
-specify if Hürthle cell (oncocytic) type		
(V) Suspicious for malignancy (SFM)	60–75	Near-total thyroidectomy or surgical lobectomy[c]
Suspicious for papillary carcinoma		
Suspicious for medullary carcinoma		
Suspicious for metastatic carcinoma		
Suspicious for lymphoma		
Other		
(VI) Malignant	97–99	Near-total thyroidectomy[c]
Papillary thyroid carcinoma		
Poorly differentiated carcinoma		
Medullary thyroid carcinoma		
Undifferentiated (anaplastic) carcinoma		
Squamous cell carcinoma		
Carcinoma with mixed features (specify)		
Metastatic carcinoma		
Non-Hodgkin lymphoma		
Other		

[a]Actual management may depend on other factors (e.g., clinical and sonographic) besides the FNA interpretation.
[b]Estimate extrapolated from histopathologic data from patients with "repeated atypicals" [7, 26].
[c]In the case of "suspicious for metastatic tumor" or a "malignant" interpretation indicating metastatic tumor rather than a primary thyroid malignancy, surgery may not be indicated.

category is linked to evidence based clinical management guidelines.

The objective of the present prospective study, done in an Indian hospital, was to report thyroid cytology smears by TBSRTC into various diagnostic categories, analyze their cytological features using TBSRTC monograph, conveying brief management plan to the clinicians, and correlate with histology of surgical specimens received.

2. Materials and Methods

This was a prospective study of all successive cases with thyroid swelling referred to the Department of Pathology, Employees State Insurance (ESI) Postgraduate Institute of Medical Sciences and Research and ESI Model Hospital, Basaidarapur, New Delhi, for FNAC during the period from March 2010 to February 2012. Relevant clinical history was taken and examination done. Pre-FNAC requirements as recommended by Committee I of the NCI State of the Science Conference, Bethesda, were followed [5]. All patients were subjected to FNA sampling under ultrasound guidance by one of the two authors using Zajdela technique 4-5 times randomly in different areas [6]. The smears were prepared using conventional methods and stained with Giemsa and Papanicolaou stains. The cytological features were evaluated and the reporting was done according to TBSRTC (Table 1). The

Table 2: Number of cases in various diagnostic categories and subcategories according to the Bethesda System for Reporting Thyroid Cytopathology (TBSRTC).

S. number	Cytological categories	Subcategories	Number of cases	Total number of cases in each category
1	Nondiagnostic/unsatisfactory (ND/UNS)	Cyst fluid only	16	16 (7.2)
		Virtually acellular specimen	0	
		Other (obscuring blood, clotting artifact, etc.)	0	
2	Benign	Consistent with benign follicular nodule (includes adenomatoid nodule, colloid nodule, etc.)	138	180 (80)
		Consistent with lymphocytic (Hashimoto) thyroiditis in the proper clinical context	36	
		Consistent with granulomatous (subacute) thyroiditis	02	
		Other	04	
3	Atypia of undetermined significance/follicular lesion of undetermined significance (AUS/FLUS)			11 (4.9)
4	Follicular neoplasm/suspicious for a follicular neoplasm (FN/SFN)			5 (2.2)
5	Suspicious for malignancy (SFM)	Suspicious for papillary carcinoma	06	8 (3.6)
		Suspicious for medullary carcinoma	0	
		Suspicious for metastatic carcinoma	0	
		Suspicious for lymphoma	01	
		Other	01	
6	Malignant	Papillary thyroid carcinoma	04	5 (2.2)
		Poorly differentiated carcinoma	0	
		Medullary thyroid carcinoma	01	
		Undifferentiated (anaplastic) carcinoma	0	
		Squamous cell carcinoma	0	
		Carcinoma with mixed features	0	
		Metastatic carcinoma	0	
		Non-Hodgkin lymphoma	0	
		Other	0	
	Total			**225 (100)**

(1) Figures in parentheses indicate percentages.
(2) "Other" subcategory in benign category consisted of cases of chronic nonspecific abscess.
(3) "Other" subcategory in suspicious for malignancy category consisted of a case of suspicious for malignancy, not otherwise specified.

morphological criteria given in the monograph of TBSRTC were used [4]. The clinicians were communicated implied risk of malignancy and recommended clinical management along with the report. Histopathological specimens, wherever available, were processed as per standard methods. Sensitivity, specificity, positive predictive value, and negative predictive value were calculated using histopathology diagnosis as gold standard. For calculating statistical parameters ND/UNS and AUS/FLUS cases were excluded as nondefinitive diagnosis and categories "SFM" and "malignant" were put together. All the parameters were calculated either excluding FN/SFN or including it with either benign or malignant diagnosis to highlight the effect on statistical values.

3. Results

The distribution of 225 cases is shown in Table 2. Benign category was the largest (80%) followed by ND/UNS category (7.2%). Malignant and SFM categories constituted 2.2% and 3.6%, respectively, making a total of 5.7%. AUS/FLUS constituted 4.9% cases, while FN/SFN had 2.2% cases.

In the ND/UNS category, all cases were subcategorized as cyst fluid only. There was no case in subcategory virtually acellular specimen or other (obscuring blood, clotting artifact, etc.).

In benign category 76.7% of total cases were consistent with benign follicular nodule (BFN). It had follicular cells

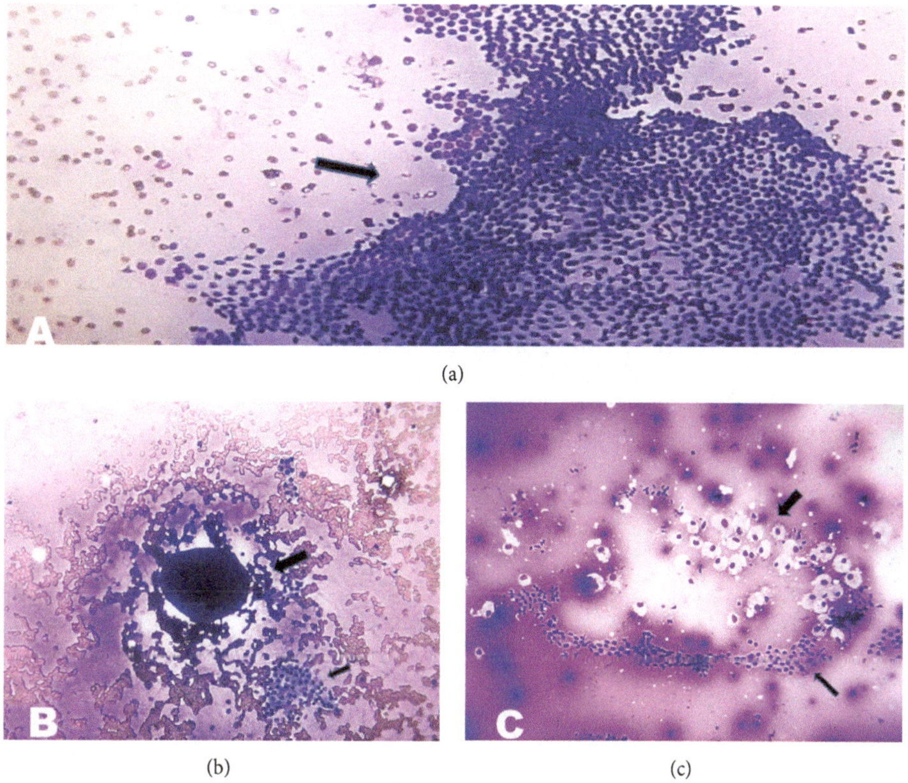

FIGURE 1: (a) Benign follicular nodule. Photomicrograph showing monolayer sheets of evenly spaced follicular cells having a honeycomb-like arrangement (arrow) (Smear, Giemsa, 400x magnification). (b) Benign follicular nodule. Photomicrograph showing globular mass of colloid with superimposed follicular cells (thick arrow) mixed with monolayer sheet of follicular cells (thin arrow) against the background of colloid and blood (Smear, Giemsa, 400x magnification). (c) Benign follicular nodule. Photomicrograph showing follicular cells arranged in sheets (honeycomb-like) (thin arrow) mixed with macrophages (thick arrow) against the background of colloid (Smear, Giemsa, 400x magnification).

which were arranged predominantly in monolayer sheets or were occasionally in intact, 3-dimensional, variably sized balls/spheres (Figures 1(a) and 1(b)). Rare microfollicles were present. Anisonucleosis was seen in some cases but there was no significant pleomorphism or nuclear atypia. Cellularity was low to moderate; low cellularity was seen in 52.2% cases and moderate cellularity in 47.8% cases. High cellularity was not seen. Pleomorphism was present only in 2.9% cases out of 138 cases. Hürthle cells were present only in 2.2% cases. Foam cells (macrophages) were present in 21.7% cases (Figure 1(c)).

Background was blood-mixed with colloid in 55.8% cases and was only colloid in 44.2% cases. Fire flare or spindle cell was not seen in any case of benign follicular nodule in this study.

The subcategory consistent with lymphocytic thyroiditis (LT) had 20% cases in benign category. All specimens were moderately cellular. The lymphoid population was moderate in amount in 88.9% cases. The lymphoid cells were polymorphic (Figure 2(a)). Intact lymphoid follicles and lymphohistiocytic (Figure 2(b)) aggregates were also seen. Hürthle cells (oncocytes) were present in all cases. Multinucleated giant cells were found in 27.8% cases and epithelioid cells in 11.1% cases.

In subcategory consistent with granulomatous thyroiditis (GT), there were 1.1% cases, which showed hypocellular smears with clusters of epithelioid histiocytes (Figure 3(a)), that is, granulomas along with many multinucleated giant cells (Figure 3(b)), lymphocytes, macrophages, and scant degenerated follicular cells. Neutrophils were present in both cases.

The subcategory "other" included cases of chronic abscess. The pus obtained was negative for acid fast bacilli and fungus.

In this study, category AUS/FLUS constituted 4.9%. 81.8% of these prominently showed microfollicles in some but not all the moderately cellular smears (Figure 4(a)), 9.1% prominently showed microfollicles with sparsely cellular smear with scant colloid (Figure 4(b)), and 9.1% showed predominantly benign appearing smear with focal features of papillary thyroid carcinoma (PTC) including nuclear grooves, enlarged nuclei with pale chromatin, and alterations in nuclear contour and shape.

There were 2.2% cases in category FN/SFN (Figure 5). There was no case of FN, Hürthle cell type.

In the category SFM, 75% were suspicious for papillary carcinoma and 12.5% were suspected for lymphoma and 12.5% were SFM, not otherwise specified (SFM, NOS). 66.6% cases of suspicious for papillary carcinoma were of Pattern A (patchy nuclear change), 16.7% cases were of Pattern B (incomplete nuclear change) and 16.7% cases were of Pattern

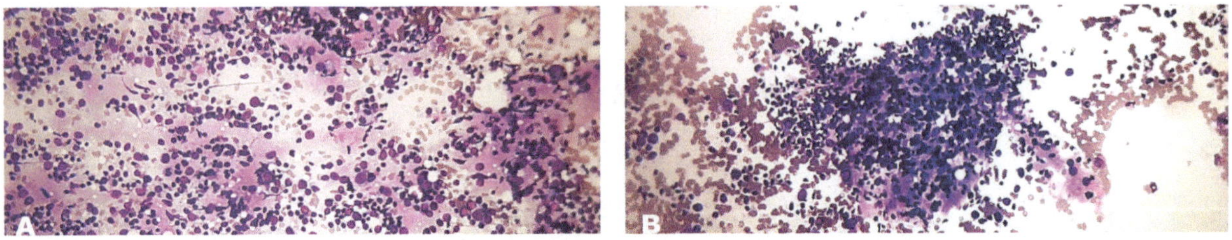

(a) (b)

Figure 2: (a) Lymphocytic (Hashimoto) thyroiditis. Photomicrograph showing polymorphous lymphoid population (Smear, Giemsa, 400x magnification). (b) Lymphocytic (Hashimoto) thyroiditis. Photomicrograph showing lymphohistiocytic aggregates in lymphocytic (Hashimoto) thyroiditis (Smear, Giemsa, 400x magnification).

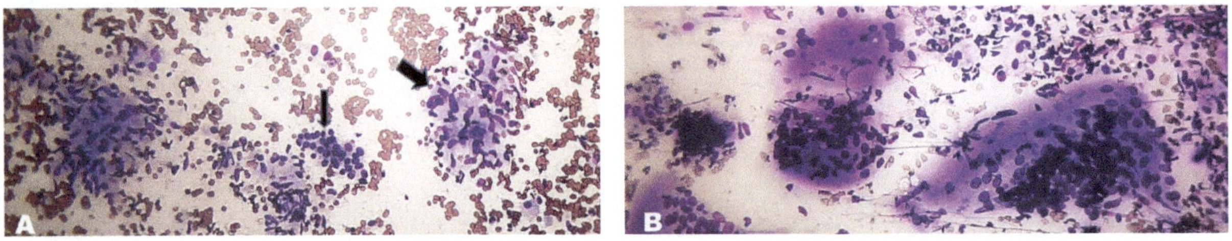

(a) (b)

Figure 3: (a) Granulomatous (subacute) thyroiditis. Photomicrograph showing clusters of epithelioid histiocytes (thick arrow) mixed with benign follicular cells (thin arrow) (Smear, Giemsa, 400x magnification). (b) Granulomatous (subacute) thyroiditis. Photomicrograph showing many multinucleated giant cells against the background of colloid and blood (Smear, Giemsa, 400x magnification).

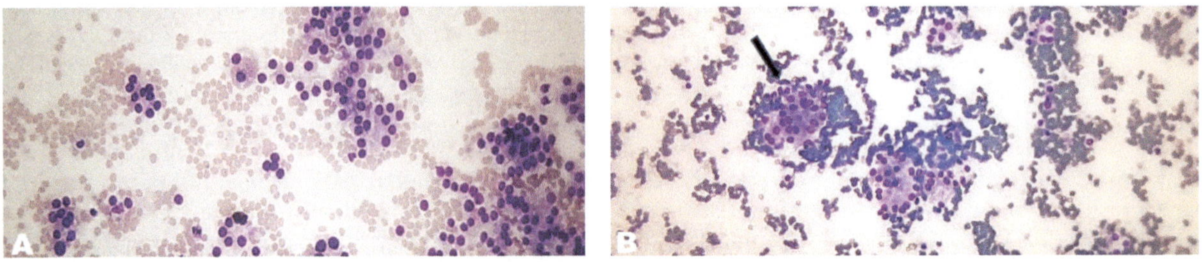

(a) (b)

Figure 4: (a) Atypia of undetermined significance. Photomicrograph showing prominent microfollicles in a moderately cellular specimen (Smear, Giemsa, 400x magnification). (b) Atypia of undetermined significance. Photomicrograph showing sparsely cellular specimen with a predominance of microfollicles (Smear, Giemsa, 400x magnification).

D (cystic degeneration). There was no case of Pattern C (sparsely cellular specimen). 1 (12.5%) case of subcategory suspicious for lymphoma cytologically showed cellular smear composed of numerous monomorphic small to intermediate sized lymphoid cells (Figure 6). In the subcategory SFM, NOS, there was only one case showing cytological features suggestive of malignancy, but they were not enough to categorize the type of malignancy.

Category malignant included, 5(2.2%) cases. The maximum number of cases 4 (80%) were of PTC (Figures 7(a)–7(e)) and 1 (20%) case of medullary thyroid carcinoma (MTC) (Figures 8(a) and 8(b)).

Out of 225 cases that were cytologically studied, histopathological specimens of 40 (17.8%) cases were received and studied (Table 3).

Surgical specimens of 2 cases, 23 cases, and 1 case, respectively, for categories ND/UNS, benign, and AUS/FLUS amounting to 12.5%, 12.8%, and 9% of cases aspirated were received.

Of 18 cases of FN/SFN, SFM, and malignant category, only 15 were surgically resected. Out of 4 cases of FN/SFN, 3 were benign (follicular adenoma) and 1 was malignant (PTC). Histopathology was received for 6 cases of SFM. Five of them were reported cytologically as being suspicious for papillary carcinoma. Histopathologically, 3 of them turned out to be papillary thyroid carcinoma, but 2 were lymphocytic (Hashimoto) thyroiditis.

In total, 27 out of 40, that is, 67.5%, cases in this study with a subsequent tissue diagnosis had a definitive cytologic diagnosis of being benign or malignant (Table 4). Twenty

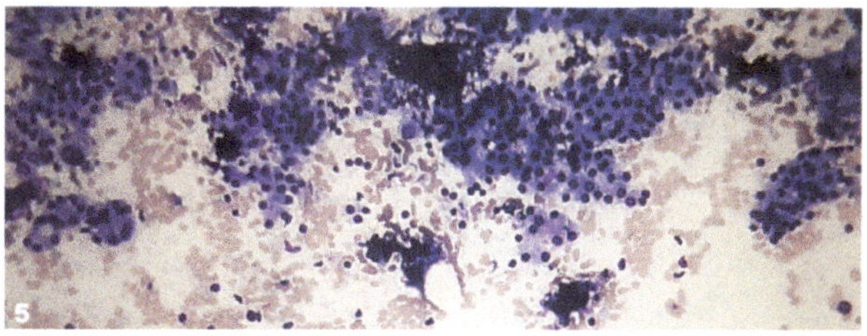

FIGURE 5: Follicular neoplasm/suspicious for a follicular neoplasm. Photomicrograph showing a highly cellular aspirate composed of uniform follicular cells arranged in crowded clusters and microfollicles (Smear, Giemsa, 400x magnification).

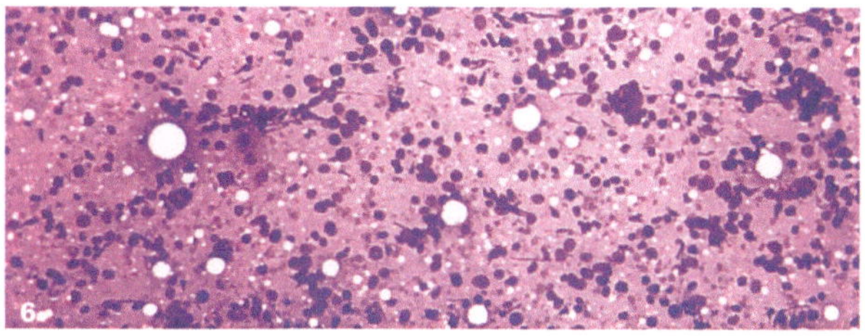

FIGURE 6: Suspicious for lymphoma. Photomicrograph showing a hemodiluted sample comprising exclusively lymphoid cells (Smear, Giemsa, 400x magnification).

cases were benign by both cytopathology and histopathology. Four cases were malignant by both cytopathology and histopathology. None of the cases with a malignant diagnosis on cytology proved to be benign on biopsy and 3 cases out of 23 that were benign on cytology proved to be malignant lesion on examination of tissue specimen.

The results of various statistical parameters are summarized in Table 5.

If FN/SFN is included in malignant group, the sensitivity increases but the specificity decreases. There is marked decrease in positive predictive value also.

4. Discussion

This paper shows the two-year experience in reporting thyroid aspirations by TBSRTC in an Indian academic institution as well as response of clinicians to the brief management plan suggested. TBSRTC does not recommend surgery for ND/UNS, benign and AUS/FLUS categories. In the FN/SFN, SFM, and malignant categories, we expected excision of nodules or partial/complete thyroidectomy in all cases as per TBSRTC recommendations.

The present study had 16 (7.2%) cases in ND/UNS category. Other recent studies had 1.2% to 16.4% cases in this group [7–14]. The guidelines for this category are very clear in TBSRTC. All of them were advised to be reaspirated after a minimum period of 3 months. The 3-month interval was recommended to prevent false positive interpretations due to reactive or reparative changes, as recommended by Committee VI (Post-FNA Technique and Treatment Options) [15]. The number of cases in this category is dependent on the aspirator's experience. The recommendations of Committee I on indications of thyroid FNA and pre-FNA and Committee II on training and credentialing are likely to bring down the number in this category in future studies [5, 16]. TBSRTC does not provide the implied risk of malignancy for this category. However a recent study found a rate of 8.9% in ND/UNS category [10]. Two histopathological specimens were received and both were nodular goiter. Clinician was not comfortable with the term ND/UNS and was not willing to wait for 3 months, thus preferred to go for surgery.

The benign category had 180 cases (80%) with BFN being the predominant group followed by LT. The "benign" category had a range of 34% to 87.5% in recent studies [7–14]. However, only one study had a percentage less than 50 and this was due a high incidence of AUS/FLUS and FN/SFN. The diagnostic criteria of all the subcategories are well characterized in TBSRTC monograph. However, TBSRTC recommendation on diagnostic terminology and morphologic criteria does not mention giant cells and epithelioid cells in LT previously described in the literature [17, 18]. 23 histopathological specimens from category diagnosed as "benign" were received. All of them were operated because of cosmetic reasons or pressure symptoms. 18 were nodular goiter, 2 follicular adenoma, and 3 PTC. The cytological appearance of nodular goiter can overlap with those of follicular adenoma and cytological criteria alone cannot reliably distinguish between the two in certain cases [19]. These 2 cases had on cytology abundant colloid in addition to follicular cells and hence were diagnosed as BFN. There were 3 cases of PTC which were incidental findings in thyroid specimen and were less than 1 cm in size and thus these nodules were not aspirated. There were no lymph nodes in these cases and ultrasound features were not suspicious. These "incidentalomas" remain indolent in most cases as implied by 30% prevalence in a study by Harach et al. in 1985 in an autopsy study [20]. One study does not consider incidental papillary carcinoma as malignant for analysis of their data [10].

The classification of "indeterminate" lesions (those not clearly benign or malignant) in thyroid cytopathology has long been a source of confusion for both pathologists and clinicians. The general category AUS/FLUS is reserved for specimens that contained cells (follicular, lymphoid, or other) with architectural and/or nuclear atypia that is not sufficient to be classified as suspicious for a follicular neoplasm or suspicious for malignancy. The atypia is more marked than can be ascribed confidently to benign changes.

We had 11 cases in group AUS/FLUS. An AUS result has been reported in 3.2–29% of thyroid cases [7–14]. TBSRTC suggests that the frequency of AUS interpretations should be in the range of approximately 7% of all thyroid FNA interpretations. This is a category of last resort and should not be used indiscriminately. Not much data exists in the literature to support the recommendation that the category should not exceed 7% of all thyroid categories [21]. The incidence also varies with experience and training of cytopathologists. The recommended management for an initial AUS/FLUS interpretation is the clinical correlation and, for most cases, a repeat FNA at an appropriate interval. A repeat FNA usually results in a more definitive interpretation; only about 20–25% of nodules are repeatedly AUS. One case of AUS/FLUS

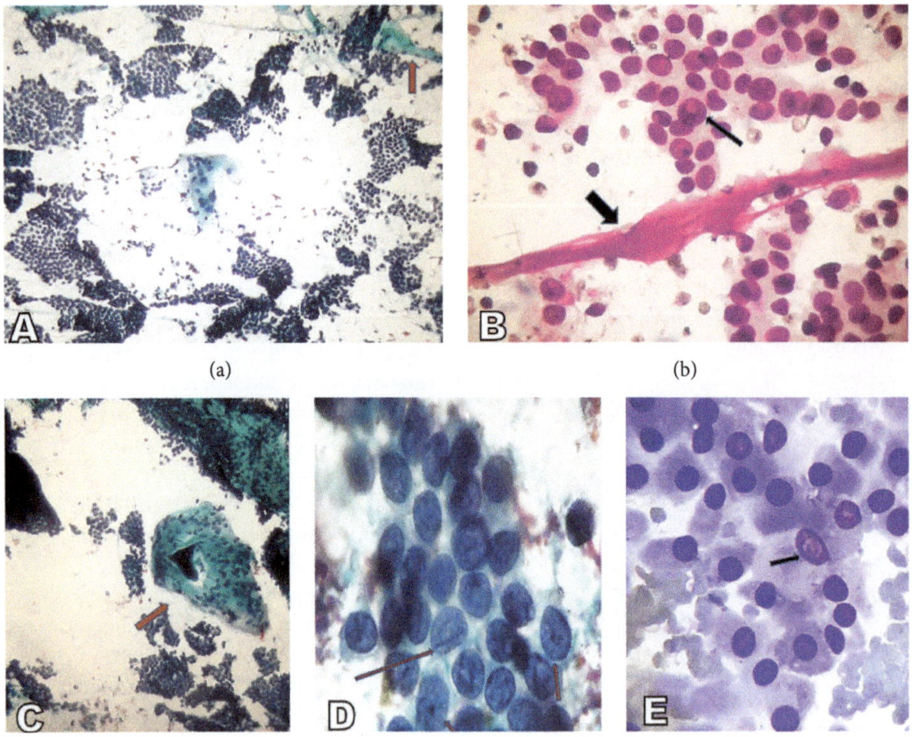

(a) (b) (c) (d) (e)

Figure 7: (a) Papillary thyroid carcinoma. Photomicrograph showing highly cellular specimen composed of numerous monolayer sheets and occasional papillary-like fragments and "stringy," "ropy" colloid (arrow) (Smear, Papanicolaou stain, 400x magnification). (b) Papillary thyroid carcinoma. Photomicrograph showing "stringy" colloid (thick arrow) and intranuclear cytoplasmic inclusions (thin arrow) (Smear, Giemsa, 1000x magnification). (c) Papillary thyroid carcinoma. Photomicrograph showing multinucleated giant cell engulfing sticky colloid (arrow) in a case of papillary thyroid carcinoma (Smear, Papanicolaou stain, 400x magnification). (d) Papillary thyroid carcinoma. Photomicrograph showing longitudinal nuclear grooves (thin long arrow) and micronucleoli (thin short arrows) (Smear, Papanicolaou stain, 1000x magnification). (e) Papillary thyroid carcinoma, oncocytic variant. Photomicrograph showing the neoplasm composed throughout of oncocytic (Hürthle-like) cells that have abundant granular cytoplasm. Intranuclear cytoplasmic inclusions are visible (arrow) (Smear, Giemsa, 1000x magnification).

Table 3: Cytological/histopathological diagnosis correlation.

Cytopathological categorization	Number of cases where surgical specimens were received (n = 40)	Percent of the category	Histopathological diagnosis	Number of cases
ND/UNS (n = 16)	2	12.5	Nodular goiter	2
Benign (n = 180)	23	12.8	Nodular goiter	18
			Follicular adenoma	2
			Papillary thyroid carcinoma	3
AUS/FLUS (n = 11)	1	9	Papillary thyroid carcinoma	1
FN/SFN (n = 5)	4	80	Follicular adenoma	3
			Papillary thyroid carcinoma	1
SFM (n = 8)	6	75	Lymphocytic thyroiditis	2
			Papillary thyroid carcinoma	3
			Follicular adenoma	1
Malignant (n = 5)	4	80	Papillary thyroid carcinoma	4

(1) ND/UNS = nondiagnostic/unsatisfactory, AUS/FLUS = atypia of undetermined significance/follicular lesion of undetermined significance, FN/SFN = follicular neoplasm/suspected for a follicular neoplasm, and SFM = suspected for malignancy.
(2) n = total number of cases.

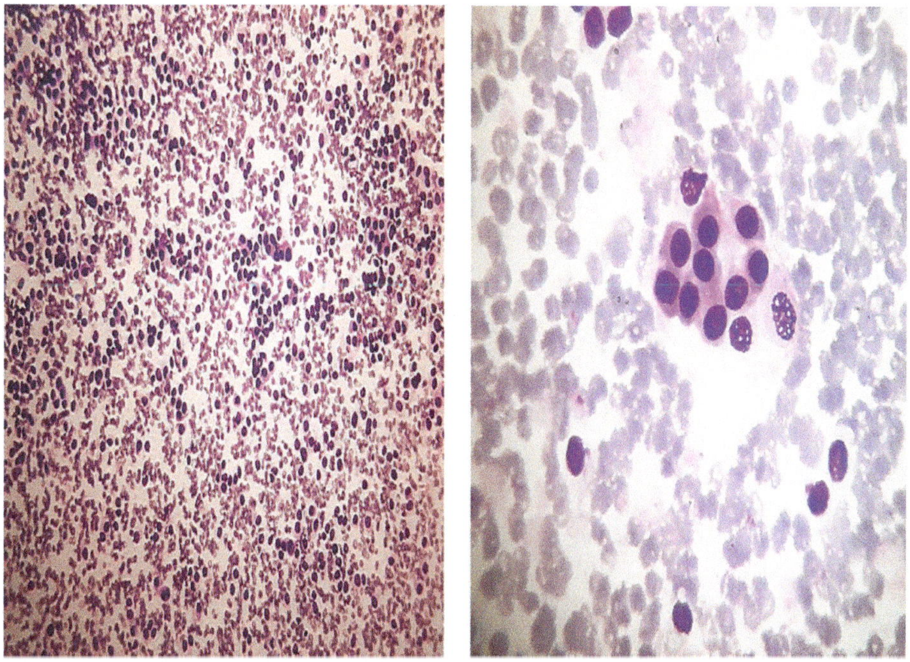

(a) (b)

FIGURE 8: (a) (100x magnification) and (b) (1000x magnification) Medullary thyroid carcinoma. Photomicrographs showing predominantly cohesive, syncytial-like clusters with few isolated plasmacytoid cells (Smear, Giemsa stain).

TABLE 4: Cytological/histopathological correlation with benign and malignant cases.

Cytodiagnosis	Histologic diagnosis	
	Benign	Malignant
ND/UNS ($n = 2$)	2	0
Benign ($n = 23$)	20	3
AUS/FLUS ($n = 1$)	0	1
FN/SFN ($n = 4$)	3	1
SFM ($n = 6$)	3	3
Malignant ($n = 4$)	0	4

(1) ND/UNS = nondiagnostic/unsatisfactory, AUS/FLUS = atypia of undetermined significance/follicular lesion of undetermined significance, FN/SFN = follicular neoplasm/suspected for a follicular neoplasm, and SFM = suspected for malignancy.
(2) n = total number of cases.

on cytology proved to be malignant on histology and was PTC. On cytology, this case showed predominantly benign appearing smear with focal features of PTC in only one of the smears and thus was put under this category.

FN/SFN category had 8 cases (2.2%). TBSRTC provides clear guidelines for this category. Recent studies have shown 2.2–16.1% cases in this group [7–14]. Four specimens were received, 1 of which was follicular variant of papillary carcinoma. Smears of the latter had predominant follicular pattern but the classic nuclear features of PTC were not present in the cytological smears.

SFM category had 8 cases (3.6%), 6 of which were suspicious for papillary carcinoma, one was suspicious for lymphoma, and one was SFM, NOS. Histopathology was received for 6 cases of SFM. It varies from 1.3 to 10% in recent studies [7–14]. Five of them were reported cytologically as suspicious for papillary carcinoma. Histopathologically 3 of them turned out to be papillary thyroid carcinoma, but 2 were lymphocytic (Hashimoto) thyroiditis. The latter were on cytology diagnosed as suspicious for papillary carcinoma because of high proportion of follicular cells and presence of intranuclear cytoplasmic inclusions (INCIs) in rare cells. INCIs are not specific for papillary thyroid carcinoma as they may be seen focally in benign thyroid nodules. Moreover, an increased incidence of PTC is well known in LT and hence a diagnosis of suspicious for papillary carcinoma was given so as not to miss out malignancy. SFM, NOS, had very high cellularity with 3D clusters of follicular cells in all the smears but could not be typed cytologically. Histologically, it turned out to be follicular adenoma.

Committee V of the NCI Thyroid Fine Needle Aspiration State of the Science Conference has provided guidelines for indications of ancillary studies, specific ancillary studies to be performed, and sample preparation for each study. Immunohistochemistry panels have been suggested for suspicious malignancies which include medullary carcinoma (calcitonin, thyroglobulin, CEA, and chromogranin), anaplastic carcinoma (pan-cytokeratin), and metastatic carcinoma (TTF-1). These are to be done on cell block from FNA, preferably including at least one dedicated pass for the study. For suspicious lymphoma, flow cytometric immunophenotyping is suggested. Dedicated passes are also needed for studies to detect genetic alterations such as BRAF mutation or RET/PTC chromosomal rearrangements, which are

Table 5: Statistical parameters when FN/SFN cases are excluded or are included with either benign or malignant cases.

Statistical Parameters	FN/SFN cases excluded	FN/SFN cases included with benign cases (%)	FN/SFN cases included with malignant cases (%)
Sensitivity	76.92 (46.20–94.69)	73.33 (44.91–92.05)	78.57 (49.21–95.09)
Specificity	88.46 (69.82–97.42)	89.66 (72.62–97.69)	81.25 (63.55–92.75)
Positive predictive value	76.92 (46.20–94.69)	78.57 (49.21–95.09)	64.71 (38.35–85.70)
Negative predictive value	88.46 (69.82–97.42)	86.67 (69.26–96.16)	89.66 (72.62–97.69)

Figures in parentheses show 95% confidence interval.

Table 6: Comparison of results of the present study and random studies over the last 30 years.

Study	Number	Sensitivity %	Specificity %	PPV %	NPV %
Al-Sayer et al. [27]	70	86	93	80	96
Silverman et al. [28]	309	93	96.5	88.9	96.5
Cusick et al. [29]	283	76	58	72	64
Altavilla et al. [30]	257	71.4	100	100	94.4
Bouvet et al. [31]	78	93.5	75	85.3	88.2
Ko et al. [32]	207	78.4	98.2	99	66.3
Kessler et al. [33]	170	79	98.5	98.7	76.6
Handa et al. [34]	66	97	100	96	100
Gupta et al. [35]	75	80	86.6	80	86.6
Present study (FN/SFN excluded)	40	76.92	88.46	76.92	88.46
Present study (FN/SFN included as benign)	40	73.33	89.66	78.57	86.67
Present study (FN/SFN included as malignant)	40	78.57	81.25	64.71	89.66

PPV = positive predictive value and NPV = negative predictive value.

very promising for the diagnosis of papillary carcinoma. Immunocytochemistry on cytospin, direct smear, or prefixed monolayer may also be utilized, but protocols should be carefully validated [22].

The category malignant had a range of 2.9% to 11% in recent studies [7–14]. The present study had 5 (2.2%) cases in the malignant category. We received 4 specimens from the category diagnosed as "malignant" cytologically. All of them were diagnosed as PTC both histopathologically and cytologically.

Table 6 shows a comparison of statistical parameters of our study and other studies over the last 30 years.

The method of data analysis can alter the results of statistical parameters. If suspicious lesions are considered positive, the sensitivity increases while the specificity decreases. If suspicious lesions are excluded, then the sensitivity decreases and the false negative rates increase. For statistical purpose we had put categories "SFM" and "malignant" in one group. "Unsatisfactory" smears were likely to be malignant or benign and putting them into a single diagnostic category automatically presents a false picture. All the parameters were calculated either excluding FN/SFN or including it with either benign or malignant diagnosis to highlight the effect on statistical values.

Articles implementing TBSRTC have started appearing in the literature [14, 23–25]. TBSRTC is a relatively recent six-category scheme to classify thyroid cytology smears. It needs to be validated by more prospective studies on larger number of cases with histopathological correlation. There is need for consensus amongst institutions in various countries to utilize TBSRTC to facilitate easy sharing of data across the world for surveys and research.

5. Conclusions

This study is a prospective analysis of reporting of thyroid aspiration smears by TBSRTC using the Bethesda monograph. It was found that the monograph is succinctly written in an easy-to-read format and has useful color images which help in making the diagnosis. The clinicians are also benefitted because of the management plan it suggests. Cases of AUS/FLUS are followed by repeat FNAC, thus reducing the incidence of surgery in our series (1/11). However, the exact incidence of malignancy in this heterogeneous category is difficult to predict as most of these cases are unlikely to be operated if the Bethesda recommendations are to be followed. There is a need for a large study with histopathological correlation for this category.

Conflict of Interests

The authors declare that there is no conflict of interests regarding the publication of this paper.

Acknowledgments

The authors acknowledge the help provided by Dr. K. S. Charak, former Head of the department of surgery, and Dr. S. Kohli, Head of the department of radiodiagnosis, for this study.

References

[1] H. H. Wang, "Reporting thyroid fine-needle aspiration: Literature review and a proposal," *Diagnostic Cytopathology*, vol. 34, no. 1, pp. 67–76, 2006.

[2] E. S. Cibas and M. A. Sanchez, "The national cancer institute thyroid fine-needle aspiration state-of-the-science conference: inspiration for a uniform terminology linked to management guidelines," *Cancer Cytopathology*, vol. 114, no. 2, pp. 71–73, 2008.

[3] Z. W. Baloch, V. A. LiVolsi, S. L. Asa et al., "Diagnostic terminology and morphologic criteria for cytologic diagnosis of thyroid lesions: a synopsis of the national cancer institute thyroid fine-needle aspiration state of the science conference," *Diagnostic Cytopathology*, vol. 36, no. 6, pp. 425–437, 2008.

[4] S. Z. Ali and E. S. Cibas, Eds., *The Bethesda System for Reporting Thyroid Cytopathology. Definitions, Criteria and Explanatory Notes*, Springer, New York, NY, USA, 2010.

[5] E. S. Cibas, E. K. Alexander, C. B. Benson et al., "Indications for thyroid FNA and pre-FNA requirements: a synopsis of the National Cancer Institute thyroid fine-needle aspiration state of the science conference," *Diagnostic Cytopathology*, vol. 36, no. 6, pp. 390–399, 2008.

[6] A. Zajdela, M. A. de Maublanc, P. Schlienger, and C. Haye, "Cytologic diagnosis of orbital and periorbital palpable tumors using fine-needle sampling without aspiration," *Diagnostic Cytopathology*, vol. 2, no. 1, pp. 17–20, 1986.

[7] J. Yang, V. Schnadig, R. Logrono, and P. G. Wasserman, "Fine-needle aspiration of thyroid nodules: a study of 4703 patients with histologic and clinical correlations.," *Cancer*, vol. 111, no. 5, pp. 306–315, 2007.

[8] R. Nayar and M. Ivanovic, "The indeterminate thyroid fine-needle aspiration: Experience from an academic center using terminology similar to that proposed in the 2007 national cancer institute thyroid fine needle aspiration state of the science conference," *Cancer Cytopathology*, vol. 117, no. 3, pp. 195–202, 2009.

[9] C. G. A. Theoharis, K. M. Schofield, L. Hammers, R. Udelsman, and D. C. Chhieng, "The bethesda thyroid fine-needle aspiration classification system: year 1 at an academic institution," *Thyroid*, vol. 19, no. 11, pp. 1215–1223, 2009.

[10] V. Y. Jo, E. B. Stelow, S. M. Dustin, and K. Z. Hanley, "Malignancy risk for fine-needle aspiration of thyroid lesions according to the Bethesda system for reporting thyroid cytopathology," *The American Journal of Clinical Pathology*, vol. 134, no. 3, pp. 450–456, 2010.

[11] M. Bonzanini, P. Amadori, L. Morelli et al., "Subclassification of the 'grey zone' of thyroid cytology; a retrospective descriptive study with clinical, cytological, and histological correlation," *Journal of Thyroid Research*, vol. 2011, Article ID 251680, 8 pages, 2011.

[12] J. T. Broome and C. C. Solorzano, "The impact of atypia/follicular lesion of undetermined significance on the rate of malignancy in thyroid fine-needle aspiration: evaluation of the Bethesda system for reporting thyroid cytopathology," *Surgery*, vol. 150, no. 6, pp. 1234–1241, 2011.

[13] M. M. Al-Shraim, O. M. Kaood, M. R. Hussein et al., "Assessment of malignancy rate in thyroid nodules according to the Bethesda system of fine-needle aspiration: report from a tertiary center in the Southwestern region of Saudi Arabia," *Saudi Medical Journal*, vol. 33, no. 2, pp. 167–171, 2012.

[14] S. K. Mondal, S. Sinha, B. Basak, D. N. Roy, and S. K. Sinha, "The Bethesda system for reporting thyroid fine needle aspirates: a cytologic study with histologic follow-up," *Journal of Cytology*, vol. 30, no. 2, pp. 94–99, 2013.

[15] L. J. Layfield, J. Abrams, B. Cochand-Priollet et al., "Post-thyroid FNA testing and treatment options: a synopsis of the national cancer institute thyroid fine needle aspiration state of the science conference," *Diagnostic Cytopathology*, vol. 36, no. 6, pp. 442–448, 2008.

[16] B.-M. E. Ljung, J. Langer, E. L. Mazzaferri, Y. C. Oertel, S. A. Wells, and J. Waisman, "Training, credentialing and re-credentialing for the performance of a thyroid FNA: a synopsis of the National Cancer Institute thyroid fine-needle aspiration state of the science conference," *Diagnostic Cytopathology*, vol. 36, no. 6, pp. 400–406, 2008.

[17] P. S. Persson, "Cytodiagnosis of thyroiditis. A comparative study of cytological, histological, immunological and clinical findings in thyroiditis, particularly in diffuse lymphoid thyroiditis," *Acta Medica Scandinavica*, vol. 483, pp. 7–100, 1968.

[18] R. Bhalotra and G. Jayaram, "Overlapping morphology in thyroiditis (Hashimoto's and subacute) and Grave's disease," *Cytopathology*, vol. 1, no. 6, pp. 371–372, 1990.

[19] S. R. Orell, G. F. Sterrett, and D. Whitaker, "Chapter 6. Thyroid," in *Fine Needle Aspiration Cytology*, pp. 125–164, Elsevier, Sydney, Australia, 2005.

[20] H. R. Harach, K. O. Franssila, and V.-M. Wasenius, "Occult papillary carcinoma of the thyroid. A 'normal' finding in Finland. A systematic autopsy study," *Cancer*, vol. 56, no. 3, pp. 531–538, 1985.

[21] L. J. Layfield, M. J. Morton, H. M. Cramer, and S. Hirschowitz, "Implications of the proposed thyroid fine-needle aspiration category of follicular lesion of undetermined significance: a five-year multi-institutional analysis," *Diagnostic Cytopathology*, vol. 37, no. 10, pp. 710–714, 2009.

[22] A. C. Filie, S. L. Asa, K. R. Geisinger et al., "Utilization of ancillary studies in thyroid fine needle aspirates: a synopsis of the national cancer institute thyroid fine needle aspiration state of the science conference," *Diagnostic Cytopathology*, vol. 36, no. 6, pp. 438–441, 2008.

[23] L. Q. Wong and Z. W. Baloch, "Analysis of the Bethesda System for reporting thyroid cytopathology and similar precursor thyroid cytopathology reporting schemes," *Advances in Anatomic Pathology*, vol. 19, no. 5, pp. 313–319, 2012.

[24] M. Bongiovanni, A. Spitale, W. C. Faquin, L. Mazzucchelli, and Z. W. Baloch, "The Bethesda system for reporting thyroid cytopathology: a meta-analysis," *Acta Cytologica*, vol. 56, no. 4, pp. 333–339, 2012.

[25] B. K. Richmond, B. A. O'Brien, W. Mangano, S. Thompson, and S. Kemper, "The impact of implementation of the Bethesda system for reporting thyroid cytopathology on the surgical treatment of thyroid nodules," *The American Surgeon*, vol. 78, no. 6, pp. 706–710, 2012.

[26] L. Yassa, E. S. Cibas, C. B. Benson et al., "Long-term assessment of a multidisciplinary approach to thyroid nodule diagnostic evaluation," *Cancer*, vol. 111, no. 6, pp. 508–516, 2007.

[27] H. M. Al-Sayer, Z. H. Krukowski, V. M. M. Williams, and N. A. Matheson, "Fine needle aspiration cytology in isolated thyroid swellings: a prospective two year evaluation," *British Medical Journal*, vol. 290, no. 6480, pp. 1490–1492, 1985.

[28] J. F. Silverman, R. L. West, and E. W. Larkin, "The role of fine-needle aspiration biopsy in the rapid diagnosis and

management of thyroid neoplasm," *Cancer*, vol. 57, no. 6, pp. 1164–1170, 1986.

[29] E. L. Cusick, C. A. MacIntosh, Z. H. Krukowski, V. M. M. Williams, S. W. B. Ewen, and N. A. Matheson, "Management of isolated thyroid swellings: a prospective six year study of fine needle aspiration cytology in diagnosis," *British Medical Journal*, vol. 301, no. 6747, pp. 318–321, 1990.

[30] G. Altavilla, M. Pascale, and I. Nenci, "Fine needle aspiration cytology of thyroid gland diseases," *Acta Cytologica*, vol. 34, no. 2, pp. 251–256, 1990.

[31] M. Bouvet, J. I. Feldman, G. N. Gill et al., "Surgical management of the thyroid nodule: patient selection based on the results of fine-needle aspiration cytology," *The Laryngoscope*, vol. 102, no. 12 I, pp. 1353–1356, 1992.

[32] H.-M. Ko, I.-K. Jhu, S.-H. Yang et al., "Clinicopathologic analysis of fine needle aspiration cytology of the thyroid: a review of 1,613 cases and correlation with histopathologic diagnoses," *Acta Cytologica*, vol. 47, no. 5, pp. 727–732, 2003.

[33] A. Kessler, H. Gavriel, S. Zahav et al., "Accuracy and consistency of fine-needle aspiration biopsy in the diagnosis and management of solitary thyroid nodules," *Israel Medical Association Journal*, vol. 7, no. 6, pp. 371–373, 2005.

[34] U. Handa, S. Garg, H. Mohan, and N. Nagarkar, "Role of fine needle aspiration cytology in diagnosis and management of thyroid lesions: a study on 434 patients," *Journal of Cytology*, vol. 25, no. 1, pp. 13–17, 2008.

[35] M. Gupta, S. Gupta, and V. B. Gupta, "Correlation of fine needle aspiration cytology with histopathology in the diagnosis of solitary thyroid nodule," *Journal of Thyroid Research*, vol. 2010, Article ID 379051, 5 pages, 2010.

9

A Compendium of Urinary Biomarkers Indicative of Glomerular Podocytopathy

Miroslav Sekulic[1,2] and Simona Pichler Sekulic[3]

[1] *Department of Laboratory Medicine and Pathology, University of Minnesota, 420 Delaware Street SE, MMC 609 Mayo D185, Minneapolis, MN 55455, USA*
[2] *Division of Nephrology, Department of Medicine, Harvard Medical School, Massachusetts General Hospital, 149 13th Street, Boston, MA 02129, USA*
[3] *University of Belgrade School of Medicine, Dr. Subotica 8, 11000 Belgrade, Serbia*

Correspondence should be addressed to Miroslav Sekulic; sekul002@umn.edu

Academic Editor: Piero Tosi

It is well known that glomerular podocyte injury and loss are present in numerous nephropathies and that the pathophysiologic consecution of disease hinges upon the fate of the podocyte. While multiple factors play a hand in glomerulopathy progression, basic logic lends that if one monitors the podocyte's status, that may reflect the status of disease. Recent investigations have focused on what one can elucidate from the noninvasive collection of urine, and have proven that certain, specific biomarkers of podocytes can be readily identified via varying techniques. This paper has brought together all described urinary biomarkers of podocyte injury and is made to provide a concise summary of their utility and testing in laboratory and clinical theatres. While promising in the potential that they hold as tools for clinicians and investigators, the described biomarkers require further comprehensive vetting in the form of larger clinical trials and studies that would give their value true weight. These urinary biomarkers are put forth as novel indicators of glomerular disease presence, disease progression, and therapeutic efficacy that in some cases may be more advantageous than the established parameters/measures currently used in practice.

1. Introduction

The glomerulus is the functional unit of the kidney that creates from the afferent blood flow an ultrafiltrate, which passes through the remainder of the nephron for further modification. The glomerulus can be compared to a selective filter in that it discerns based on size and charge what passes on through to become the formed ultrafiltrate. This selectivity is intrinsic to the glomerular filtration apparatus and is dictated by the structural integrity of the three main components of which it is made: the capillary endothelium, the glomerular basement membrane (GBM), and the visceral epithelium overlying the GBM. Material that navigates through the glomerular filter must pass through these three components in that order to attain passage from the vascular capillary side into Bowman's space. The visceral epithelial layer of the glomerulus is made up of podocytes: terminally differentiated cells that have formed foot processes that encircle the GBM. The foot processes interdigitate between one another, with the space between each laying the slit diaphragm: described as a zipper-like interaction of membrane proteins between adjacent podocyte foot processes [1]. The slit diaphragm is considered to be the size limiting component of the glomerular filtration apparatus: permitting material approximately under the size of albumin, while limiting the passage of molecules the size of serum albumin—70 kilodaltons (kDa)—and larger [2]. The visceral epithelial layer is continuous with the parietal epithelial layer—the layer that constitutes Bowman's capsule—and there are phenotypic characteristics displayed by the two that allow for differentiation [3, 4]. A novel concept poses that there may be additional layers to designate within the glomerular filtration apparatus: an endothelial surface layer and a subpodocyte space, which gives new insight on the generally accepted structure of the glomerulus [5].

Further, more detailed discussion of the components of the glomerulus will be limited in this paper; however, there are numerous reviews that pour over the details of each [6–17].

As described before, the visceral epithelial layer of the glomerulus is made up of podocytes. The podocyte cell itself is comprised of a cell body, major processes which are large projections from the cell body, and long foot processes that adhere to the GBM. Three surfaces of a foot process can be described as apical, lateral, and basal, and while each surface is characterized by distinctive functional and structural roles, they are intertwined through intracellular associations. The apical surface faces Bowman's space, and with anionic surface proteins such as podocalyxin and podoplanin localized on the podocyte cell membrane, it is partially responsible for the repulsion of anionic molecules passing through the glomerular filtration apparatus [18–20]. Also on the apical membrane there is a protein tyrosine kinase phosphatase receptor named glomerular epithelial protein 1 (GLEPP-1), which is noted to regulate podocyte structure and function [21]. This negative charge lining the membrane surface of podocytes is also considered to be responsible for the maintenance of separation between adjacent foot processes [22]. The lateral surface of the foot process is comprised of the slit diaphragm, which is made up of many proteins, most notably the transmembrane protein nephrin that has numerous intracellular associations with both structural and signaling roles for the podocyte [23]. In mature podocytes, the slit diaphragm is also the only interaction between adjacent foot processes, and loss of this normal cell-cell interaction can be noted in the diseased state [9]. The basal surface of the podocyte foot process is attached to the GBM by the way of integrins, dystroglycans, and tetraspanins [24, 25]. Of the integrins that relate the podocyte to the GBM, $\alpha3\beta1$ integrins are the most numerous [16]. The highly specialized structure of the podocyte is essential for its ability to function as part of the glomerular filtering unit, and when its structural integrity is compromised, so is its ability to parse out what material from the blood may pass through to form the ultrafiltrate. Much of the structure of the podocyte is based on its actin cytoskeleton, whose numerous interactions with surface proteins such as podocalyxin and nephrin highlight the fact that though the surfaces of the foot processes may seem to have separate roles and constitutional make-up, they are in fact highly related. Figure 1 illustrates the basic cellular organization of the podocyte foot process, with specific emphasis upon the localization and the protein-protein associations amongst the soon to be discussed biomarkers of podocytopathy.

Podocytes are responsible for maintaining normal glomerular filtration in a number of ways: both in mechanical and functional fashions. Via the slit diaphragm, the podocytes (as previously described) act as barrier to protein based upon size. By way of the negatively charged surface of the podocyte foot processes, they serve as a barrier based on charge thus impairing passage of anionic proteins/material [12]. As a pericyte-like cell that encircles glomerular capillaries, a podocyte physically influences its vascular neighbors. Podocytes act as both a maintainer of glomerular capillary lumen patency and as a counteracting support against the intracapillary hydrostatic pressure (approximately 60 mmHg, a pressure that is greater than that found in most capillary networks) that would otherwise cause bulging [26]. It is notable in the pathogenesis of glomerulosclerosis that when podocytes are lost due to injury, the intracapillary pressure is no longer held in check by the podocyte counter-pressure, allowing the nude glomerular capillary to bulge and abut the parietal epithelium [10, 22]. Adhesions between the glomerular capillary and parietal epithelium are histologically evident in states when podocyte loss occurs [4]. In a functional manner, podocytes also lend to normal glomerular integrity by way of the elaboration of vascular endothelial growth factor-A (VEGF-A), which is necessary for the maintenance of the glomerular endothelium. VEGF-A has been considered to play a role in the pathogenesis of preeclampsia, with reduced expression of VEGF-A resulting in proteinuria and endotheliosis: both are pathognomonic renal findings in preeclampsia. The connection between preeclampsia and podocytes has been enlightened by findings that podocytes can be found in urine of women with preeclampsia and may be a diagnostic tool in diagnosing this gestational pathology [27]. Further glomerular capillary maintenance by podocytes is evident by their expression of angiopoietins (specifically Angl) and the presence of Angl receptors (protein tyrosine kinase 2-Tie2) on glomerular capillary endothelium [28, 29]. The relationship between the podocyte and the underlying GBM is more than a static physical relationship. It has been shown that while both the glomerular endothelium and podocyte are responsible for production of the GBM in the developing kidney, there is a transition where podocytes resume responsibility and continue to add material to the GBM even at the stage of the adult glomerulus [30]. In addition, podocytes clear material that may deposit in the GBM, aiding in our understanding of how this filtering apparatus remains unclogged from debris over time [31]. Podocytes have also been shown to produce platelet-derived growth factor (PDGF), which has trophic properties for neighboring mesangial cells [32]. There is also evidence that podocytes may have a hand in immune response, with localization and isolation of CD80 and complement receptor 1 (CRl) from podocytes [33, 34]. The podocyte plays not simply a static, mechanical role, but it also has paracrine activity through elaboration of factors necessary for maintaining glomerular homeostasis and may have an active role in immune mediated functions within the glomerulus.

There are numerous etiologies for which podocyte injury manifests as clinically evident disease: most notably as proteinuria. When injured, podocytes undergo histologically notable changes in structure that directly relate to a reduction of normal filtrating function. Most characteristically, podocytes can undergo a process termed effacement, where the normal cellular architecture of the foot process is altered and results in flattening and spreading of the foot process along the GBM and disruption of the slit diaphragm. Effacement can manifest whenever the following occurs: when the slit diaphragm and its related protein-protein interactions are disrupted, when there is interference in the normal association of the foot processes with the underlying GBM, when there is reorganization of the actin cytoskeleton and its related protein-protein interactions, or when there is

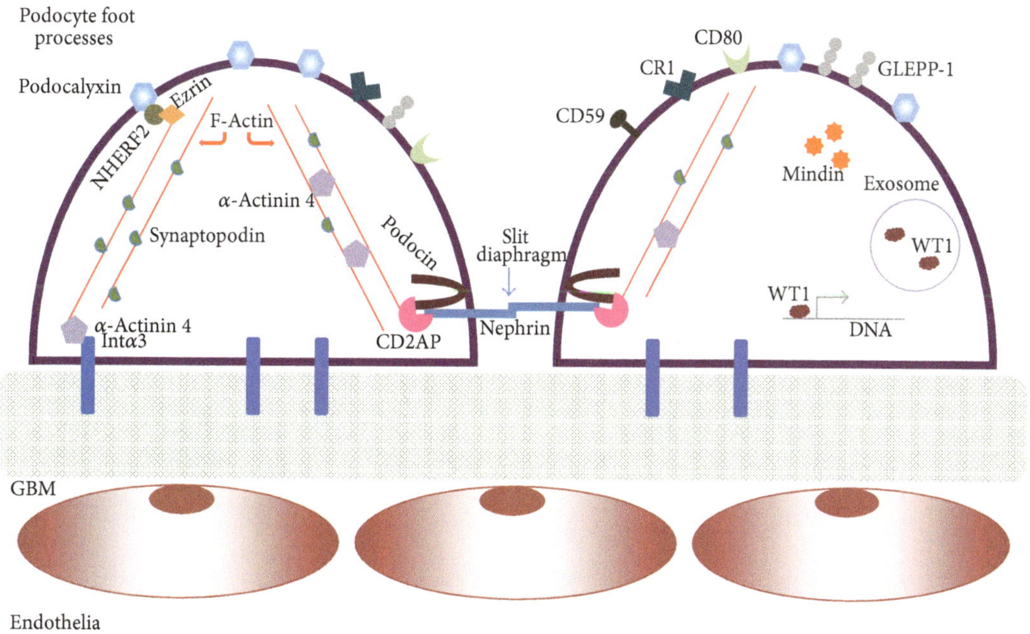

FIGURE 1: The protein biomarkers discussed in the paper are highlighted in this figure to show their cellular localization and the protein-protein associations that occur in glomerular podocyte foot processes. The podocyte is situated upon the glomerular basement membrane (GBM) and is anchored to it in part by alpha 3 integrins (Intα3). The slit diaphragm is illustrated with nephrin from adjacent foot processes interacting and forming a "zipper-like" structure. One can appreciate how the actin cytoskeleton (composed of F-actin) brings together the apical, lateral, and basal surfaces of the foot process: membrane proteins (podocalyxin, nephrin, alpha 3 integrin, etc.) via adaptor proteins (CD2AP, α-actinin 4, etc.) interact with actin, and as such they can modulate it. Wilms tumor protein 1 (WT1) has been identified as a transcription factor and is also localized within exosomes. Mindin has been localized within glomeruli, specifically to podocytes, and in cell culture found to be secreted into culture medium. Further details of each protein can be found in their respective sections within the paper.

disruption of the normal negatively charged apical surface of the foot processes [14]. Effacement can be accompanied by progressive changes in podocyte structure characterized by vacuolization, formation of pseudocysts, apical membrane microvillus formation, disruption of podocyte foot processes from the underlying GBM, and consequentially, in appropriate conditions, loss of podocytes [8, 35]. Figure 2 depicts a simplified view of the glomerular filtration apparatus and the consequences of podocyte injury.

Glomerular pathology that includes injury to podocytes has been classically diagnosed by the analysis of biomarkers related to renal dysfunction and structural damage: blood urea nitrogen (BUN), creatinine in urine and blood, measure of creatinine clearance, and qualitative/quantitative measures of proteinuria. Though these measures are generally cheap and noninvasive, the final diagnosis of any patient with a suspected glomerulopathy is based upon the histologic findings from a kidney biopsy: a procedure that is not without risk [36]. The integrity of the slit diaphragm—a zipper-like interaction of membrane proteins between adjacent podocyte foot processes—is necessary for the inhibition of abnormal passage of proteins which have the size of and larger than albumin into the ultrafiltrate, and once the slit diaphragm is disrupted by way of podocyte injury, one can note the states of proteinuria that can range from inconspicuous to that of a florid nephrotic state (>3 g/day protein in urine). It should be added that while proteinuria is commonly associated with podocyte/slit diaphragm disruption, injury to the GBM or the glomerular capillary endothelium also results in proteinuria and thus brings to attention the lack of specificity of proteinuria for podocyte damage [37]. The level of proteinuria has also been found to be limited as a measure of monitoring disease progression as well as being limited for the monitoring of disease response to therapy [38]. Quantification of proteinuria is, however, still recognized as a simple and useful measure of glomerular injury and has been shown to correlate with progression of chronic kidney disease and as an indicator for increased cardiovascular morbidity/mortality [39]. To be curt, this paper is not aiming to dispel the proven worth of utilizing proteinuria as an indicator of glomerular/podocyte injury, but instead it aims to highlight the advantages—or weaknesses—of novel markers of podocytopathy and the potential they hold for clinical utility. While the strengths, weaknesses, and proper usage of measuring protein in the urine for diagnostic purposes has been discussed in many papers [40–43], as with any instrument in medicine, there comes a time when better tools come to be and advance the ability of the clinician to more confidently care for a patient. The fact that proteinuria can be measured noninvasively and relatively cheap with a urine dipstick argues for the continuing usage of it as a biomarker of glomerular injury, at least until more advantageous tools fall

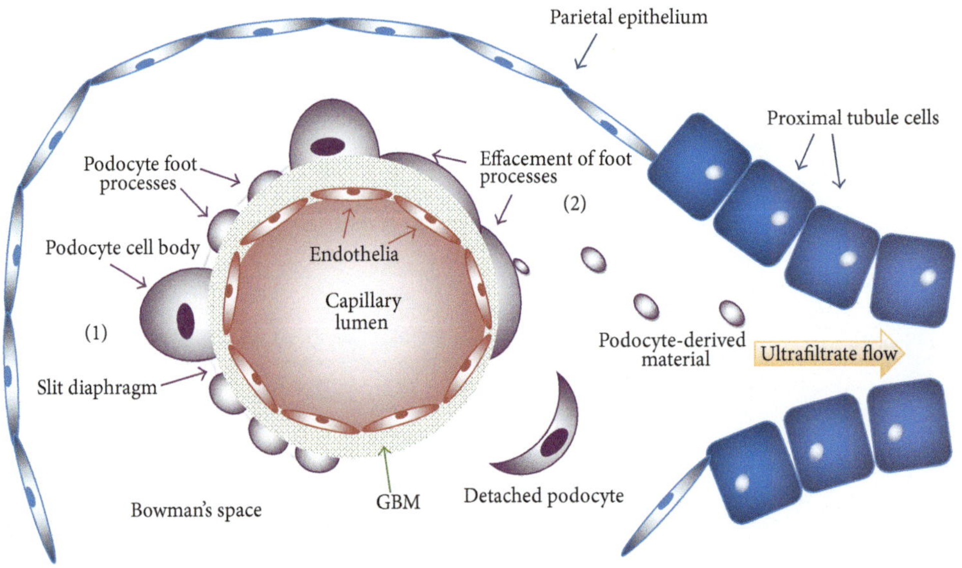

FIGURE 2: A simplified glomerulus and initial segment of the nephron are depicted; mesangia and the interweaved, capillary tuft structure are not shown to focus upon a single capillary and its related glomerular filtration apparatus. Also not depicted is the continuity between the visceral and parietal epithelial layers of the glomerulus. A glomerular capillary is lined by the fenestrated endothelia, which is intimately associated with the glomerular basement membrane (GBM). Also associated with the GBM is the visceral epithelial layer consisting of podocytes; the podocyte is made up of a cell body and processes that allow it to wrap finger-like projects about glomerular capillaries. Interposed between podocyte foot processes is a space spanned by the slit diaphragm—a key structure in the limitation of particles (based on size) from passing into the ultrafiltrate. Material/fluid that passes through the endothelia, GBM, and podocyte/slit diaphragm (these three constitute the glomerular filtration apparatus) makes it into Bowman's space, and the fluid at this point is termed ultrafiltrate. The ultrafiltrate from here passes through the length of the nephron—with modification possible—and urinary tract. The podocytes that lay on the left side of the shown capillary (1) are shown in a normal, healthy state: foot processes exist with developed slit diaphragms in between. In contrast, the right side of the capillary exhibits podocytes of an injured phenotype (2) effacement is present (other manifestations of an injured podocyte are not depicted, but can be read about in the paper), and at times podocytes may shed material later to be found in urine. If the podocyte is injured to a certain degree, it may detach from the underlying GBM and be observed in collected urine. A GBM denuded of podocytes may develop and lend itself as a surface for adherence with the parietal epithelium.

into hand. With that, we shall proceed with the discussion of some potentially more efficacious indicators of podocyte injury.

Over the last two decades, investigations have shed light on the fact that podocytes are present in the urine in concurrence with a renal disease state and that podocyturia and biomarkers specific for podocytes themselves can relate to disease progression. Figure 1 depicts a simplified view of the glomerular filtration apparatus and consequences of podocyte injury. It has also been noted that the level of podocyturia is a more sensitive indicator of disease activity than the level of proteinuria [44]. Notice should be taken of the fact that culture-viable podocytes can be isolated from the urine of healthy volunteers, so the specificity of podocyturia for glomerulopathies is not perfect [45]. In the urine of patients with certain glomerulopathies, evidence of podocyte injury can be found with the presence of viable podocytes (capable for the usage in primary cell culture), apoptotic podocytes, and podocyte derived exosomes and granular structures—all which have the possibility of being utilized as potential biomarkers of podocyte injury [46]. Urinary biomarkers that have been found to be specific for podocyte injury include proteins (podocalyxin, nephrin, podocin, CR1, CD80, synaptopodin, GLEPP-1, mindin, alpha 3 integrin, CD59, and Wilms tumor protein 1-WT1), podocyte specific messenger ribonucleic acid (mRNA) (nephrin, podocin, synaptopodin, podocalyxin, CD2-associated protein-*CD2AP*, *ACTN4*-encodes for α-actinin 4, *PTPRO*-encodes for GLEPP-1, *WT1*, and *B7-1*-encodes for CD80), an exosomal transcription factor (WT1), and podocalyxin positive granular structures (PPGS). Utilizing immunofluorescent staining, Western blot, enzyme-linked immunosorbent assay (ELISA), flow cytometry, and mass spectrometry, protein-based biomarkers are elucidated from urine samples of patients with glomerular disease, while polymerase chain reaction (PCR) is utilized to quantify the presence of podocyte specific mRNA. Figure 3 illustrates the premise of the following urinary biomarkers in podocytopathies.

This review will describe the urinary biomarkers of podocyte injury that have been investigated to date: proteins, podocyte specific mRNA, an exosomal transcription factor, and PPGS. A brief characterization of each biomarker in normal and injured podocyte states shall be discussed along with an overview of how each has been examined as a urinary biomarker of podocyte injury.

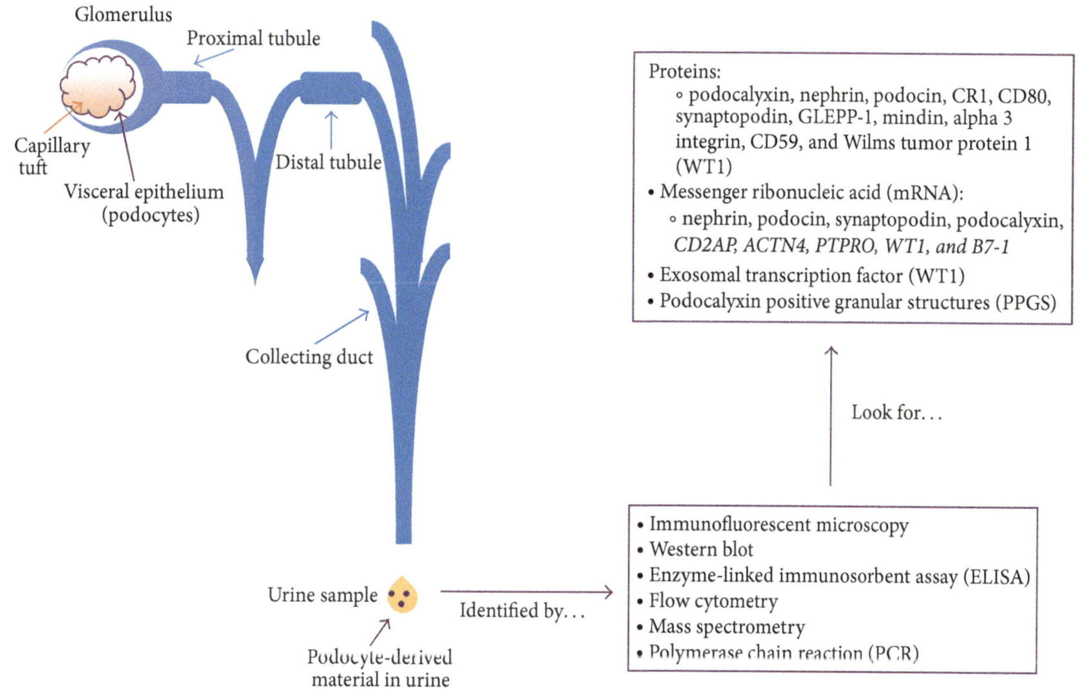

FIGURE 3: Podocytes envelop the capillary tuft of the glomerular body and are an integral part of the glomerular filtration apparatus. If podocytes are injured or lost via any number of mechanisms, podocyte specific material or whole podocytes themselves may traverse the length of the nephron and urinary tract to be collected/observed in the excreted urine product. With such material in hand, a number of noted techniques can be used to identify the podocyte derivations. More poignantly, investigations to date have described that such techniques can identify podocyte specific proteins, mRNA, an exosomal transcription factor, and podocalyxin positive granular structures.

2. Podocalyxin

Podocalyxin is an anionic, transmembrane protein that localizes to the apical membrane of glomerular podocytes. Aside from the kidney, podocalyxin is also localized in hematopoietic progenitor cells, vascular endothelium, and certain neurons [47–49]. Structurally, podocalyxin's extracellular portion consists of O-glycosylated, sialylated (providing the anionic charge), and N-glycosylated domains, along with a globular domain and a juxtamembrane stalk [50]. Intracellularly, podocalyxin has putative sites for phosphorylation along with a PDZ-binding domain. It is this PDZ domain that allows for podocalyxin's interaction with Na^+/H^+ exchanger regulatory factors 1 and 2 (NHERFl and NHERF2) [51, 52]. Podocalyxin also interacts with ezrin—a protein that is found to be complex with NHERF2 and that binds actin—and thus relates podocalyxin to the cytoskeletal network that dictates podocyte structure [53]. Podocalyxin is also important in normal development of glomeruli, for knockout mice that do not express podocalyxin, and normal podocyte architecture is disrupted with histologic evidence of absence of foot processes and slit diaphragms [54]. It seems that in the glomerular podocyte, podocalyxin plays a role as the main contributor to the anionic surface of foot processes, and via its relation with the actin cytoskeleton it is involved in the normal formation and maintenance of podocyte structure.

Hara et al. first noted that podocalyxin in urine was related directly to podocyte injury in patients with IgA nephropathy and Henoch-Schönlein purpura nephritis [55, 56]. Many papers thereafter used their technique of immunostaining against podocalyxin in urine samples to detect podocyte material. Hara had also noted that when podocalyxin was tested as a urinary biomarker for detecting the presence of varying glomerular diseases, it had a sensitivity of 88.4% and specificity of 100% [57]. When urine from patients with diabetes mellitus was examined, subjects with more severe disease (determined by severity of albuminuria) had significantly more podocalyxin positive podocytes in the urine than diabetic patients with less severe disease (defined as microalbuminuria equaling 20–200 μg/min urine albumin excreted) and compared to healthy controls [58]. The same study also showed that treatment with trandolapril (an angiotensin converting enzyme inhibitor) reduced albuminuria and podocalyxin positive podocyturia in diabetic patients: a proof that podocalyxin and podocyturia are biomarkers that can be used to monitor therapeutic efficacy and disease progression. To further substantiate urinary podocalyxin's ability to reflect change in disease status with therapy, the adriamycin rat model of nephropathy induced increases proteinuria, podocyturia (detected via podocalyxin immunofluorescent staining), and foot process width. Treatment with 1,25-dihydroxyvitamin D_3 reduced all mentioned parameters, showing that efficacy of therapy could be followed with the monitoring of urinary podocalyxin [59]. An investigation of adult patients with IgA nephropathy revealed that the severity of acute extracapillary abnormalities correlated with the level of urinary podocalyxin and that some patients with lower proteinuria and high urinary podocalyxin had poorer prognoses. The latter finding exhibits that in some cases proteinuria does not necessarily reflect the severity of disease but that the urinary level of podocalyxin does [60]. When podocytes, casts, and granules from the urine of children diagnosed with IgA nephropathy were immunofluorescently stained for podocalyxin, the degree of fluorescence directly correlated with the degree of glomerular epithelial injury as noted through renal biopsy histologic examination of the same patients [61]. These results would tend to allow one to believe that in children—and possibly adults—with IgA nephropathy, the degree of glomerular involvement and injury could be anticipated before renal biopsy through quantification of podocalyxin positive urine material, as well as a possible biomarker to follow disease progression. In a study examining patients diagnosed with focal segmental glomerular sclerosis (FSGS), it was shown that patients that were significant excreters of podocalyxin positive cells in the urine had a fall of serum creatinine in follow-up, lending to recovery [62]. Podocalyxin has been utilized as a urinary biomarker in studies examining podocyturia in preeclamptic women [63]. When podocalyxin was compared with podocin and nephrin in women with preeclampsia, it was found that podocin had superior diagnostic accuracy [64]. A separate study showed that levels of urinary podocalyxin were significantly greater in women with preeclampsia than normal pregnant women [65]. So where podocalyxin lies in the panel of podocyte biomarkers in the diagnosis of preeclampsia is yet to be decided. Urinary podocalyxin has also been detected—utilizing ELISA—in the urine of patients with acute kidney injury, and it was notable that urinary podocalyxin levels were greatest, whilst creatinine levels were recovering [66]. This group utilized the same assay to detect urinary podocalyxin in diabetic patients with glomerulopathy and found that there was a significant difference in control, healthy subjects and normoalbuminuric, diabetic patients [67]. This illustrates how a urinary biomarker specific for podocytes can detect disease otherwise passed over by the conventional monitoring of albuminuria. Early detection of podocyte lesions in diabetic glomerulopathy could give the clinician a chance to revert kidney disease by way of implementing appropriate therapeutic measures—a chance missed if one relied solely on the level of albuminuria. In order to create a more objective measure of urinary podocalyxin, a recent investigation used flow cytometry to detect the biomarker in the presence of glomerular disease [68].

Urinary podocalyxin mRNA expression has been illustrated to be significantly greater in patients with diabetic nephropathy compared to healthy controls, the level of mRNA increased with progression of disease, and the level of urinary podocalyxin mRNA positively correlated with urinary albumin excretion, BUN, and with serum creatinine [69]. Results from the same investigation showed that urinary podocalyxin mRNA negatively correlated with estimated glomerular filtration rate (eGFR). It should be noted that the quantitative analysis of urinary podocalyxin mRNA—and not just qualitative—should be recommended for clinical analysis, for podocalyxin mRNA has been shown to be expressed in urine of healthy, human volunteers [45]. All in all, it can be seen from the summary of studies utilizing podocalyxin as a urinary biomarker of podocyte injury—incurred through numerous different pathologies—that there is potential for its usage in the clinical setting to guide diagnosis and follow disease progression.

3. Nephrin

Nephrin is a 180 kDa transmembrane protein localized on the lateral surface of the podocyte foot process and is a major component of the slit diaphragm. Aside from podocytes, nephrin can be found in central nervous system tissue and pancreas, specifically in the β-cells of the islets of the Langerhans [70]. In the capillary loop stage of nephron development, nephrin can be localized at junctures of incipient podocyte foot processes, while nephrin mRNA expression can be detected in the S-shaped bodies of the developing nephron [71]. Nephrin—the product of the *NPHS1* gene—was discovered when mutations in *NPHS1* were found in patients with congenital nephrotic syndrome of the Finnish type [72]. Examination of kidney samples from patients with congenital nephrotic syndrome of the Finnish type shows thinning of the lamina densa layer of the GBM, yet otherwise insignificantly different from healthy, control kidneys [73]. An experiment utilizing a murine model, in which the *Nphs1* gene is inactivated, presents histologic evidence of podocyte foot process effacement and absence of a slit diaphragm, along with proteinuria and the immediate death soon after parturition [70]. Nephrin associates and colocalizes with podocin and the actin cytoskeleton, and the interaction of nephrin with the actin cytoskeleton is done so through an association with CD2AP [74, 75]. In addition, nephrin forms complexes—as proven through coimmunoprecipitation and pull-down assays—with cadherins, p120 catenin, and scaffolding proteins zonula occludens protein 1 (ZO-1), CD2AP, and calcium/calmodulin-dependent serine protein kinase (CASK) [76]. There is also a proof that nephrin and the slit diaphragm can be a source of intracellular signaling mechanisms in podocytes. This was made evident by the fact that nephrin expression triggers cellular activation via protein kinase p38 and the c-Jun N-terminal kinase in HEK293T cells [23]. Cellular activation was enhanced in the presence of podocin, and this would suggest that signaling involving the slit diaphragm requires normal interaction of nephrin and podocin. Nephrin's interaction with the actin cytoskeleton via CD2AP might also lend to the idea that nephrin's role in intracellular signaling may be transmissible to the cytoskeleton and result in structural changes. It can be appreciated that nephrin has a significant role as a constituent of the slit diaphragm, a role in maintaining normal podocyte foot process architecture, and an additional position in intra-podocyte signaling.

Urinary nephrin protein and mRNA have also been examined in patients with a number of glomerulopathies and hold potential as clinically useful biomarkers of podocyte injury. A study of patients with type 1 diabetes noted that while microalbuminuria was used for the early detection of kidney involvement in disease, advanced glomerulopathy was already present and presented that 30% of normoalbuminuric patients had nephrinuria; all healthy controls in the study were found to be negative for urinary nephrin [77]. The detection of urinary nephrin from type 2 diabetic patients determined to be normoalbuminuric also showed that urinary nephrin was a more sensitive marker of nephropathy in diabetes than the measure of urinary albumin [78]. Relatedly, observation of the FVB/NJ Akita mouse model of diabetic nephropathy noted that urinary nephrin could be detected before detectable albuminuria develops [79]. These data again highlight how a urinary biomarker specific for podocytes can detect disease otherwise passed over by the conventional monitoring of albuminuria. Investigators have recently shown that preeclamptic women had significantly higher levels of urinary nephrin than healthy pregnant women [65] and that there was a correlation between urinary nephrin levels and urinary protein, serum creatinine, and diastolic blood pressure in preeclamptic women [80]. Utilizing Heymann nephritis model, immunohistochemistry and PCR showed a decrease in both urinary nephrin protein and mRNA expression compared to healthy controls, and this decrease was noted before the onset of proteinuria was detected [81]. As part of the same study, it was shown that urinary nephrin could be quantified by Western blot and that healthy animals did not excrete detectable nephrin in their urine.

A second study utilizing a passive Heymann nephritis model found that nephrin protein and mRNA could be quantified from cells isolated from collected urine samples [46]. In a study using a streptozotocin model, it was noted that urinary cells could be stained against nephrin and that, in healthy controls, cells could not be detected in urine [82]. The same investigation showed that the cells collected from streptozotocin-treated rats were viable for primary culture. Aaltonen et al. noted similarly that urinary nephrin could be detected early in the streptozotocin rat model [83]. Podocyturia determined via nephrin staining did not significantly predict preeclampsia; however, the study noted that the urine of some women with severe disease was positive for podocyturia by nephrin staining [84]. Urinary nephrin mRNA levels increased after instigation of glomerular injury in models utilizing human diphtheria toxin receptor (hDTR) transgenic rats (expressing hDTR specifically on podocytes); however, on follow-up urine analysis, nephrin mRNA could not be detected [85]. Another study using hDTR transgenic rats showed that the podocin : nephrin mRNA ratio correlated with the renal histologic state [86]. The same study showed that human patients diagnosed with systemic lupus erythematosus (SLE) with associated glomerular disease had measurable levels of urinary nephrin mRNA. Urinary nephrin mRNA expression significantly correlated with the degree of proteinuria in patients with diabetic nephropathy, showing that nephrin mRNA in the urine could possibly be clinically used as a biomarker to follow glomerulopathy progression in diabetic patients [87]. In patients with lupus nephritis, urinary nephrin mRNA could be measured and was found to correlate with the level of proteinuria [88]. Urinary nephrin mRNA was found to correlate with the decline of renal function and degree of proteinuria in a study examining the progression of disease in a group of patients with diagnoses of diabetic glomerulosclerosis, IgA nephropathy, minimal change disease, and membranous nephropathy [89]. Further, supporting the strength of urinary nephrin mRNA in clinical utility, the level of mRNA was significantly greater in the urine of patients with glomerular kidney disease than healthy controls, and the level of urinary nephrin mRNA could differentiate between proliferative and nonproliferative disease [90]. Urinary nephrin mRNA levels could differentiate between preeclamptic women and healthy controls, as well as being used to differentiate between preeclamptic women and women with gestational diabetes [91]. Quantitative analysis of urinary nephrin mRNA—and not just qualitative—should be recommended for clinical analysis, since nephrin mRNA was expressed in urine of healthy, human volunteers [45]. It can be seen that the evidence for urinary nephrin (protein and mRNA) being used as a biomarker of podocyte injury is building, and in a number of different glomerulopathies could be of clinical use.

4. Podocin

Podocin is a 42 kDa membrane-associated protein that has a hairpin structure resulting with both N- and C-terminal ends located in the cytoplasm. The *NPHS2* gene—the product being podocin—is mutated in certain patients with autosomal recessive steroid resistant nephrotic syndrome, with disease manifesting early in childhood and progression to end-stage renal failure [92]. In development, podocin mRNA is first expressed in the S-shaped body of the incipient nephron, while podocin protein is first expressed in the capillary loop stage. In the mature kidney, podocin mRNA expression is only detectable in podocytes [93]. Localized to the lateral membrane of the podocyte foot process at the insertion of the slit diaphragm, podocin can be found in an oligomeric formation within lipid rafts and interacts with nephrin and CD2AP by way of a COOH-terminal domain [75]. Podocin plays an integral role in nephrin mediated cellular signaling, and thus it has a putative role in podocyte structure and function [23].

In a number of studies to date, podocin protein and mRNA have been shown to be quantifiable in the urine of both animal models of glomerulopathies and humans with renal disease. In a concerted effort to objectively measure a urinary podocyte biomarker, a recent study used mass spectrometry to detect podocin in urine samples of preeclamptic women [94]. It would be highly interesting to follow up with further studies detecting other discussed podocyte biomarkers with mass spectrometry. Nakatsue and colleagues have shown that while urinary nephrin was detectable by Western blot in diseased Heymann nephritis animals, podocin could not be detected in the urine of the same animals [81]. However, a different study from a second group had shown that podocin protein and mRNA could in fact be quantified from cells isolated from collected urine samples in passive

Heymann nephritic rats [46]. Whether podocin protein can be quantified from urine of Heymann nephritis animals or the human equivalent of membranous nephropathy is still to be determined. As previously described in the podocalyxin section, in women, podocin had greater diagnostic accuracy compared to the utilization of podocalyxin and nephrin as biomarkers of podocytes in urine for determining the presence of preeclampsia [64]. A separate study noted similarly that urinary derived podocin mRNA was significantly elevated from preeclamptic women compared to healthy controls [91]. In a study using a streptozotocin model, it was noted that urinary cells could be stained against podocin and that in healthy controls cells couldnot be detected in urine [82]. Urinary podocin mRNA levels increased after the instigation of glomerular injury in models utilizing hDTR transgenic rats, and on follow-up urine analysis podocin mRNA could still be detected—in contrast to urinary nephrin mRNA which could not be detected [85]. Data from the same study showed that urinary podocin mRNA levels were found to positively correlate to the level of proteinuria, and human patients diagnosed with SLE with associated glomerular disease had measurable levels of urinary podocin mRNA. An investigation using hDTR transgenic rats illustrated that the podocin : nephrin mRNA ratio correlated with the renal pathohistologic state [86]. In patients with lupus nephritis, urinary podocin mRNA could be measured, and as the patients are followed over time, urinary podocin mRNA decreased along with a worsening glomerular filtration rate (GFR) [88]. This may be the evidence to support that urinary podocin mRNA could be a clinically useful biomarker for following disease progression in patients with lupus nephritis since it seems to trend along with the GFR, a measure of glomerular function. Urinary podocin mRNA expression was significantly greater in patients with diabetic nephropathy compared to healthy controls, the level of mRNA increased with progression of disease, and the level of urinary podocin mRNA positively correlated with levels of urinary albumin excretion, BUN, and with serum creatinine [69]. Urinary podocin mRNA could also be collected from some dogs with chronic kidney disease, but this study did not contain a healthy control group, so the significance of these findings is yet to be determined [95]. Urinary podocin mRNA was found to correlate with the decline of renal function in a study that examined the progression of disease in a group of patients with diagnoses of diabetic glomerulosclerosis, IgA nephropathy, minimal change disease, and membranous nephropathy [89]. Thus it can be seen that urinary podocin protein and mRNA have been found to be viable biomarkers of podocyte injury, though further investigations will be necessary to see their efficacy as a clinical tools.

5. Complement Receptor 1 (CR1)

Complement receptor 1 (CR1)—also known as CD35 or C3bR—is a 200 kDa membrane bound receptor that within the adult glomerulus is expressed only in podocytes [96, 97]. Outside of the glomerulus, CR1 expression is found in follicular dendritic cells, the Langerhans cells in the skin, the Küpffer cells, circulating erythrocytes, neutrophils, monocytes, and T-lymphocytes [98, 99]. CR1 protein is expressed in both fetal podocytes of the developing kidney and in the mature, adult kidney. In the fetal kidney, CR1 mRNA is detectable in immature podocytes in early stages of glomerular differentiation, specifically after vascularization of the developing glomerulus [33, 100]. By binding C3b—the active form of C3—CR1 regulates complement activation on the cell membrane by inhibiting activation of the complement pathway [101]. The specific role that CR1 plays on the surface of podocytes has yet to be fully elucidated, but one may assume that it may hold a protective role for podocytes from immune attack.

CR1 positive vesicles have been found by Western blot in the urine of healthy patients, and in comparison, urinary CR1 expression was decreased in patients with more advanced cases of SLE [102]. In a study by Hara, the diagnostic sensitivity and specificity of urinary CR1 for patients with an amalgam of glomerulopathies were determined to be 51.4% and 100%, respectively [57]. CR1 was also noted to have been localized to PPGS found in the urine of patients with active glomerulonephritis and nephrotic syndrome [103]. It has been shown that CR1 can be found in the urine of both healthy subjects and patients afflicted by glomerulopathies, but more work must be done in order to understand the expression of urinary CR1 in individual glomerular disease states. With the evidence in hand, it appears that CR1's utility in monitoring podocyte injury is lacking.

6. CD80

CD80 (also referred to as B7-1) is a 53 kDa membrane-associated protein that in the glomerulus is localized exclusively in podocytes, but it can also be found in renal tubules [104, 105]. It is better known for its role in the immune system as a costimulatory receptor involved in T-lymphocyte activation [104]. CD80 activation by puromycin in cultured podocytes is found to attenuate expression of nephrin and results in foot process effacement and retraction, providing insight on how CD80 can influence podocyte structure and function [106]. The ability of CD80 to regulate podocytes' filtering capacity is also shown when lipopolysaccharide is injected in mice, resulting in increased CD80 expression and proteinuria, and in mice that are knockouts for CD80, proteinuria does not occur [105]. Therefore, the immune stimulatory role of CD80 within the glomerular milieu would support the idea that it may modulate immune mediated injury to podocytes.

CD80 and its mRNA (*B7-1*) can be detected and measured in collected urine and may be potential biomarkers of podocyte injury. Urinary levels of CD80 in patients with relapsed minimal change disease were significantly greater when compared to those in patients with minimal change disease in remission, SLE (with and without proteinuria), other glomerulopathies (FSGS, membranoproliferative glomerulonephritis, IgA nephropathy, and membranous nephropathy), and healthy control patients [104]. Data from a second study by the same group showed that urinary CD80 was increased in patients with minimal change disease in relapse compared to patients with minimal change disease in remission or those with FSGS [34]. These results support that urinary CD80 could be used clinically to differentiate between patients with the relapsed minimal change disease and FSGS. Additionally, the level of urinary *B7-1* mRNA was found to be enhanced in patients with glomerular kidney disease compared to that of healthy subjects [90]. Promising data is presented for the utility of urinary CD80 for a biomarker of podocytopathy; however, much more work is needed to substantiate confidence in its clinical usage, and the fact that CD80 can also be derived from tubular epithelium reduces confidence in its specificity.

7. Synaptopodin

Synaptopodin (also referred to as podocyte protein 44-pp44) is an actin binding protein, and through this interaction it can modulate the podocyte actin cytoskeleton and resultant cellular function [107]. Synaptopodin is immunohistochemically expressed in podocyte foot processes and colocalizes with actin within the cytoplasm, and in the central nervous system synaptopodin mRNA expression is positive in the olfactory bulb, cerebral cortex, striatum, and hippocampus [108]. Synaptic plasticity in the hippocampus seems to be reliant on the activity of synaptopodin and its interaction with calcium stores [109]. During renal development, synaptopodin is first identified in the incipient glomerulus during the capillary loop stage—the stage at which foot processes formulate [110]. Synaptopodin—in the fully developed glomerulus—is exclusively expressed in podocytes [111]. More specifically, synaptopodin is a marker of the well-differentiated podocytes, as an investigation into the culturing of podocytes noted that synaptopodin expression is synonymous with the development of foot processes and a phenotype similar to that found *in vivo* [108]. It has been shown that synaptopodin is proteolytically downregulated by cathepsin L—a protease that is induced in the diseased state—resulting in actin reorganization, podocyte architecture change, and proteinuria [107, 112]. Thus the role that synaptopodin plays in maintaining the actin cytoskeleton is evident when its activity is attenuated, with subsequent podocyte dysfunction.

There are a number of studies that have examined the presence and utility of urinary synaptopodin protein and mRNA to determine podocyte damage. It was found in diabetic nephropathy patients that urinary synaptopodin mRNA significantly correlated with glomerular podocyte number observed in histologic examination, showing that urinary synaptopodin mRNA may be clinically applicative in monitoring disease progression in these patients [113]. Data from another study examining patients with diagnosed diabetic nephropathy presented that urinary synaptopodin mRNA correlated with the degree of proteinuria [87]. In patients with lupus nephritis, urinary synaptopodin mRNA was measured, and as the patients were followed over time, urinary synaptopodin mRNA decreased along with the GFR [88]. This may be the evidence to support that urinary synaptopodin mRNA could be a clinically useful biomarker for following disease progression in patients with lupus nephritis since it seems to trend along with the GFR. Urinary synaptopodin mRNA expression was significantly greater in patients with diabetic nephropathy compared to healthy controls, the level of mRNA increased with progression of disease, and the level of urinary synaptopodin mRNA positively correlated with the level of urinary albumin excretion and BUN [69]. Using a streptozotocin model of diabetic nephropathy, urinary cells could be stained against synaptopodin; however, in healthy controls, urinary cells stained for synaptopodin could not be detected [82]. The same group has also shown that synaptopodin protein and mRNA could be quantified from cells isolated from urine samples of passive Heymann nephritic rats [46]. Urinary synaptopodin mRNA was found not to correlate with the decline of renal function in a study examining the progression of disease in a group of patients with diagnoses of diabetic glomerulosclerosis, IgA nephropathy, minimal change disease, and membranous nephropathy [89]. In addition, synaptopodin mRNA was found in urinary podocytes of both FSGS patients and healthy humans [45]. Data from a study that included patients with a number of different glomerulopathies showed that urine sediment did not stain for synaptopodin [57]. Urinary synaptopodin is also noted to be a poor indicator of the preeclamptic state, as it was found to have diagnostic sensitivity of only 38% and specificity of 70% [114]. It is difficult to conclude from the collected studies if urinary synaptopodin protein or mRNA can be utilized regularly with confidence in clinical practice as biomarkers of podocyte injury.

8. Glomerular Epithelial Protein 1 (GLEPP-1)

GLEPP-1 (also referred to as protein tyrosine phosphatase receptor type-O—PTPRO) is an apical-membrane-associated protein tyrosine phosphatase found on glomerular podocytes [115, 116]. Central nervous system expression of *Ptpro* (encodes for GLEPP-1 protein) is localized to the olfactory bulb, developing neocortex, thalamus, and hippocampus [117]. In the developing kidney, GLEPP-1 protein expression is first detected during the S-shaped stage of the glomerular anlage, with increasing expression noted in podocytes through development and into maturity [118]. GLEPP-1's importance in the maintenance of normal glomerular filtration has been shown in patients diagnosed with idiopathic nephrotic syndrome, steroid resistant subtype, that different mutations in *PTPRO* are to blame in resultant phenotypic changes of podocytes and massive proteinuria [119]. In *Ptpro* knockout mice, altered podocyte architecture can be observed with foot processes shorter and broader, and functionally these mice have reduced glomerular filtration function (25–50% lower GFR than wild-type) and a propensity for hypertension if the kidney is placed under increased functional stress (as exhibited in the animal model after nephrectomy) [21]. GLEPP-1 has an important role to play in normal podocyte function and the maintenance of glomerular integrity, and its activity as a phosphatase lends to the hypothesis for a putative role in intracellular signaling.

Urinary GLEPP-1 protein and *Ptpro* mRNA have been examined for usage as biomarkers of podocyte injury.

Using a streptozotocin model of diabetic nephropathy, urinary cells could be stained against GLEPP-1; however, in healthy controls, urinary cells stained for GLEPP-1 could not be observed [82]. The same group also presented that GLEPP-1 protein and *Ptpro* mRNA could be quantified from cells isolated from urine samples of passive Heymann nephritic rats [46]. Utilizing a puromycin aminonucleoside (PAN) nephrosis model, *Ptpro* mRNA was found in the urine of rats after insult, but not in untreated, healthy rats [120]. It is obvious that there is a paucity of data relating to GLEPP-1's usage as a urinary biomarker of podocytopathy, and evaluation of its efficacy clinically is not possible at this time as thus.

9. Mindin

Mindin (also known as spondin-2) is a secreted protein that becomes a constituent of extracellular matrix, as it was first observed in the zebrafish floor plate [121]. Mindin mRNA is found in the brain, liver, spleen, placenta, lung, heart, kidney, muscle, and thymus, and in the central nervous system mindin has been implicated as a promoter of hippocampal neuron development [121, 122]. In the kidney, the immunohistochemistry shows that mindin localizes predominately to podocytes within the glomerulus and that secretion of mindin is appreciated in podocyte cell culture [123]. Inflammatory reactions are also mediated by mindin, and this has been illustrated in mindin knockout mice that are resistant to lipopolysaccharide-induced septic shock, and the same mice are not as capable in clearing bacterial infections *in vivo* [124]. Mindin is found to bind neutrophils through the involvement of integrins, and with localization in the glomerulus mindin may have a role as a recruiter of inflammatory cells in the pathogenesis of glomerular lesions [125].

While mindin has not previously been utilized as a biomarker of podocyte injury, a recent study by Murakoshi et al. has shed light upon mindin's histologic and urinary expression in diabetic nephropathy [123]. The study presented that mice fed on high calorie diets expressed augmented levels of glomerular mindin protein and mRNA than mice fed on a standard diet. As well, mice fed on high calorie diets were also found to have greater amount of mindin protein in their urine than their standard diet counterparts. In podocyte cell culture, glucose administration was found to accentuate mindin secretion. In humans with type II diabetes, the level of urinary mindin was greater than that measured in healthy controls, and the amount of urinary mindin increased in concert with progression of diabetic nephropathy disease. Thus, it can be appreciated that urinary mindin can function as a biomarker of podocyte injury in diabetic nephropathy; however, its general usage will be limited until further investigations can determine its efficacy in this and other glomerulopathies.

10. Alpha 3 Integrin (Intα3)

Intα3 is a heterodimeric, podocyte basal-membrane surface protein that is responsible for the attachment of the foot processes to the underlying GBM. During renal development, Intα3 is necessary for normal organogenesis, for in mice with a mutated Itga3 gene abnormal collecting duct, proximal tubule, and glomerular histology can be observed [24, 126]. The same mutated mice show a disrupted GBM and an immature phenotype of podocytes lacking formation of foot processes. Intα3 is also shown to be necessary for normal pulmonary organogenesis, with abnormal branching of bronchi being observed. In patients found to be homozygous for mutations in the gene encoding Intα3, basement membrane disruption was notable in numerous tissues and presented clinically with congenital nephrotic syndrome, interstitial lung disease, and epidermolysis bullosa [127]. Intα3 is an important contributor to the development and the maintenance of the GBM-podocyte interaction.

Urinary Intα3 has been examined to determine if it can be utilized in the clinical setting as a biomarker of podocyte injury. Data from an investigation examining Intα3 as a urinary biomarker for detecting the presence of varying glomerular diseases concluded that it had a diagnostic sensitivity of 18.6% and specificity of 100% [57]. The data from this one reported study and a lack of any other investigations do not support the utilization of Intα3 as a diagnostic urinary biomarker for glomerulopathies.

11. CD59

CD59 (also referred to as protectin or 20 kDa homologous restriction factor—HRF20) is a glycosylphosphatidylinositol-anchored membrane bound protein that regulates the formation of the terminal complement complex of the immune complement cascade [128]. Regulation of the formation of the terminal complement complex is done so by the inhibition of the binding of C9 to the C5b–C8 complex. In the developing kidney, CD59 protein and mRNA are expressed in the ureteric duct epithelium, while in the mature, adult kidney expression they are found in the collecting ducts [96]. CD59 immunofluorescent expression is also notable in frozen sections of renal cortex—specifically in podocytes, tubular epithelium, and endothelial cells—and in cultured podocytes [129]. The role of CD59 in renal development is not clear, though it may act through inhibition of formation of the terminal complement complexes which could otherwise attenuate normal cellular growth. Regulation of the complement cascade within the glomerulus by CD59 is suggested by its ability to inhibit the complement mediated immune response to subepithelial immune complex deposition [130].

CD59 has not been utilized widely as a biomarker of podocyte injury, but a single study did present data supporting further investigations. When the CD59 immunofluorescent expression in renal tissue samples from patients diagnosed with membranous glomerulonephritis was compared to that in healthy controls, membranous glomerulonephritis patients had lower CD59 expression [131]. CD59 concentration in the urine of patients with membranous glomerulonephritis was higher in comparison to urinary CD59 from healthy controls and patients with diabetic nephropathy. The same investigation presented that urinary CD59 levels did not correlate to serum creatinine, urinary protein concentration, or duration of disease. With a paucity of data in hand, conclusions on CD59's usefulness as a histologic or urinary biomarker of podocyte injury are constrained.

12. Wilms Tumor Protein 1 (WT1)

A podocyte transcription factor—WT1—can been found in urine (associated with cells or exosomes) and as thus is a novel biomarker for recognizing podocyte injury. As any other typical transcription factor, WT1 activity is upregulated by certain stimuli, and its activity is responsible for the promotion of selective gene expression. WT1 regulates the expression of *Nphs1* and *Podxl* in mice, as both transcripts are reduced in *Wt1* knockouts [132]. In the same *Wt1* knockout mice, crescentic glomerulonephritis or mesangial sclerosis can be observed. WT1 has been shown to directly bind to the *Podxl* gene promoter, and through this mechanism it influences expression [133]. WT1 is first noted in the C- and S-shaped glomerular bodies of the developing kidney, and in the mature kidney, WT1 can be found in glomerular podocytes and arteriole endothelium [111]. *WT1* is mutated in patients with the Denys-Drash syndrome and the Frasier syndrome, both which are present with nephrotic syndrome and extra-renal malformations within the genital urinary system [132]. It should be noted that while WT1 is a proven histologic biomarker of podocytes [4, 118, 134], in a number of glomerulopathies WT1 protein is immunohistochemically expressed in glomerular parietal epithelium; therefore, WT1 as a biomarker of podocytes may not be exclusive and specific in diseased states [4, 135].

Urinary WT1 protein as a biomarker of podocyte injury has been described in one study, and thus this is an initial presentation of its utility. Data showed that by utilizing a passive Heymann nephritis model, WT1 protein and *Wt1* mRNA could be quantified from cells isolated from collected urine samples [46]. Unfortunately with only one study in hand, not much can be made in terms of deduction on the efficacy of WT1 protein as a biomarker of podocyte injury; however, investigation of WT1 from urinary exosomes shall be discussed in the following section.

13. Podocyte Specific mRNA

Podocyte specific mRNA has been detected in urine, and its usefulness as a biomarker of podocytopathy has been described. Nephrin, podocin, synaptopodin, podocalyxin, *CD2AP*, *ACTN4* (encodes for α-actinin 4), *PTPRO* (encodes for GLEPP-1), and *WT1* mRNA have been isolated from urine of patients with varying glomerulopathies. Review of urinary nephrin, podocin, synaptopodin, podocalyxin, *B7-1*, and *PTPRO* mRNA has already been described and can be found in their respective sections above. *CD2AP*, *ACTN4*, and *WT1* urinary mRNA shall be discussed as follows.

Urinary WT1 protein and *Wt1* mRNA expression were observed and analyzed from cells isolated from urine samples of passive Heymann nephritic rats, and there was a concomitant decrease in glomerular podocyte quantity as proteinuria worsened [46]. This data would lend to the hypothesis that glomerular podocytes in certain glomerulopathies are shed and lost in the urine, and those podocytes in urine could directly relate to the severity of podocyte/glomerular injury. *CD2AP* and *WT1* mRNA were found in urinary derived podocytes of both FSGS patients and healthy humans; therefore, quantitative analysis should be recommended in determining if disease is present [45]. Urinary *WT1* and *ACTN4* mRNA could also be collected from some dogs and cats with chronic kidney disease, but this study did not contain healthy control groups, so the significance of these findings has yet to be determined [95]. Urinary *CD2AP* and *ACTN4* mRNA expression were significantly increased in patients with diabetic nephropathy compared to healthy controls, the level of mRNA increased with progression of disease, and the levels of urinary *CD2AP* and *ACTN4* mRNA positively correlated with levels of urinary albumin excretion, BUN, and with serum creatinine [69]. With the data presented in this and previous sections, along with the fact that very little sample is necessary for the quantification of mRNA transcript, there is promising evidence supporting podocyte specific urinary mRNA as a biomarker of injury.

14. Exosomal Transcription Factor WT1

Exosomes are vesicles that can be attained from urine via differential centrifugation, and they are excreted through the length of the nephron, including from podocytes. Generally they are found to be 50–100 nm in diameter and have been seen to contain a number of cytosolic and membrane proteins as shown with proteomic profiling [136]. The origin of exosomes can be described as such: endocytic vesicles fuse with multivesicular bodies, and thereafter multivesicular bodies can undergo invagination—taking into the new vesicles matter that may be within the cytosolic milieu (e.g., WT1). At this stage, there is a multivesicular body that contains vesicles, and at some point the multivesicular body can fuse with the cellular plasma membrane and exocytose the vesicles contained within it. Methods of urinary exosome preparation and storage have been fine-tuned so that under proper conditions the protein profile of exosomes remains intact over time for analysis [137].

Data from one study presented that podocyte specific urinary exosomes could be quantified from patients and animal models of glomerulopathies: the podocyte specific aspect of these exosomes as being the transcription factor WT1 [138]. In animal models for FSGS and collapsing glomerulopathy, urinary exosomal WT1 quantity significantly increased after insult, and in control animals urinary exosomal WT1 was undetectable. Likewise, in human patients with diagnosed FSGS urinary exosomal WT1 could be identified, while exosomal WT1 couldnot be detected in the urine of healthy volunteers. Thus, with the given data, urinary exosomal WT1 is specific for a diagnosis of glomerulopathy; however, more work will have to be done to elaborate on the usefulness of urinary exosomal WT1 as a biomarker of podocyte injury.

15. Podocalyxin Positive Granular Structures (PPGS)

Under microscopic examination of urine, granular structures can be identified, and if they are immunoreactive for the podocyte specific antigen podocalyxin are termed PPGS. PPGS have been proven to originate from podocytes via podocalyxin immunostaining and are thought to form through a process of tip vesiculation from microvillus formations of injured podocytes. PPGS can be differentiated from podocyte exosomes on three points: PPGS are found not to contain exosomal specific markers (CD24 and CD63), PPGS are larger than 100 nm in diameter (exosomes are typically smaller), and in kidney samples from patients with PPGS found in urine, histologic evidence of exocytosis—the mechanism of by which exosomes are excreted—is not prevalent [103, 139]. While PPGS are immunoreactive for podocalyxin, there is weak staining against other podocyte apical membrane specific proteins (GLEPP-1 and CR1), and there was no observed staining against slit diaphragm specific ZO-1 and podocyte basal membrane specific Intα3 [103]. This further supports that PPGS originate from the apical membrane of podocytes. It is also notable that urinary supernatant has greater amount of podocalyxin protein than urinary sediment (this is true for urine of both healthy and patients with diagnosed glomerulopathies) and that within the sediment PPGS are found within casts. Therefore, quantification of PPGS from supernatant would be of higher yield than from centrifuged urinary sediment. When urine of patients with active glomerulonephritis and nephrotic syndrome was compared to that from healthy controls, greater amount of excreted PPGS could be observed in the urine of diseased patients [139]. Healthy controls excreted low levels of PPGS, and it may be explained by normal turnover of podocytes. In glomerulonephritis patients (diagnosed with IgA nephropathy, Henoch-Schönlein purpura nephritis, or lupus nephritis) and patients with a diagnosis of nephrotic syndrome, urinary sedimentary podocalyxin (which PPGS was a constituent) was greater than in healthy controls, and podocalyxin concentration was significantly greater in the urinary sediment of glomerulonephritis patients than that of the nephrotic patients [103]. PPGS could also be observed in the urine of glomerulonephritis patients that did not exhibit podocyturia, therefore showing that PPGS may be more sensitive in detecting glomerulopathy and podocyte injury [57]. The described data shows that PPGS are a more focused biomarker than general podocalyxin in the urine—keeping in mind that podocalyxin may be present in the urine additionally in association with whole podocytes. Utilization of PPGS as a biomarker of podocyte injury seems promising; however, as with all of the discussed biomarkers above, thorough clinical studies it would be needed to strengthen the argument for its clinical usage.

16. Conclusion

It has been found that podocyte injury can be diagnosed and monitored through the utilization of urinary derived biomarkers. The findings that podocalyxin and nephrin proteins can be detected in the urine of a significant percentage of normoalbuminuric, diabetic patients highlight the screening utility that these two podocyte specific proteins carry. Since monitoring urinary albumin potentially results in the passing over of a significant segment of diabetic patients—a fraction of today's population that cannot be dismissed—the medical field may wish to examine closely the earlier detection of diabetic nephropathy garnered from utilizing a podocyte specific marker. One could also monitor glomerulopathy progression with a urinary derived biomarker, diverting the need for follow-up renal biopsy if the patient was not physiologically stable or did not desire for such a procedure. Monitoring urinary biomarkers of podocyte injury also holds the capacity to be a cheaper method of diagnosis than the renal biopsy—a concept that we cannot ignore as the financial environment pressures the budget of healthcare. With respect to other biomarkers used in clinical practice, urinary biomarkers could be utilized in such manners as supplemental evidence of disease (as troponins are used alongside electrocardiography to aid in the diagnosis of myocardial infarction) or for the monitoring of disease progression with analysis of therapeutic efficacy (as hemoglobin A1C is used in patients with diabetes mellitus). The strength of urinary podocyte biomarkers in clinical utility would be measured the best in their combination with the clinical picture of the patient and other determinants of renal function, and they most likely will not themselves usurp the quantification of proteinuria as a measure of glomerular function. The utilization of the podocyte specific urinary biomarkers has not yet translated into common clinical practice, while the age-old quantification of proteinuria and renal biopsy are the mainstays that clinicians have at hand and will probably continue to rely on. However, with further investigations of the podocyte biomarkers discussed this stance could change, and attest to their utility. The reader is referred to Table 1 as a synoptic of the discussed urinary biomarkers and their prognostic correlation to specifically studied glomerulopathies.

By definition, a biomarker is any parameter of a patient/animal model that can be quantified, and through its quantification a normal physiologic state, a pathologic state, or disease response to initiated therapy can be indicated [140]. Before any of the described urinary biomarkers of podocyte injury can be used in the clinical setting, they should express a number of characteristics. Characteristics of a renal biomarker satisfactory for regular usage would include the following: that its quantification is simple, accurate, and reproducible; it is a sensitive indicator of kidney injury or a sensitive indicator of disease response to treatment; it gives clinicians a budget-sensitive tool; it provides the clinician additional information not yet attained by other tests/examinations; it diagnoses and differentiates between renal pathologies; it is clinically applicable in differing demographics [38, 141]. Since the classic monitoring of proteinuria/albuminuria does not meet all of the described characteristics of an ideal biomarker, possibly the novel biomarkers in this paper may complement data gleaned from such conventional tests and provide the clinician more information on the presence of a glomerulopathy.

Table 1: Urinary biomarkers of podocytopathy in patients: increased urinary levels correlate with the presence or the advancement of glomerular disease (except when otherwise noted*).

Protein		mRNA		Exosomal transcription factor		PPGS
Podocalyxin	IgAN [55, 56, 60, 61] HSPN [55, 56] DN [58, 67] FSGS—increased u-podocalyxin correlates with better prognosis [62]* AKI—increased u-podocalyxin in recovering patients [66]* PE [65]	Podocalyxin	DN [69]	WT1	FSGS [138]	AcGN [139] NS [103, 139] IgAN [103] HSPN [103] LN [103]
Nephrin	DN [77, 78] PE [65, 80]	Nephrin	DN [87, 89] PE [91] FSGS [90] LN [86, 88] IgAN [89] MCD [89] MN [89]			
Podocin	PE [64]	Podocin	PE [91] DN [69, 89] IgAN [89] MCD [89] MN [89] LN [85] and—decrease in u-podocin mRNA follows decrease in GFR [88]*			
CR1	AuGN [103] NS [103] LN [57] and—lower u-CR1 in advanced cases [102]* MN [57] MPGN [57] AS [57] PSAGN [57] HSPN [57] IgAN [57]	*CD2AP*	DN [69]			
CD80	Relapsed MCD [104]	*B7-1*[a]	FSGS [90]			
Mindin	DN [123]	Synaptopodin	DN [69, 87, 113] LN—decrease of u-synaptopodin mRNA follows decrease in GFR [88]*			
CD59	MG [131]	*ACTN4*[b]	DN [69]			

Numbers in parentheses refer to citations that can be noted in the References section of this paper.

Abbreviations: messenger ribonucleic acid (mRNA), complement receptor 1 (CR1), Wilms tumor protein 1 (WT1), CD-2-associated protein (CD2AP), podocalyxin positive granular structures (PPGS), urinary podocalyxin (u-podocalyxin), urinary CR1 (u-CR1), urinary podocin mRNA (u-podocin mRNA), urinary synaptopodin mRNA (u-synaptopodin mRNA), IgA nephropathy (IgAN), Henoch-Schönlein purpura nephritis (HSPN), diabetic nephropathy (DN), focal segmental glomerulosclerosis (FSGS), acute kidney injury (AKI), preeclampsia (PE), lupus nephritis (LN), minimal change disease (MCD), membranous nephropathy (MN), nephrotic syndrome (NS), acute glomerulonephritis (AuGN), active glomerulonephritis (AcGN), membranoproliferative glomerulonephritis (MPGN), Alport syndrome (AS), and poststreptococcal acute glomerulonephritis (PSAGN).

*This table summarizes that the majority of studies presented direct correlation of increased urinary levels of a biomarker with the incident or worsening of a specific glomerular disease; however, some studies (as noted with an asterisk and a short explanation) presented opposite findings and are thus highlighted.

[a] *B7-1* encodes for CD80.

[b] *ACTN4* encodes for α-actinin 4.

It is also obvious from this review of the literature that more work will be needed to determine if the discussed urinary biomarkers of podocyte injury are suitable for clinical use. In addition for the need for further investigation of the already mentioned biomarkers, there are other possible podocyte specific biomarkers that could be quantified in urine. For example, neurexin-1 is a slit diaphragm protein that also has indirect interaction with the podocyte actin cytoskeleton and therefore may be influential in regulating both podocyte function and architecture [142, 143]. Another potential candidate for usage as a urinary biomarker of podocyte injury is myosin heavy chain 9 (MYH9), which is a subunit of a larger protein named nonmuscle myosin IIA [8]. Mutation in the gene that encodes for MYH9 is found to be responsible for Fechtner's syndrome, and in addition, MYH9 has been identified in urine samples [136, 144]. There are potentially other components of podocytes that could be identified in the urine of patients afflicted with glomerulopathies useful as biomarkers, and as such this provides a number of possible routes of investigation to follow.

Confict of Interests

The authors declare that they have no conflict of interests.

Acknowledgments

The authors would like to thank Dr. Dusan Cemerikic for his professional advice regarding this paper. Miroslav Sekulic would like to specifically thank Dr. Sanja Sever for introducing him to the basic science realm of podocyte biology and allowing him to train in the field within the confines of her laboratory.

References

[1] R. Rodewald and M. J. Karnovsky, "Porous substructure of the glomerular slit diaphragm in the rat and mouse," *Journal of Cell Biology*, vol. 60, no. 2, pp. 423–433, 1974.

[2] J. Wartiovaara, L. G. Ofverstedt, J. Khoshnoodi et al., "Nephrin strands contribute to a porous slit diaphragm scaffold as revealed by electron microscopy," *The Journal of Clinical Investigation*, vol. 114, pp. 1475–1483, 2004.

[3] J. Bariety, G. S. Hill, C. Mandet et al., "Glomerural epithelial-mesenchymal transdifferentiation in pauci-immune crescentic glomerulonephritis," *Nephrology Dialysis Transplantation*, vol. 18, no. 9, pp. 1777–1784, 2003.

[4] G. S. Hill, K. E. Karoui, A. Karras et al., "Focal segmental glomerulosclerosis plays a major role in the progression of IgA nephropathy. I. Immunohistochemical studies," *Kidney International*, vol. 79, no. 6, pp. 635–642, 2011.

[5] A. H. J. Salmon, C. R. Neal, and S. J. Harper, "New aspects of glomerular filtration barrier structure and function: five layers (at least) not three," *Current Opinion in Nephrology and Hypertension*, vol. 18, no. 3, pp. 197–205, 2009.

[6] L. Barisoni and J. B. Kopp, "Update in podocyte biology: putting one's best foot forward," *Current Opinion in Nephrology and Hypertension*, vol. 12, no. 3, pp. 251–258, 2003.

[7] L. Barisoni and P. Mundel, "Podocyte biology and the emerging understanding of podocyte diseases," *American Journal of Nephrology*, vol. 23, no. 5, pp. 353–360, 2003.

[8] H. Cheng and R. C. Harris, "The glomerulus—a view from the outside—the podocyte," *International Journal of Biochemistry and Cell Biology*, vol. 42, no. 9, pp. 1380–1387, 2010.

[9] J. R. de Zoysa and P. S. Topham, "Podocyte biology in human disease," *Nephrology*, vol. 10, no. 4, pp. 362–367, 2005.

[10] J. A. Jefferson, C. E. Alpers, and S. J. Shankland, "Podocyte biology for the bedside," *American Journal of Kidney Diseases*, vol. 58, no. 5, pp. 835–845, 2011.

[11] J. Ly, M. Alexander, and S. E. Quaggin, "A podocentric view of nephrology," *Current Opinion in Nephrology and Hypertension*, vol. 13, no. 3, pp. 299–305, 2004.

[12] S. Menzel and M. J. Moeller, "Role of the podocyte in proteinuria," *Pediatric Nephrology*, vol. 26, no. 10, pp. 1775–1780, 2011.

[13] P. Mundel and J. Reiser, "Proteinuria: an enzymatic disease of the podocyte," *Kidney International*, vol. 77, no. 7, pp. 571–580, 2010.

[14] P. Mundel and S. J. Shankland, "Podocyte biology and response to injury," *Journal of the American Society of Nephrology*, vol. 13, no. 12, pp. 3005–3015, 2002.

[15] J. S. Nielsen and K. M. McNagny, "The role of podocalyxin in health and disease," *Journal of the American Society of Nephrology*, vol. 20, no. 8, pp. 1669–1676, 2009.

[16] J. Patrakka and K. Tryggvason, "Molecular make-up of the glomerular filtration barrier," *Biochemical and Biophysical Research Communications*, vol. 396, no. 1, pp. 164–169, 2010.

[17] H. Pavenstädt, W. Kriz, and M. Kretzler, "Cell biology of the glomerular podocyte," *Physiological Reviews*, vol. 83, no. 1, pp. 253–307, 2003.

[18] S. Breiteneder-Geleff, K. Matsui, A. Soleiman et al., "Podoplanin, novel 43-kd membrane protein of glomerular epithelial cells, is down-regulated in puromycin nephrosis," *American Journal of Pathology*, vol. 151, no. 4, pp. 1141–1152, 1997.

[19] T. W. Huang and J. C. Langlois, "Podoendin. A new cell surface protein of the podocyte and endothelium," *Journal of Experimental Medicine*, vol. 162, no. 1, pp. 245–267, 1985.

[20] E. Schnabel, G. Dekan, A. Miettinen, and M. G. Farquhar, "Biogenesis of podocalyxin—the major glomerular sialoglycoprotein—in the newborn rat kidney," *European Journal of Cell Biology*, vol. 48, no. 2, pp. 313–326, 1989.

[21] B. L. Wharram, M. Goyal, P. J. Gillespie et al., "Altered podocyte structure in GLEPP1 (Ptpro)-deficient mice associated with hypertension and low glomerular filtration rate," *The Journal of Clinical Investigation*, vol. 106, no. 10, pp. 1281–1290, 2000.

[22] S. J. Shankland, "The podocyte's response to injury: role in proteinuria and glomerulosclerosis," *Kidney International*, vol. 69, no. 12, pp. 2131–2147, 2006.

[23] T. B. Huber, M. Köttgen, B. Schilling, G. Walz, and T. Benzing, "Interaction with podocin facilitates nephrin signaling," *Journal of Biological Chemistry*, vol. 276, no. 45, pp. 41543–41546, 2001.

[24] N. Sachs, M. Kreft, M. A. van den Bergh Weerman et al., "Kidney failure in mice lacking the tetraspanin CD151," *Journal of Cell Biology*, vol. 175, no. 1, pp. 33–39, 2006.

[25] N. P. J. Vogtländer, H. Dijkman, M. A. H. Bakker, K. P. Campbell, J. van der Vlag, and J. H. M. Berden, "Localization of α-dystroglycan on the podocyte: from top to toe," *Journal of Histochemistry and Cytochemistry*, vol. 53, no. 11, pp. 1345–1353, 2005.

[26] S. J. Shankland, H. Ly, K. Thai, and J. W. Scholey, "Increased glomerular capillary pressure alters glomerular cytokine expression," *Circulation Research*, vol. 75, no. 5, pp. 844–853, 1994.

[27] S. A. Karumanchi and M. D. Lindheimer, "Preeclampsia and the kidney: footprints in the urine," *American Journal of Obstetrics and Gynecology*, vol. 196, no. 4, pp. 287–288, 2007.

[28] S. C. Satchell, S. J. Harper, J. E. Tooke, D. Kerjaschki, M. A. Saleem, and P. W. Mathieson, "Human podocytes express

angiopoietin 1, a potential regulator of glomerular vascular endothelial growth factor," *Journal of the American Society of Nephrology*, vol. 13, no. 2, pp. 544–550, 2002.

[29] M. Yang, M. Zhang, J. Chen et al., "Angiopoietin-1 inhibits mouse glomerular endothelial cell senescence via Tie2 receptor-modulated ERK1/2 signaling," *American Journal of Nephrology*, vol. 31, no. 6, pp. 490–500, 2010.

[30] D. R. Abrahamson, "Structure and development of the glomerular capillary wall and basement membrane," *American Journal of Physiology—Renal Fluid and Electrolyte Physiology*, vol. 253, no. 5, pp. F783–F794, 1987.

[31] S. Akilesh, T. B. Huber, H. Wu et al., "Podocytes use FcRn to clear IgG from the glomerular basement membrane," *Proceedings of the National Academy of Sciences of the United States of America*, vol. 105, no. 3, pp. 967–972, 2008.

[32] C. R. C. van Roeyen, F. Eitner, P. Boor et al., "Induction of progressive glomerulonephritis by podocyte-specific overexpression of platelet-derived growth factor-D," *Kidney International*, vol. 80, no. 12, pp. 1292–1305, 2011.

[33] M.-D. Appary, M. D. Kazatchkine, M. Levi-Strauss, N. Hinglais, and J. Bariety, "Expression of CR1 (CD35) mRNA in podocytes from adult and fetal human kidneys," *Kidney International*, vol. 38, no. 2, pp. 289–293, 1990.

[34] E. H. Garin, W. Mu, J. M. Arthur et al., "Urinary CD80 is elevated in minimal change disease but not in focal segmental glomerulosclerosis," *Kidney International*, vol. 78, no. 3, pp. 296–302, 2010.

[35] D. Kerjaschki, "Dysfunctions of cell biological mechanisms of visceral epithelial cell (podocytes) in glomerular diseases," *Kidney International*, vol. 45, no. 2, pp. 300–313, 1994.

[36] C. Manno, G. F. M. Strippoli, L. Arnesano et al., "Predictors of bleeding complications in percutaneous ultrasound-guided renal biopsy," *Kidney International*, vol. 66, no. 4, pp. 1570–1577, 2004.

[37] A. Konvalinka, J. W. Scholey, and E. P. Diamandis, "Searching for new biomarkers of renal diseases through proteomics," *Clinical Chemistry*, vol. 58, no. 2, pp. 353–365, 2012.

[38] G. H. Tesch, "Review: serum and urine biomarkers of kidney disease: a pathophysiological perspective," *Nephrology*, vol. 15, no. 6, pp. 609–616, 2010.

[39] J. L. Gorriz and A. Martinez-Castelao, "Proteinuria: detection and role in native renal disease progression," *Transplantation Reviews*, vol. 26, no. 1, pp. 3–13, 2012.

[40] J. Barratt and P. Topham, "Urine proteomics: the present and future of measuring urinary protein components in disease," *Canadian Medical Association Journal*, vol. 177, no. 4, pp. 361–368, 2007.

[41] M. Cirillo, "Evaluation of glomerular filtration rate and of albuminuria/proteinuria," *Journal of Nephrology*, vol. 23, no. 2, pp. 125–132, 2010.

[42] J.-Y. Guh, "Proteinuria versus albuminuria in chronic kidney disease," *Nephrology*, vol. 15, no. 2, pp. 53–56, 2010.

[43] T. Wada, M. Shimizu, T. Toyama, A. Hara, S. Kaneko, and K. Furuichi, "Clinical impact of albuminuria in diabetic nephropathy," *Clinical and Experimental Nephrology*, vol. 16, no. 1, pp. 96–101, 2012.

[44] D. Yu, A. Petermann, U. Kunter, S. Rong, S. J. Shankland, and J. Floege, "Urinary podocyte loss is a more specific marker of ongoing glomerular damage than proteinuria," *Journal of the American Society of Nephrology*, vol. 16, no. 6, pp. 1733–1741, 2005.

[45] T. Sakairi, Y. Abe, H. Kajiyama et al., "Conditionally immortalized human podocyte cell lines established from urine," *American Journal of Physiology—Renal Physiology*, vol. 298, no. 3, pp. F557–F567, 2010.

[46] A. T. Petermann, R. Krofft, M. Blonski et al., "Podocytes that detach in experimental membranous nephropathy are viable," *Kidney International*, vol. 64, no. 4, pp. 1222–1231, 2003.

[47] R. Doyonnas, J. S. Nielsen, S. Chelliah et al., "Podocalyxin is a CD34-related marker of murine hematopoietic stem cells and embryonic erythroid cells," *Blood*, vol. 105, no. 11, pp. 4170–4178, 2005.

[48] C. Sassetti, K. Tangemann, M. S. Singer, D. B. Kershaw, and S. D. Rosen, "Identification of podocalyxin-like protein as a high endothelial venule ligand for L-selectin: parallels to CD34," *Journal of Experimental Medicine*, vol. 187, no. 12, pp. 1965–1975, 1998.

[49] N. Vitureira, K. McNagny, E. Soriano, and F. Burgaya, "Pattern of expression of the podocalyxin gene in the mouse brain during development," *Gene Expression Patterns*, vol. 5, no. 3, pp. 349–354, 2005.

[50] D. Kerjaschki, D. J. Sharkey, and M. G. Farquhar, "Identification and characterization of podocalyxin—the major sialoprotein of the renal glomerular epithelial cell," *Journal of Cell Biology*, vol. 98, no. 4, pp. 1591–1596, 1984.

[51] Y. Li, J. Li, S. W. Straight, and D. B. Kershaw, "PDZ domain-mediated interaction of rabbit podocalyxin and Na^+/H^+ exchange regulatory factor-2," *American Journal of Physiology—Renal Physiology*, vol. 282, no. 6, pp. F1129–F1139, 2002.

[52] S. Schmieder, M. Nagai, R. A. Orlando, T. Takeda, and M. G. Farquhar, "Podocalyxin activates RhoA and induces actin reorganization through NHERF1 and Ezrin in MDCK cells," *Journal of the American Society of Nephrology*, vol. 15, no. 9, pp. 2289–2298, 2004.

[53] R. A. Orlando, T. Takeda, B. Zak et al., "The glomerular epithelial cell anti-adhesin podocalyxin associates with the actin cytoskeleton through interactions with ezrin," *Journal of the American Society of Nephrology*, vol. 12, no. 8, pp. 1589–1598, 2001.

[54] R. Doyonnas, D. B. Kershaw, C. Duhme et al., "Anuria, omphalocele, and perinatal lethality in mice lacking the CD34-related protein podocalyxin," *Journal of Experimental Medicine*, vol. 194, no. 1, pp. 13–27, 2001.

[55] M. Hara, T. Yamamoto, T. Yanagihara et al., "Urinary excretion of podocalyxin indicates glomerular epithelial cell injuries in glomerulonephritis," *Nephron*, vol. 69, no. 4, pp. 397–403, 1995.

[56] M. Hara, T. Yanagihara, and I. Kihara, "Cumulative excretion of urinary podocytes reflects disease progression in IgA nephropathy and Schönlein-Henoch purpura nephritis," *Clinical Journal of the American Society of Nephrology*, vol. 2, no. 2, pp. 231–238, 2007.

[57] M. Hara, T. Yanagihara, M. Itoh, M. Matsuno, and I. Kihara, "Immunohistochemical and urinary markers of podocyte injury," *Pediatric Nephrology*, vol. 12, no. 1, pp. 43–48, 1998.

[58] T. Nakamura, C. Ushiyama, S. Suzuki et al., "Urinary excretion of podocytes in patients with diabetic nephropathy," *Nephrology Dialysis Transplantation*, vol. 15, no. 9, pp. 1379–1383, 2000.

[59] M.-S. Zou, J. Yu, J.-H. Zhou et al., "1,25-dihydroxyvitamin D3 ameliorates podocytopenia in rats with adriamycin-induced nephropathy," *Internal Medicine*, vol. 49, no. 24, pp. 2677–2686, 2010.

[60] R. Asao, K. Asanuma, F. Kodama et al., "Relationships between levels of urinary podocalyxin, number of urinary podocytes,

and histologic injury in adult patients with IgA nephropathy," *Clinical Journal of the American Society of Nephrology*, vol. 7, no. 9, pp. 1385–1393, 2012.

[61] S. Okubo, "A study of urinary podocalyxin in children with IgA nephropathy," *Japanese Journal of Nephrology*, vol. 37, no. 7, pp. 357–365, 1995.

[62] J. Mueller-Deile, P. Kümpers, J. Achenbach et al., "Podocalyxin-positive glomerular epithelial cells in urine correlate with a positive outcome in FSGS," *Journal of Nephrology*, vol. 25, pp. 802–809, 2012.

[63] K. Aita, M. Etoh, H. Hamada et al., "Acute and transient podocyte loss and proteinuria in preeclampsia," *Nephron—Clinical Practice*, vol. 112, no. 2, pp. c65–c70, 2009.

[64] V. D. Garovic, S. J. Wagner, S. T. Turner et al., "Urinary podocyte excretion as a marker for preeclampsia," *American Journal of Obstetrics and Gynecology*, vol. 196, no. 4, pp. 320.e1–320.e7, 2007.

[65] Y. Wang, S. Zhao, S. Loyd, and L. J. Groome, "Increased urinary excretion of nephrin, podocalyxin, and βig-h3 in women with preeclampsia," *American Journal of Physiology—Renal Physiology*, vol. 302, no. 9, pp. F1084–F1089, 2012.

[66] K. Matsui, A. Kamijo-Ikemori, M. Hara et al., "Clinical significance of tubular and podocyte biomarkers in acute kidney injury," *Clinical and Experimental Nephrology*, vol. 15, no. 2, pp. 220–225, 2011.

[67] M. Hara, K. Yamagata, Y. Tomino et al., "Urinary podocalyxin is an early marker for podocyte injury in patients with diabetes establishment of a highly sensitive ELISA to detect urinary podocalyxin," *Diabetologia*, vol. 55, no. 11, pp. 2913–2919, 2012.

[68] P. Habara, H. Marečková, K. Maličková et al., "Novel flow cytometric method for the detection of podocalyxin-positive elements in urine of patients with glomerulonephritides—first promising results," *Folia Biologica*, vol. 58, pp. 57–63, 2012.

[69] M. Zheng, L.-L. Lv, J. Ni et al., "Urinary podocyte-associated mRNA profile in various stages of diabetic nephropathy," *PLoS ONE*, vol. 6, no. 5, Article ID e20431, 2011.

[70] H. Putaala, R. Soininen, P. Kilpeläinen, J. Wartiovaara, and K. Tryggvason, "The murine nephrin gene is specifically expressed in kidney, brain and pancreas: inactivation of the gene leads to massive proteinuria and neonatal death," *Human Molecular Genetics*, vol. 10, no. 1, pp. 1–8, 2001.

[71] C. Li, V. Ruotsalainen, K. Tryggvason, A. S. Shaw, and J. H. Miner, "CD2AP is expressed with nephrin in developing podocytes and is found widely in mature kidney and elsewhere," *American Journal of Physiology—Renal Physiology*, vol. 279, no. 4, pp. F785–F792, 2000.

[72] M. Kestilä, U. Lenkkeri, M. Männikkö et al., "Positionally cloned gene for a novel glomerular protein—nephrin—is mutated in congenital nephrotic syndrome," *Molecular Cell*, vol. 1, no. 4, pp. 575–582, 1998.

[73] H. Autio-Harmainen and J. Rapola, "The thickness of the glomerular basement membrane in congenital nephrotic syndrome of the Finnish type," *Nephron*, vol. 34, no. 1, pp. 48–50, 1983.

[74] M. A. Saleem, L. Ni, I. Witherden et al., "Co-localization of nephrin, podocin, and the actin cytoskeleton: evidence for a role in podocyte foot process formation," *American Journal of Pathology*, vol. 161, no. 4, pp. 1459–1466, 2002.

[75] K. Schwarz, M. Simons, J. Reiser et al., "Podocin, a raft-associated component of the glomerular slit diaphragm, interacts with CD2AP and nephrin," *The Journal of Clinical Investigation*, vol. 108, no. 11, pp. 1621–1629, 2001.

[76] S. Lehtonen, E. Lehtonen, K. Kudlicka, H. Holthöfer, and M. G. Farquhar, "Nephrin forms a complex with adherens junction proteins and CASK in podocytes and in Madin-Darby canine kidney cells expressing nephrin," *American Journal of Pathology*, vol. 165, no. 3, pp. 923–936, 2004.

[77] A. Pätäri, C. Forsblom, M. Havana, H. Taipale, P.-H. Groop, and H. Holthöfer, "Nephrinuria in diabetic nephropathy of type 1 diabetes," *Diabetes*, vol. 52, no. 12, pp. 2969–2974, 2003.

[78] D. P. K. Ng, B.-C. Tai, E. Tan et al., "Nephrinuria associates with multiple renal traits in type 2 diabetes," *Nephrology Dialysis Transplantation*, vol. 26, no. 8, pp. 2508–2514, 2011.

[79] J.-H. Chang, S.-Y. Paik, L. Mao et al., "Diabetic kidney disease in FVB/NJ akita mice: temporal pattern of kidney injury and urinary nephrin excretion," *PLoS ONE*, vol. 7, no. 4, Article ID e33942, 2012.

[80] G. H. Son, J. Y. Kwon, S. Lee et al., "Comparison of serum and urinary nephrin levels between normal pregnancies and severe preeclampsia," *European Journal of Obstetrics & Gynecology and Reproductive Biology*, vol. 166, no. 2, pp. 139–144, 2013.

[81] T. Nakatsue, H. Koike, G. D. Han et al., "Nephrin and podocin dissociate at the onset of proteinuria in experimental membranous nephropathy," *Kidney International*, vol. 67, no. 6, pp. 2239–2253, 2005.

[82] A. T. Petermann, J. Pippin, R. Krofft et al., "Viable podocytes detach in experimental diabetic nephropathy: potential mechanism underlying glomerulosclerosis," *Nephron—Experimental Nephrology*, vol. 98, no. 4, pp. e114–e123, 2004.

[83] P. Aaltonen, P. Luimula, E. Åström et al., "Changes in the expression of nephrin gene and protein in experimental diabetic nephropathy," *Laboratory Investigation*, vol. 81, no. 9, pp. 1185–1190, 2001.

[84] T. A. Facca, G. M. Kirsztajn, A. R. Pereira et al., "Renal evaluation in women with preeclampsia," *Nephron Extra*, vol. 2, no. 1, pp. 125–132, 2012.

[85] Y. Sato, B. L. Wharram, S. K. Lee et al., "Urine podocyte mRNAs mark progression of renal disease," *Journal of the American Society of Nephrology*, vol. 20, no. 5, pp. 1041–1052, 2009.

[86] A. Fukuda, L. T. Wickman, M. P. Venkatareddy et al., "Urine podocin:nephrin mRNA ratio (PNR) as a podocyte stress biomarker," *Nephrology Dialysis Transplantation*, vol. 27, no. 11, pp. 4079–4087, 2012.

[87] G. Wang, F. M.-M. Lai, K.-B. Lai, K.-M. Chow, K.-T. P. Li, and C.-C. Szeto, "Messenger RNA expression of podocyte-associated molecules in the urinary sediment of patients with diabetic nephropathy," *Nephron—Clinical Practice*, vol. 106, no. 4, pp. c169–c179, 2007.

[88] G. Wang, F. M.-M. Lai, L.-S. Tam et al., "Messenger RNA expression of podocyte-associated molecules in urinary sediment of patients with lupus nephritis," *Journal of Rheumatology*, vol. 34, no. 12, pp. 2358–2364, 2007.

[89] C.-C. Szeto, K.-B. Lai, K.-M. Chow et al., "Messenger RNA expression of glomerular podocyte markers in the urinary sediment of acquired proteinuric diseases," *Clinica Chimica Acta*, vol. 361, no. 1-2, pp. 182–190, 2005.

[90] M. Navarro-Muñoz, M. Ibernon, V. Pérez et al., "Messenger RNA expression of B7-1 and NPHS1 in urinary sediment could be useful to differentiate between minimal-change disease and focal segmental glomerulosclerosis in adult patients," *Nephrology Dialysis Transplantation*, vol. 26, no. 12, pp. 3914–3923, 2011.

[91] T. P. Kelder, M. E. Penning, H. W. Uh et al., "Quantitative polymerase chain reaction-based analysis of podocyturia is

a feasible diagnostic tool in preeclampsia," *Hypertension*, vol. 60, pp. 1538–1544, 2012.

[92] N. Boute, O. Gribouval, S. Roselli et al., "NPHS2, encoding the glomerular protein podocin, is mutated in autosomal recessive steroid-resistant nephrotic syndrome," *Nature Genetics*, vol. 24, no. 4, pp. 349–354, 2000.

[93] S. Roselli, O. Gribouval, N. Boute et al., "Podocin localizes in the kidney to the slit diaphragm area," *American Journal of Pathology*, vol. 160, no. 1, pp. 131–139, 2002.

[94] V. D. Garovic, I. M. Craici, S. J. Wagner et al., "Mass spectrometry as a novel method for detection of podocyturia in preeclampsia," *Nephrology, Dialysis, Transplantation*, vol. 28, no. 6, pp. 1555–1561, 2013.

[95] O. Ichii, A. Yabuki, N. Sasaki et al., "Pathological correlations between podocyte injuries and renal functions in canine and feline chronic kidney diseases," *Histology and Histopathology*, vol. 26, no. 10, pp. 1243–1255, 2011.

[96] D. J. V. Bridgewater, A. Mok, and D. G. Matsell, "Expression of complement regulatory proteins in the developing human kidney," *Pediatric Nephrology*, vol. 15, no. 1-2, pp. 36–42, 2000.

[97] M. D. Kazatchkine, D. T. Fearon, M. D. Appay, C. Mandet, and J. Bariety, "Immunohistochemical study of the human glomerular C3b receptor in normal kidney and in seventy-five cases of renal diseases. Loss of C3b receptor antigen in focal hyalinosis and in proliferative nephritis of systemic lupus erythematosus," *The Journal of Clinical Investigation*, vol. 69, no. 4, pp. 900–912, 1982.

[98] E. Fung, L. Esposito, J. A. Todd, and L. S. Wicker, "Multiplexed immunophenotyping of human antigen-presenting cells in whole blood by polychromatic flow cytometry," *Nature Protocols*, vol. 5, no. 2, pp. 357–370, 2010.

[99] N. Hinglais, M. D. Kazatchkine, C. Mandet, M.-D. Appay, and J. Bariety, "Human liver Kupffer cells express CR1, CR3, and CR4 complement receptor antigens. An immunohistochemistry study," *Laboratory Investigation*, vol. 61, no. 5, pp. 509–514, 1989.

[100] E. Fischer, M. D. Appay, J. Cook, and M. D. Kazatchkine, "Characterization of the human glomerular C3 receptor as the C3b/C4b complement type one (CR1) receptor," *Journal of Immunology*, vol. 136, no. 4, pp. 1373–1377, 1986.

[101] T. S. Puri and R. J. Quigg, "The many effects of complement C3- and C5-binding proteins in renal injury," *Seminars in Nephrology*, vol. 27, no. 3, pp. 321–337, 2007.

[102] M. Pascual, G. Steiger, S. Sadallah et al., "Identification of membrane-bound CR1 (CD35) in human urine: evidence for its release by glomerular podocytes," *Journal of Experimental Medicine*, vol. 179, no. 3, pp. 889–899, 1994.

[103] M. Hara, T. Yanagihara, I. Kihara, K. Higashi, K. Fujimoto, and T. Kajita, "Apical cell membranes are shed into urine from injured podocytes: a novel phenomenon of podocyte injury," *Journal of the American Society of Nephrology*, vol. 16, no. 2, pp. 408–416, 2005.

[104] E. H. Garin, L. N. Diaz, W. Mu et al., "Urinary CD80 excretion increases in idiopathic minimal-change disease," *Journal of the American Society of Nephrology*, vol. 20, no. 2, pp. 260–266, 2009.

[105] J. Reiser, G. von Gersdorff, M. Loos et al., "Induction of B7-1 in podocytes is associated with nephrotic syndrome," *The Journal of Clinical Investigation*, vol. 113, no. 10, pp. 1390–1397, 2004.

[106] N. Eto, T. Wada, R. Inagi et al., "Podocyte protection by darbepoetin: preservation of the cytoskeleton and nephrin expression," *Kidney International*, vol. 72, no. 4, pp. 455–463, 2007.

[107] C. Faul, M. Donnelly, S. Merscher-Gomez et al., "The actin cytoskeleton of kidney podocytes is a direct target of the antiproteinuric effect of cyclosporine A," *Nature Medicine*, vol. 14, no. 9, pp. 931–938, 2008.

[108] P. Mundel, H. W. Heid, T. M. Mundel, M. Krüger, J. Reiser, and W. Kriz, "Synaptopodin: an actin-associated protein in telencephalic dendrites and renal podocytes," *Journal of Cell Biology*, vol. 139, no. 1, pp. 193–204, 1997.

[109] A. Vlachos, E. Korkotian, E. Schonfeld, E. Copanaki, T. Deller, and M. Segal, "Synaptopodin regulates plasticity of dendritic spines in hippocampal neurons," *Journal of Neuroscience*, vol. 29, no. 4, pp. 1017–1033, 2009.

[110] P. Mundel, P. Gilbert, and W. Kriz, "Podocytes in glomerulus of rat kidney express a characteristic 44 KD protein," *Journal of Histochemistry and Cytochemistry*, vol. 39, no. 8, pp. 1047–1056, 1991.

[111] C. A. Batchelder, C. C. I. Lee, M. L. Martinez, and A. F. Tarantal, "Ontogeny of the kidney and renal developmental markers in the rhesus monkey (Macaca mulatta)," *Anatomical Record*, vol. 293, no. 11, pp. 1971–1983, 2010.

[112] S. Yaddanapudi, M. M. Altintas, A. D. Kistler et al., "CD2AP in mouse and human podocytes controls a proteolytic program that regulates cytoskeletal structure and cellular survival," *The Journal of Clinical Investigation*, vol. 121, no. 10, pp. 3965–3980, 2011.

[113] G. Wang, F. M.-M. Lai, K.-B. Lai et al., "Intra-renal and urinary mRNA expression of podocyte-associated molecules for the estimation of glomerular podocyte loss," *Renal Failure*, vol. 32, no. 3, pp. 372–379, 2010.

[114] B. Jim, P. Jean-Louis, A. Qipo et al., "Podocyturia as a diagnostic marker for preeclampsia amongst high-risk pregnant patients," *Journal of Pregnancy*, vol. 2012, Article ID 984630, 5 pages, 2012.

[115] C. Pyke, P. Kristensen, P. B. Østergaard, P. S. Oturai, and J. Rømer, "Proteoglycan expression in the normal rat kidney," *Nephron*, vol. 77, no. 4, pp. 461–470, 1997.

[116] P. E. Thomas, B. L. Wharram, M. Goyal, J. E. Wiggins, L. B. Holzman, and R. C. Wiggins, "GLEPP1, a renal glomerular epithelial cell (podocyte) membrane protein- tyrosine phosphatase. Identification, molecular cloning, and characterization in rabbit," *Journal of Biological Chemistry*, vol. 269, no. 31, pp. 19953–19961, 1994.

[117] M. Tagawa, T. Shirasawa, Y.-I. Yahagi et al., "Identification of a receptor-type protein tyrosine phosphatase expressed in postmitotic maturing neurons: its structure and expression in the central nervous system," *Biochemical Journal*, vol. 321, no. 3, pp. 865–871, 1997.

[118] L. Barisoni, W. Kriz, P. Mundel, and V. D'Agati, "The dysregulated podocyte phenotype: a novel concept in the pathogenesis of collapsing idiopathic focal segmental glomerulosclerosis and HIV-associated nephropathy," *Journal of the American Society of Nephrology*, vol. 10, no. 1, pp. 51–61, 1999.

[119] F. Ozaltin, T. Ibsirlioglu, E. Z. Taskiran et al., "Disruption of PTPRO causes childhood-onset nephrotic syndrome," *American Journal of Human Genetics*, vol. 89, no. 1, pp. 139–147, 2011.

[120] Y. H. Kim, M. Goyal, D. Kurnit et al., "Podocyte depletion and glomerulosclerosis have a direct relationship in the PAN-treated rat," *Kidney International*, vol. 60, no. 3, pp. 957–968, 2001.

[121] S.-I. Higashijima, A. Nose, G. Eguchi, Y. Hotta, and H. Okamoto, "Mindin/F-spondin family: novel ECM proteins expressed in the zebrafish embryonic axis," *Developmental Biology*, vol. 192, no. 2, pp. 211–227, 1997.

[122] Y. Feinstein, V. Borrell, C. Garcia et al., "F-spondin and mindin: two structurally and functionally related genes expressed in the hippocampus that promote outgrowth of embryonic hippocampal neurons," *Development*, vol. 126, no. 16, pp. 3637–3648, 1999.

[123] M. Murakoshi, M. Tanimoto, T. Gohda et al., "Mindin: a novel marker for podocyte injury in diabetic nephropathy," *Nephrology Dialysis Transplantation*, vol. 26, no. 7, pp. 2153–2160, 2011.

[124] Y.-W. He, H. Li, J. Zhang et al., "The extracellular matrix protein mindin is a pattern-recognition molecule for microbial pathogens," *Nature Immunology*, vol. 5, no. 1, pp. 88–97, 2004.

[125] W. Jia, H. Li, and Y.-W. He, "The extracellular matrix protein mindin serves as an integrin ligand and is critical for inflammatory cell recruitment," *Blood*, vol. 106, no. 12, pp. 3854–3859, 2005.

[126] J. A. Kreidberg, M. J. Donovan, S. L. Goldstein et al., "Alpha 3 beta 1 integrin has a crucial role in kidney and lung organogenesis," *Development*, vol. 122, no. 11, pp. 3537–3547, 1996.

[127] C. Has, G. Spartà, D. Kiritsi et al., "Integrin $\alpha 3$ mutations with kidney, lung, and skin disease," *The New England Journal of Medicine*, vol. 366, no. 16, pp. 1508–1514, 2012.

[128] Y. Sugita and Y. Masuho, "CD59: its role in complement regulation and potential for therapeutic use," *Immunotechnology*, vol. 1, no. 3-4, pp. 157–168, 1995.

[129] I. A. Rooney, A. Davies, D. Griffiths et al., "The complement-inhibiting protein, protectin (CD59 antigen), is present and functionally active on glomerular epithelial cells," *Clinical and Experimental Immunology*, vol. 83, no. 2, pp. 251–256, 1991.

[130] P. N. Cunningham, B. K. Hack, G. Ren, A. W. M. Minto, B. P. Morgan, and R. J. Quigg, "Glomerular complement regulation is overwhelmed in passive Heymann nephritis," *Kidney International*, vol. 60, no. 3, pp. 900–909, 2001.

[131] T. Lehto, E. Honkanen, A.-M. Teppo, and S. Meri, "Urinary excretion of protectin (CD59), complement SC5b-9 and cytokines in membranous glomerulonephritis," *Kidney International*, vol. 47, no. 5, pp. 1403–1411, 1995.

[132] J.-K. Guo, A. L. Menke, M.-C. Gubler et al., "WT1 is a key regulator of podocyte function: reduced expression levels cause crescentic glomerulonephritis and mesangial sclerosis," *Human Molecular Genetics*, vol. 11, no. 6, pp. 651–659, 2002.

[133] R. E. Palmer, A. Kotsianti, B. Cadman, T. Boyd, W. Gerald, and D. A. Haber, "WT1 regulates the expression of the major glomerular podocyte membrane protein Podocalyxin," *Current Biology*, vol. 11, no. 22, pp. 1805–1809, 2001.

[134] K. Schwab, D. P. Witte, B. J. Aronow, P. Devarajan, S. S. Potter, and L. T. Patterson, "Microarray analysis of focal segmental glomerulosclerosis," *American Journal of Nephrology*, vol. 24, no. 4, pp. 438–447, 2004.

[135] T. Ohse, M. R. Vaughan, J. B. Kopp et al., "De novo expression of podocyte proteins in parietal epithelial cells during experimental glomerular disease," *American Journal of Physiology—Renal Physiology*, vol. 298, no. 3, pp. F702–F711, 2010.

[136] T. Pisitkun, R.-F. Shen, and M. A. Knepper, "Identification and proteomic profiling of exosomes in human urine," *Proceedings of the National Academy of Sciences of the United States of America*, vol. 101, no. 36, pp. 13368–13373, 2004.

[137] H. Zhou, P. S. T. Yuen, T. Pisitkun et al., "Collection, storage, preservation, and normalization of human urinary exosomes for biomarker discovery," *Kidney International*, vol. 69, no. 8, pp. 1471–1476, 2006.

[138] H. Zhou, A. Cheruvanky, X. Hu et al., "Urinary exosomal transcription factors, a new class of biomarkers for renal disease," *Kidney International*, vol. 74, no. 5, pp. 613–621, 2008.

[139] M. Hara, T. Yanagihara, Y. Hirayama et al., "Podocyte membrane vesicles in urine originate from tip vesiculation of podocyte microvilli," *Human Pathology*, vol. 41, no. 9, pp. 1265–1275, 2010.

[140] S. M. Hewitt, J. Dear, and R. A. Star, "Discovery of protein biomarkers for renal diseases," *Journal of the American Society of Nephrology*, vol. 15, no. 7, pp. 1677–1689, 2004.

[141] J. Malyszko, "Biomarkers of acute kidney injury in different clinical settings: a time to change the paradigm?" *Kidney and Blood Pressure Research*, vol. 33, no. 5, pp. 368–382, 2010.

[142] T. Biederer and T. C. Südhof, "CASK and protein 4.1 support F-actin nucleation on neurexins," *Journal of Biological Chemistry*, vol. 276, no. 51, pp. 47869–47876, 2001.

[143] A. Saito, N. Miyauchi, T. Hashimoto et al., "Neurexin-1, a presynaptic adhesion molecule, localizes at the slit diaphragm of the glomerular podocytes in kidneys," *American Journal of Physiology—Regulatory Integrative and Comparative Physiology*, vol. 300, no. 2, pp. R340–R348, 2011.

[144] G. M. Ghiggeri, G. Caridi, U. Magrini et al., "Genetics, clinical and pathological features of glomerulonephrites associated with mutations of nonmuscle myosin IIA (Fechtner syndrome)," *American Journal of Kidney Diseases*, vol. 41, no. 1, pp. 95–104, 2003.

10

Expression of Prostanoid EP3 Receptors in Oral Squamous Epithelium and Oral Squamous Cell Carcinoma

Muhammad Kashif,[1] Muhammad Ishfaq,[2] and A. H. Nagi[1]

[1]*Department of Morbid Anatomy and Histopathology, University of Health Sciences, Lahore 54000, Pakistan*
[2]*Oral & Maxillofacial Surgery Department, Nishtar Institute of Dentistry, Multan 60000, Pakistan*

Correspondence should be addressed to Muhammad Kashif; drkashifazam@gmail.com

Academic Editor: Naila Kayani

Objectives. To carry out a descriptive analysis of the expression of the EP3 receptors of PGE2 in different histological grades of OSCC and adjacent normal epithelium. *Material and Methods.* A total of 46 patients presenting with various histological subtypes and grades of OSCC were recruited from Maxillofacial Surgery Department of Nishtar Institute of Dentistry Multan. Microscopically tumour subtyping and histological grading according to Anneroth's grading system were carried out. Immunohistochemical staining with rabbit polyclonal EP3 receptor antibody was performed and sections were scored for intensity and proportion of positive adjacent squamous epithelial and tumour cells. *Results.* Out of 46 patients $n = 28$ (60.9%) were well differentiated, $n = 15$ (32.6%) were moderately differentiated, and only $n = 3$ (6.5%) were poorly differentiated. All $n = 46$ cases of OSCC were positive for EP3 receptor antibody, $n = 14$ (30.4%) cases had strong intensity of anti EP3 antibody staining in tumour tissue, $n = 17$ (37%) cases showed moderate intensity, and $n = 15$ (32.6%) cases showed weak intensity. *Conclusion.* Prostanoid EP3 receptors are widely but variably expressed in OSCC. Most of well differentiated OSCC cases show a moderate to strong expression of EP3 receptors. However, insignificant statistical relation to histological grades of OSCC has been observed. This might be due to small sample size of the study.

1. Introduction

Globally, oral cancer is the eighth most common cause of cancer-related deaths, but in spite of this fact most of the people are unaware of its presence [1]. Squamous cell carcinomas (SCC) comprise more than 90% of these oral cancers arising in the mucous membranes of the oral cavity and oropharynx [2]. OSCC is manifested in various clinical forms. It may resemble leukoplakia, verrucous leukoplakia, or an erythroleukoplakia. The erythroplakia may eventually develop into a necrotic ulcer with irregular, raised indurated edges or as an exophytic broad-based mass with warty surface. When traumatised, OSCC bleeds easily and frequently becomes secondarily infected at the surface. It is usually painless unless secondarily infected. Larger lesions can interfere with normal speech, chewing, or swallowing [3, 4].

OSCC arises from various molecular pathways that progress from the mutual effects of susceptibility and vulnerability to environmental carcinogens. These carcinogens are snuff, chemical carcinogens, alcohol, microorganisms, and ultraviolet or ionizing radiation. Damage to genes and chromosomes may occur due to prolonged exposure to these carcinogens [5].

For decades, no change in mortality rate has been observed. Even with advancements in surgery and radiotherapy, mortality still is very high with a 5-year survival rate of only 50% [6]. Currently, targeted molecular therapy such as monoclonal antibody therapy and gene therapy has been applied to patients with oral cancer. This treatment modality has limited or minimal side effects in normal cells of the body, in contrast to surgery, chemotherapy, and radiotherapy. The important molecular targets in cancer chemotherapy are progesterone receptor, cyclooxygenase-2 (COX-2), peroxisome proliferator-activated receptor (PPAR), and epidermal growth factor receptor (EGFR). These molecular targets are related with the proliferation and the differentiation of OSCC [7].

Among the prostanoids, the E-type PGs, particularly PGE2 derived from arachidonic acid, are produced in the body. PGE2 is found in most animal species and exhibits the multipurpose actions. There are four different receptors labelled EP1, EP2, EP3, and EP4 for the E-type PGs [8]. The probable involvement of PGs in the carcinogenesis is reinforced by the presence of enhanced expression of cyclooxygenase-2 in both premalignant and malignant tissues. There is also evidence that growth factors, cytokines, oncogenes, and tumour promoters stimulate COX-2 transcription via protein kinase C (PKC) and Ras-mediated signaling [9]. Further evidence of the role of PGs in carcinogenesis is evident from the plentiful epidemiological studies showing that continued consumption of drugs, especially aspirin, prevents the development of cancer [10, 11]. PGs play a vital role in numerous mechanisms that have been involved in carcinogenesis such as cell proliferation, angiogenesis, apoptosis, and mutagenesis [12]. Regardless of the fact that prostaglandin E2 is a notable carcinogenic agent and that PGE2 modifiers have a potential beneficial role, very few studies have so far fully investigated the components that are involved in synthesis and action of PGE2. The objective of the present study was to carry out a descriptive analysis of the expression of the EP3 receptors of PGE2 in different histological grades of OSCC. To our knowledge no such study elaborating the relationship between expression of PGE2 receptors EP3 in oral squamous cell carcinomas of various histological differentiation and adjacent normal tissue has so far been carried out in Pakistan. The results of this study may also help in assessing the presumptive prognostic role of PGE2 receptors EP3 in oral squamous cell carcinoma especially in terms of targeted therapy.

2. Methodology

2.1. Materials and Methods. After informed consent, biopsy specimens from 46 patients having undergone various diagnostic and/or surgical resection procedures for OSCC were acquired from Maxillofacial Surgical Department of NID, Multan. Sociodemographic information (name, age, gender, occupation, full address, history of smoking or using any form of smokeless tobacco, and family history of any cancer and oral cancer) was obtained along with relevant clinical, laboratory, and radiological information. To confirm the diagnosis 5 μm thick, paraffin embedded sections were cut and mounted on glass slides and sections were stained with haematoxylin and eosin stain and examined by light microscope. Anneroth's histological grading system had been used to grade OSCC cases on H&E staining [13].

2.2. Immunohistochemistry. About 4 μm thick sections were cut from all specimens and mounted on positively charged glass slides. Sections were deparaffinized in xylene and rehydrated in graded ethyl alcohol, followed by immersion in citrate buffer solution of pH 6.0, and were put in the microwave oven before staining procedures. For immunostaining, Universal Kit (Lab Vision) employing the streptavidin biotin system was used to carry out the peroxidase-antiperoxidase method of immunohistochemistry staining. Sections were then incubated with a primary polyclonal anti-EP3 receptor antibody (anti-PTGER3 antibody; ABCAM) and DAB chromogen was applied to the sections followed by counterstaining with haematoxylin [14].

The intensity and proportion of positive tumour cells of the EP3 immunohistochemical staining were evaluated using a light microscope. The intensity of cytoplasmic staining was graded from 0 to 3 (0: negative, 1: weak, 2: moderate, and 3: strong) and the tumour was also scored according to the proportion of positive tumour cells (0: 0–10% positive cells, 1: 11–25% positive cells, 2: 26–50% positive cells, 3: 51–75% positive cells, and 4: 76–100% positive cells) [15, 16]. The data was entered and analysed using SPSS 20.0. Data was expressed as mean ± SD. Comparisons between clinical and microscopic parameters were performed with the sample t-test. A difference of $P < 0.05$ was considered to be significant. The present study was certified by the Ethical Review Committee and Advanced Studies and Research Board of University of Health Sciences Lahore.

3. Results

A total of 46 cases of OSCC had been collected in accordance with inclusion and exclusion criteria. The overall mean age was 52.74 ± 14.14. The age range in males was 30 to 80 years (mean age 53.48±13.27) while in females the age range was 25 to 95 years (mean age 51.68 ± 15.61). This data shows that age of incidence was similar in both genders; however, most of the patients were in the range of 40 to 70 years of age ($n = 36$). In the present study male to female ratio was found to be 1.4 : 1 (Table 1).

Patients clinically presented most commonly with ulceration which was noted in 35 (76.1%) cases, fungating mass in 8 (17.4%) cases, and plaque-like lesion in 3 (6.5%) cases. Regarding the site of involvement of oral cavity, the occurrence of OSCC was found significantly higher on buccal mucosa where 23 (50%) cases were present. There were 13 (28.3%) cases that involved the tongue (mostly lateral border of tongue). When site of specimen was corelated with gender, the most number of cases in both genders were located on buccal mucosa but in females $n = 9$ (47%) cases were located on tongue while in males only $n = 4$ (14.8%) cases were located on tongue. When t-test was applied to observe the statistical relation it was significant ($P = 0.01$) (Figure 1).

A total of 60.9% were well differentiated (WD) (Figures 9 and 11), 32.6% were moderately differentiated (MD) (Figure 13), and only 6.5% were poorly differentiated (PD) cases of OSCC (Figure 15). Lymphovascular invasion was present in 61.8% of cases.

Among 46 cases of OSCC, 31 cases had attached non-tumorous epithelium. Out of these 31 cases of OSCC with attached epithelium, 11 (23.9%) had strong intensity (Score +3) of EP3 antibody staining, 17 (37%) had moderate intensity (Score +2) of antibody staining, and only 3 (6.5%) cases had

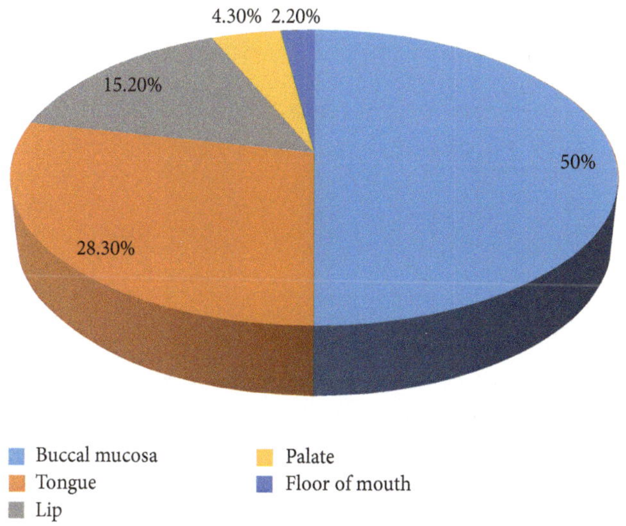

FIGURE 1: Distribution of OSCC cases at different sites of oral cavity.

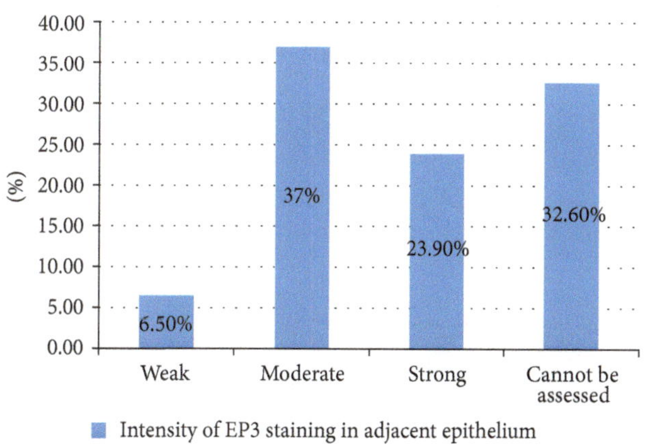

FIGURE 2: Intensity of EP3 staining in adjacent epithelium.

TABLE 1: Gender frequency in study cases.

Gender	Frequency	Percent
Male	27	58.7%
Female	19	41.3%
Total	46	100.0%

weak intensity (Score +1) of EP3 antibody staining (Figures 2, 5, 6, 7 and 8).

Among 46 cases of OSCC, 14 (30.4%) cases had strong intensity (+3) of anti-EP3 antibody staining in tumour tissue, 17 (37%) cases showed moderate intensity (+2), and 15 (32.6%) cases showed weak intensity (+1) (Figure 3).

The statistical relation between intensity of antibody staining and histological grade of OSCC was insignificant ($P = 0.486$). Table 2 shows the comparison between intensity of antibody staining and histological grade of OSCC (Table 2).

The number of cases showing weak intensity EP3 antibody in adjacent epithelium was $n = 3$ (6.5%) while the number of cases showing weak intensity in tumorous tissue

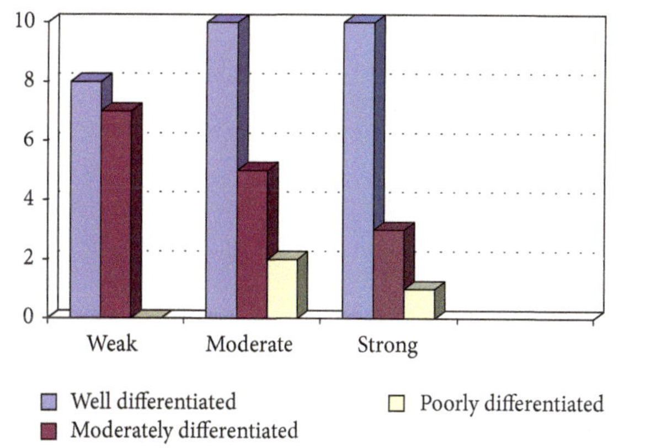

FIGURE 3: Comparison between intensity of EP3 staining in tumour tissue and histological grades of OSCC.

TABLE 2: Proportions of positive adjacent epithelial cells.

Proportion of positive epithelial cells	Frequency	Percent
11–25% positive epithelial cells (Score +1)	1	2.2%
26–50% positive epithelial cells (Score +2)	8	17.4%
51–75% positive epithelial cells (Score +3)	11	23.9%
76–100% positive epithelial cells (Score +4)	11	23.9%
Cannot be assessed	15	32.6%
Total	46	

was $n = 15$ (32.6%) in the present study (Figures 14 and 16). This difference in intensity of EP3 antibody staining in both of these tissues is statistically significant ($P = 0.042$).

As already stated above that a total of 31 cases had attached nontumorous epithelium, 11 (23.9%) cases had 76–100% (Score +4) positive epithelial cells for EP3 antibody, 11 (23.9%) cases had 51–75% (Score +3) positive epithelial cells, 26–50% (Score +2) epithelial cells were positive in 8 (17.4%) cases, and only 1 (2.2%) had 11–25% (Score +1) positive epithelial cells.

Among 46 cases of OSCC, 15 (32.6%) cases had 76–100% (Score +4) positive tumour cells for EP3 antibody, 21 (45.7%) cases had 51–75% (Score +3) positive tumour cells, and 10 (21.7%) cases had 26–50% (Score +2) positive tumour cells (Figure 4).

When we applied t-test to observe the statistical relation between histological grade and proportion of positive tumour cells for EP3 antibody, it was found to be insignificant ($P = 0.843$). It was also insignificant when it was applied to find the relation between proportion of positive adjacent epithelial and tumour cells for EP3 antibody ($P = 0.213$).

In summary, all 46 cases of OSCC were positive for EP3 receptor antibody. The maximum intensity and proportion score of EP3 in WDOSCC were +3 (35.5%) and +3 (45.6%); similarly 46.6% of MD exhibited +1 and +3, while 66% of each of PD tumours demonstrates +2 and +3 of intensity and proportion score, respectively. So most cases of well differentiated OSCC (71%) showed moderate to strong intensity of staining ($P = 0.486$). A total of 31 cases had attached nontumorous epithelium, 54.8% showing (+2)

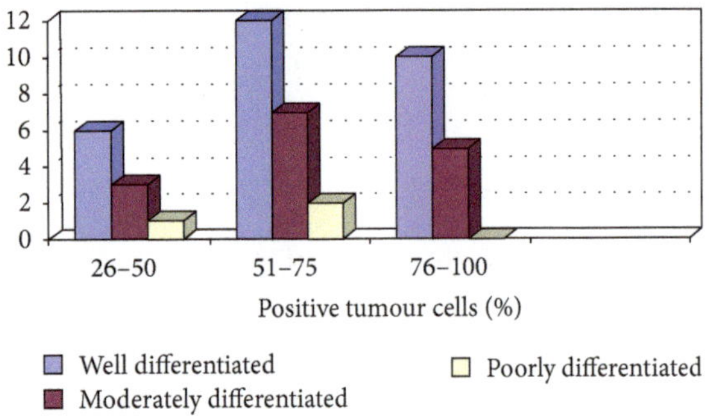

FIGURE 4: Comparison between histological grade and proportion of positive tumour cells.

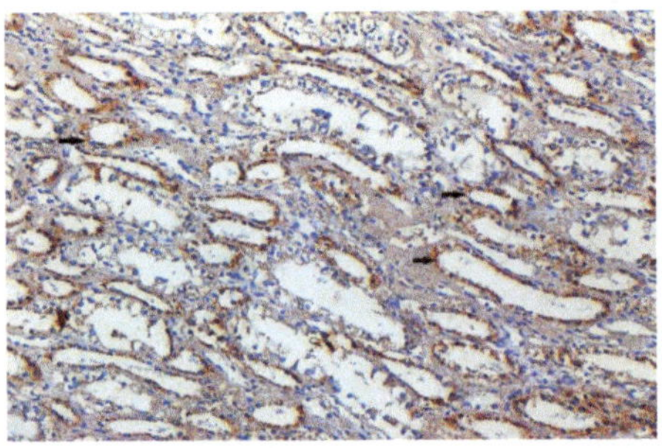

FIGURE 5: Human kidney tubules (control tissue) lining epithelial cells IHC staining (EP3 IHC, 20x).

intensity score, 35.4% cases showing (+4) proportion score for EP3 antibody (Figures 10, 12, 14 and 16).

4. Discussion

The likelihood of developing oral SCC increases with the period of exposure to risk factors and increasing age adds to the dimension of the mutagenic and epigenetic changes associated with age. In the present study 1.4 : 1 male to female ratio was noted, showing male predominance. The overall mean age was 52.74±14.14. These findings are consistent with certain European studies which reported male predominance in patients of OSCC [17]. Most of local studies from Pakistan also reported male predominance [18, 19]. A morphological study of OSCC carried out in Pakistan by Ayaz et al. also reported 1.5 : 1 male to female ratio with 53 (SD ± 15.16) years of mean age of incidence [20]. The exception to gender related findings of this present study is a study from Lahore which reported female predominance with a ratio of 1.5 : 1 [21]. Another study carried out in India on 80 cases of OSCC reported a prevalence of cancer in 61.25% of males [22] and Yazdi and Khalili in their study in Iran on 48 cases of OSCC of tongue also reported male prevalence of 60.4%. The present study is also consistent with both of these studies. The high proportion of cases among men may be due to the high prevalence of snuff consumption habits in them, combined with cigarette smoking, whereas in our society females less commonly indulge in tobacco smoking [23].

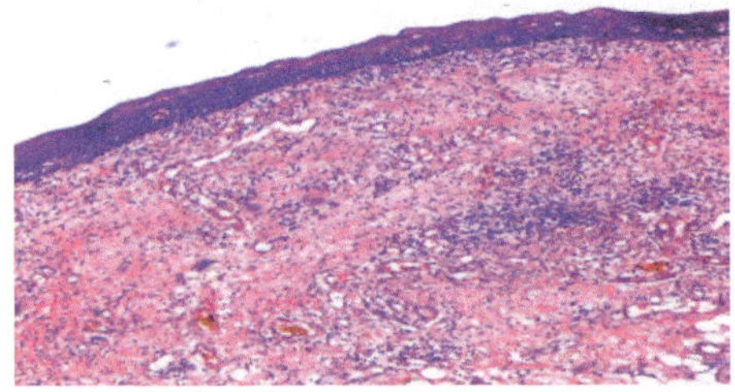

FIGURE 6: Oral epithelium with atrophy of rete ridges and inflammatory infiltrate in underlying connective tissue (H&E, 10x).

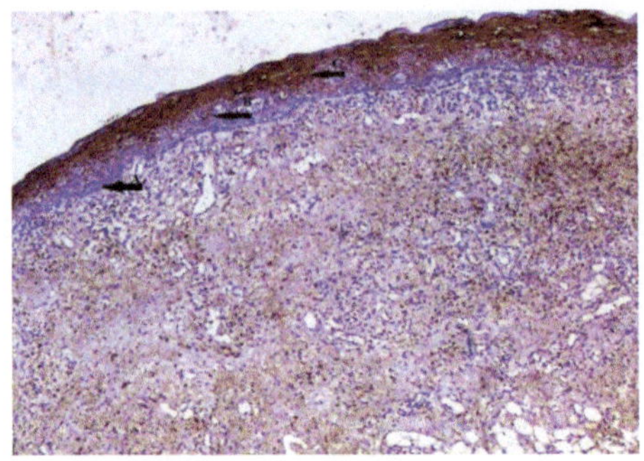

FIGURE 7: Oral epithelium showing differing staining intensity: (↑A) basal epithelial cells negative staining, (↑B) moderate, and (↑C) strong (EP3 IHC, 10x).

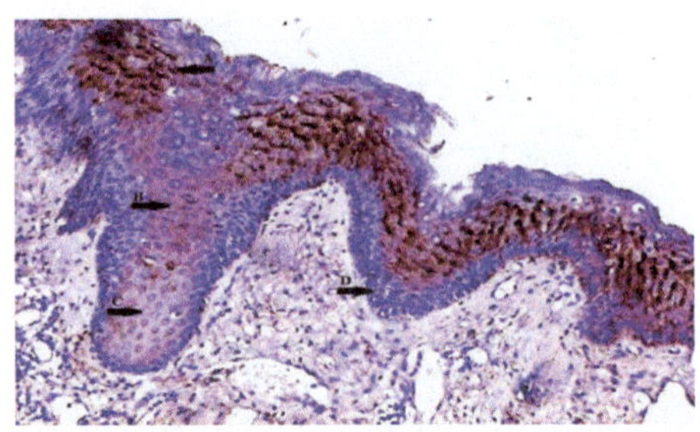

FIGURE 8: Normal oral epithelium showing differing staining intensity: (↑A) strong, (↑B) moderate, (↑C) weak, and (↑D) basal epithelial cells negative staining (EP3 IHC, 20x).

Considering the site of involvement in the oral cavity, the occurrence of OSCC was significantly higher on buccal mucosa where 23 (50%) cases were present followed by 13 (28.3%) cases that involved the tongue (mostly lateral border of tongue). A study by Tahir et al. on OSCC reported results which were similar to the present study regarding the site of involvement. The most frequent location of OSCC in that study was also buccal mucosa (32.4%) (slightly higher in the present study which was 50%) followed by tongue (21.6%); this value is also comparable to the present study (28.3%) [24]. Many studies carried out in the USA and Europe reported quite different findings. In Western countries OSCC involves the tongue in 20%–40% of cases and the floor of the mouth in 15%–20% of the cases, and together these sites represent

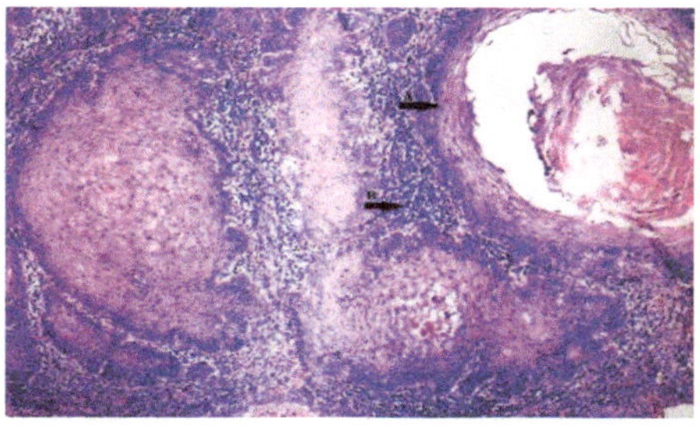

FIGURE 9: Photomicrograph of well differentiated OSCC: (↑A) keratin pearl, (↑B) intense inflammatory infiltrate (H&E, 20x).

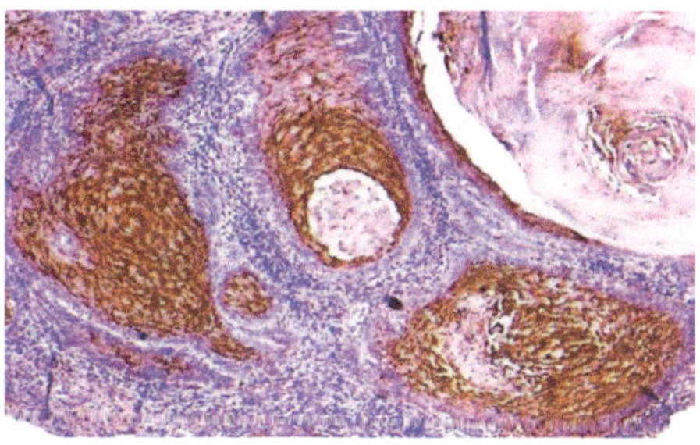

FIGURE 10: Photomicrograph of well differentiated OSCC showing strong intensity of staining (EP3 IHC, 20x).

approximately 50% of all cases of OSCC. The gums, palate, retromolar area, and the buccal and labial mucosa are oral sites affected less frequently [4, 25, 26].

Tumours can grow to a size that exceeds its blood supply, leading to tumour necrosis and ulceration. In the present study the most frequent presenting symptom was ulcerating lesion on buccal mucosa ($P = 0.049$). This is comparable to another study carried out in Pakistan in the recent past in which the most common clinical presentation of OSCC was a nonhealing indurated ulcer (51.4%) and it was also significantly common on the buccal mucosa ($P = 0.001$) [24]. Another study carried out in Canada by Mirbod and his coworker also reported that ulceration was the most common finding in OSCC patients; this finding is consistent with the present study [27].

In the current study out of 46 cases, lymphovascular invasion was found in 33 (71.7%) while 13 cases showed no lymphovascular invasion. In another study carried out in Japan Nomura et al. reported 57.5% lymphovascular invasion in cases of OSCC, which is slightly lower than the present study [28]. In the present study, among all the 46 cases of OSCC, 31 had attached nontumorous epithelium. Adjacent epithelium showed reactivity of varying intensity and proportion in all of these 31 cases of OSCC with attached epithelium in the present study. A few studies carried out in Japan reported that EP3 receptor is extensively expressed in all the human body organ systems. More or less all tissues in mice and rats express its mRNA [8]. Shoji and his associates also reported that EP3 receptors may play a vital role in skin carcinogenesis. They demonstrated this fact in EP3 receptors knockout mice by observing two-stage skin carcinogenesis [29]. All these studies validate our findings that squamous

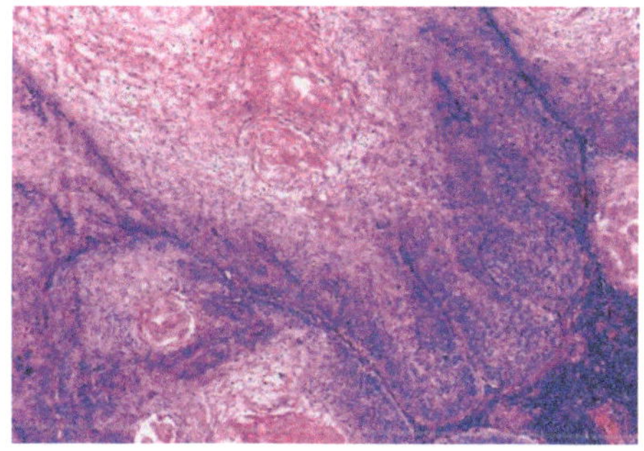

FIGURE 11: Verrucous variant of SCC with tonguelike projections, abundant keratinization, and mild degree of lymphocytic infiltrate (H&E, 20x).

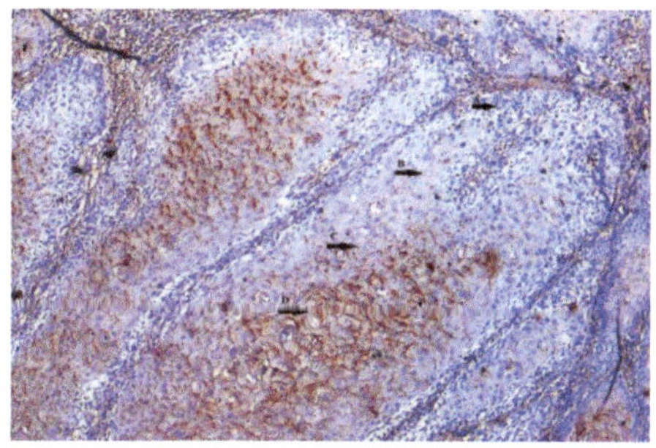

FIGURE 12: Photomicrograph of verrucous variant of OSCC showing differing staining intensity: (↑A) negative, (↑B) weak, (↑C) moderate, and (↑D) strong (EP3 IHC, 20x).

epithelium expresses the EP3 receptors normally. Similarly, in present study, all 46 cases of OSCC were variably positive for EP3 receptor antibody. As shown in Results, the number of cases showing weak intensity of EP3 antibody staining in attached epithelium was 3 (6.5%) while the number of cases showing weak intensity in tumorous tissue was 15 (32.6%) in the present study which is five times higher frequency of intensity of EP3 staining in tumorous tissue than frequency in attached epithelium. This difference in intensity of EP3 antibody staining in both of these tissues is statistically significant ($P = 0.042$). This finding suggests that as the squamous epithelial cell becomes less differentiated it loses its ability to express prostanoid EP3 receptors. This was also observed during the histological examination of OSCC cases stained with EP3 antibody: as the squamous cell is more differentiated it shows more intense staining and as the cell gradually loses its differentiation, it also loses its property to express prostanoid EP3 receptors and the intensity of staining with EP3 antibody becomes weak. When we applied Fisher's exact test to observe the statistical relation between intensity of antibody staining and histological grade of OSCC, it was found to be insignificant ($P = 0.486$), because overall intensity of staining was randomly distributed among different grades of OSCC.

A similar study carried out in Brazil by Ryott et al. reported that 94% of cases of OSCC were positive for EP3 receptor antibody and most of the cases in that study were of moderately differentiated histological grade [15]. While

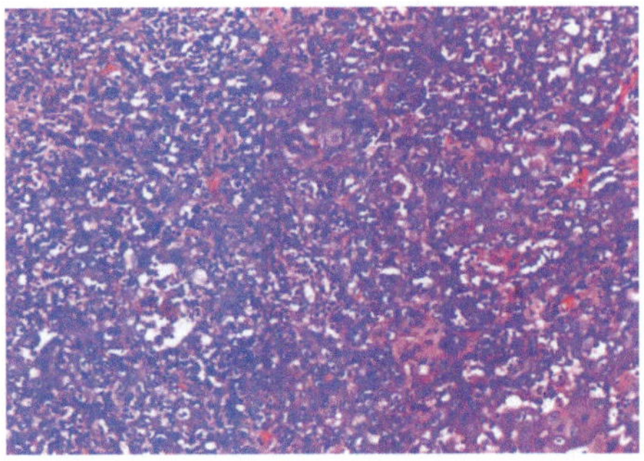

FIGURE 13: Photomicrograph of moderately differentiated OSCC (H&E, 20x).

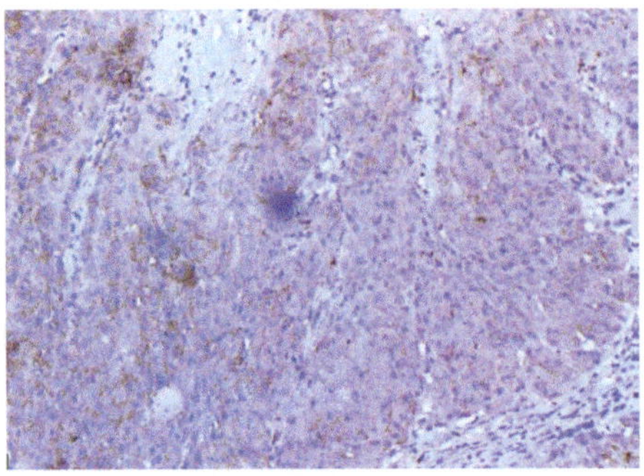

FIGURE 14: Photomicrograph of moderately differentiated OSCC showing weak to moderate intensity of staining (EP3 IHC, 20x).

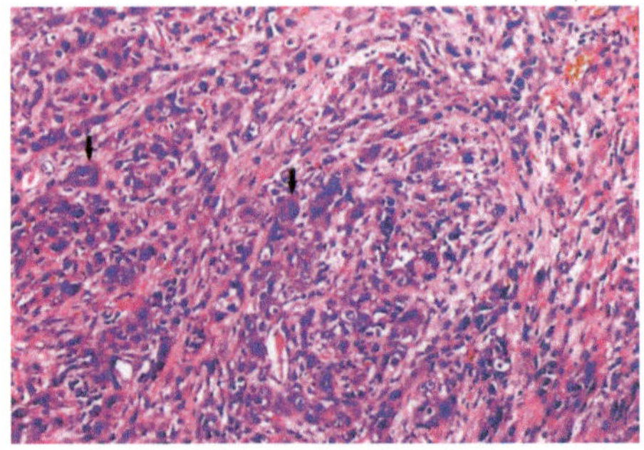

FIGURE 15: Photomicrograph of poorly differentiated OSCC with high degree of cytological and nuclear pleomorphism (↑) (H&E, 20x).

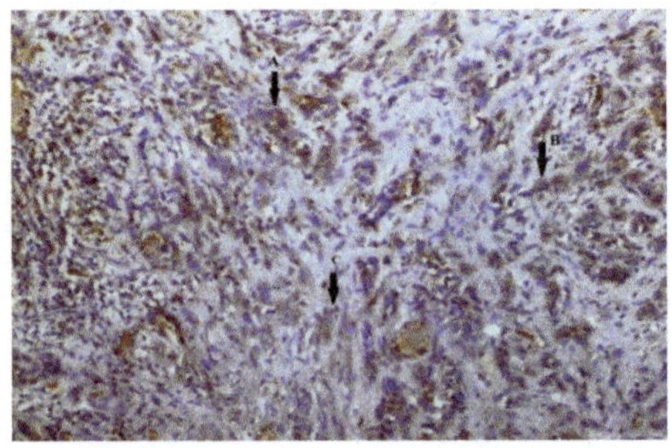

FIGURE 16: Photomicrograph of poorly differentiated OSCC showing weak intensity of staining (EP3 IHC, 20x).

in lung and colon carcinogenesis the role of prostaglandin E2 receptors is well established by many researches, a small number of studies have assessed their involvement in HNSCC and described that EP3 and EP4 receptors were expressed in cancer cell lines but Very weak EP1 and EP2 receptors expression was noticed [30]. Hoshikawa et al. also showed antiproliferative effects of EP3 receptor signalling pathway in cancer lines and EP3 receptor antagonist decreases the PGE2 level in vitro and stops the cell cycle in Go/G1 phase of cell cycle [31]. The growth and proliferation of head and neck squamous cell carcinoma cells were shown to reduce by the application of EP3 receptor antagonists [31].

Knowledge of the molecular mechanisms underlying dysregulated growth and progression of OSCC may provide a rational basis for exploring new treatment modalities and can prove valuable in the development of new molecular therapies and targeting tools. Since PGE2 is likely to pile up at high levels in the tumour microenvironment and can be produced by the action of the COX-2 expressed in both cancer and stromal cells [15], PGE2 may play an important role in OSCC carcinogenesis via acting on EP3 receptors. Prostaglandin E2 can also play a vital role in increasing the proliferative capability of OSCC cell lines. As depicted from these studies, targeted therapies against prostaglandin E2 and EP receptors may represent valuable adjuvant modalities in treatment of the initial phases of development of OSCC.

To our knowledge no such documented immunohistochemical study elaborating the role of prostanoid receptor EP3 in OSCC has been carried in Pakistan or any other South Asian country so there is a lack of data comparison in this aspect. Further studies on large sample size are now needed to elucidate the underlying molecular and genetic mechanisms to assess the tumour related effects of PGE2 and its receptors in vivo. This area of future research undoubtedly will further improve our understanding of carcinogenesis of OSCC and the role played by EP3 receptors and prostaglandin E2.

5. Conclusion

Prostanoid EP3 receptors are widely but variably expressed in OSCC. Most of well differentiated OSCC cases show a moderate to strong expression of EP3 receptors (Figure 10). However insignificant statistical relation to histological grades of OSCC has been observed. This might be due to small sample size of the study. By acting on EP3 receptors expressed on OSCC cells, PGE2 may contribute to increase of OSCC cell proliferative potential. In this regard, PGE2 blocking therapies, as well as EP3-specific treatment modalities, may represent helpful approaches as adjuvants in OSCC treatment for patients at the initial stages of OSCC development. Immunohistochemical findings of the present study may predict that expression of EP3 receptors in OSCC may play a significant role in the carcinogenic progression of squamous epithelial cells. Further studies are needed on a larger sample size that may focus on molecular and genetic pathways to completely define the role of PGE2 receptors in oral carcinogenesis.

Conflict of Interests

The authors declare that they have no conflict of interests regarding the publication of this paper.

Acknowledgments

The authors acknowledge the encouragement extended by the Vice-Chancellor of UHS, laboratory staff of Histopathology Department, and all the staff of Maxillofacial Surgery Department of NID for their technical and logistic support.

References

[1] V. A. Papadimitrakopoulou, J. J. Lee, W. N. William Jr. et al., "Randomized trial of 13-cis retinoic acid compared with retinyl palmitate with or without beta-carotene in oral premalignancy," *Journal of Clinical Oncology*, vol. 27, no. 4, pp. 599–604, 2009.

[2] C. Scully and J. Bagan, "Oral squamous cell carcinoma overview," *Oral Oncology*, vol. 45, no. 4-5, pp. 301–308, 2009.

[3] B. W. Neville, D. O. Darnrn, C. M. Allen, and J. Bouqout, *Oral and Maxillofacial Pathology*, Saunders, Philadelphia, Pa, USA, 3rd edition, 2009.

[4] J. Bagan, G. Sarrion, and Y. Jimenez, "Oral cancer: clinical features," *Oral Oncology*, vol. 46, no. 6, pp. 414–417, 2010.

[5] J. Califano, P. van der Riet, W. Westra et al., "Genetic progression model for head and neck cancer: implications for field cancerization," *Cancer Research*, vol. 56, no. 11, pp. 2488–2492, 1996.

[6] D. Marsh, K. Suchak, K. A. Moutasim et al., "Stromal features are predictive of disease mortality in oral cancer patients," *The Journal of Pathology*, vol. 223, no. 4, pp. 470–481, 2011.

[7] H. Hamakawa, K.-I. Nakashiro, T. Sumida et al., "Basic evidence of molecular targeted therapy for oral cancer and salivary gland cancer," *Head & Neck*, vol. 30, no. 6, pp. 800–809, 2008.

[8] S. Narumiya, Y. Sugimoto, and F. Ushikubi, "Prostanoid receptors: structures, properties, and functions," *Physiological Reviews*, vol. 79, no. 4, pp. 1193–1226, 1999.

[9] R. A. Gupta and R. N. DuBois, "Colorectal cancer prevention and treatment by inhibition of cyclooxygenase-2," *Nature Reviews Cancer*, vol. 1, no. 1, pp. 11–21, 2001.

[10] T. F. Imperiale, "Aspirin and the prevention of colorectal cancer," *The New England Journal of Medicine*, vol. 348, no. 10, pp. 879–880, 2003.

[11] M. J. Thun, M. M. Namboodiri, and C. W. Heath Jr., "Aspirin use and reduced risk of fatal colon cancer," *The New England Journal of Medicine*, vol. 325, no. 23, pp. 1593–1596, 1991.

[12] A. Zarghi and S. Arfaei, "Selective COX-2 inhibitors: a review of their structure-activity relationships," *Iranian Journal of Pharmaceutical Research*, vol. 10, no. 4, pp. 655–683, 2011.

[13] M. Akhter, S. Hossain, Q. Rahman, and M. Molla, "A study on histological grading of oral squamous cell carcinoma and its co-relationship with regional metastasis," *Journal of Oral and Maxillofacial Pathology*, vol. 15, no. 2, pp. 168–176, 2011.

[14] *Anti-PTGER3 antibody: ab115667*, ABCAM, Cambridge, Mass, USA, 2013, http://www.abcam.com/ptger3-antibody-ab11 5667.html.

[15] M. Ryott, L. Marklund, D. Wangsa, G. Elmberger, and E. Munck-Wikland, "Cyclooxygenase-2 expression in oral tongue squamous cell carcinoma," *Journal of Oral Pathology and Medicine*, vol. 40, no. 5, pp. 385–389, 2011.

[16] A. C. Abrahao, R. M. Castilho, C. H. Squarize, A. A. Molinolo, D. D. Santos-Pinto Jr., and J. S. Gutkind, "A role for COX2-derived PGE2 and PGE2-receptor subtypes in head and neck squamous carcinoma cell proliferation," *Oral Oncology*, vol. 46, no. 12, pp. 880–887, 2010.

[17] C. L. B. Lavelle and C. Scully, "Criteria to rationalize population screening to control oral cancer," *Oral Oncology*, vol. 41, no. 1, pp. 11–16, 2005.

[18] J. S. Isaac, N. R. Qureshi, and U. Isaac, "Report on oral cancers patients at atomic energy medical center, Jamshoro during the year 2002: a pilot study," *Journal of Pakistan Dental Association*, vol. 12, no. 3, pp. 176–178, 2003.

[19] M. Alamgir, Q. Jamal, N. A. Jafarey, and T. Mirza, "Clinico-pathological parameters of 50 oral squamous cell carcinoma cases in Karachi," *Pakistan Journal of Medicine and Dentistry*, vol. 2, no. 2, pp. 3–8, 2013.

[20] B. Ayaz, K. Saleem, W. Azim, and A. Shaikh, "A clinicopathological study of oral cancers," *Biomedica*, vol. 27, pp. 29–32, 2011.

[21] M. Ali, A. H. Bhatti, M. Tariq et al., "An epidemiological study of 202 cases of oral cavity cancer (OCC) in Pakistani subjects," *Biomedica*, vol. 14, pp. 27–31, 1998.

[22] S. P. Khandelkarl and P. S. Bagdey, "Oral cancer and some emiological factors: a hospital based study," *Indian Journal of Community Medicine*, vol. 31, no. 3, pp. 157–162, 2006.

[23] D. Yazdi and M. Khalili, "Grading of oral cancer: comparison of different systems with respect to lymph n ode metastasis in tongue SCC," Original Article, http://www.ams.ac.ir/AIM/9922/yazdi9922.html.

[24] A. Tahir, A. H. Nagi, E. Ullah, and O. S. Janjua, "The role of mast cells and angiogenesis in well-differentiated oral squamous cell carcinoma," *Journal of Cancer Research and Therapeutics*, vol. 9, no. 3, pp. 387–391, 2013.

[25] S. Warnakulasuriya, "Causes of oral cancer—an appraisal of controversies," *British Dental Journal*, vol. 207, no. 10, pp. 471–475, 2009.

[26] I. O. Bello, Y. Soini, and T. Salo, "Prognostic evaluation of oral tongue cancer: means, markers and perspectives (I)," *Oral Oncology*, vol. 46, no. 9, pp. 630–635, 2010.

[27] S. M. Mirbod and S. I. Ahing, "Tobacco-associated lesions of the oral cavity: part II. Malignant lesions," *Journal of the Canadian Dental Association*, vol. 66, pp. 308–311, 2000.

[28] H. Nomura, K. Uzawa, Y. Yamano et al., "Overexpression and altered subcellular localization of autophagy-related 16-like 1 in human oral squamous-cell carcinoma: correlation with lymphovascular invasion and lymph-node metastasis," *Human Pathology*, vol. 40, no. 1, pp. 83–91, 2009.

[29] Y. Shoji, M. Takahashi, N. Takasuka et al., "Prostaglandin E receptor EP_3 deficiency modifies tumor outcome in mouse two-stage skin carcinogenesis," *Carcinogenesis*, vol. 26, no. 12, pp. 2116–2122, 2005.

[30] R. T. Dorsam and J. S. Gutkind, "G-protein-coupled receptors and cancer," *Nature Reviews Cancer*, vol. 7, no. 2, pp. 79–94, 2007.

[31] H. Hoshikawa, R. Goto, T. Mori, T. Mitani, and N. Mori, "Expression of prostaglandin E2 receptors in oral squamous cell carcinomas and growth inhibitory effects of an EP3 selective antagonist, ONO-AE3-240," *International Journal of Oncology*, vol. 34, no. 3, pp. 847–852, 2009.

11

Comparative Study of Cytomorphological Robinson's Grading for Breast Carcinoma with Modified Bloom-Richardson Histopathological Grading

Neelam Sood, Jitendra Singh Nigam, Poonam Yadav, Shivani Rewri, Ankit Sharma, Anita Omhare, and Jaya Malhotra

Department of Pathology, D.D.U. Hospital, Harinagar, New Delhi 110066, India

Correspondence should be addressed to Jitendra Singh Nigam; nigamjs@gmail.com

Academic Editor: Luigi M. Terracciano

Objective. To study the correlation of cytomorphological Robinson's grading for breast cancers with a modified Bloom-Richardson histopathological grading. *Materials and Methods.* One hundred sixteen cytologically malignant breast tumour cases were included in this study and correlated with paraffin embedded sections. Breast lumps were varied from less than 1 cm to 11 cm in greatest dimension. FNA was performed from different sites of the breast lump, and smears were stained with Giemsa and H&E stain and evaluated for cytological grading according to Robinson's grading system. Paraffin embedded tissue sections were stained with hematoxylin and eosin stain and graded according to modified Bloom-Richardson grading system. Comparison between these two grading systems was done. *Results.* Cytologically grade I, grade II, and grade III cases were 13.8%, 64.65%, and 21.55%, respectively. Histologically 25%, 54.31%, and 20.69% cases were grade I, grade II, and grade III, respectively. Concordance rate between cytology and histology of grade I, grade II, and grade III tumors was 75%, 70.67%, and 60% respectively. The absolute concordance rate was 68.97%. *Conclusion.* In the era of multiple treatment modalities and neoadjuvant therapy, cytological grading can be used as a prognostic factor for better management of patients.

1. Introduction

Breast cancer is the commonest cancer in urban Indian women and the second commonest cancer in the rural women next to cervical carcinoma. Due to general indifference towards the health of females in the Indian society, lack of an organized breast cancer screening program, and paucity of diagnostic aids, majority of breast cancers are diagnosed at a relatively advanced stage [1]. Since last decade, cytodiagnosis has gained importance due to rapid results at low cost and may help in early diagnosis in country like India. FNAB is a reliable method for the initial evaluation and diagnosis of palpable masses of the breast. In addition, it also has the ability of providing necessary prognostic/predictive information, particularly for patients that may undergo neoadjuvant therapy [2]. The standard prognostic factors, recognized by the National Cancer Institute in 1990, include lymph node status, tumor size, nuclear grade, steroid receptor content, tumor type, and cellular proliferation rate and recommend that for patients who undergo preoperative chemotherapy or radiotherapy, breast fine-needle aspirates can be used to provide prognostic information [3]. The grading of breast cancer on fine-needle aspiration help in understanding of the biology of the disease, to predict the outcome, select the appropriate treatment modality, explain variations in treatment outcome, plan specific therapeutic interventions, and, occasionally, alleviate patient anxiety [3]. Elston's modified Bloom and Richardson method is a widely accepted tumor grading system and has been found to have good prognostic correlations [4]. Histological grade forms part of the multifactorial Nottingham prognostic index, together with tumour size and lymph node stage and used to stratify individual patients for appropriate therapy [4]. Various studies correlate the cytological grading with Elston's modified Bloom and Richardson method. Robinson's cytological grading (RCG) to correlate with Elston's modified Bloom and Richardson

TABLE 1: Cytological features on FNAC grading and histological grading.

	Cytological features on FNAC grading			Cytological features on histological grading		
	Grade I	Grade II	Grade III	Grade I	Grade II	Grade III
Cell dissociation						
Mostly clusters	2	2		2	18	
Single cells and clusters	12	71	20	21	44	15
Mostly single cells	2	2	5	6	1	9
Nuclear size						
1-2x RBC	5			7	10	2
3-4x RBC	11	50	3	21	48	5
5x or more RBC		25	22	1	5	17
Cell uniformity						
Monomorphic	9			8	10	2
Mildly pleomorphic	7	45		20	48	5
Pleomorphic		30	25	1	5	17
Nucleoli						
Indistinct/small	12	19		14	20	3
Noticeable	4	51	14	13	39	8
Abnormal		5	11	2	4	13
Nuclear margin						
Smooth	8			8	10	2
Slightly irregular/folds and grooves	8	67	19	20	50	9
Buds and clefts		8	6	1	3	13
Chromatin pattern						
Vesicular	9	3		10	12	2
Granular	7	70	20	19	48	7
Clumping and clearing		2	5		3	15
Total cases	16	75	25	29	63	24

method because of better concordance rate than other cytological grading systems. Also RCG has more objective set of criteria and easy reproducibility [5–7].

In present study, Robinson's cytological grading was done on cytology and compared with modified Bloom-Richardson system on paraffin embedded sections.

2. Materials and Methods

One hundred sixteen cytologically malignant breast tumour cases were included in this study and correlated with paraffin embedded sections. Breast lumps were varied from less than 1 cm to 11 cm in greatest dimension. 60 cases were in left breast, and 56 cases, in right breast with commonest age group were 56 to 60 years. 54 cases were premenopausal, and 62 cases were postmenopausal. FNA was performed from different sites of the breast lump using a 10 mL disposable syringe and 22/23-gauge needle without local anesthesia. FNA smears were stained with Giemsa and H&E stain and evaluated for cytological grading according to Robinson's grading system. Paraffin embedded tissue sections obtained from mastectomy specimens were stained with hematoxylin and eosin stain and graded according Elston-Ellis modification of Bloom-Richardson grading system. Comparison between these two grading systems was, done and concordance rates between each grade were calculated separately, and absolute concordance was calculated between all three corresponding grades. Kappa coefficient was used to compare the agreement for each grade.

3. Results

All cases were graded cytologically and histologically using cytologic Robinson's grading system and modified bloom-Richardson histologic grading system, respectively. Comparison between both grading systems was done. The details of all cytological features are evaluated according to histological grading, and cytological grading is shown in Table 1. In this study, 13.8%, 64.65%, 21.55% cases were cytologically grade I (Figure 1(a)), grade II (Figure 1(c)), and grade III (Figure 2(a)) respectively. Histologically 25%, 54.31%, 20.69% cases were grade I (Figure 1(b)), grade II (Figure 1(d)), and grade III (Figure 2(b)), respectively. Concordance rate between grade I tumors in cytology and histology was 75%, for grade II tumors, it was 70.67%, and for grade III tumors it was 60%. The absolute concordance rate between all three corresponding grades was 68.97% (Table 2).

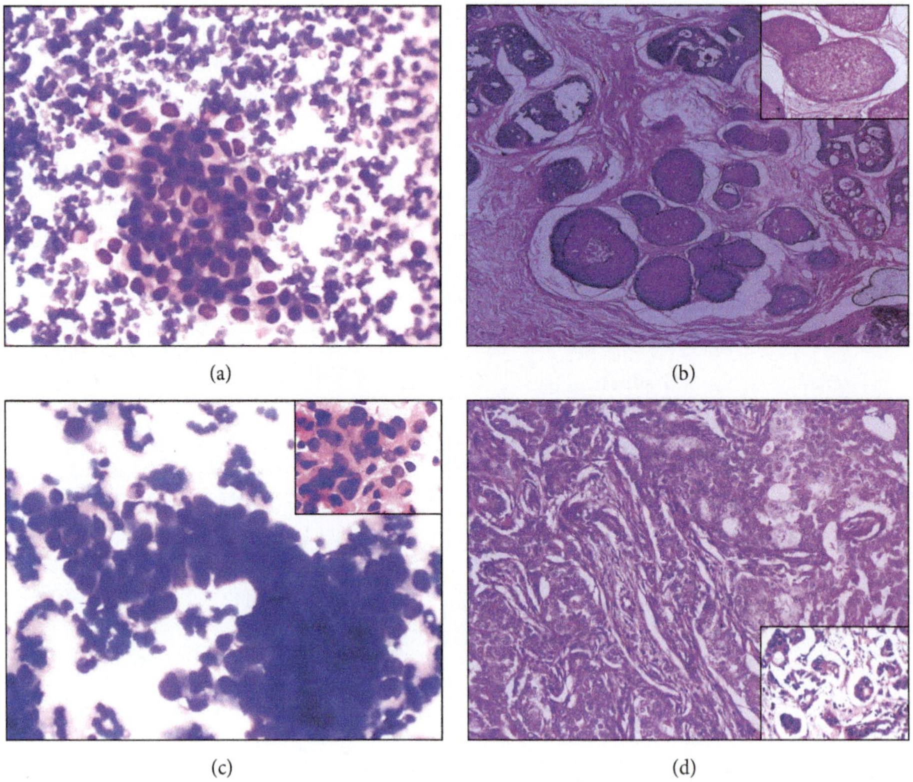

FIGURE 1: (a) Loosely cohesive cluster of mild pleomorphic ductal cells with smooth nuclear membrane and indistinct nucleoli—cytologic grade I (Giemsa ×400). (b) Invasive breast carcinoma with tubular/glandular differentiation, little increase in size, regular outlines, and uniform nuclear chromatin—histological grade I (H&E ×100, inset, H&E ×400). (c) Loosely cohesive cluster as well as single cells with moderate pleomorphism, slightly irregular nuclear membrane, and noticeable nucleoli. Nuclei are three to four times the erythrocytes—cytologic grade II (Giemsa ×400) (inset, H&E ×1000). (d) Invasive breast carcinoma with cords, islands with tubular differentiation, moderate variability in size and shape, open vesicular nuclei, and visible nucleoli—histological grade II (H&E ×100, inset, H&E ×400).

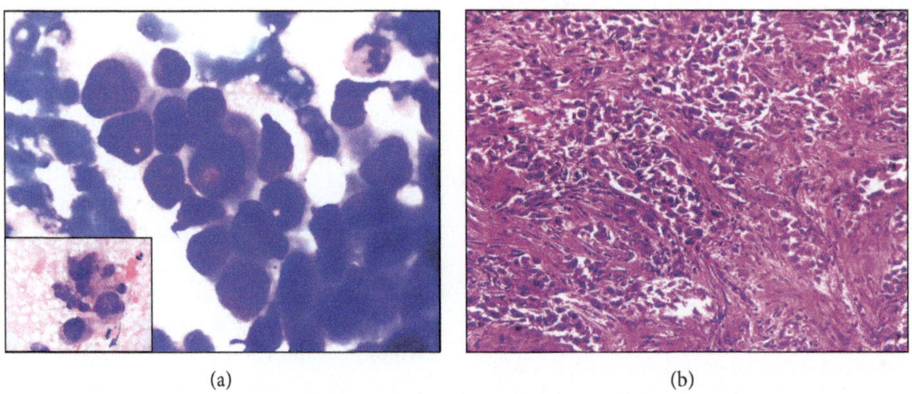

FIGURE 2: (a) Markedly pleomorphic ductal cells irregular nuclear margin and prominent nucleoli, coarse chromatin, and mitosis—cytologic grade III (Giemsa ×1000) (inset, H&E ×1000). (b) Invasive breast carcinoma infiltrative islands, with minimal tubular differentiation, marked variability in size and shape, open vesicular nuclei, visible nucleoli, and mitosis is seen histological grade III (H&E ×400).

Discordance between cytological and histological grading was seen in 36 (31.03%) cases only. Most mismatching cases were seen in tumour size ranging from 2 cm to 5 cm (Table 3), and most the common age group was 36–60 years (58.33%) followed by 25–35 years (27.78%). 79 cases were of borderline cytological scoring, that is, scoring between 11 and 12 and between 14 and 15. Sixteen cases with discordance belonged to borderline cytological grades.

The kappa statistics was done to measure the strength of agreement between cytological and histologic grades. Kappa value for grade I tumors, grade II, and grade III tumors was 0.43, 0.43, and 0.51, respectively which indicates

TABLE 2: Comparison of Robinson's cytological grading with modified Bloom-Richardson grade.

		Histological grading			Concordance rate
		Grade I	Grade II	Grade III	
Cytological grading	Grade I	12	3	1	75%
	Grade II	14	53	8	70.67%
	Grade III	3	7	15	60%
		Absolute concordance rate			68.97%

TABLE 3: Cytological and histological grading with tumour size.

Tumour size	FNAC grading			Histological grade		
	Grade I	Grade II	Grade III	Grade I	Grade II	Grade III
1-2 cm	6	15	3	8	13	2
2–5 cm	8	42	14	16	38	9
5 cm or more	2	18	8	5	12	11

moderate agreement between cytological and histological grading systems.

The nuclear features of histology mirrored the cytological grading. Cytological grading of histology of grade I showed 22 cases of grade I, 6 cases of grade II, and one case of grade III. On cytological grading of histology grade II, cytological features of grade III were seen in 9 cases and 3 cases of cytological grade I. On cytological grading of histology grade III, cytological features of grade II were seen in 7 cases, and cytological features of grade I were seen in one case.

4. Discussion

A palpable breast lump is a common clinical problem that is presented to surgeons, gynaecologists, and general practitioners and a multidisciplinary approach based on the "triple test," analyzing clinical and radiologic findings in conjunction with the pathologic features to diagnose the lesion and determine the best treatment plan for the patient [8]. Preoperative biopsy is also used for hormone receptor analysis and for the evaluation of other prognostic parameters by various ancillary techniques [8]. There are many cytologic grading systems for breast carcinoma, and they have good correlation with Elston-Ellis grading system. Because of more sensitivity, simplicity, more objective set of criteria and easy reproducibility, Robinson's method was considered better than the other methods [5–7, 9]. The concordance rate of histological and cytological grading was ranging from 56.9% to 89.1% [9]. In the present study, absolute concordance rate was 68.97% and observed predominance of grade II tumours, which is in corroboration with previous studies by Khan et al. [10], Das et al. [11], and Wani et al. [6, 12], Yu et al. correlated the Robinson's cytological grading with Bloom-Richardson's histopathological grading in 59 cases and observed substantial strength of agreement for grade I and grade II tumours with nearly perfect concordance in grade III tumours between cytology and histopathology [13]. In the present study, Highest of discordance was observed in grade III tumours followed by grade II and grade I. Discordance may be due to subjectivity when assessing cytological features that are not included in histological grading. Yu et al. observed discordance between cytological and histological grading due to difficulties in detecting mitoses or tubules in the cytology of breast carcinoma while nuclear features have contributed more to cytological grading which is one of the criteria in histopathological grading [14]. The extent of tubule formation, number of mitotic figures and degree of nuclear pleomorphism are the important factors of MBR histological grading systems but several features like nuclear margin, chromatin pattern and nucleoli that are included in cytological grading are not of much importance in histopathological grading [5]. Cangiarella and Simsir observed that cytological features, dissociation, cell size, cell uniformity, nucleoli, nuclear margin, and chromatin show a strong correlation with cytological grade and found that cell dissociation, cell uniformity, and nucleoli are the most influential features [7]. The features like cellular arrangement, degree of cellular pleomorphism, degree of nuclear pleomorphism, and absence of myoepithelial cells are important to diagnose carcinoma on histopathology [5]. The degree of cell dissociation indicates cell cohesion status, to an extent, and the degree of expression of the E-cadherin/catenin complex. Several studies showed that neoplasm with greater cell dissociation shows a higher incidence of regional lymph node metastasis [15–17]. Cytological grading before surgery is important because preoperative neoadjuvant chemotherapy is becoming common for the treatment of breast cancer and helps in the selection of appropriate regime [17]. The cytological prognostic grading system helps in identifying fast growing tumors (grade III), which are more likely to respond to chemotherapy than the low grade tumors; slow growing tumors may be better suited to pretreatment with Tamoxifen [18]. The high accuracy rate, rapid diagnosis, negligible risk of tumor spread, minimal subjective discomfort, insignificant complications, and utility for multiple lesions of FNAC; FNAC grading is compared with histology grading and is useful in assessing the tumor behaviour and prognosis and guiding neo adjuvant chemotherapy. Various attempts have been made to determine various prognostic parameters on FNA materials [9]. The National Cancer Institute (NCI), Bethesda, MD, USA, sponsored conference had also recommended that tumor grading on FNA material should be incorporated in FNA reports for prognostication [16].

5. Conclusion

In the era of multiple treatment modalities and neoadjuvant therapy, cytological grading helps in evaluating the aggressiveness of tumour, neo adjuvant chemotherapy and can be used as a prognostic factor for better management of patients.

Disclosure

On behalf of all the contributors, Jitendra Singh Nigam will act and guarantor as will correspond with the journal from this point onward. The authors hereby transfer, assign, or otherwise convey all copyright ownership, including any and all rights incidental thereto, exclusively to the journal, in the event that such work is published by the journal.

Conflict of Interests

The authors declare that they have no conflict of interests.

References

[1] G. Agarwal and P. Ramakant, "Breast cancer care in India: the current scenario and the challenges for the future," *Breast Care*, vol. 3, no. 1, pp. 21–27, 2008.

[2] M. Rosa, A. Mohammadi, and S. Masood, "The value of fine needle aspiration biopsy in the diagnosis and prognostic assessment of palpable breast lesions," *Diagnostic Cytopathology*, vol. 40, no. 1, pp. 26–34, 2012.

[3] S. Masood, "Assessment of prognostic factor in breast FNA," *American Journal of Clinical Pathology*, vol. 113, supplement 1, pp. s84–s96, 2000.

[4] C. W. Elston and I. O. Ellis, "Pathological prognostic factors in breast cancer. I. The value of histological grade in breast cancer: experience from a large study with long-term follow-up," *Histopathology*, vol. 19, no. 5, pp. 403–410, 1991.

[5] T. S. Rekha, N. M. Nandini, and M. Dhar, "Validity of different cytological grading systems of breast carcinoma-a hospital-based study in South India," *Asian Pacific Journal of Cancer Prevention*, vol. 12, no. 11, pp. 3013–3016, 2011.

[6] F. A. Wani, S. Bhardwaj, D. Kumar, and P. Katoch, "Cytological grading of breast cancers and comparative evaluation of two grading systems," *Journal of Cytology*, vol. 27, no. 2, pp. 55–58, 2010.

[7] J. Cangiarella and A. Simsir, "Breast," in *Orell & Sterrett's Fine Needle Aspiration Cytology*, S. R. Orell and G. F. Sterrett, Eds., pp. 156–161, Churchill Livingstone, Philadelphia, Pa, USA; Elsevier Limited, Beijing, China, 5th edition, 2012.

[8] A. K. Das, K. Kapila, A. K. Dinda, and K. Verma, "Comparative evaluation of grading of breast carcinomas in fine needle aspirates by two methods," *Indian Journal of Medical Research*, vol. 118, pp. 247–250, 2003.

[9] A. N. Pandya and N. P. Shah, "Comparative evaluation of Robinson's cytological grading with Elston and Ellis' Nottingham modification of bloom Richardson histopathology grading for breast carcinoma," *National Journal of Community Medicine*, vol. 3, no. 3, pp. 491–495, 2012.

[10] N. Khan, N. Afroz, F. Rana, and M. A. Khan, "Role of cytologic grading in prognostication of invasive breast carcinoma," *Journal of Cytology*, vol. 26, no. 2, pp. 65–68, 2009.

[11] S. Das, Kalyani, and H. Kumar, "Breast carcinoma aspirates: a study on cytological grading," *International Journal of Basic and Applied Medical Sciences*, vol. 2, no. 2, pp. 189–195, 2012.

[12] R. Yoshida, N. Kimura, Y. Harada, and N. Ohuchi, "The loss of E-cadherin, alpha- and beta-catenin expression is associated with metastasis and poor prognosis in invasive breast cancer," *International Journal of Oncology*, vol. 18, no. 3, pp. 513–520, 2001.

[13] G. H. Yu, R. S. Cajulis, and D. V. S. De Frias, "Tumor cell (dys)cohesion as a prognostic factor in aspirate smears of breast carcinoma," *American Journal of Clinical Pathology*, vol. 109, no. 3, pp. 315–319, 1998.

[14] G. H. Yu, T. J. Lawton, T. L. Pasha, and C. Reynolds, "Intercellular adhesion molecule expression in ductal carcinoma of the breast: correlation of immunohistochemical staining with cytologic smear pattern," *Diagnostic Cytopathology*, vol. 23, no. 2, pp. 73–76, 2000.

[15] V. Bhargava, M. Jain, K. Agarwal, S. Thomas, and S. Singh, "Critical appraisal of cytological nuclear grading in carcinoma of the breast and its correlation with ER/PR expression," *Journal of Cytology*, vol. 25, no. 2, pp. 58–61, 2008.

[16] A. Abati, J. Abele, S. S. Bacus et al., "The uniform approach to breast fine needle aspiration biopsy," *Diagnostic Cytopathology*, vol. 16, no. 4, pp. 295–311, 1997.

[17] I. A. Robinson, G. McKee, A. Nicholson et al., "Prognostic value of cytological grading of fine-needle aspirates from breast carcinomas," *The Lancet*, vol. 343, no. 8903, pp. 947–949, 1994.

[18] R. L. Katz, "Editorial: a turning point in breast cancer cytology reporting: moving from callowness to maturity," *Acta Cytologica*, vol. 38, no. 6, pp. 881–883, 1994.

12

Cytohistopathological Study of Salivary Gland Lesions in Bundelkhand Region, Uttar Pradesh

Anita Omhare,[1] Sanjeev Kumar Singh,[2] Jitendra Singh Nigam,[3] and Ankit Sharma[4]

[1] *Department of Pathology, GSVM Medical College, Kanpur, Uttar pradesh 208012, India*
[2] *Department of Pathology, M.L.B. Medical College, Jhansi, Uttar Pradesh 284128, India*
[3] *Department of Pathology, Saraswathi Institute of Medical Sciences, Anwarpur, Pilkhuwa, Hapur, Uttar Pradesh 245304, India*
[4] *Department of Pathology, D.D.U. Hospital, Harinagar, New Delhi 110066, India*

Correspondence should be addressed to Jitendra Singh Nigam; nigamjs@gmail.com

Academic Editor: Oscar W. Cummings

Background. FNAC is a useful method for evaluating suspicious salivary glands lesions due to its low cost, minimum morbidity, rapid turnaround time, high specificity, and sensitivity. *Aim.* To know the frequency of the salivary gland lesions and cytohistological correlation in the Jhansi region, Uttar Pradesh, India. *Material and Methods.* In present study 124 cases were included and cytohistological correlation was made in 86 cases only. FNA was performed by using a 23/24-gauge needle without local anaesthesia. Air dried and 95% ethyl alcohol fixed wet smears were stained with Giemsa stain and Papanicolaou stain, respectively. Paraffin embedded tissue sections were stained with Haematoxylin and Eosin. *Results.* Parotid gland was the most commonly involved salivary gland. The commonest age group was 20 to 29 years, 30 to 39 years, and 60 to 69 years for nonneoplastic lesions, benign tumours, and malignant tumours, respectively. The overall male to female ratio was 1.17 : 1. The diagnostic accuracy of FNAC was 100%, 93.3%, and 88.2% for nonneoplastic lesions, benign tumours, and malignant tumours, respectively. *Conclusion.* The high accuracy, sensitivity, and specificity of FNAC confirm that preoperative cytology is a useful, quick, reliable diagnostic technique for rapid diagnosis and suitable for developing countries.

1. Introduction

Salivary glands are exocrine organs responsible for production and secretion of saliva and consist of the parotid, submandibular, sublingual, and the minor glands that are numerous and widely distributed throughout the mouth and oropharynx [1]. Salivary glands neoplasms account for 6% of all head and neck tumors [1]. Fine needle aspiration cytology (FNAC) is a useful method for evaluating suspicious salivary glands lesions due to its low cost, minimum morbidity, rapid turnaround time, high specificity, and sensitivity [2]. By cytological examination, lesions can be divided into inflammatory, reactive, benign, or malignant and, if possible, specific diagnosis is given which helps the clinicians in planning the management of the lesion [3]. The present study was taken to know the frequency of the salivary gland lesions especially in reference to malignancy in the Jhansi region, cytological evaluation of salivary gland masses by FNAC methods with regard to sensitivity, specificity and accuracy, and cytohistopathological correlation of salivary glands masses.

2. Material and Methods

Present study was carried out in the Department of Pathology, MLB Medical College, Jhansi, retrospectively and prospectively. Cases were selected from the patients attending ENT department or were admitted in the wards and also from the records presented with salivary gland swelling in the parotid, submandibular, and submental region. In the present study, 132 cases of salivary gland swelling are included in which cytological and histological studies were done. Eight cases were excluded due to scanty, inadequate aspirate on FNAC; thus only 124 cases were included in this study and cytohistological correlation was made in 86 cases only and in the remaining 38 cases either cytology or histology was available. All patients were clinically evaluated by detailed history, clinical examination, and haematological and radiological investigations. FNA was performed from different sites of the salivary gland swelling using a 10 mL disposable syringe and 23/24-gauge needle without local anaesthesia. FNA air-dried smears were stained with Giemsa stain and wet smears fixed in 95% ethyl alcohol were stained with Papanicolaou stain. Paraffin embedded tissue sections obtained from salivary gland tissue were stained with haematoxylin and eosin and few special stains were performed whenever required. Salivary gland lesions were studied under the three groups including nonneoplastic lesions and benign and malignant tumors.

3. Results

In the present study, nonneoplastic lesions accounted for 53.22% (66/124), followed by 31.45% (39/124) benign tumours and 15.32% (19/124) malignant tumours. Commonest gland involved was parotid (48.3%, 60/124), followed by submandibular gland (41.2%, 51/124) and minor salivary glands (10.4%, 13/124) whereas no case of sublingual salivary gland lesion was observed in the present study. Age range for nonneoplastic lesions was 8 years to 68 years with commonest age group being 20 to 29 years. Male : female ratio was 3.7 : 1. Age range for neoplastic lesions was 18 years to 78 years with commonest age group for benign neoplasms being 30 to 39 years, and, for malignant neoplasms, it was 60 to 69 years. Male : female ratio was 0.34 : 1. The overall male to female ratio was 1.17 : 1. In nonneoplastic lesions, 38 lesions involved the submandibular gland (57.5%, 38/66), 20 lesions involved the parotid gland (30.35%, 20/66), and 8 lesions involved the minor salivary gland (12.1%, 8/66). Chronic sialadenitis was the commonest lesion Figures 1(a) and 1(b) (63.64%, 42/66) followed by benign cysts (16.67%, 11/66), suppurative sialadenitis (7.57%, 5/66), and tubercular sialadenitis (6%, 4/66). In neoplastic lesions, most commonly involved site was the parotid gland (68.9%, 40/58) followed by submandibular gland (22.42%, 13/58) and minor salivary gland (8.62%, 5/58). In benign tumours, pleomorphic adenoma accounted for maximum number of cases (66.6%, 26/39), followed by monomorphic adenoma (25.6%, 10/39), haemangioma (5.1%, 2/39), and Warthin's tumour (2.5%, 1/39) Figures 1(c)–1(f), 2(a), and 2(b). In malignant lesions, mucoepidermoid Figures 2(c) and 2(d) carcinoma was the most common malignant tumour (42.1%, 8/19) followed by malignant mixed tumour (21%, 4/19), acinic cell carcinoma (21%, 4/19), adenoid cystic carcinoma (10.5%, 2/19), and adenocarcinoma (5.3%, 1/19). In the present study, both cytology and histology were carried out in 86 cases only and a correlation was done for sensitivity, specificity, and diagnostic accuracy. The diagnostic accuracy of FNAC for the nonneoplastic lesions, benign tumours, and malignant tumours was 100%, 93.3%, and 88.2%, respectively, and overall diagnostic accuracy was 95.3%. Positive predictive value and negative predictive value for neoplastic tumours were 88.2% and 97.1%, respectively. In nonneoplastic lesions, the specific diagnosis of all 39 cases by FNAC was correlated with histopathological findings. In benign tumours (30 cases) cytological diagnosis of 28 cases was consistent with histopathological diagnosis. Two cases reported as pleomorphic adenoma and Warthin's tumor on FNAC turn to malignant mixed tumour and low grade mucoepidermoid carcinoma, respectively, on histopathological examination. In malignant group, cytological diagnosis of 15 cases was consistent with histopathological diagnosis. In 2 cases cytological diagnosis of malignant mixed tumors turns to pleomorphic adenoma on histopathological examination.

4. Discussion

In the diagnosis of salivary gland lesions, FNAC has gained the popularity as diagnostic tool due to its low cost and safe procedure with minimal risk to the patient [4] and aid to the clinicians in the management planning. The rate of unsatisfactory samples on FNAC is varied from 3% to 12% [5–8]. In present study it was 6.4%. This difference may be due to inexperience of the pathologist and sampling errors. Nguansangiam et al. observed the age range from 6 to 100 years with mean age 53 years and female predominance [5]. As opposed to this, present study observed the age range of 8 to 68 years with mean age of 40 years with male predominance which was similar to the study done by Choudhury et al. [9]. The rate of nonneoplastic lesion in this study was 53.22%. It is in concordance with those of other studies, ranging from 20% to 72.9% [5, 10–12]. In the present study most common age group for nonneoplastic lesions was 20 to 40 years and male to female ratio was 3.7 : 1. Most common nonneoplastic lesion was chronic sialadenitis followed by benign cyst and most of the nonneoplastic lesions involved the submandibular gland and this similar finding is also observed by Atula et al. [13]. In the present study, benign neoplasms accounted for 39 cases (31.45%). The rate of benign neoplasm was lower than other reports which ranged from 49 to 83% [5–9]. We observed the pleomorphic adenoma as the commonest benign neoplasm followed by monomorphic adenoma and the predominance of these two benign neoplasms was similar to those previously reported number of studies [5, 10–12]. Various authors have reported that the incidence of malignant tumours ranged from 15% to 32% [10, 11], and in the present study it accounted for 15.32% whereas Nguansangiam et al. have found the lower rate of malignant neoplasms [5]. In our study, the most common malignant salivary gland tumor was mucoepidermoid carcinoma which accounted for 42.1% of all malignant neoplasms followed by malignant mixed tumours. As compared to this, Nguansangiam et al. have found that lymphoma is the commonest primary malignant salivary gland tumors followed by mucoepidermoid carcinoma [5]. Parotid gland was observed as the commonest site of salivary gland neoplasms; 68.9% (40/58) of all salivary gland neoplasms involved the parotid gland in this series. Almost similar distribution of salivary gland neoplasms in the parotid gland has also been described by Choudhury et al. [9]. The present study showed a false positive rate of 2.3%; it is in keeping with those of other studies, ranging from 0 to 4.7% [4, 14]. The false negative rate in the present study

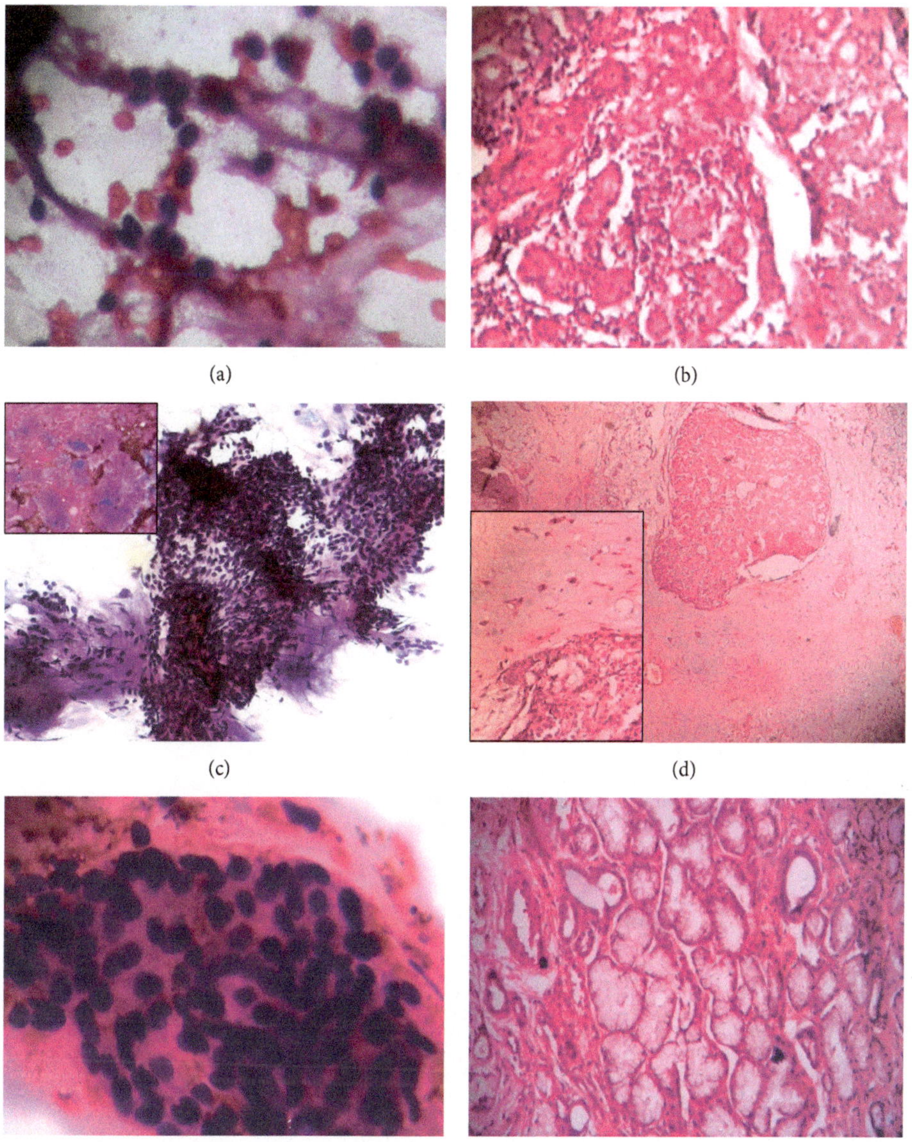

(a) (b) (c) (d) (e) (f)

FIGURE 1: (a) Chronic sialadenitis: hypocellular smear with background lymphocytes and small cohesive group of ductal cells (Giemsa ×400). (b) Chronic sialadenitis: periductal fibrosis accompanied by chronic inflammatory cell infiltrate and acinar atrophy (H&E ×400). (c) Pleomorphic adenoma: the matrix is in slight magenta colour with myoepithelial cells present individually and in clusters (Giemsa ×400). (d) Pleomorphic adenoma: ductal structures are surrounded by abluminal myoepithelial cells and hyalinized, myxoid, and chondromyxoid stroma (H&E ×400). (e) Monomorphic adenoma: fragmented groups of haphazard arranged cells as squamous morules and intercellular matrix droplets (Giemsa ×400). (f) Monomorphic adenoma: aggregates of tumor cells were arranged as an inner layer of luminal epithelial cells and surrounded by an outer layer of myoepithelial cells (H&E ×400).

was also 2.3%, which was in concordance with other studies, reporting a range of 2.2% to 24.5% [5, 14, 15]. Diagnosis of low grade mucoepidermoid carcinoma is difficult because it may be misdiagnosed as chronic sialadenitis, Warthin's tumor, mucous retention cysts, and adenomatoid hyperplasia of the mucous salivary gland as observed in the present study [15]. In our study, sensitivity, specificity, positive predictive value (PPV), and negative predictive value (NPV) of preoperative FNA cytology of salivary gland tumours were 88.2%, 97.1%, 88.2%, and 97.1%, respectively; however, overall diagnostic accuracy for all salivary gland lesions was 95.3%, indicating good results compared with those previously reported in various studies [2, 6, 7, 11, 14].

5. Conclusion

The high accuracy, sensitivity, and specificity of FNAC confirm that preoperative cytology is a useful, quick, reliable diagnostic technique for rapid and early diagnosis and we also

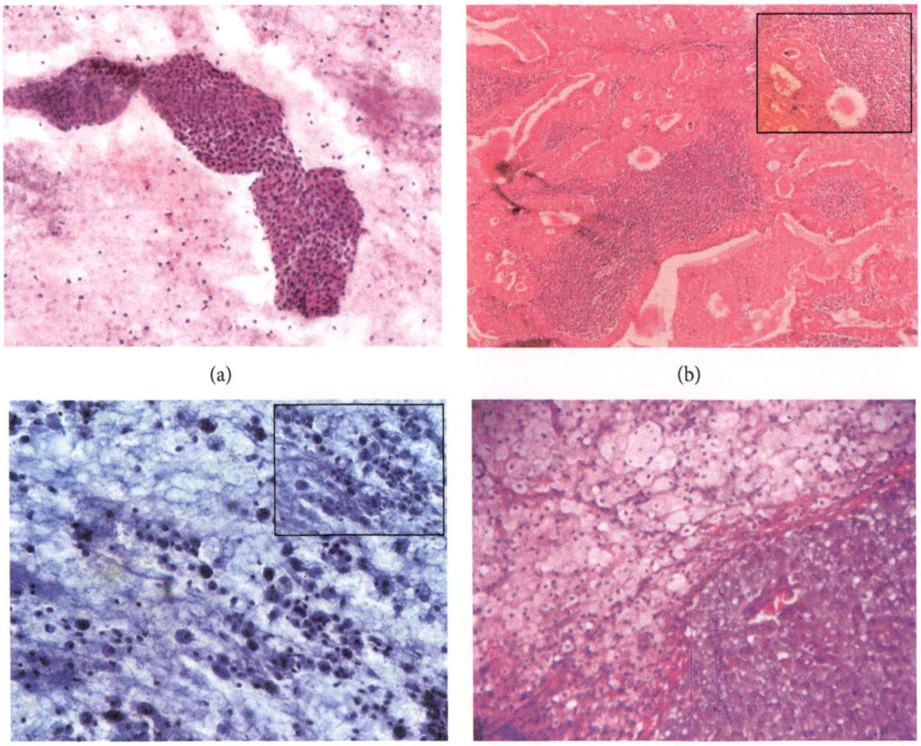

FIGURE 2: (a) Warthin tumor: the characteristic findings include cohesive flat sheets of oncocytes, lymphocytes, and a granular proteinaceous background (Giemsa ×400). (b) Warthin tumor: oncocytic epithelium with cuboidal basal cell to columnar luminal cell dense lymph node-like stroma (H&E ×400, Inset, H&E ×400). (c) Mucoepidermoid carcinoma: cells with abundant squamoid to vacuolated cytoplasm and large nuclei with a prominent nucleoli and necrotic background (Giemsa ×400). (d) Mucoepidermoid carcinoma: cluster of epidermoid cells with numerous clear cells (H&E ×400).

conclude that it is simple and cost-effective diagnostic tool suitable for developing countries.

Conflict of Interests

The authors declare that there is no conflict of interests regarding the publication of this paper.

References

[1] L. Barnes, J. W. Eveson, P. Reichart, and D. Sidransky, "Pathology and genetics of head and neck tumors," in *World Health Organization Classification of Tumors*, P. Kleihues and L. H. Sobin, Eds., p. 210, IARC Press, Lyon, France, 2005.

[2] M. A. S. Frable and W. J. Frable, "Fine-needle aspiration biopsy of salivary glands," *Laryngoscope*, vol. 101, no. 3, pp. 245–249, 1991.

[3] M. W. Stanley, R. H. Bardales, C. E. Farmer et al., "Primary and metastatic high-grade carcinomas of the salivary glands: a cytologic-histologic correlation study of twenty cases," *Diagnostic Cytopathology*, vol. 13, no. 1, pp. 37–43, 1995.

[4] A. H. Qizilbash, J. Sianos, J. E. M. Young, and S. D. Archibald, "Fine needle aspiration biopsy cytology of major salivary glands," *Acta Cytologica*, vol. 29, no. 4, pp. 503–512, 1985.

[5] S. Nguansangiam, S. Jesdapatarakul, N. Dhanarak, and K. Sosrisakorn, "Accuracy of fine needle aspiration cytology of salivary gland lesions: routine diagnostic experience in Bangkok, Thailand," *Asian Pacific Journal of Cancer Prevention*, vol. 13, no. 4, pp. 1583–1588, 2012.

[6] L. G. Tan and M. L. Khoo, "Accuracy of fine needle aspiration cytology and frozen section histopathology for lesions of the major salivary glands," *Annals of the Academy of Medicine Singapore*, vol. 35, no. 4, pp. 242–248, 2006.

[7] H. Mihashi, A. Kawahara, M. Kage et al., "Comparison of preoperative fine-needle aspiration cytology diagnosis and histopathological diagnosis of salivary gland tumors," *Kurume Medical Journal*, vol. 53, no. 1-2, pp. 23–27, 2006.

[8] I. S. Jan, P. Chung, M. Weng et al., "Analysis of fine-needle aspiration cytology of the salivary gland," *Journal of the Formosan Medical Association*, vol. 107, no. 5, pp. 364–370, 2008.

[9] A. A. Choudhury, T. Sultana, B. H. Siddique, and A. S. A. Amin, "Diagnosis of parotid gland mass by the fine needle aspiration cytology (FNAC) and its histopathological correlation—2 years study in BSMMU, Dhaka," *Bangabandhu Sheikh Mujib Medical University Journal*, vol. 4, no. 2, pp. 65–69, 2011.

[10] R. S. Cajulis, S. T. Gokaslan, G. H. Yu, and D. Frias-Hidvegi, "Fine needle aspiration biopsy of the salivary glands: a five-year experience with emphasis on diagnostic pitfalls," *Acta Cytologica*, vol. 41, no. 5, pp. 1412–1420, 1997.

[11] P. Boccato, G. Altavilla, and S. Blandamura, "Fine needle aspiration biopsy of salivary gland lesions: a reappraisal of

pitfalls and problems," *Acta Cytologica*, vol. 42, no. 4, pp. 888–898, 1998.

[12] D. K. Das, M. A. Petkar, N. M. Al-Mane, Z. A. Sheikh, M. K. Mallik, and J. T. Anim, "Role of fine needle aspiration cytology in the diagnosis of swellings in the salivary gland regions: a study of 712 cases," *Medical Principles and Practice*, vol. 13, no. 2, pp. 95–106, 2004.

[13] T. Atula, R. Grenman, and P. Laippala, "Fine-needle aspiration cytology of submandibular gland lesions," *The Journal of Laryngology & Otology*, vol. 109, no. 9, pp. 853–858, 1995.

[14] P. O'Dwyer, W. B. Farrar, A. G. James, W. Finkelmeier, and D. P. McCabe, "Needle aspiration biopsy of major salivary gland tumors: its value," *Cancer*, vol. 57, pp. 554–557, 1986.

[15] L. J. Layfield and B. J. Glasgow, "Diagnosis of salivary gland tumors by fine-needle aspiration cytology: a review of clinical utility and pitfalls," *Diagnostic Cytopathology*, vol. 7, no. 3, pp. 267–272, 1991.

13

Outcomes in Ovarian Cancer among Hispanic Women Living in the United States: A Population-Based Analysis

Okechukwu A. Ibeanu and Teresa P. Díaz-Montes

Division of Gynecologic Oncology, Department of Gynecology and Obstetrics, The Kelly Gynecologic Oncology Service, The Johns Hopkins Medical Institutions, Baltimore, MD 21287, USA

Correspondence should be addressed to Okechukwu A. Ibeanu; oibeanul@jhmi.edu

Academic Editor: Paulette Mhawech-Fauceglia

Introduction. Ovarian cancer is the deadliest gynecologic cancer in the United States. There is limited data on presentation and outcomes among Hispanic women with ovarian cancer. *Objective.* To investigate how ovarian cancer presents among Hispanic women in the USA and to analyze differences in presentation, staging, and survival between Hispanic and non-Hispanic women with ovarian cancer. *Methods.* Data from January 1, 2000 to December 31, 2004 were extracted from the National Cancer Institute's Surveillance, Epidemiology and End Results (SEER) database. *Results.* The study sample comprised 1215 Hispanics (10%), 10 652 non-Hispanic whites (83%), and 905 non-Hispanic blacks (7%). Hispanic women were diagnosed with ovarian cancer at a younger age and earlier stage when compared to non-Hispanic whites, non-Hispanic blacks; $P < 0.001$. Similar proportion of Hispanics (33%), non-Hispanic whites (32%), and non-Hispanic blacks (24%) underwent lymphadenectomy; $P < 0.001$. Hispanics with epithelial ovarian cancer histology had longer five-year survival of 30.6 months compared to non-Hispanic whites (22.8 months) and non-Hispanic blacks (23.3 months); $P = 0.001$. *Conclusion.* Hispanic women with ovarian cancer have a statistically significantly longer median survival compared to whites and blacks. This survival difference was most apparent in patients with epithelial cancers and patients with stage IV disease.

1. Introduction

Ovarian cancer is the leading cause of mortality among gynecologic cancers diagnosed in the United States (USA) [1]. The American Cancer Society has estimated that approximately 22,280 new cases of ovarian cancer will be diagnosed during 2012 making it the ninth most common cancer diagnosed among women living in the USA. It is also estimated that 15,500 women will die of this disease, making it the fifth most common cause of cancer-related deaths among women in the USA during 2012 [2]. Sporadic ovarian cancer has a peak age of incidence of 60–70 years [1]. The disease is typically diagnosed in advanced stage (stage III/IV), partly because there is no routine screening procedure for ovarian cancer among women in the general population [3], and as yet, no reliable screening biomarker has been detected. Cancer Antigen (CA 125) measurements do not have adequate sensitivity and specificity to satisfy requirements for use as a screening tool [4]. Overall 5-year survival rate in women with ovarian cancer is 46% and is related to stage of disease at diagnosis. Five-year survival rates are 93%, 71%, and 31% for local, regional, and distant disease, respectively [5]. Important prognostic factors for ovarian cancer are age, histology (serous versus nonserous), stage of disease, and the volume of residual disease after cytoreductive surgery [3]. Current standard treatment is primary cytoreductive surgery and adjuvant platinum-based chemotherapy.

Ovarian cancer trends have previously been evaluated among several ethnic groups in the USA. A review of the Surveillance, Epidemiology, and End Results (SEER) data from 2005 showed that Caucasian women had the highest incidence rate of ovarian cancer (12.9 per 100,000 population) followed by Hispanics (10.9 per 100,000 population), African-Americans (9.3 per 100,000 population), Asian/Pacific Islander (8.7 per 100,000 population), and American Indian/Alaska Natives (7.0 per 100,000 population)

[6]. Caucasian women also had the highest mortality rates (9.0 per 100,000 population) followed by African-Americans (7.2 per 100,000 population), Hispanics, and American Indian/Alaska Natives (6.0 per 100,000 population) and Asian/Pacific Islander (5.0 per 100,000 population) [6].

Hispanics currently make up the largest and fastest-growing minority ethnic group in the USA, constituting 12.5% of the population and are expected to make up one quarter of the total population by 2050 [7]. At present, there is a paucity of data regarding age at diagnosis, histology, stage of disease, grading, treatment offered, and prognosis among Hispanic women diagnosed with ovarian cancer. Given the huge healthcare costs in the USA, and the expected increase in cancer cases diagnosed in the coming decades, it is important to have accurate knowledge of the distribution of disease, disparities in risk factor prevalence, treatments, and outcomes among various subgroups of the population, in order to use healthcare resources efficiently.

The goals of this study are to investigate how ovarian cancer presents among Hispanic women living in the USA and to evaluate the differences in presentation, staging, and survival between Hispanic and non-Hispanic women diagnosed with ovarian cancer.

2. Methods

Demographic, clinico-pathological, treatment and survival information from women with ovarian cancer from January 1, 2000 to December 31, 2004 was extracted from the National Cancer Institute's Surveillance, Epidemiology and End Results (SEER) Program database. The SEER Program is an authoritative source of information on cancer incidence and survival in the USA, which collects information and publishes cancer incidence and survival from 12 population-based cancer registries and 3 supplemental registries that encompass nearly 14% of the total USA population [8]. Included in the analysis were all women identified as Hispanic, Non-Hispanic black, and non-Hispanic white under the race coding with a diagnosis of ovarian cancer under the primary site coding for cancer (183.0 ICD-O) [9]. Any cases that did not meet all of the above criteria were excluded from our analysis. The study was exempt from Institutional Review Board (IRB) approval because the information obtained is not individually identifiable and was not collected by direct contact with participants specifically for this study. The SEER Program database is of public use and is federally funded by the National Cancer Institute.

Statistical analysis was performed using the SPSS version 17.0 statistical software program (SPSS Inc, Chicago, IL, USA). Descriptive statistics were used to present demographic data. Chi-square test was used to analyze the differences between the groups with respect to demographic variables, disease and treatment characteristics. Kaplan-Meier survival analysis was performed and log-rank tests were used to compare survival among racial groups. Cox regression method was used to analyze independent factors that were related to survival. A two-sided P value < 0.05 was considered statistically significant.

3. Results

A total of 12,772 women were included in the study. Overall, the mean age at diagnosis among the cohort of women was 62.6 years. Hispanic women were diagnosed with ovarian cancer at a younger age (54.5 years) when compared to the non-Hispanic groups (non-Hispanic whites: 63.8 years, non-Hispanic blacks: 59.8 years; $P < 0.001$). Sixty-nine percent of the women in the cohort were 55 years of age or older. Whereas 51% of the ovarian cancer cases among Hispanic women presented at age 55 years or younger, only 28% of non-Hispanic white and 37% of non-Hispanic black women were in this age group ($P < 0.001$) (Table 1). Hispanic women also had a lower frequency of ovarian cancer being diagnosed at 65 years and older when compared to the non-Hispanic groups (Hispanics: 32%, non-Hispanic whites: 50%, and non-Hispanic blacks: 43%; $P < 0.001$) (Table 1).

Fifty-three percent of the women in the cohort were diagnosed with advanced stage (III-IV) disease and 26% with early stage (I-II) at the time of initial presentation. Hispanic women had a higher proportion of ovarian cancer being diagnosed at an earlier stage (I-II) when compared to the non-Hispanic groups (Hispanics: 32%, non-Hispanic whites: 26% and non-Hispanic blacks: 26%, $P < 0.001$). The majority of the women (60%) in the cohort were diagnosed with epithelial ovarian cancer. This trend was noted among the different ethnic groups (Hispanics: 57%, non-Hispanic whites: 61%, and non-Hispanic blacks: 49%) (Table 1).

Only 31% of the overall study population underwent a lymphadenectomy during the initial surgical staging. Similar proportion of Hispanics and non-Hispanic whites underwent a lymphadenectomy, as compared to non-Hispanic blacks (Hispanics: 33%, non-Hispanic-whites: 32%, and non-Hispanic blacks: 24%) ($P < 0.001$) (Table 1).

The overall median survival of the study population was 36 months. Hispanics had a median survival of 45 months, which was statistically significantly longer when compared to 36 months for non-Hispanic whites and 24 months for non-Hispanic blacks ($P < 0.001$). As expected, age at diagnosis of 54 years or younger, early stage (I-II) disease, low-grade histology, and negative lymph node status were associated with longer median survival across all groups (Table 2). Hispanics with an epithelial histology had a survival of 30.6 months which was longer when compared to non-Hispanic whites (22.8 months) and non-Hispanic blacks (23.3 months) ($P = 0.001$) (Table 2).

Kaplan-Meier survival curves are shown in Figure 1, illustrating 5-year survival values for overall survival and median survival for Hispanic patients. The differences were not statistically significant.

4. Discussion

In 2005, immigrants represented twelve percent of the total USA population. Fifty-three percent of all foreign-born individuals in the USA were from Latin America [10]. Hispanics currently make up the largest minority ethnic group in the United States and are expected to grow to one-fourth of the USA population by 2050 [7]. Unfortunately, there are few

Table 1: Age at diagnosis, histology, and extent of disease among Hispanic, non-Hispanics white, and non-Hispanics black women diagnosed with ovarian cancer, US SEER Data 2000–2004.

Characteristics	Non-Hispanic white	Non-Hispanic black	Hispanic	Overall	*P* value
Age categories		*n* (%)			
<23 years	125 (1.2)	29 (3.2)	68 (5.6)	222 (1.7)	
24–54 years	2860 (26.8)	308 (34)	555 (45.7)	3723 (29.1)	
55–64 years	2329 (21.9)	183 (20.2)	208 (17.1)	2720 (21.3)	<0.001
65–74 years	2313 (21.7)	194 (21.4)	207 (17.0)	2714 (21.2)	
>74 years	3025 (28.4)	191 (21.9)	177 (14.6)	3393 (26.6)	
Histology					
Epithelial	6483 (60.9)	440 (48.6)	693 (57)	7616 (59.6)	
Nonepithelial	333 (3.1)	46 (5.1)	111 (9.2)	490 (3.9)	<0.001
Other	3836 (36.0)	4.9 (46.3)	411 (33.8)	4666 (36.5)	
Stage					
I	2059 (19.3)	169 (18.9)	308 (25.3)	2536 (19.4)	
II	735 (6.9)	63 (7.0)	83 (6.8)	881 (6.9)	
III	2873 (27.0)	208 (23.0)	311 (25.6)	3392 (28.6)	<0.001
IV	2575 (24.4)	263 (29.1)	253 (20.8)	3111 (24.4)	
Unknown	2390 (22.4)	202 (22.3)	260 (21.4)	2852 (22.3)	

Table 2: Showing factors related to survival at 5 years among Hispanic, non-Hispanics white, and non-Hispanics black women diagnosed with ovarian cancer, US SEER Data 2000–2004.

Characteristics	Non-Hispanic white survival (months)	Non-Hispanic black survival (months)	Hispanic survival (months)	Overall survival (months)	*P* value
Median	36	24	45	36	<0.001
Age at diagnosis (years)					
<54	47.4	42.8	46.6	46.9	
55–64	39.2	29.8	36.2	38.4	
65–74	32.3	24.6	28.8	31.5	
>74	18.4	12.0	12.8	17.9	
Stage					
I-II	52.2	51.0	52.7	52.0	<0.001
III-IV	29.1	23.0	30.5	28.7	
Grade					
1	50.8	47.1	51.0	50.7	
2	43.0	34.8	40.2	42.3	0.02
3	35.2	30.2	35.1	34.9	
unclassified	26.6	32.3	34.3	34.2	
Histology					
Epithelial	22.8	23.3	30.6	23.6	0.001
Nonepithelial	41.3	37.1	42.0	41.2	

studies reporting on the outcomes of gynecologic malignancies among Hispanics. In addition, the demographic factors that influence the presentation, management, and prognosis among Hispanic women with ovarian cancer remain underreported.

On average, Hispanics were diagnosed at an age 9.3 years younger than non-Hispanic whites and 5.3 years earlier than non-Hispanic blacks. These findings may be related to the larger proportion of younger age group individuals in the Hispanic subpopulation, according to USA census data [3]. It is also observed that the incidence of epithelial ovarian cancers is lower among Hispanics than Caucasian women [3]. The lower incidence rate of epithelial tumors could be partly linked to the fact that Hispanic women have higher numbers of offspring and practice breastfeeding more commonly than Caucasian women; both of which are protective factors against the development of ovarian cancer [11].

Uncharacterized genetic factors could also be involved in ovarian carcinogenesis among this Hispanic cohort. Ovarian cancer occurs at a younger age among BRCA mutation carriers. Some investigators have reported on hereditary ovarian cancer-related genetic mutations among certain clusters of Hispanic women showing that BRCA 1/2 mutations exist among Hispanic probands in the United States and Latin America [12–14].

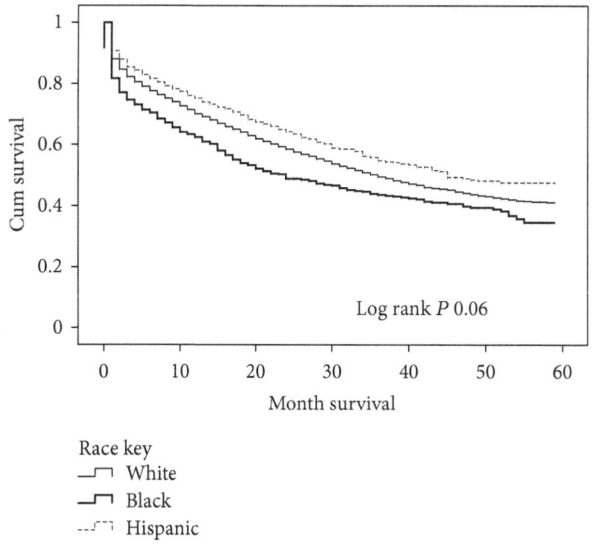

FIGURE 1: Kaplan-Meier survival curve of all patients based on ethnicity.

More Hispanic women in this analysis had early stage disease (32.2%) than Caucasians (26.2%) and blacks (25.9%). This difference was statistically significant. The reasons for this are not clear; however, one clinically relevant consequence is that earlier age at presentation among Hispanics may have influenced the use of aggressive primary surgical treatments with the expectation of lower surgery-related morbidity in younger aged patients. Further analysis of the cohort shows that a statistically significantly larger proportion of Hispanic women underwent staging lymphadenectomy as part of their treatment. The prognostic effect of lymphadenectomy in early stage ovarian cancer is well known [15]. The higher frequency of lymphadenectomy in Hispanics is unexplained but suggests more frequent use of complete staging procedures among Hispanics as a proxy measure of health process measure. Process-related measures and outcomes merit further study in this group of women.

Overall, our data indicate that Hispanics with ovarian cancer have a statistically significantly longer median survival compared to whites and blacks. This survival difference was most apparent in the patients with epithelial cancers and those with stage IV disease. Stage for stage, Hispanic patients had a more favorable survival profile than the rest of the cohort. The survival difference was not statistically significant.

The current study has several limitations that must be considered when interpreting the results. First, the use of the SEER database as our source of patients lacks external validity. The SEER database only represents 14% of the USA population. The configuration of the SEER data set does not allow stratification of different Hispanic subgroups in order to evaluate whether the diagnosis of ovarian cancer at a younger age is a Hispanic characteristic or whether it is more strongly related to the subethnicity within the Hispanic community. There is incomplete followup, and also, the self-reporting of race and ethnicity may be subjective. The information in the SEER database does not provide information on provider specialization.

Despite these limitations, the current study provides the most extensive comparison of ovarian cancer patterns between Hispanic and non-Hispanic women in the United States. The observation that Hispanic women are diagnosed with ovarian cancer at an earlier age than non-Hispanic groups underscores the need for additional studies to explore this trend. The information obtained from this study is useful given the anticipated changes in the USA population over the next few decades. This could influence the allocation of health care resources and guide the provision of specialized cancer care to at-risk demographic groups.

References

[1] P. C. Nasca and H. Pastides, Eds., *Fundamentals of Cancer Epidemiology*, Jones and Bartlett, Sudbury, Mass, USA, 2nd edition, 2008.

[2] R. Siegel, D. Naishadham, and A. Jemal, "Cancer Statistics 2012," *CA—A Cancer Journal for Clinicians*, vol. 62, pp. 10–29, 2012.

[3] "Cancer Statistics," American Cancer Society, 2008.

[4] D. Badgwell and R. C. Bast, "Early detection of ovarian cancer," *Disease Markers*, vol. 23, no. 5-6, pp. 397–410, 2007.

[5] L. Ries, D. Melbert, M. Krapcho et al., "SEER Cancer Statistics Review, 1975," National Cancer Institute, Bethesda, Md, USA, 2005, http://seer.cancer.gov/csr/1975_2005/.

[6] "United States Cancer Statistics: 1999–2005 Incidence and Mortality Web-based Report. Atlanta," U.S. Department of Health and Human Services, Centers of Disease Control and Prevention and National Cancer Institute, 2009, http://www.cdc.gov/uscs.

[7] I. De Alba and J. M. Sweningson, "English proficiency and physicians' recommendation of Pap smears among Hispanics," *Cancer Detection and Prevention*, vol. 30, no. 3, pp. 292–296, 2006.

[8] "Surveillance, Epidemiology, and End Results (SEER) Program. SEER*Stat Database: Incidence-SEER 12 Regs Public-Use. November 2007 Sub (1973–2005)," National Cancer Institute, 2008, http://www.seer.cancer.gov/.

[9] A. Fritz, C. Percy, A. Jack et al., Eds., *International Classification of Diseases for Oncology*, World Health Organization, Geneva, Switzerland, 3rd edition, 2000.

[10] K. P. Derose, J. J. Escarce, and N. Lurie, "Immigrants and health care: sources of vulnerability," *Health Affairs*, vol. 26, no. 5, pp. 1258–1268, 2007.

[11] M. Schiff, T. M. Becker, H. O. Smith, F. D. Gilliland, and C. R. Key, "Ovarian cancer incidence and mortality in American Indian, Hispanic, and non-Hispanic white women in New Mexico," *Cancer Epidemiology Biomarkers and Prevention*, vol. 5, no. 5, pp. 323–327, 1996.

[12] J. N. Weitzel, V. Lagos, K. R. Blazer et al., "Prevalence of BRCA mutations and founder effect in high-risk Hispanic families," *Cancer Epidemiology Biomarkers and Prevention*, vol. 14, no. 7, pp. 1666–1671, 2005.

[13] D. Torres, M. U. Rashid, F. Gil et al., "High proportion of BRCA1/2 founder mutations in Hispanic breast/ovarian cancer families from Colombia," *Breast Cancer Research and Treatment*, vol. 103, no. 2, pp. 225–232, 2007.

[14] S. M. Eisenkop, N. M. Spirtos, and W. C. M. Lin, “”Optimal” cytoreduction for advanced epithelial ovarian cancer: a commentary,” *Gynecologic Oncology*, vol. 103, no. 1, pp. 329–335, 2006.

[15] J. K. Chan, M. Zhang, J. M. Hu, J. Y. Shin, K. Osann, and D. S. Kapp, “Racial disparities in surgical treatment and survival of epithelial ovarian cancer in United States,” *Journal of Surgical Oncology*, vol. 97, no. 2, pp. 103–107, 2008.

14

Molecular Mechanisms of Liver Injury and Hepatocarcinogenesis: Focusing on the Role of Stress-Activated MAPK

Hayato Nakagawa[1, 2] and Shin Maeda[3]

[1] *Department of Gastroenterology, University of Tokyo, 7-3-1 Hongo, Bunkyo-ku, Tokyo 113-8655, Japan*
[2] *Laboratory of Gene Regulation and Signal Transduction, Departments of Pharmacology and Pathology, School of Medicine, University of California, La Jolla, CA 92093, USA*
[3] *Department of Gastroenterology, Yokohama City University, 3-9 Fukuura, Kanazawa-ku, Yokohama 236-0004, Japan*

Correspondence should be addressed to Hayato Nakagawa, n-hayato@yf7.so-net.ne.jp

Academic Editor: P. J. Van Diest

Hepatocellular carcinoma (HCC) is the third most common cause of cancer mortality. Short-term prognosis of patients with HCC has improved recently due to advances in early diagnosis and treatment, but long-term prognosis is still unsatisfactory. Therefore, obtaining a further understanding of the molecular carcinogenic mechanisms and the unique pathogenic biology of HCC is important. The most characteristic process in hepatocarcinogenesis is underlying chronic liver injury, which leads to repeated cycles of hepatocyte death, inflammation, and compensatory proliferation and subsequently provides a mitogenic and mutagenic environment leading to the development of HCC. Recent *in vivo* studies have shown that the stress-activated mitogen-activated protein kinase (MAPK) cascade converging on c-Jun NH_2-terminal kinase (JNK) and p38 plays a central role in these processes, and it has attracted considerable attention as a therapeutic target. However, JNK and p38 have complex functions and a wide range of cellular effects. In addition, crosstalk with each other and the nuclear factor-kappaB pathway further complicate these functions. A full understanding is essential to bring these observations into clinical settings. In this paper, we discuss the latest findings regarding the mechanisms of liver injury and hepatocarcinogenesis focusing on the role of the stress-activated MAPK pathway.

1. Introduction

Hepatocellular carcinoma (HCC) is the fifth most common cancer and the third most common cause of cancer mortality worldwide [1]. The age-adjusted incidence rate of HCC varies geographically, with high rates in East Asia and moderate rates in Europe, North/South America, and Oceania. In addition, a definite increase in HCC incidence has recently been reported in Europe and North America [2].

Although the etiology of background liver disease varies geographically, chronic hepatitis B virus (HBV) or hepatitis C virus (HCV) infection is the main cause of HCC in most areas. Other major etiologies include alcoholic hepatitis, hemochromatosis, and nonalcoholic steatohepatitis (NASH) [1, 3]. Accumulating evidence indicates that a sustained inflammatory reaction in the liver is the major contributing factor to the development of HCC. For example, in chronic hepatitis C, the host immune responses to HCV are often not strong enough to completely clear the infection, resulting in chronic stimulation of an antigen-specific immune response [4]. Hepatocyte damage is induced by the continued expression of cytokines and recruitment of activated inflammatory cells to the liver, which is followed by hepatocyte regeneration. This persistent cycle of necroinflammation and hepatocyte regeneration is thought to provide a mitogenic and mutagenic environment leading to the development of HCC [5–7].

Effective treatments for HCC include surgical resection, percutaneous ablation, and liver transplantation. Although liver transplantation results in a better survival rate [8], its application is limited by the scarcity of donor organs. Surgical resection and percutaneous ablation also provide a high rate of complete responses [9, 10], but long-term prognosis is not satisfactory, as indicated by the low overall survival of 22%–35% at 10 years [2]. This is due to frequent recurrence and lack of effective treatment for advanced HCC. Transarterial chemoembolization, radiotherapy, and conventional chemotherapy have been performed for advanced HCC, but their efficacies are limited [11].

Recently, molecular-targeted therapy was developed for the treatment of HCC. Sorafenib is a small molecule multikinase inhibitor targeting the Raf serine/threonine kinases, vascular endothelial growth factor receptor (VEGFR) and platelet-derived growth factor receptor (PDGFR) pathway. In the SHARP (Sorafenib HCC Assessment Randomized Protocol) trial, sorafenib significantly prolonged median overall survival compared to placebo (10.7 *versus* 7.9 months, resp.) [12]. However, median survival was not satisfactory even in the sorafenib group. Although other molecular-targeting agents are currently under investigation, only limited improvements in survival benefit have been reported [13].

Eradication of the cause of chronic inflammation, such as hepatitis viruses, is the most beneficial means of preventing HCC [14]. Recent advances in antiviral treatment have made the eradication of HCV or significant suppression of HBV replication possible [15–17]. However, these therapies are not effective for all patients, and the development of HCC will not be prevented completely, especially in patients with advanced fibrosis. In addition, in patients with HCC based on metabolic syndrome including NASH, the incidence rate of which is increasing, dietary modifications and exercise are fundamental, but these approaches are sometimes ineffective and genetic background may also be important in such cases. Furthermore, once HCC has developed, the recurrence rate does not decline with time regardless of background liver disease, suggesting that most cases of late-phase recurrence are due to metachronous multicentric carcinogenesis [11]. Thus, gaining further understanding of the molecular mechanisms of carcinogenesis in HCC is important to discover new molecular targets, especially for preventing the occurrence or recurrence of HCC and systemic therapy for patients in the advanced stage.

Several molecular pathways have been reported to play important roles in hepatocarcinogenesis. As mentioned above, inflammation-mediated liver injury and compensatory hepatocyte proliferation are indispensable components during HCC development. Recent high-quality *in vivo* studies have shown that stress-activated mitogen-activated protein kinase (MAPK) signaling converging on c-Jun NH_2-terminal kinase (JNK) and p38 plays a central role in these processes, and it has attracted considerable attention as a therapeutic target [18–24]. In this paper, we discuss the mechanisms of liver injury and hepatocarcinogenesis focusing on the role of the stress-activated MAPK pathway.

2. General Role of JNK in the Liver

2.1. Stress-Activated MAPK. MAPK cascades are signaling systems that transmit stimuli from outside the cell to the nucleus [25, 26]. Three major MAPK cascades have been characterized in detail, converging on ERKs, JNKs, and p38 MAPKs; each consists of three classes of serine/threonine kinases, MAPK, MAPK kinase (MAPKK), and MPKK kinase (MAP3K). MAP3K phosphorylates and thereby activates MAPKK, and activated MAPKK in turn phosphorylates and activates MAPK (Figure 1). Among the three MAPKs, ERKs are activated by various cytokines and growth factors and play a central role in cell growth and differentiation. JNKs and p38 MAPKs, also called stress-activated MAPKs, are preferentially activated by proinflammatory cytokines, such as tumor necrosis factor α (TNFα) and environmental and genotoxic stresses. After activation, stress-activated MAPKs phosphorylate specific serine/threonine residues of target substrates and exert a variety of cellular functions, such as cell death, survival, proliferation, migration, and inflammation.

2.2. JNK Signaling. JNK has three isoforms (JNK1, JNK2, and JNK3) encoded by three different genes. JNK1 and JNK2 are expressed in almost all organs, including the liver, whereas JNK3 is a neuronal-specific isoform [27]. JNK is phosphorylated and activated by two MAPKKs, MKK4, and MKK7. Activated JNK phosphorylates and thereby activates c-Jun, JunD, ATF, and other transcription factors, which are involved in the formation and activation of the AP-1 complex [28]. In addition, JNK also modulates the function of other proteins by phosphorylation, such as Bcl-2 family members, which are closely related to apoptotic cell death factors [29]. Furthermore, although JNK1 and JNK2 isoforms play redundant roles in many physiological processes, they also have distinct biological activities in some situations [30]. For example, JNK1-deficient $CD8^+$ T cells are unable to undergo antigen-stimulated expansion, whereas JNK2-deficient $CD8^+$ T cells are hyperproliferative [31]. Therefore, the role of JNK in controlling diverse cellular functions, such as cell proliferation, differentiation, and apoptosis, is based on the phosphorylation and functional modification of downstream molecular targets in a stimulus- and cell-type-dependent manner.

2.3. Role of JNK in TNFα-Mediated Liver Injury. Underlying liver injury, which leads to repeated cycles of hepatocyte death, inflammation, and compensatory proliferation, is an indispensable factor in the development of most liver cancers. Therefore, determining the mechanism of liver injury is a basic requirement for understanding hepatocarcinogenesis.

The proinflammatory cytokine TNFα plays a pivotal role in various inflammatory liver diseases [32]. Serum and hepatic TNFα levels are increased in patients with acute and chronic viral hepatitis, alcoholic hepatitis, and NASH [33–36]. Although TNFα can kill hepatocytes during such liver diseases, the healthy liver usually has defense systems against TNFα-induced cell death. In fact, TNFα stimulates proliferation rather than death through DNA synthesis in the normal hepatocyte, which is required for liver regeneration after partial hepatectomy [37, 38]. However, once antiapoptotic response is inhibited, TNFα signaling is converted from proliferation to apoptosis. Thus, TNFα has the capacity to

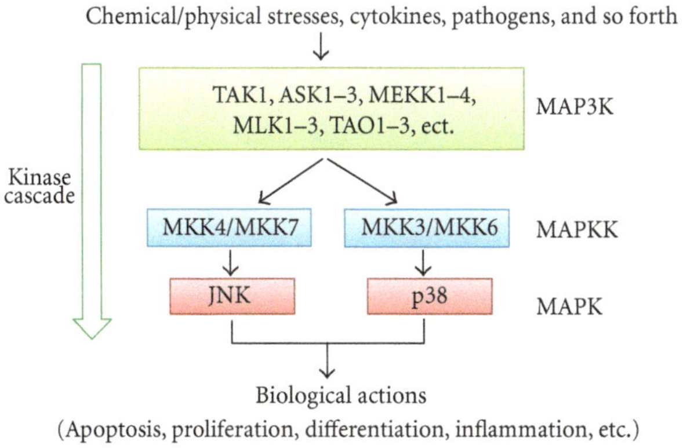

FIGURE 1: Stress-activated MAPK signaling pathway. This pathway consists of three classes of protein kinase—MAP3K, MAPKK, and MAPK—and converges on JNK and p38 through a kinase cascade. Only representative molecules are shown in MAP3K.

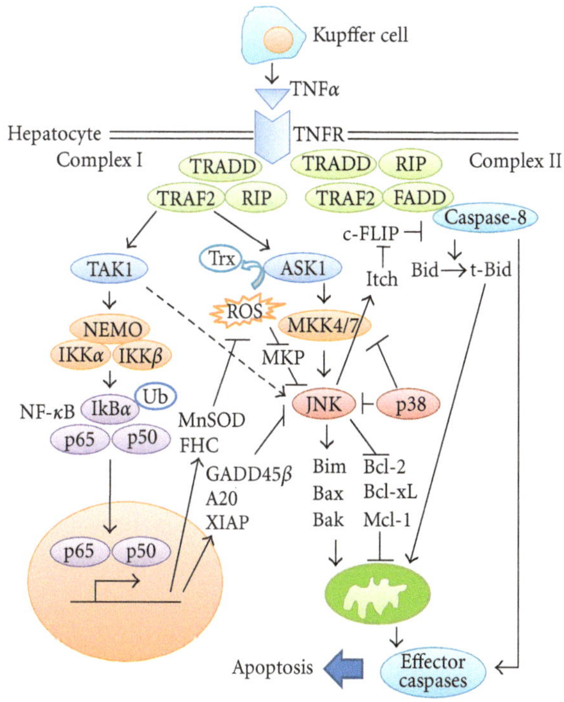

FIGURE 2: Signaling pathways of TNFα-induced hepatocyte death. After binding of TNFα to TNF-R1, complexes I and II are formed. As the amount of caspase-8 activation in complex II is not sufficient to induce cell death of hepatocytes, activation of the mitochondrial apoptotic pathway is essential. Activated caspase-8 initiates the mitochondrial apoptotic pathway by cleaving Bid to tBid. In addition, JNK can also activate the mitochondrial apoptotic pathway though modulation of Bcl-2 family members or degradation of c-FLIP. These pathways cooperate to induce cell death, while NF-κB and p38 inhibit TNFα-induced hepatocyte death by suppressing JNK activation through various mechanisms.

induce hepatocyte death as well as hepatocyte proliferation, and plays a crucial role in preserving liver homeostasis [39]. Recent studies have uncovered the important role of the cross talk between JNK and nuclear factor-kappaB (NF-κB) pathways in these processes, as described later.

TNFα is produced mainly by Kupffer cells in the liver and exerts biological effects by binding to two plasma membrane receptors, TNF-receptor 1 (TNF-R1) and TNF-R2 [40]. The majority of the biological effects of TNFα are mediated by TNF-R1. Upon binding of TNFα to TNF-R1, the signaling molecule TNF-R-associated death domain (TRADD), TNF-R-associated factor 2 (TRAF2), and receptor interacting protein 1 (RIP1) are recruited to form the so-called complex I [41] (Figure 2). Assembly of this complex is essential to activate two key players, JNK and NF-κB pathways.

In addition to the formation of complex I, TNFα binding to TNF-R1 simultaneously recruits Fas-associated death domain (FADD) and caspase-8, thus forming another complex, the so-called complex II [41] (Figure 2). Here, caspase-8 is activated through autocatalytic cleavage and active caspase-8 is then able to proteolytically activate several effector caspases such as caspase-3. However, in the case of hepatocytes, the amount of active caspase-8 generated by complex II is too small for activation of effector caspases, requiring an amplification loop through mitochondria [42]. Caspase-8 cleaves Bid to a truncated form, tBid, which translocates to the mitochondria, causing activation of Bak/Bax and subsequent activation of the mitochondrial apoptotic pathway. This mitochondrial pathway involves the release of numerous apoptogenic factors from the mitochondrial intermembrane space into the cytosol, including cytochrome *c*, which activates effector caspases and then induces cell death and amplification of caspase-8 activation.

The importance of JNK in TNFα-mediated liver injury has been confirmed by many *in vitro* and *in vivo* studies. In an *in vitro* study, TNFα-induced apoptosis was blocked by the small molecule JNK inhibitor SP600125 in mouse and rat primary hepatocytes [43]. *In vivo*, NF-κB-deficient embryos, which normally die due to TNFα-mediated hepatocyte apoptosis, were shown to survive longer when the JNK1 gene was also disrupted [44]. In addition, JNK1 knockout ($JNK1^{-/-}$) and JNK2 knockout ($JNK2^{-/-}$) mice were resistant to concanavalin-A-(Con-A-) induced liver injury, which is primarily TNFα dependent [45]. In another study, $JNK2^{-/-}$ mice, but not $JNK1^{-/-}$, mice were shown to be resistant to lipopolysaccharide (LPS)/D-galactosamine (GalN)-induced liver injury, which is also a TNFα-dependent liver injury model [46]. A recent study showed that both $JNK1^{-/-}$, and $JNK2^{-/-}$, mice are resistant to LPS/GalN-induced liver injury, and JNK2 plays a more prominent role in TNFα-induced hepatocyte death [47]. Despite the discrepancies among studies concerning which of the JNK isoforms is more important in hepatocyte death, they all support the concept that JNK plays a key role in controlling TNFα signaling toward cell death.

As TNFα-mediated hepatocyte death is also important for acute liver injury, JNK is considered to be a promising therapeutic target for acute liver injury. In fact, SP600125 and another JNK inhibitor D-JNKi, which is a peptide inhibitor of JNK, exert protective effects on LPS/GalN-induced fulminant hepatitis [44, 48].

2.4. Reactive Oxygen Species as Upstream Activators of JNK in TNFα Signaling. TNFα binding to TNF-R1 leads to the formation of complex I and then activates a member of the MAP3K family, transforming growth factor β-activated kinase 1 (TAK1). Activated TAK1 activates MKK4 and MKK7, which leads to JNK activation [49]. However, transient activation of JNK is not sufficient to induce cell death. Reactive-oxygen-species-(ROS-) mediated prolongation of JNK activation is considered important for the proapoptotic function of JNK. This concept was supported by the higher levels of intracellular ROS observed in TNFα-treated cells and the observation that antioxidants, such as *N*-acetyl-L-cysteine which is precursor of glutathione and butylated hydroxyanisole which is synthetic antioxidant authorized as a food additive, can suppress TNFα-induced prolonged JNK activation and subsequent apoptosis [30].

In TNFα signaling, two mechanisms have been proposed for ROS-mediated prolongation of JNK activation. One study indicated that ROS extended JNK activation by inactivating MAPK phosphatases (MKPs), which are essential for dephosphorylation of activated JNK [50]. TNFα-induced ROS oxidize critical Cys residues in the catalytic sites of various MKPs, leading to their inactivation, and ROS-mediated oxidation of MKP-1 rapidly leads to its degradation by the ubiquitin-proteasome pathway. Another study demonstrated an important role of apoptosis signal-regulating kinase 1 (ASK1), one of the major MAP3Ks, in the regulation of stress-activated MAPK [51]. TNFα-induced sustained activation of JNK is lost in $ASK1^{-/-}$ embryonic fibroblasts, and $ASK1^{-/-}$ cells are resistant to TNFα-induced apoptosis. While TAK1 is activated directly by TNF-R1-induced signaling, activation of ASK1 is secondary to the generation of ROS. The involvement of ASK1 in ROS-mediated JNK activation is based on links between ASK1 and thioredoxin (Trx), a reduction/oxidation regulatory protein [52]. In the absence of oxidative stress, Trx inhibits ASK1 kinase activity via direct binding to the N-terminal region of ASK1. Excess oxidative stress converts Trx to its oxidized form, resulting in its dissociation from ASK1 and subsequent ASK1 kinase activation. This system has been confirmed to function in the liver *in vivo* using an acetaminophen-induced liver injury model, which is a typical ROS-mediated liver injury model [53]. In addition, a recent study showed that $ASK1^{-/-}$ mice are resistant to LPS/GalN-induced liver injury [54]. Furthermore, Trx transgenic mice are also resistant to LPS/GalN-induced liver injury [55]. Thus, TNFα-induced ROS prolongs JNK activity by blocking the inhibitory MKPs and simultaneously promoting the activation of ASK1, then shifting the balance from cell survival toward cell death.

Viral proteins, including HCV core proteins, are also capable of ROS accumulation in hepatocytes, and ROS-mediated JNK activation in the liver is linked not only to liver disease but also to systemic disorders, such as insulin resistance and metabolic syndrome. Therefore, further elucidation of this process is very important [56–58].

2.5. Downstream Targets of JNK in TNFα-Induced Cell Death. Several targets of JNK in TNFα-induced cell death have been proposed. The primary question is whether JNK is or is not involved in caspase-8 activation. JNK was initially suggested to induce caspase-8-independent cleavage of Bid at a site distinct from the Bid cleavage product jBid, which translocates to mitochondria and subsequently amplifies caspase-8 activation [59]. However, this finding has not been confirmed in an *in vivo* liver injury model. In the LPS/GalN-induced liver injury model, $JNK2^{-/-}$ mice showed significant attenuation of caspase-8 activation and subsequent Bid cleavage, suggesting that JNK2 acts at the level of caspase-8 activation [46]. However, the detailed mechanism remains unclear and attenuated caspase-8 activation may be the indirect result of a lack of amplification by the mitochondrial release of proapoptotic factors. JNK may also be involved in caspase-8 activation through regulation of the caspase-8 inhibitor c-$FLIP_L$ [44]. Prolonged activation of JNK1 leads to phosphorylation of Itch, thereby activating its ubiquitin ligase activity, which results in polyubiquitination and subsequent degradation of c-$FLIP_L$. As c-$FLIP_L$ competes with caspase-8 for binding to complex II and impairs caspase-8 activation, JNK1-mediated c-$FLIP_L$ degradation results in full activation of caspase-8 and cell death. These studies support the suggestion that JNK is located upstream of caspase-8 activation.

Other studies support the alternative suggestion that JNK plays an apoptotic role at a level farther downstream through the regulation of Bcl-2 family activation. Activated JNK has been shown to phosphorylate and inactivate the anti-apoptotic proteins Bcl-2 and Bcl-xL [60–62]. Furthermore, activated JNK promotes Bax translocation to mitochondria through phosphorylation of 14-3-3, a cytoplasmic anchor of Bax. Phosphorylation of 14-3-3 leads to dissociation of Bax from this protein [63]. A more recent study showed that JNK contributes to TNFα-induced cell death through phosphorylation of the pro-apoptotic BH-3-only protein Bim, rather than Bid [64]. JNK-mediated Bim phosphorylation triggers the proapoptotic activity of Bim by causing its release from sequestration to the microtubular dynein motor complex and then activates the mitochondrial apoptotic pathway [65, 66]. These studies indicated that JNK acts in parallel and independent of caspase-8. Thus, although the downstream targets of JNK in TNFα signaling are not fully understood, most studies have demonstrated that JNK is required for activation of the mitochondrial apoptotic pathway.

2.6. Crosstalk between JNK and NF-κB. As prolonged JNK activation is closely related to cell death, systems for the regulation of JNK activity are mandatory for tissue homeostasis. The crosstalk between NF-κB and JNK is considered to be a major determinant in the fate of hepatocytes, including TNFα signaling.

NF-κB is a transcription factor that consists of homodimers and heterodimers composed of five members, that is, p65 (RelA), c-Rel, RelB, p50, and p52 [67]. Each NF-κB dimer has a different DNA-binding affinity and controls specific targets. Additionally, transcriptional activity of NF-κB is regulated by transcription coactivators such as SRC family and corepressors such as HDAC family [68]. The p50/p65 heterodimer, the most abundant form of the NF-κB, is regulated by so-called canonical pathway. Without stimulation, this heterodimer is bound to specific inhibitory factors, such as inhibitor of NF-κB (IκB) proteins in the cytoplasm. TNFα signaling complex I activates canonical NF-κB pathway via the IKK complex, which consists of two catalytic subunits, IKKα and IKKβ, and a regulatory component, IKKγ/NEMO (Figure 2). The IKK complex phosphorylates and subsequently induces degradation of IκB. Once activated, NF-κB dimers translocate into the nucleus and stimulate transcription of various genes, such as those encoding cytokines and antiapoptotic factors.

Hepatocyte-specific IKKβ or NEMO knockout mice are more sensitive to the hepatotoxic effects of injecting Con-A or LPS, respectively, suggesting a crucial role of NF-κB activation in protection from TNFα-induced liver injury [45, 69]. Also note that the extent of TNFα-induced JNK activation is strengthened and prolonged in these mice.

Several mechanisms have been proposed by which NF-κB activation controls the level of JNK activation. At least three NF-κB-dependent genes have been identified as potential candidates, that is, growth arrest DNA damage-inducible gene 45β (Gadd45β), X-linked inhibitor of apoptosis (XIAP), and the zinc finger protein A20 [70–76]. However, the precise implications and detailed mechanisms of action of these molecules in the regulation of TNFα-induced JNK activation and cell death remain unclear, especially *in vivo*. In addition to the expression of JNK inhibitory proteins, NF-κB also inhibits JNK activation by controlling intracellular ROS levels. NF-κB activation leads to expression of the antioxidants ferritin heavy chain (FHC) and manganese-dependent superoxide dismutase (MnSOD), both of which prevent accumulation of ROS, thus inhibiting prolongation of JNK activation [77, 78].

2.7. Crosstalk between JNK and Other MAPK Signaling Molecules. p38α also plays an important role in inhibiting TNFα induced JNK activation and liver injury. Hepatocyte-specific p38α knockout mice showed much stronger JNK activation after administration of LPS [79]. Although p38α ablation is not sufficient to induce hepatocyte death after LPS administration, hepatocyte-specific p38α, and IKKβ double-knockout mice show severe liver injury, suggesting that p38α and IKKβ act synergistically to protect the liver from TNFα-induced toxicity. Unlike in the case of NF-κB, pretreatment with antioxidants could not reduce LPS-induced JNK activation in hepatocyte-specific p38α knockout mice. Furthermore, the levels of MKPs were similar between hepatocyte-specific p38α knockout mice and wild-type controls. Therefore, the detailed mechanisms of action of p38α in regulating TNFα-induced JNK activation and cell death remain unclear. However, hepatocyte-specific p38α knockout mice showed increased MKK4 activation, so targets of p38α are considered to be upstream of JNK, such as MAPKKs and MAP3Ks. Interestingly, not only MKK4 but also MKK3 and MKK6 activation, all of which are involved in p38 activation, are increased in hepatocyte-specific p38α knockout mice, suggesting that there might be negative feedback mechanism in p38 signaling pathway in the liver. In fact, p38 has been reported to negatively regulate upstream MAP3Ks such as TAK1 and MLK3 in other cells [80, 81].

Two recent studies have introduced MAP3K TAK1 into the complex field of NF-κB/JNK interaction in the liver [82, 83]. In TNFα signaling, TAK1 is recruited into complex I and phosphorylated through TRAFs. Then, phosphorylated TAK1 activates IKK and MKK4/7. Therefore, TAK1 can activate both NF-κB and JNK, which play opposing roles in cell death. Inokuchi et al. reported that hepatocyte-specific TAK1 knockout mice generated by intercrossing TAK1 floxed mice with Alb-Cre mice showed spontaneous hepatocyte death, which was partially canceled by further genetic deletion of TNF-R1, suggesting that TAK1-deficient hepatocytes are sensitive to endogenous TNFα [82]. They also reported that hepatocyte-specific TAK1-deficient mice showed enhanced JNK activation *in vivo*. Primary hepatocytes derived from these mice also demonstrated enhanced cell death by TNFα stimulation, and not only NF-κB activation but also JNK activation were inhibited *ex vivo*. Bettermann et al. reported that liver-specific TAK1 knockout mice generated by intercrossing TAK1 floxed mice with Alfp-Cre mice showed strong JNK activation, lack of NF-κB activation, and massive hepatocyte apoptosis after LPS injection [83]. This enhanced JNK activation may occur through activation of other MAP3K TAO2. Furthermore, they showed that TAK1 is required for the prevention of cholangiocyte apoptosis. Thus, although the role of TAK1 in the regulation of TNFα-mediated JNK activation has not been fully elucidated, TAK1 plays an antiapoptotic role in the liver mainly through NF-κB activation.

2.8. Implication of JNK in Other Types of Liver Injury. JNK signaling has also been implicated in hepatocyte injury due to other causes, including lipotoxicity, ER stress, ischemia-reperfusion, and drug toxicity, such as from acetaminophen [53, 84–87]. Although the role of JNK in these types of hepatocyte death cannot be discussed here in detail due to space limitations, JNK is generally considered to play an important role in cell death induction through similar mechanisms as seen in TNFα signaling. Therefore, JNK is a possible candidate therapeutic target for various types of liver injury.

3. JNK in Hepatocarcinogenesis

3.1. General Function of JNK in Carcinogenesis. Although this review has mainly discussed the pro-apoptotic function of JNK, this molecule has various functions in carcinogenesis. First, JNK plays an important role in cell proliferation. JNK is considered to be involved in cell cycle progression mostly through interaction with the transcription factor c-Jun, which is a well-established cell cycle regulator. A previous study using $JNK1^{-/-}$ or $JNK2^{-/-}$ fibroblasts showed that $JNK2^{-/-}$ fibroblasts proliferate faster with increased c-Jun expression, whereas $JNK1^{-/-}$ fibroblasts proliferate slower with decreased c-Jun expression, suggesting that JNK1 might play a major role in c-Jun-mediated cell cycle progression [88]. However, another study using fibroblasts from mice with a knockin mutation in the *JNK2* gene showed that JNK2 is also involved in c-jun expression and cellular proliferation

[89]. Thus, in general, both JNK1 and JNK2 play important roles in cell cycle progression.

In the liver, JNK1 has been shown to be a major player in cell cycle regulation using a partial hepatectomy model. Hui et al. reported that the number of Ki67-positive proliferating hepatocytes in $JNK1^{-/-}$ mice was significantly reduced compared to wild-type controls after partial hepatectomy [20]. The impaired proliferation in $JNK1^{-/-}$ mice was caused by increased expression of p21, a cell cycle inhibitor, and reduced expression of c-Myc, a negative regulator of p21. In contrast, $JNK2^{-/-}$ mice showed similar hepatocyte proliferation rates to wild-type controls. Another study showed that administration of the pan-JNK inhibitor SP600125 inhibited hepatocyte proliferation after partial hepatectomy through reduced expression of cyclin D1 [90]. Thus, JNK plays an important role in hepatocyte proliferation *in vivo*.

In addition to its roles in cell proliferation, JNK has been shown to also have various oncogenic functions. For example, the JNK pathway is involved in HCC cell migration and tumor invasion through matrix metalloproteinase (MMP) production [91]. A recent study showed that JNK is required for Ras-induced suppression of contact growth inhibition by regulating e-cadherin expression [92]. Furthermore, JNK facilitates cancer progression by interacting with other oncogenic pathways, such as Wnt/β-catenin signaling [93–95]. Thus, although JNK is generally considered to play oncogenic roles, it also plays roles in tumor suppression in some cases through p53 activation and induction of apoptosis [96–98].

3.2. Role of JNK in Hepatocarcinogenesis. In general, induction of cell death acts as a tumor-suppressing function. However, this function does not always act as a tumor suppressor, but instead acts as a tumor promoter in the liver, because the loss of hepatic mass due to hepatocyte death activates the proliferation of residual hepatocytes that may provide a promoting environment for tumor formation. Recent *in vivo* studies strongly implicated JNK as a key regulator in this process.

Diethylnitrosamine (DEN) is a chemical carcinogen commonly used to induce HCC in rodents. Administration of DEN causes acute liver injury and DNA damage in the hepatocytes, and subsequently leads to inflammation, liver regeneration, and neoplastic lesions in the liver. A study using hepatocyte-specific IKKβ knockout mice demonstrated a critical concept with regard to the role of cross talk between NF-κB and JNK in hepatocytes in DEN-induced HCC [78] (Figure 3). Hepatocyte-specific knockout of IKKβ markedly enhanced DEN-induced HCC. The ablation of hepatocyte IKKβ induces greater DEN-induced JNK activation and greater cell death during the acute reaction to DEN administration. The absence of NF-κB induces prolonged JNK activation by enhancing ROS production, and prolonged JNK activation plays a critical role in DEN-induced hepatocyte death, as seen in TNFα-mediated liver injury. Subsequently, the elevated hepatocyte death rate enhances compensatory proliferation. Thus, the hepatocyte-specific deletion of IKKβ augments DEN-induced hepatocyte death, compensatory proliferation, and increased tumorigenesis, probably through enhanced JNK activation. Similar findings were obtained in mice lacking NEMO, the hepatocyte-specific deletion of which results in spontaneous liver damage, hepatosteatosis, fibrosis, and the development of HCC [69]. To further investigate the role of JNK in this process, $JNK1^{-/-}$ mice were interbred with hepatocyte-specific IKKβ knockout mice, and the double-knockout mice developed significantly fewer tumors compared to IKKβ knockout mice [18]. In addition, $JNK1^{-/-}$ mice showed a significant reduction of tumor development compared to wild-type controls. In addition to the involvement in DEN-induced acute liver injury, JNK1 has tumor-promoting functions by enhancing cancer cell proliferation and neovascularization through the increased expression of cyclin D1 and VEGF, respectively. Another group also reported the critical role of JNK1 in hepatocarcinogenesis using the DEN and phenobarbital-induced HCC model [20]. They showed that cancer cell proliferation decreases significantly in $JNK1^{-/-}$ mice due to increased p21 expression and reduced c-Myc expression. In addition, pharmacological inhibition of JNK by D-JNKi reduced the growth of xenografted human HCC cells and chemically induced mouse liver cancers, suggesting that JNK is a promising therapeutic target for HCC. Their study, however, also showed that JNK2 is not involved in hepatocarcinogenesis. About 50%–60% of human HCC show strong activation of JNK1 compared to adjacent nontumor tissue, whereas JNK2 activation is similar between HCC and non-tumor tissue [20, 99]. These results suggest that JNK, especially JNK1, plays an important role in the development of HCC.

JNK activation is also implicated in HCC based on viral hepatitis. *In vitro* studies showed that several HBV and HCV proteins can activate the JNK pathway [100, 101]. In addition, JNK-mediated enhanced cell proliferation is involved in hepatocarcinogenesis of HCV core protein transgenic mice and HBx protein transgenic mice, both of which spontaneously develop HCC [102, 103].

However, a more recent study using conditional knockout mice of both JNK isoforms, JNK1 and JNK2, suggested that JNK may play dual roles in hepatocarcinogenesis [104]. In their study, JNK deficiency in hepatocytes increased DEN-induced HCC. In contrast, JNK deficiency in both hepatocytes and myeloid cells reduced hepatic inflammation and the development of HCC. Although the detailed mechanisms remain unclear, this study suggested that JNK in hepatocytes may act as a tumor suppressor, whereas that in myeloid cells may act as a tumor promoter in the development of HCC.

JNK is also wellknown as a critical regulator of obesity and metabolic syndrome through inhibition of insulin signaling in the liver and muscle, and modulation of adipokine secretion from adipocytes [105, 106]. Recent studies have suggested that obesity-induced insulin resistance and dysregulation of adipokines play important roles in hepatocarcinogenesis [107–110]. As the incidence rate of this metabolic syndrome-associated hepatocarcinogenesis is likely to increase in the near future, investigating whether JNK activation also contributes to hepatocarcinogenesis under this condition is critical.

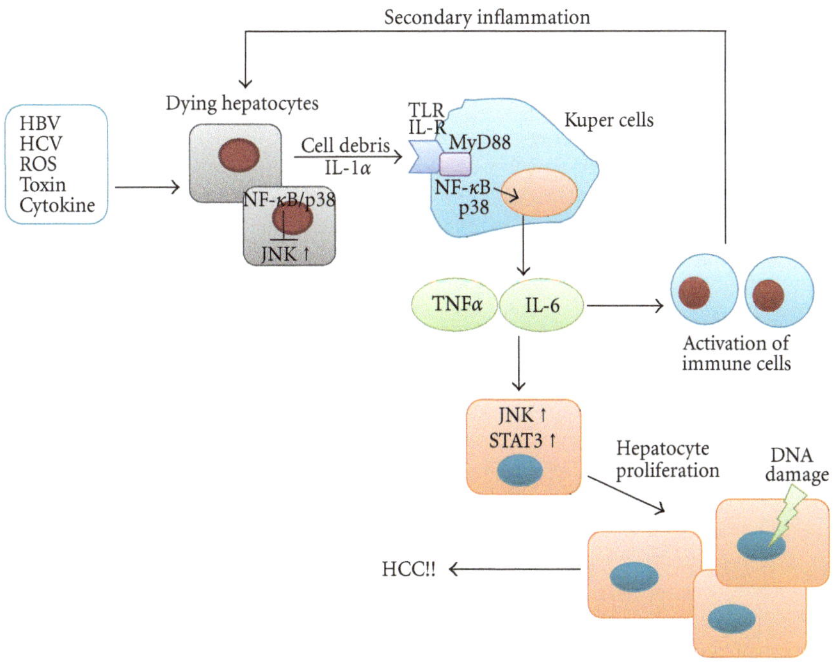

FIGURE 3: Current model of the role of stress-activated MAPK and NF-κB in inflammation-mediated hepatocarcinogenesis. In chronic liver injury, hepatitis virus, ROS, toxins, and cytokines kill hepatocytes. JNK promotes cell death, while NF-κB and p38 promote cell survival. Dying hepatocytes activate Kupffer cells via TLR or IL-1R. Activated Kupffer cells secrete cytokines, such as IL-6 and TNFα, through a mechanism mediated by NF-κB and p38. Subsequently, these cytokines induce recruitment of activated inflammatory cells to the liver, which is followed by hepatocyte regeneration. JNK and STAT3 promote cytokine-mediated hepatocyte proliferation. This persistent cycle of necroinflammation and hepatocyte regeneration provides a mitogenic and mutagenic environment, leading to the development of HCC.

4. p38 and MAP3Ks in Hepatocarcinogenesis

4.1. p38 Signaling. The p38 MAPK group consists of four members: p38α, p38β, p38γ, and p38δ [111]. p38α and p38β are universally expressed and closely related proteins that have overlapping functions. Whereas p38α is highly abundant in most cell types, p38β seems to be expressed at very low levels. p38γ and p38δ have more restricted expression patterns and are likely to have specialized functions [23]. Most of the published literature on p38 MAPKs refers to p38α, and we mainly discuss p38α in this paper. MKK3 and MKK6 are the primary upstream MAPKKs of p38, but MKK4 has also been shown to activate p38 in response to certain stimuli. p38 can also be activated independently of the MAP3K/MAPKK cascade by autophosphorylation [112]. Substrates of p38 include protein kinases, such as MAPKAP kinase 2 (MK2) and MK5, and transcription factors, such as ATF2, p53, and Mitf [113]. These diverse targets mediate the activated p38 signal to various types of cellular functions such as differentiation, apoptosis, cytokine production, and cell cycle control.

4.2. General Function of p38 in Carcinogenesis. Although p38 was first recognized as a regulator of inflammatory cytokine production, recent studies uncovered a role of p38α as an essential inhibitor of cell proliferation. p38α negatively regulates cell cycle progression both at the G1/S and G2/M transitions by several mechanisms, including the downregulation of cyclins, upregulation of cyclin-dependent kinase (CDK) inhibitors, and modulation of the tumor suppressor p53 [114]. p38α also acts as an inhibitor of hepatocyte proliferation after partial hepatectomy, and inactivation of p38α is seen during liver regeneration [115, 116]. This effect of p38α is partially mediated by negative regulation of the JNK/c-Jun pathway [19].

In addition to the suppression of cell proliferation, p38 exerts tumor-suppressing effects through oncogene-induced senescence (OIS), contact inhibition, and DNA damage responses [111]. In particular, recent studies demonstrated a major role of p38 in OIS caused by oncogenic Ras or its downstream effector Raf-1. The Ras-Raf-MEK-ERK signaling cascade increases the intracellular ROS level and subsequently activates the p38 pathway [117]. Activated p38 phosphorylates multiple residues on p53, leading to increased transcriptional activity of p53 and induction of p21 [111, 118]. Active p38 also induces the expression of p16 and p14/p19, which together with the p53-p21 cascade, cause senescence that serves as a tumor-suppressing defense mechanism [119]. Thus, a great deal of evidence supports a role of p38 as a tumor suppressor. However, p38 may also have oncogenic effects by facilitating cell invasion, inflammation, and angiogenesis [120, 121].

4.3. Role of p38 in Hepatocarcinogenesis. The role of p38 in hepatocarcinogenesis has also been investigated using the DEN-induced mouse HCC model. Similar to hepatocyte-specific IKKβ knockout mice, hepatocyte-specific p38α knockout mice showed enhanced DEN-induced ROS accumulation, JNK activation, liver damage, and subsequent hepatocyte proliferation, which resulted in enhanced carcinogenesis [21]. In addition, hepatocyte-specific p38α ablation leads to enhanced IL-1α release from necrotic hepatocytes. IL-1α can activate Kupffer cells, and activated Kupffer cells produce various cytokines, such as TNFα, IL-6, and hepatocyte growth factor, which promote proliferation of residual hepatocytes (Figure 3). The activation of p38 and NF-κB in Kupffer cells plays an important role in this process because mice with p38α or IKKβ knockout in both hepatocytes and myeloid cells, including Kupffer cells, showed markedly reduced hepatic expression of these cytokines after DEN challenge, resulting in reduced future HCC development [21, 78]. Thus, p38α and NF-κB in the hepatocytes act as tumor suppressors by conferring protection against DEN-induced cell death, whereas p38α and NF-κB in the Kupffer cells act as tumor promoters by enhancing cytokine production. Another study using hepatocyte-specific p38α knockout mice indicated its role in tumor suppression by focusing on the antiproliferative function at the advanced stage [19]. Ablation of p38α in the hepatocytes results in upregulation of the JNK/c-Jun pathway, which plays an important role in the increased proliferation of tumor cells.

In human samples, the activity of the MKK6-p38 pathway is decreased in HCC tissues compared to adjacent nontumor tissues [122]. In particular, its activity is significantly lower in larger HCC tissues, suggesting that the p38 pathway may play an antiproliferative role in human HCC.

4.4. Role of MAP3Ks in Hepatocarcinogenesis. The evidence presented to date suggests that JNK generally acts as a tumor promoter and p38 generally acts as a tumor suppressor in hepatocarcinogenesis. However, as JNK and p38 have complex functions and modulate a wide range of cellular effect, some studies showed dual roles of these molecules in hepatocarcinogenesis. Furthermore, cross talk among JNK and p38, and molecules involved in other signaling pathways such as NF-κB, further complicate their roles. Several recent studies have uncovered the roles of MAP3Ks in the regulation of stress-activated MAPK signaling in hepatocarcinogenesis.

One player is TAK1, which can activate NF-κB as well as JNK and p38 in response to the signaling of Toll-like receptors, IL-1 receptor, TNF receptor, and TGF-β receptor. As mentioned above, hepatocyte-specific TAK1 knockout mice show spontaneous hepatocyte death, which is partially mediated by endogenous TNFα [82, 83]. This spontaneous cell death subsequently causes compensatory hepatocyte proliferation, inflammation, and fibrosis. Furthermore, about 80%–90% of these mice spontaneously develop HCC at 9 months of age. These phenomena, which resembled the phenotype observed in hepatocyte-specific NF-κB knockout mice, are considered to occur through attenuated NF-κB activation and elevated JNK activation. The p38 pathway, however, seems not to be involved in this phenotype. Thus, TAK1 in the hepatocytes acts as a tumor suppressor mainly by regulating activation of the NF-κB pathway. Unexpectedly, crossing hepatocyte-specific TAK1 knockout mice with NEMO knockout mice attenuates JNK activation and prevents hepatocyte death and the development of HCC, suggesting that NEMO has a tumor-promoting function in the setting of TAK1 deletion [83]. Furthermore, this function of NEMO is considered to be independent of NF-κB.

Another player is ASK1, which selectively activates JNK and p38 signaling in response to a variety of stimuli, including ROS and cytokines [123]. The role of ASK1 in hepatocarcinogenesis has been investigated using the DEN-induced HCC model [54]. The number of tumors in $ASK1^{-/-}$ mice is three times higher than that in wild-type controls, and cancer cell apoptosis is significantly suppressed in $ASK1^{-/-}$ HCC. JNK activation and hyperphosphorylation of BimEL, which are required for death receptor-mediated apoptosis, including TNF-R and Fas, are attenuated in $ASK1^{-/-}$ HCC but not in non-tumor tissues, suggesting escape from the antitumor immune response. In contrast, tumor-promoting functions of JNK, such as cell proliferation and neovascularization, are preserved in $ASK1^{-/-}$ mice. Therefore, ASK1 is considered to play a major part in the tumor-suppressing role of JNK in hepatocarcinogenesis. In addition, activation of the p38 pathway is also attenuated in $ASK1^{-/-}$ mice, and DNA damage-induced p21 upregulation via the p38 pathway is inhibited. Thus, ASK1 controls the tumor-suppressing function of stress-activated MAPK signaling through induction of apoptosis and the DNA damage response, and acts as a tumor suppressor in hepatocarcinogenesis (Figure 4). Furthermore, another recent study indicated that ASK1 and Bim are also required for sorafenib-induced apoptosis in HCC cells [124]. Therefore, ASK1 may play important roles in not only hepatocarcinogenesis but also in the therapeutic effects of anticancer drugs.

In some cases, MAP3K may be a better therapeutic target than MAPK. To date, more than ten molecules have been identified as MAP3K in stress-activated MAPK signaling, which is much more than the number of the downstream MAPK (Figure 1) [125]. This fact indicates that the MAP3Ks are activated by various stimuli, and function as signaling hubs, integrating these signals into a unique pattern of MAPK activation, and eventually leading to a specific function of MAPK to the stimulus. Thus, blocking MAP3K may be able to inhibit specific function of MAPK. In addition, inhibition of JNK or p38 causes compensatory activation of another stress-activated MAPK, whereas inhibition of some MAP3Ks such as ASK1 does not cause such compensation, which may be advantageous in the clinical settings as discussed in the next section. However, which MAP3K is important in growth factor-mediated JNK activation in HCC remains unclear, especially *in vivo*, although MEKK1 and MLK3 have been reported to be involved in this role of JNK in non-HCC cells such as colon cancer [126, 127]. Therefore, further understanding of the regulatory system of stress-activated MAPK signaling by MAP3Ks is important.

5. Future Perspectives

These recent studies have gradually clarified the roles and regulation systems of stress-activated MAPK in hepatocarcinogenesis, but some issues remain to be elucidated.

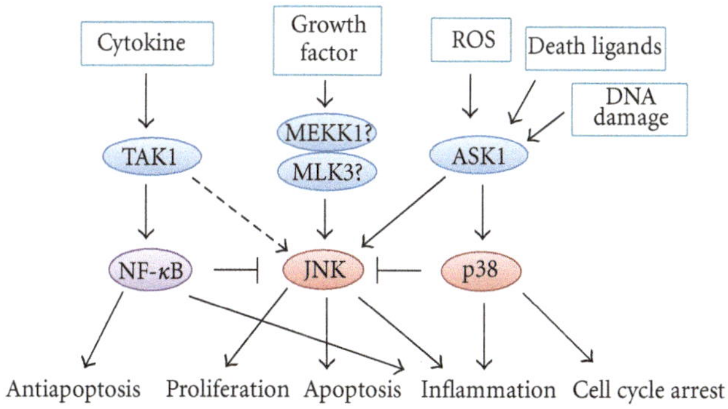

FIGURE 4: Roles of MAP3Ks in controlling the function of stress-activated MAPK and NF-κB in hepatocarcinogenesis. TAK1 can activate NF-κB and JNK, but TAK1 mainly regulates NF-κB activation and acts as a tumor suppressor in hepatocarcinogenesis. ASK1 controls the tumor-suppressing function of JNK and p38 through apoptosis induction and DNA damage response, and thus acts as a tumor suppressor. MEKK1 and MLK3 may be involved in JNK-mediated tumor cell proliferation in hepatocarcinogenesis, but no supporting *in vivo* evidence exists to support this contention at present. Furthermore, the roles of these molecules may differ according to the disease model and timing.

One issue is that the role of these molecules may change according to the disease model. A good example is NF-κB. As mentioned above, DEN-induced HCC is increased in hepatocyte-specific IKKβ knockout mice and spontaneous HCC development is seen in hepatocyte-specific NEMO knockout mice, suggesting a role of NF-κB as a tumor suppressor [69, 78]. However, experiments crossing transgenic mice expressing a nondegradable IκBα mutant with MDR2 knockout mice, which show chronic inflammation in the portal area and subsequent cancer development, indicated a tumor-promoting role of NF-κB [128]. These results indicate the dual roles of NF-κB in hepatocarcinogenesis depending on the disease model. Thus, more appropriate models mimicking human chronic hepatitis and hepatocarcinogenesis are required. In this sense, TAK1 knockout mice may be a promising candidate because TAK1-deficient HCC develops in the context of chronic inflammation and fibrosis, as commonly found in human HCC [82, 83]. Furthermore, the time manipulation is also an important problem. For example, studies in TAK1 knockout and ASK1 knockout mice confirmed that too much apoptosis in the chronic inflammatory phase facilitates hepatocarcinogenesis, whereas too little apoptosis in already initiated cells also aggravates cancer progression, suggesting that the apoptotic function plays dual roles in a stage-dependent manner [54, 82, 83]. Therefore, therapeutic targets may need to be redefined according to the carcinogenic stage.

The critical role of stress-activated MAPK signaling in hepatocarcinogenesis prompts their introduction (especially JNK1) into the clinical settings as therapeutic targets. Several inhibitors targeting JNK or p38 have entered clinical trials for other diseases. In particular, p38 inhibitors for inflammatory diseases, such as rheumatoid arthritis and inflammatory bowel disease, have been studied extensively [129, 130]. However, few have progressed beyond phase I clinical trials and none have yet appeared in clinical settings. One reason for this is the occurrence of side effects, such as liver toxicity. Although whether these are due to target inhibition or to the effects of the drugs on additional targets is unclear, cross talk among signaling pathways is considered to be one explanation because p38 inhibition induces compensatory JNK activation. Therefore, alternative strategies, such as the targeting of particular MAPK isoforms, including JNK1, upstream regulators, including MAP3K, and downstream effectors, including Bcl-2 family members, will be more beneficial than targeting the whole pathway. Note that the roles of these molecules differ among cell types, such as hepatocytes and myeloid cells, including Kupffer cells. Therefore, one must take into account its total function in disease progression. Furthermore, combination therapies are likely to be more important in the future. Hence, further understanding of these pathways will help to develop novel treatment strategies for advanced HCC or prevention of HCC development.

6. Conclusion

Recent studies have indicated that MAPK signaling pathways play key roles and have potential as therapeutic targets in liver injury and hepatocarcinogenesis. Among them, JNK signaling is a promising therapeutic target. However, these pathways have a wide range of functions and show complex cross talk. In addition, their roles differ between cell types and disease processes. Our final goal is to establish them as new diagnostic markers and targets for therapies or prevention of liver diseases. In fact, recent report showed that activation of JNK in noncancerous liver tissue predicted a high risk of HCC recurrence after surgical resection, suggesting that testing JNK activation in the liver might be useful for the risk assessment of HCC occurrence or recurrence [131]. Thus, further understanding of these very important and complicated pathways, including surrounding modulators, is essential for application in clinical settings.

Abbreviations

ASK1:	Apoptosis signal-regulating kinase 1
DEN:	Diethylnitrosamine
GalN:	Galactosamine
HBV:	Hepatitis B virus
HCC:	Hepatocellular carcinoma
HCV:	Hepatitis C virus
JNK:	c-Jun NH_2-terminal kinase
LPS:	Lipopolysaccharide
MAPK:	Mitogen-activated protein kinase
MAP3K:	Mitogen-activated protein kinase kinase kinase
NASH:	Nonalcoholic steatohepatitis
NF-κB:	Nuclear factor-kappa B
OIS:	Oncogene-induced senescence
ROS:	Reactive oxygen species
TAK1:	Transforming growth factor β-activated kinase 1
TNF-α:	Tumor necrosis factor-α
TNF-R1:	TNF-receptor 1
Trx:	Thioredoxin.

Acknowledgments

This work was supported by a fellowship from the Daiichi Sankyo Foundation of Life Science (to H. Nakagawa).

References

[1] H. B. El-Serag and K. L. Rudolph, "Hepatocellular carcinoma: epidemiology and molecular carcinogenesis," *Gastroenterology*, vol. 132, no. 7, pp. 2557–2576, 2007.

[2] R. Masuzaki, H. Yoshida, R. Tateishi, S. Shiina, and M. Omata, "Hepatocellular carcinoma in viral hepatitis: improving standard therapy," *Best Practice and Research*, vol. 22, no. 6, pp. 1137–1151, 2008.

[3] M. C. Yu and J. M. Yuan, "Environmental factors and risk for hepatocellular carcinoma," *Gastroenterology*, vol. 127, pp. S72–S78, 2004.

[4] A. Budhu and W. W. Xin, "The role of cytokines in hepatocellular carcinoma," *Journal of Leukocyte Biology*, vol. 80, no. 6, pp. 1197–1213, 2006.

[5] M. Levrero, "Viral hepatitis and liver cancer: the case of hepatitis C," *Oncogene*, vol. 25, no. 27, pp. 3834–3847, 2006.

[6] A. M. Elsharkawy and D. A. Mann, "Nuclear factor-κB and the hepatic inflammation-fibrosis-cancer axis," *Hepatology*, vol. 46, no. 2, pp. 590–597, 2007.

[7] H. Nakagawa, S. Maeda, H. Yoshida et al., "Serum IL 6 levels and the risk for hepatocarcinogenesis in chronic hepatitis C patients: an analysis based on gender differences," *International Journal of Cancer*, vol. 125, no. 10, pp. 2264–2269, 2009.

[8] V. Mazzaferro, E. Regalia, R. Doci et al., "Liver transplantation for the treatment of small hepatocellular carcinomas in patients with cirrhosis," *The New England Journal of Medicine*, vol. 334, no. 11, pp. 693–699, 1996.

[9] J. M. Llovet, M. Schwartz, and V. Mazzaferro, "Resection and liver transplantation for hepatocellular carcinoma," *Seminars in Liver Disease*, vol. 25, no. 2, pp. 181–200, 2005.

[10] R. Tateishi, S. Shiina, T. Teratani et al., "Percutaneous radiofrequency ablation for hepatocellular carcinoma: an analysis of 1000 cases," *Cancer*, vol. 103, no. 6, pp. 1201–1209, 2005.

[11] R. Masuzaki, H. Yoshida, and M. Omata, "Does chemotherapy prevent HCV-related hepatocellular carcinoma? Pros," *Digestive and Liver Disease*, vol. 42, supplement 3, pp. 281–286, 2010.

[12] J. M. Llovet, S. Ricci, V. Mazzaferro et al., "Sorafenib in advanced hepatocellular carcinoma," *The New England Journal of Medicine*, vol. 359, no. 4, pp. 378–390, 2008.

[13] A. Villanueva and J. M. Llovet, "Targeted therapies for hepatocellular carcinoma," *Gastroenterology*, vol. 140, no. 5, pp. 1410–1426, 2011.

[14] H. Yoshida, Y. Shiratori, M. Moriyama et al., "Interferon therapy reduces the risk for hepatocellular carcinoma: national surveillance program of cirrhotic and noncirrhotic patients with chronic hepatitis C in Japan. IHIT Study Group. Inhibition of Hepatocarcinogenesis by Interferon Therapy," *Annals of Internal Medicine*, vol. 131, pp. 174–181, 1999.

[15] M. W. Fried, M. L. Shiffman, K. Rajender Reddy et al., "Peginterferon alfa-2a plus ribavirin for chronic hepatitis C virus infection," *The New England Journal of Medicine*, vol. 347, no. 13, pp. 975–982, 2002.

[16] T. T. Chang, R. G. Gish, R. De Man et al., "A comparison of entecavir and lamivudine for HBeAg-positive chronic hepatitis B," *The New England Journal of Medicine*, vol. 354, no. 10, pp. 1001–1010, 2006.

[17] J. G. McHutchison, G. T. Everson, S. C. Gordon et al., "Telaprevir with peginterferon and ribavirin for chronic HCV genotype 1 infection," *The New England Journal of Medicine*, vol. 360, no. 18, pp. 1827–1838, 2009.

[18] T. Sakurai, S. Maeda, L. Chang, and M. Karin, "Loss of hepatic NF-κB activity enhances chemical hepatocarcinogenesis through sustained c-Jun N-terminal kinase 1 activation," *Proceedings of the National Academy of Sciences of the United States of America*, vol. 103, no. 28, pp. 10544–10551, 2006.

[19] L. Hui, L. Bakiri, A. Mairhorfer et al., "p38α suppresses normal and cancer cell proliferation by antagonizing the JNK-c-Jun pathway," *Nature Genetics*, vol. 39, no. 6, pp. 741–749, 2007.

[20] L. Hui, K. Zatloukal, H. Scheuch, E. Stepniak, and E. F. Wagner, "Proliferation of human HCC cells and chemically induced mouse liver cancers requires JNK1-dependent p21 downregulation," *The Journal of Clinical Investigation*, vol. 118, no. 12, pp. 3943–3953, 2008.

[21] T. Sakurai, G. He, A. Matsuzawa et al., "Hepatocyte necrosis induced by oxidative stress and IL-1 alpha release mediate carcinogen-induced compensatory proliferation and liver tumorigenesis," *Cancer Cell*, vol. 14, no. 2, pp. 156–165, 2008.

[22] S. Maeda, "NF-κB, JNK, and TLR signaling pathways in hepatocarcinogenesis," *Gastroenterology Research and Practice*, vol. 2010, Article ID 367694, 10 pages, 2010.

[23] E. F. Wagner and A. R. Nebreda, "Signal integration by JNK and p38 MAPK pathways in cancer development," *Nature Reviews Cancer*, vol. 9, no. 8, pp. 537–549, 2009.

[24] L. Min, B. He, and L. Hui, "Mitogen-activated protein kinases in hepatocellular carcinoma development," *Seminars in Cancer Biology*, vol. 21, no. 1, pp. 10–20, 2011.

[25] J. M. Kyriakis and J. Avruch, "Mammalian mitogen-activated protein kinase signal transduction pathways activated by stress and inflammation," *Physiological Reviews*, vol. 81, no. 2, pp. 807–869, 2001.

[26] L. Chang and M. Karin, "Mammalian MAP kinase signalling cascades," *Nature*, vol. 410, no. 6824, pp. 37–40, 2001.

[27] R. J. Davis, "Signal transduction by the JNK group of MAP kinases," *Cell*, vol. 103, no. 2, pp. 239–252, 2000.

[28] E. Shaulian and M. Karin, "AP-1 as a regulator of cell life and death," *Nature Cell Biology*, vol. 4, no. 5, pp. E131–E136, 2002.

[29] C. R. Weston and R. J. Davis, "The JNK signal transduction pathway," *Current Opinion in Genetics and Development*, vol. 12, no. 1, pp. 14–21, 2002.

[30] H. M. Shen and Z. G. Liu, "JNK signaling pathway is a key modulator in cell death mediated by reactive oxygen and nitrogen species," *Free Radical Biology and Medicine*, vol. 40, no. 6, pp. 928–939, 2006.

[31] D. Conze, T. Krahl, N. Kennedy et al., "c-Jun NH2-terminal kinase (JNK)1 and JNK2 have distinct roles in CD8+ T cell activation," *Journal of Experimental Medicine*, vol. 195, no. 7, pp. 811–823, 2002.

[32] R. F. Schwabe and D. A. Brenner, "Mechanisms of liver injury. I. TNF-α-induced liver injury: role of IKK, JNK, and ROS pathways," *American Journal of Physiology*, vol. 290, no. 4, pp. G583–G589, 2006.

[33] D. R. Nelson, H. L. Lim, C. G. Marousis et al., "Activation of tumor necrosis factor-α system in chronic hepatitis C virus infection," *Digestive Diseases and Sciences*, vol. 42, no. 12, pp. 2487–2494, 1997.

[34] N. Sheron, J. Lau, H. Daniels et al., "Increased production of tumour necrosis factor alpha in chronic hepatitis B virus infection," *Journal of Hepatology*, vol. 12, no. 2, pp. 241–245, 1991.

[35] G. L. A. Bird, N. Sheron, A. K. J. Goka, G. J. Alexander, and R. S. Williams, "Increased plasma tumor necrosis factor in severe alcoholic hepatitis," *Annals of Internal Medicine*, vol. 112, no. 12, pp. 917–920, 1990.

[36] M. H. Jarrar, A. Baranova, R. Collantes et al., "Adipokines and cytokines in non-alcoholic fatty liver disease," *Alimentary Pharmacology and Therapeutics*, vol. 27, no. 5, pp. 412–421, 2008.

[37] K. R. Feingold, M. Soued, C. Grunfeld, A. H. Moser, J. A. Verdier, and H. G. DoVale, "Tumor necrosis factor stimulates DNA synthesis in the liver of intact rats," *Biochemical and Biophysical Research Communications*, vol. 153, no. 2, pp. 576–582, 1988.

[38] Y. Yamada, I. Kirillova, J. J. Peschon, and N. Fausto, "Initiation of liver growth by tumor necrosis factor: deficient liver regeneration in mice lacking type I tumor necrosis factor receptor," *Proceedings of the National Academy of Sciences of the United States of America*, vol. 94, no. 4, pp. 1441–1446, 1997.

[39] A. Wullaert, G. Van Loo, K. Heyninck, and R. Beyaert, "Hepatic tumor necrosis factor signaling and nuclear factor-κB: effects on liver homeostasis and beyond," *Endocrine Reviews*, vol. 28, no. 4, pp. 365–386, 2007.

[40] S. Papa, C. Bubici, F. Zazzeroni, and G. Franzoso, "Mechanisms of liver disease: cross-talk between the NF-κB and JNK pathways," *Biological Chemistry*, vol. 390, no. 10, pp. 965–976, 2009.

[41] O. Micheau and J. Tschopp, "Induction of TNF receptor I-mediated apoptosis via two sequential signaling complexes," *Cell*, vol. 114, no. 2, pp. 181–190, 2003.

[42] C. A. Bradham, T. Qian, K. Streetz, C. Trautwein, D. A. Brenner, and J. J. Lemasters, "The mitochondrial permeability transition is required for tumor necrosis factor alpha-mediated apoptosis and cytochrome c release," *Molecular and Cellular Biology*, vol. 18, no. 11, pp. 6353–6364, 1998.

[43] R. F. Schwabe, H. Uchinami, T. Qian, B. L. Bennett, J. J. Lemasters, and D. A. Brenner, "Differential requirement for c-Jun NH2-terminal kinase in TNFalpha- and Fas-mediated apoptosis in hepatocytes.," *The FASEB Journal*, vol. 18, no. 6, pp. 720–722, 2004.

[44] L. Chang, H. Kamata, G. Solinas et al., "The E3 ubiquitin ligase itch couples JNK activation to TNFα-induced cell death by inducing c-FLIPL turnover," *Cell*, vol. 124, no. 3, pp. 601–613, 2006.

[45] S. Maeda, L. Chang, Z. W. Li, J. L. Luo, H. Leffert, and M. Karin, "IKKβ is required for prevention of apoptosis mediated by cell-bound but not by circulating TNFα," *Immunity*, vol. 19, no. 5, pp. 725–737, 2003.

[46] Y. Wang, R. Singh, J. H. Lefkowitch, R. M. Rigoli, and M. J. Czaja, "Tumor necrosis factor-induced toxic liver injury results from JNK2-dependent activation of caspase-8 and the mitochondrial death pathway," *The Journal of Biological Chemistry*, vol. 281, no. 22, pp. 15258–15267, 2006.

[47] H. M. Ni, X. Chen, Y. H. Shi et al., "Genetic delineation of the pathways mediated by bid and JNK in tumor necrosis factor-α-induced liver injury in adult and embryonic mice," *The Journal of Biological Chemistry*, vol. 284, no. 7, pp. 4373–4382, 2009.

[48] M. Takamura, Y. Matsuda, S. Yamagiwa et al., "An inhibitor of c-Jun NH2-terminal kinase, SP600125, protects mice from d-galactosamine/lipopolysaccharide-induced hepatic failure by modulating BH3-only proteins," *Life Sciences*, vol. 80, no. 14, pp. 1335–1344, 2007.

[49] C. Wang, L. Deng, M. Hong, G. R. Akkaraju, J. I. Inoue, and Z. J. Chen, "TAK1 is a ubiquitin-dependent kinase of MKK and IKK," *Nature*, vol. 412, no. 6844, pp. 346–351, 2001.

[50] H. Kamata, S. I. Honda, S. Maeda, L. Chang, H. Hirata, and M. Karin, "Reactive oxygen species promote TNFα-induced death and sustained JNK activation by inhibiting MAP kinase phosphatases," *Cell*, vol. 120, no. 5, pp. 649–661, 2005.

[51] K. Tobiume, A. Matsuzawa, T. Takahashi et al., "ASK1 is required for sustained activations of JNK/p38 MAP kinases and apoptosis," *EMBO Reports*, vol. 2, no. 3, pp. 222–228, 2001.

[52] M. Saitoh, H. Nishitoh, M. Fujii et al., "Mammalian thioredoxin is a direct inhibitor of apoptosis signal-regulating kinase (ASK) 1," *The EMBO Journal*, vol. 17, no. 9, pp. 2596–2606, 1998.

[53] H. Nakagawa, S. Maeda, Y. Hikiba et al., "Deletion of apoptosis signal-regulating kinase 1 attenuates acetaminophen-induced liver injury by inhibiting c-Jun N-terminal kinase activation," *Gastroenterology*, vol. 135, no. 4, pp. 1311–1321, 2008.

[54] H. Nakagawa, Y. Hirata, K. Takeda et al., "Apoptosis signal-regulating kinase 1 inhibits hepatocarcinogenesis by controlling the tumor-suppressing function of stress-activated mitogen-activated protein kinase," *Hepatology*, vol. 54, no. 1, pp. 185–195, 2011.

[55] H. Okuyama, H. Nakamura, Y. Shimahara et al., "Overexpression of thioredoxin prevents acute hepatitis caused by thioacetamide or lipopolysaccharide in mice," *Hepatology*, vol. 37, no. 5, pp. 1015–1025, 2003.

[56] K. Moriya, K. Nakagawa, T. Santa et al., "Oxidative stress in the absence of inflammation in a mouse model for hepatitis C virus-associated hepatocarcinogenesis," *Cancer Research*, vol. 61, no. 11, pp. 4365–4370, 2001.

[57] H. Kaneto, Y. Nakatani, T. Miyatsuka et al., "Possible novel therapy for diabetes with cell-permeable JNK-inhibitory peptide," *Nature Medicine*, vol. 10, no. 10, pp. 1128–1132, 2004.

[58] H. Nakagawa, A. Isogawa, R. Tateishi et al., "Serum gamma-glutamyltransferase level is associated with serum superoxide dismutase activity and metabolic syndrome in a Japanese population," *Journal of Gastroenterology*, vol. 47, no. 2, pp. 187–194, 2012.

[59] Y. Deng, X. Ren, L. Yang et al., "A JNK-dependent pathway is required for TNFalpha-induced apoptosis," *Cell*, vol. 115, pp. 61–70, 2003.

[60] K. Yamamoto, H. Ichijo, and S. J. Korsmeyer, "BCL-2 is phosphorylated and inactivated by an ASK1/Jun N-terminal protein kinase pathway normally activated at G2/M," *Molecular and Cellular Biology*, vol. 19, no. 12, pp. 8469–8478, 1999.

[61] X. Deng, L. Xiao, W. Lang et al., "Novel role for JNK as a stress-activated Bcl2 kinase," *The Journal of Biological Chemistry*, vol. 276, pp. 23681–23688, 2001.

[62] M. Fan, M. Goodwin, T. Vu, C. Brantley-Finley, W. A. Gaarde, and T. C. Chambers, "Vinblastine-induced phosphorylation of Bcl-2 and Bcl-X(L) is mediated by JNK and occurs in parallel with inactivation of the Raf-1/MEK/ERK cascade," *The Journal of Biological Chemistry*, vol. 275, no. 39, pp. 29980–29985, 2000.

[63] F. Tsuruta, J. Sunayama, Y. Mori et al., "JNK promotes Bax translocation to mitochondria through phosphorylation of 14-3-3 proteins," *The EMBO Journal*, vol. 23, no. 8, pp. 1889–1899, 2004.

[64] T. Kaufmann, P. J. Jost, M. Pellegrini et al., "Fatal hepatitis mediated by tumor necrosis factor TNFalpha requires caspase-8 and involves the BH3-only proteins Bid and Bim," *Immunity*, vol. 30, no. 1, pp. 56–66, 2009.

[65] K. Lei and R. J. Davis, "JNK phosphorylation of Bim-related members of the Bcl2 family induces Bax-dependent apoptosis," *Proceedings of the National Academy of Sciences of the United States of America*, vol. 100, no. 5, pp. 2432–2437, 2003.

[66] R. J. Youle and A. Strasser, "The BCL-2 protein family: opposing activities that mediate cell death," *Nature Reviews Molecular Cell Biology*, vol. 9, no. 1, pp. 47–59, 2008.

[67] A. Hoffmann and D. Baltimore, "Circuitry of nuclear factor κB signaling," *Immunological Reviews*, vol. 210, pp. 171–186, 2006.

[68] Z. Gao, P. Chiao, X. Zhang et al., "Coactivators and corepressors of NF-κB in IκBα gene promoter," *The Journal of Biological Chemistry*, vol. 280, no. 22, pp. 21091–21098, 2005.

[69] T. Luedde, N. Beraza, V. Kotsikoris et al., "Deletion of NEMO/IKKgamma in liver parenchymal cells causes steatohepatitis and hepatocellular carcinoma," *Cancer Cell*, vol. 11, no. 2, pp. 119–132, 2007.

[70] E. De Smaele, F. Zazzeroni, S. Papa et al., "Induction of gadd4β by NF-κB downregulates pro-apoptotic JNK signalling," *Nature*, vol. 414, no. 6861, pp. 308–313, 2001.

[71] S. Papa, F. Zazzeroni, C. Bubici et al., "Gadd45β mediates the NF-κB suppression of JNK signalling by targeting MKK7/JNKK2," *Nature Cell Biology*, vol. 6, no. 2, pp. 146–153, 2004.

[72] S. Papa, F. Zazzeroni, Y. X. Fu et al., "Gadd45β promotes hepatocyte survival during liver regeneration in mice by modulating JNK signaling," *The Journal of Clinical Investigation*, vol. 118, no. 5, pp. 1911–1923, 2008.

[73] S. Kaur, F. Wang, M. Venkatraman, and M. Arsura, "X-linked inhibitor of apoptosis (XIAP) inhibits c-Jun N-terminal kinase 1 (JNK1) activation by transforming growth factor β1 (TGF-β1) through ubiquitin-mediated proteosomal degradation of the TGF-β1-activated kinase 1 (TAK1)," *The Journal of Biological Chemistry*, vol. 280, no. 46, pp. 38599–38608, 2005.

[74] E. G. Lee, D. L. Boone, S. Chai et al., "Failure to regulate TNF-induced NF-κB and cell death responses in A20-deficient mice," *Science*, vol. 289, no. 5488, pp. 2350–2354, 2000.

[75] U. Lademann, T. Kallunki, and M. Jäättelä, "A20 zinc finger protein inhibits TNF-induced apoptosis and stress response early in the signaling cascades and independently of binding to TRAF2 or 14-3-3 proteins," *Cell Death and Differentiation*, vol. 8, no. 3, pp. 265–272, 2001.

[76] M. B. Arvelo, J. T. Cooper, C. Longo et al., "A20 protects mice from D-galactosamine/lipopolysaccharide acute toxic lethal hepatitis," *Hepatology*, vol. 35, no. 3, pp. 535–543, 2002.

[77] C. G. Pham, C. Bubici, F. Zazzeroni et al., "Ferritin heavy chain upregulation by NF-κB inhibits TNFα-induced apoptosis by suppressing reactive oxygen species," *Cell*, vol. 119, no. 4, pp. 529–542, 2004.

[78] S. Maeda, H. Kamata, J. L. Luo, H. Leffert, and M. Karin, "IKKβ couples hepatocyte death to cytokine-driven compensatory proliferation that promotes chemical hepatocarcinogenesis," *Cell*, vol. 121, no. 7, pp. 977–990, 2005.

[79] J. Heinrichsdorff, T. Luedde, E. Perdiguero, A. R. Nebreda, and M. Pasparakis, "p38α MAPK inhibits JNK activation and collaborates with IκB kinase 2 to prevent endotoxin-induced liver failure," *EMBO Reports*, vol. 9, no. 10, pp. 1048–1054, 2008.

[80] P. C. F. Cheung, D. G. Campbell, A. R. Nebreda, and P. Cohen, "Feedback control of the protein kinase TAK1 by SAPK2a/p38α," *The EMBO Journal*, vol. 22, no. 21, pp. 5793–5805, 2003.

[81] H. Muniyappa and K. C. Das, "Activation of c-Jun N-terminal kinase (JNK) by widely used specific p38 MAPK inhibitors SB202190 and SB203580: a MLK-3-MKK7-dependent mechanism," *Cellular Signalling*, vol. 20, no. 4, pp. 675–683, 2008.

[82] S. Inokuchi, T. Aoyama, K. Miura et al., "Disruption of TAK1 in hepatocytes causes hepatic injury, inflammation, fibrosis, and carcinogenesis," *Proceedings of the National Academy of Sciences of the United States of America*, vol. 107, no. 2, pp. 844–849, 2010.

[83] K. Bettermann, M. Vucur, J. Haybaeck et al., "TAK1 suppresses a NEMO-dependent but NF-kappaB-independent pathway to liver cancer," *Cancer Cell*, vol. 17, no. 5, pp. 481–496, 2010.

[84] H. Malhi, S. F. Bronk, N. W. Werneburg, and G. J. Gores, "Free fatty acids induce JNK-dependent hepatocyte lipoapoptosis," *The Journal of Biological Chemistry*, vol. 281, no. 17, pp. 12093–12101, 2006.

[85] H. Malhi and G. J. Gores, "Molecular mechanisms of lipotoxicity in nonalcoholic fatty liver disease," *Seminars in Liver Disease*, vol. 28, no. 4, pp. 360–369, 2008.

[86] T. Uehara, B. Bennett, S. T. Sakata et al., "JNK mediates hepatic ischemia reperfusion injury," *Journal of Hepatology*, vol. 42, no. 6, pp. 850–859, 2005.

[87] B. K. Gunawan, Z. X. Liu, D. Han, N. Hanawa, W. A. Gaarde, and N. Kaplowitz, "c-Jun N-terminal kinase plays a major role in murine acetaminophen hepatotoxicity," *Gastroenterology*, vol. 131, no. 1, pp. 165–178, 2006.

[88] K. Sabapathy, K. Hochedlinger, S. Y. Nam, A. Bauer, M. Karin, and E. F. Wagner, "Distinct roles for JNK1 and JNK2 in regulating JNK activity and c-Jun-dependent cell proliferation," *Molecular Cell*, vol. 15, no. 5, pp. 713–725, 2004.

[89] A. Jaeschke, M. Karasarides, J. J. Ventura et al., "JNK2 is a positive regulator of the cJun transcription factor," *Molecular Cell*, vol. 23, no. 6, pp. 899–911, 2006.

[90] R. F. Schwabe, C. A. Bradham, T. Uehara et al., "c-Jun-N-terminal kinase drives cyclin D1 expression and proliferation during liver regeneration," *Hepatology*, vol. 37, no. 4, pp. 824–832, 2003.

[91] Y. Sugioka, T. Watanabe, Y. Inagaki et al., "c-Jun NH2-terminal kinase pathway is involved in constitutive matrix metalloproteinase-1 expression in a hepatocellular carcinoma-derived cell line," *International Journal of Cancer*, vol. 109, no. 6, pp. 867–874, 2004.

[92] C. Cellurale, G. Sabio, N. J. Kennedy et al., "Requirement of c-Jun NH2-terminal kinase for Ras-initiated tumor formation," *Molecular and Cellular Biology*, vol. 31, no. 7, pp. 1565–1576, 2011.

[93] A. S. Nateri, B. Spencer-Dene, and A. Behrens, "Interaction of phosphorylated c-Jun with TCF4 regulates intestinal cancer development," *Nature*, vol. 437, no. 7056, pp. 281–285, 2005.

[94] X. Wu, X. Tu, K. S. Joeng, M. J. Hilton, D. A. Williams, and F. Long, "Rac1 activation controls nuclear localization of beta-catenin during canonical Wnt signaling," *Cell*, vol. 133, no. 2, pp. 340–353, 2008.

[95] R. Sancho, A. S. Nateri, A. G. De Vinuesa et al., "JNK signalling modulates intestinal homeostasis and tumourigenesis in mice," *The EMBO Journal*, vol. 28, no. 13, pp. 1843–1854, 2009.

[96] C. Cellurale, C. R. Weston, J. Reilly et al., "Role of JNK in a Trp53-dependent mouse model of breast cancer," *PLoS One*, vol. 5, no. 8, Article ID e12469, 2010.

[97] D. Schramek, A. Kotsinas, A. Meixner et al., "The stress kinase MKK7 couples oncogenic stress to p53 stability and tumor suppression," *Nature Genetics*, vol. 43, no. 3, pp. 212–219, 2011.

[98] N. K. Saxena, P. P. Fu, A. Nagalingam et al., "Adiponectin modulates C-Jun N-terminal kinase and mammalian target of rapamycin and inhibits hepatocellular carcinoma," *Gastroenterology*, vol. 139, no. 5, pp. 1762–e1765, 2010.

[99] Q. Chang, Y. Zhang, K. J. Beezhold et al., "Sustained JNK1 activation is associated with altered histone H3 methylations in human liver cancer," *Journal of Hepatology*, vol. 50, no. 2, pp. 323–333, 2009.

[100] A. Erhardt, M. Hassan, T. Heintges, and D. Häussinger, "Hepatitis C virus core protein induces cell proliferation and activates ERK, JNK, and p38 MAP kinases together with the MAP kinase phosphatase MKP-1 in a HepG2 Tet-Off cell line," *Virology*, vol. 292, no. 2, pp. 272–284, 2002.

[101] Y. Tanaka, F. Kanai, T. Ichimura et al., "The hepatitis B virus X protein enhances AP-1 activation through interaction with Jab1," *Oncogene*, vol. 25, no. 4, pp. 633–642, 2006.

[102] T. Tsutsumi, T. Suzuki, K. Moriya et al., "Alteration of intrahepatic cytokine expression and AP-1 activation in transgenic mice expressing hepatitis C virus core protein," *Virology*, vol. 304, no. 2, pp. 415–424, 2002.

[103] M. Murata, K. Matsuzaki, K. Yoshida et al., "Hepatitis B virus X protein shifts human hepatic transforming growth factor (TGF)-β signaling from tumor suppression to oncogenesis in early chronic hepatitis B," *Hepatology*, vol. 49, no. 4, pp. 1203–1217, 2009.

[104] M. Das, D. S. Garlick, D. L. Greiner, and R. J. Davis, "The role of JNK in the development of hepatocellular carcinoma," *Genes and Development*, vol. 25, no. 6, pp. 634–645, 2011.

[105] J. Hirosumi, G. Tuncman, L. Chang et al., "A central, role for JNK in obesity and insulin resistance," *Nature*, vol. 420, no. 6913, pp. 333–336, 2002.

[106] G. Sabio, M. Das, A. Mora et al., "A stress signaling pathway in adipose tissue regulates hepatic insulin resistance," *Science*, vol. 322, no. 5907, pp. 1539–1543, 2008.

[107] T. Ohki, R. Tateishi, S. Shiina et al., "Visceral fat accumulation is an independent risk factor for hepatocellular carcinoma recurrence after curative treatment in patients with suspected NASH," *Gut*, vol. 58, no. 6, pp. 839–844, 2009.

[108] F. Marra and C. Bertolani, "Adipokines in liver diseases," *Hepatology*, vol. 50, no. 3, pp. 957–969, 2009.

[109] E. J. Park, J. H. Lee, G. Y. Yu et al., "Dietary and genetic obesity promote liver inflammation and tumorigenesis by enhancing IL-6 and TNF expression," *Cell*, vol. 140, no. 2, pp. 197–208, 2010.

[110] T. Arano, H. Nakagawa, R. Tateishi et al., "Serum level of adiponectin and the risk of liver cancer development in chronic hepatitis C patients," *International Journal of Cancer*, vol. 129, no. 9, pp. 2226–2235, 2011.

[111] J. Han and P. Sun, "The pathways to tumor suppression via route p38," *Trends in Biochemical Sciences*, vol. 32, no. 8, pp. 364–371, 2007.

[112] B. Ge, H. Gram, F. Di Padova et al., "MAPKK-independent activation of p38α mediated by TAB1-dependent autophosphorylation of p38α," *Science*, vol. 295, no. 5558, pp. 1291–1294, 2002.

[113] L. Hui, L. Bakiri, E. Stepniak, and E. F. Wagner, "p38α: a suppressor of cell proliferation and tumorigenesis," *Cell Cycle*, vol. 6, no. 20, pp. 2429–2433, 2007.

[114] T. M. Thornton and M. Rincon, "Non-classical p38 map kinase functions: cell cycle checkpoints and survival," *International Journal of Biological Sciences*, vol. 5, no. 1, pp. 44–52, 2009.

[115] E. Stepniak, R. Ricci, R. Eferl et al., "c-Jun/AP-1 controls liver regeneration by repressing p53/p21 and p38 MAPK activity," *Genes and Development*, vol. 20, no. 16, pp. 2306–2314, 2006.

[116] J. S. Campbell, G. M. Argast, S. Y. Yuen, B. Hayes, and N. Fausto, "Inactivation of p38 MAPK during liver regeneration," *International Journal of Biochemistry and Cell Biology*, vol. 43, no. 2, pp. 180–188, 2011.

[117] I. Dolado, A. Swat, N. Ajenjo, G. De Vita, A. Cuadrado, and A. R. Nebreda, "p38alpha MAP kinase as a sensor of reactive oxygen species in tumorigenesis," *Cancer Cell*, vol. 11, no. 2, pp. 191–205, 2007.

[118] P. Sun, N. Yoshizuka, L. New et al., "PRAK is essential for ras-induced senescence and tumor suppression," *Cell*, vol. 128, no. 2, pp. 295–308, 2007.

[119] D. V. Bulavin, C. Phillips, B. Nannenga et al., "Inactivation of the Wip1 phosphatase inhibits mammary tumorigenesis through p38 MAPK-mediated activation of the p16Ink4a-p19 Arf pathway," *Nature Genetics*, vol. 36, no. 4, pp. 343–350, 2004.

[120] Y. H. Hsieh, T. T. Wu, C. Y. Huang, Y. S. Hsieh, J. M. Hwang, and J. Y. Liu, "p38 mitogen-activated protein kinase pathway is involved in protein kinase Cα-regulated invasion in human hepatocellular carcinoma cells," *Cancer Research*, vol. 67, no. 9, pp. 4320–4327, 2007.

[121] M. S. Kim, E. J. Lee, H. R. C. Kim, and A. Moon, "p38 kinase is a key signaling molecule for H-ras-induced cell motility and invasive phenotype in human breast epithelial cells," *Cancer Research*, vol. 63, no. 17, pp. 5454–5461, 2003.

[122] K. Iyoda, Y. Sasaki, M. Horimoto et al., "Involvement of the p38 mitogen-activated protein kinase cascade in hepatocellular carcinoma," *Cancer*, vol. 97, no. 12, pp. 3017–3026, 2003.

[123] H. Ichijo, E. Nishida, K. Irie et al., "Induction of apoptosis by ASK1, a mammalian MAPKKK that activates SAPK/JNK and p38 signaling pathways," *Science*, vol. 275, no. 5296, pp. 90–94, 1997.

[124] H. Huynh, S. P. Choo, H. C. Toh et al., "Comparing the efficacy of sunitinib with sorafenib in xenograft models of human hepatocellular carcinoma: mechanistic explanation," *Current Cancer Drug Targets*, vol. 11, no. 8, pp. 944–953, 2011.

[125] C. Runchel, A. Matsuzawa, and H. Ichijo, "Mitogen-activated protein kinases in mammalian oxidative stress responses," *Antioxidants and Redox Signaling*, vol. 15, no. 1, pp. 205–218, 2011.

[126] G. R. Fanger, N. L. Johnson, and G. L. Johnson, "MEK kinases are regulated by EGF and selectively interact with Rac/Cdc42," *The EMBO Journal*, vol. 16, no. 16, pp. 4961–4972, 1997.

[127] D. N. Chadee and J. M. Kyriakis, "MLK3 is required for mitogen activation of B-Raf, ERK and cell proliferation," *Nature Cell Biology*, vol. 6, no. 8, pp. 770–776, 2004.

[128] E. Pikarsky, R. M. Porat, I. Stein et al., "NF-κB functions as a tumour promoter in inflammation-associated cancer," *Nature*, vol. 431, no. 7007, pp. 461–466, 2004.

[129] R. J. Mayer and J. F. Callahan, "p38 MAP kinase inhibitors: a future therapy for inflammatory diseases," *Drug Discovery Today*, vol. 3, no. 1, pp. 49–54, 2006.

[130] S. Kumar, J. Boehm, and J. C. Lee, "P38 MAP kinases: key signalling molecules as therapeutic targets for inflammatory diseases," *Nature Reviews Drug Discovery*, vol. 2, no. 9, pp. 717–726, 2003.

[131] S. Hagiwara, M. Kudo, H. Chung et al., "Activation of c-Jun N-terminal kinase in non-cancerous liver tissue predicts a high risk of recurrence after hepatic resection for hepatocellular carcinoma," *Hepatology Research*, vol. 42, no. 4, pp. 394–400, 2012.

15

Calretinin as a Diagnostic Adjunct for Ameloblastoma

Chitra Anandani,[1] Rashmi Metgud,[1] and Karanprakash Singh[2]

[1] *Department of Oral and Maxillofacial Pathology, Pacific Dental College and Hospital, PAHER University, Udaipur, Rajasthan 313024, India*

[2] *Department of Public Health Dentistry, Genesis Institute of Dental Sciences and Research, Ferozepur, Punjab 152001, India*

Correspondence should be addressed to Chitra Anandani; drchitraanandani@gmail.com

Academic Editor: Gary Tse

Background. Calretinin is a 29 kDa calcium-binding protein of the EF-hand family which is expressed in a variety of normal and tumorigenic tissues. Its expression in odontogenic epithelium during odontogenesis and in neoplastic odontogenic tissues has been demonstrated. Unicystic ameloblastoma poses a diagnostic challenge, as its histologic presentation can be sometimes mistaken for keratocystic odontogenic tumor (KCOT). This study was performed to assess the usefulness of calretinin as a confirmatory marker for ameloblastic tissue. *Methodology.* Total of 40 cases: 16 unicystic ameloblastoma, 4 multicystic ameloblastoma, and 20 KCOT, were evaluated immunohistochemically for the presence, localization, distribution, and intensity of calretinin expression. Statistical analysis was done using Chi-square test to intercompare the expression between ameloblastoma and KCOT. *Results.* Sixteen cases of ameloblastoma (12 unicystic, 4 multicystic) showed positive calretinin staining of ameloblastic epithelium and only one case of KCOT was positive for calretinin, with the positivity restricted to the stellate reticulum like epithelium. Intercomparison between two groups revealed statistically significant difference ($P = 0.000$). *Conclusion.* Calretinin appears to be a specific immunohistochemical marker for neoplastic ameloblastic epithelium and may be an important diagnostic adjunct in the differential diagnosis of ameloblastoma and KCOT.

1. Introduction

Calcium ions (Ca^{2+}) regulate a large number of biological processes such as metabolism, contraction, secretion, cell division, cell growth, and memory storage—either directly or indirectly. Elevated cytoplasmic calcium levels found in several tumor cells might contribute to the increased motility and hence invasiveness of these cells.

The calcium signal is transmitted into the intracellular response, in part via interactions with a wide variety of intracellular calcium-binding proteins that are involved in the regulation of many cellular activities. One class of these proteins shares a common calcium-binding motif, the EF-hand [1]. The EF-hand homologue family contains more than 200 different calcium-binding proteins, among them being 29 kDa calretinin, which was isolated initially from a cDNA clone from the chick retina, and it is most homologous to another important member of the EF-hand family, that is, 28 kDa calbindin [2].

Calretinin is widely expressed in central and peripheral neural tissues, particularly in the retina and in neurons of sensory pathways. Outside the central nervous system, it is expressed in normal and reactive mesothelial lining of all serosal membranes, the pilar infundibulum, eccrine glands, convoluted tubules of the kidney, leydig and sertoli cells of the testis, endometrium and ovarian stromal cells, adrenal cortex, epithelial cells of the thymus, and adipocytes [2, 3].

Studies in rats have demonstrated calretinin expression in neural elements of the tooth pulp, periodontal ligament and viscerosensory nerve fibres of oral and pharyngeal tissues [4], as well as in epithelium-derived tissues during odontogenesis in rat molar tooth germs, suggesting that this protein may play a part in enamel formation [2]. The exact biological function of calretinin remains unknown but its possible roles as a calcium buffer and/or calcium sensor and regulator of apoptosis have been postulated [5]. Calretinin also seems to share with calbindin certain features such as regulation of expression by growth factors and involvement in cell proliferation, differentiation, and neoplastic transformation [6].

Apart from its expression in normal human tissues, calretinin has been shown to be expressed in a wide variety of tumors [7]. Calretinin has recently emerged as an immunohistochemical marker with great utility for delineating mesothelioma and adenocarcinomas of lung, as its diagnostic sensitivity for mesothelioma is nearly 100% [8].

Odontogenic tumors comprise a group of heterogeneous lesions ranging from hamartomatous or nonneoplastic tissue proliferations to benign neoplasms to malignant tumors with metastatic potential [9]. The odontogenic cysts, which may be intimately associated with the development of certain of the odontogenic tumors, also represent an aberration at some stage of odontogenesis [10]. Keratocystic odontogenic tumor (KCOT) has been recently classified by World Health Organization (WHO) in 2005 as a benign tumor of odontogenic epithelium to emphasize its neoplastic nature [9].

Unicystic ameloblastoma is considered at best an in situ or superficially invasive form of ameloblastoma [11]. Unicystic ameloblastomas are well known to be lined by a variable epithelium ranging from one that has typical ameloblastic characteristics to one that is metaplastic and which appears completely nondescript consisting of several layers of nonkeratinizing squamous cells. In such cases, the differentiation of odontogenic cysts from the unicystic ameloblastoma can be problematic [12].

The histologic presentation of ameloblastoma, especially unicystic type, can be, in some instances, mistaken for keratocystic odontogenic tumor (KCOT). Overlapping clinical and radiographic presentation further adds to this diagnostic difficulty [3].

Hence, the present study was carried out to evaluate and intercompare the expression of calretinin in ameloblastoma and keratocystic odontogenic tumor in order to assess its usefulness as a confirmatory marker for ameloblastic tissue that would aid in the differential diagnosis of such lesions.

2. Materials and Methods

2.1. Case Selection. Formalin-fixed paraffin-embedded tissue blocks of ameloblastoma (unicystic and multicystic variants) and KCOT (parakeratinized type) were retrieved from the archives of Department of Oral and Maxillofacial Pathology, Pacific Dental College and Hospital, Udaipur. Re-evaluation of all cases was performed according to the World Health Organization histological typing of odontogenic tumors [9] by two oral pathologists on light microscopy using hematoxylin and eosin sections. The study protocol was reviewed by the Ethical Committee of Pacific Dental College and Hospital and was granted ethical clearance.

2.2. Immunohistochemistry. Formalin-fixed paraffin-embedded tissue blocks were cut into 4 μm thick sections and placed on organosilane-pretreated slides. Immunohistochemical staining was performed using the primary antibody for calretinin using supersensitive one-step polymer-HRP technique (Biogenex Life Sciences, San Ramon, CA, USA). The sections were deparaffinized and rehydrated through xylene and descending grades of alcohol, respectively. Antigen retrieval was carried out using commercial microwave antigen retrieval system where the sections were immersed in 10 mM sodium citrate buffer (pH 6.0) at 800, 420, and 320°F for three cycles of 10 min each (EZ-Retriever System, Biogenex Life Sciences). After rinsing in tris buffer (pH 7.2), the sections were incubated with 3% hydrogen peroxide in water for 15 min to block the endogenous peroxidase activity. This was followed by a power block for 10 min at room temperature to block any nonspecific antigenic sites. The sections were then incubated with optimally prediluted rabbit polyclonal antibody against calretinin protein (Biogenex, CA, USA) for 30 min at room temperature in a moist chamber. After washing with tris buffer (pH 7.2) for 5 min, the sections were then incubated with super enhancer for 20 min at room temperature, followed by secondary antibody incubation with one-step polymer-HRP reagent for 30 min at room temperature in a moist chamber. Visualization was performed using freshly prepared 3,3′-diaminobenzidine hydrochloride (DAB) substrate (Sigma) for 5 min. The slides were counterstained with Mayer's hematoxylin for 3 min, subsequent to which sections were dehydrated, cleared, and mounted with dibutyl phthalate xylene (DPX) (Rankem, RFCL Ltd.). For each batch of staining, positive and negative controls were run simultaneously with the study specimens. Human mesothelioma which is known to have a high level of calretinin expression served as the positive control, while the primary antibodies were replaced by nonimmune mouse serum at the same dilutions for the negative controls.

2.3. Evaluation of Slides. The evaluation of the stained slides was carried out using a binocular research microscope (Lawrence & Mayo) under 100x and 400x magnification. The sections stained with calretinin antibody were evaluated for the presence, localization, distribution, and intensity of the immunoreactive cells [4]. *Presence* was evaluated to estimate whether the staining was positive or negative and, if positive, which epithelial layer was stained. *Localization* was evaluated to estimate whether the staining was nuclear (N), cytoplasmic (C), or both. *Distribution* was evaluated as being either focal (involving <50% of positive cells) or diffuse (involving >50% of positive cells). The *intensity* was graded based on the number of positive cells seen: 0 = no staining; 1 = weak staining; 2 = moderate staining; 3 = intense staining.

The Chi-square test was applied to intercompare the calretinin expression between ameloblastoma and KCOT and for the comparison between the variants of ameloblastoma (unicystic and multicystic). P values <0.05 were considered to be statistically significant.

3. Results

A total of 40 cases (20 each) of ameloblastoma and KCOT were studied. Out of the 20 cases of ameloblastoma, 16 were of unicystic type and the remaining 4 were of solid/multicystic type [2 follicular, 1 plexiform, and 1 granular cell ameloblastoma].

TABLE 1: Intercomparison of calretinin presence in ameloblastoma and KCOT.

Presence	Ameloblastoma ($n = 20$)		KCOT ($n = 20$)	
	Frequency	Percent	Frequency	Percent
+	12	30%	1	2.5%
−	8	20%	19	47.5%
P^* value		0.000		

$^*P$ value < 0.05: statistically significant.

3.1. Unicystic Ameloblastoma. Out of the 16 cases of unicystic ameloblastoma, positive calretinin expression of the ameloblastic epithelium was seen in 8 (50%) cases. In all the immunopositive cases, reactivity was observed in both the nucleus and cytoplasm of the cells. The distribution of calretinin was focal in 5 and diffuse in 3 cases and was limited to the stellate reticulum like area. The luminal layer of ameloblast-like cells did not stain, except for the few single basal cells that were positive in 2 cases only. Four cases showed weak staining, 3 showed moderate, and 1 showed severe staining of the ameloblastic epithelium (Figure 1).

3.2. Solid/Multicystic Ameloblastoma. All the 4 cases showed weak positive staining of stellate reticulum like areas whereas only one case showed focal positivity in the basal cell layer also. Immunoreactivity was observed in both the nucleus and cytoplasm of the cells. Staining was focally distributed in 3 cases while one case stained diffusely (Figure 2).

In addition, all the cases of ameloblastoma also showed scattered positive cells within the stroma, which were thought to be nonepithelial in type and could represent mast cells.

3.3. Keratocystic Odontogenic Tumor. Nineteen (95%) cases showed negative staining of calretinin in the epithelial lining of the cyst, except for some scattered, darkly stained individual cells in the fibrous connective tissue wall. Only one case that showed positivity to calretinin revealed a highly inflamed odontogenic keratocyst with one bit of tissue depicting stellate reticulum like epithelium overlying the palisaded basal cell layer in the hematoxylin and eosin stained sections. The calretinin staining for the same bit showed uniform diffuse immunopositivity of the nucleus and cytoplasm of the stellate reticulum like epithelium (Figure 3).

The intercomparison of calretinin positivity between ameloblastoma and KCOT revealed a statistically significant difference at $P = 0.000$ (Table 1).

4. Discussion

Odontogenic cysts and tumors are a group of lesions arising from the tooth-producing apparatus or its remnants. They may originate from odontogenic epithelium and/or ectomesenchyme with varying degrees of inductive tissue interaction [13]. They are rare and lack of familiarity with these lesions and their variable appearance may lead to difficulties in diagnosis with occasional serious confusion with more sinister lesions [14].

Different odontogenic cysts and tumors have variable clinical and biological behaviors. Ameloblastoma is a benign, locally aggressive epithelial odontogenic tumor that has the potential to become malignant and produce metastasis to distant sites such as lungs and kidneys. KCOT is an aggressive cyst with neoplastic behaviour while unicystic ameloblastoma is a neoplasm with cyst like behaviour [15, 16]. KCOT also arises from cell rests of the dental lamina, same origin as ameloblastoma, and there are clinical and radiographic similarities between KCOT and unicystic ameloblastoma, as both present as ordinary cysts in the dentate areas [17]. Histologically, unicystic ameloblastoma is lined in some areas, but rarely entirely, by odontogenic epithelium of ameloblastoma appearance and stratified squamous epithelium in the remaining areas [18]. In fact, such squamous metaplasia is a relatively frequent phenomenon in unicystic ameloblastoma and many of these lesions are lined by such nondescript epithelium, which can create diagnostic confusion with odontogenic cysts [12].

KCOT is characterized, histologically, by a palisaded basal cell layer of basophilic columnar cells and a surface of corrugated parakeratin, sometimes with spongiosis, resembling closely the stellate like reticulum and the acanthomatous differentiation of ameloblastoma. If the tissue sample is small and if the neoplastic epithelium displays reactive changes induced by inflammation, it can closely resemble unicystic ameloblastoma histologically [3]. Thus, at times, both lesions become histologically indistinguishable.

Many techniques have been used in an attempt to distinguish odontogenic cysts (including KCOT) from ameloblastomas (especially unicystic type), which include demonstration of cell surface carbohydrates with blood group specificity; determination of alkaline phosphatase activity in the stroma; distribution of lectins and involucrin in the epithelium; characterization of cytokeratin profiles; counting of AgNORs and quantification of cell proliferation markers such as PCNA and Ki67. While differences have been shown to occur between various cysts and ameloblastomas, considerable overlap exists and none of the above techniques can be used to routinely distinguish these lesions from one another [5].

Also, a number of studies have reported the immunohistochemical expression of intermediate filaments, growth factors, basement membrane components, cell cycle regulating factors, and apoptotic proteins in ameloblastomas but calcium-binding proteins have not been investigated to a greater extent in these tumors [19].

The present study assessed the expression of calretinin in 20 cases each of ameloblastoma and keratocystic odontogenic tumor and the results demonstrated frequent expression of calretinin in the epithelium of both unicystic and solid multicystic ameloblastomas. Positive staining was seen in 50% (8 cases) of unicystic ameloblastoma and 100% (4 cases) of multicystic ameloblastoma, whereas only 1 out of 20 cases of KCOT lining showed positive staining for calretinin. The intercomparison between both groups revealed a statistically significant difference at $P = 0.000$. Also, the immunopositivity was seen exclusively in the stellate reticulum like epithelium in both the unicystic and multicystic ameloblastomas,

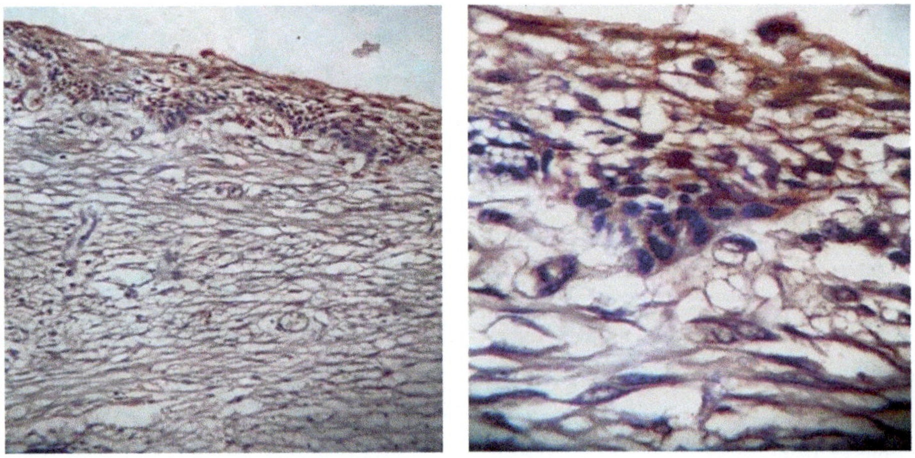

(a) 100x (b) 400x

FIGURE 1: Photomicrograph showing calretinin staining in unicystic ameloblastoma in (a) 100x and (b) 400x.

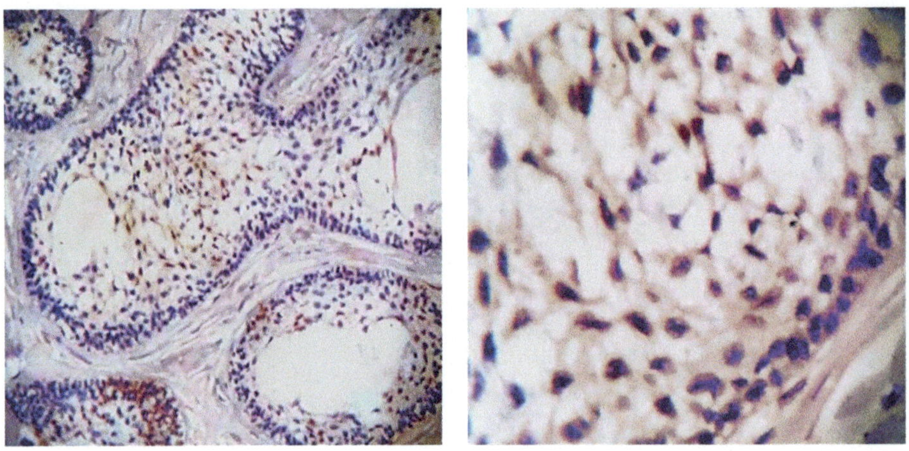

(a) 100x (b) 400x

FIGURE 2: Photomicrograph showing calretinin staining in solid multicystic ameloblastoma in (a) 100x and (b) 400x.

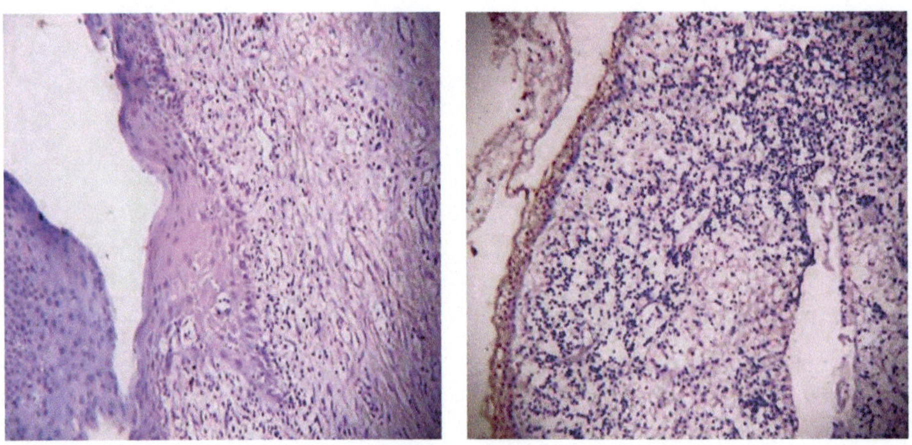

(a) (b)

FIGURE 3: Photomicrograph showing (a) negative calretinin staining in keratocystic odontogenic tumor (100x) and (b) positive calretinin staining in keratocystic odontogenic tumor (100x).

and the ameloblast-like basal cells were positive in only 1 of the multicystic and 2 of the unicystic variants, where single cell expressing calretinin was observed.

These findings were in accordance with earlier studies which also observed calretinin positive cells restricted to the neoplastic stellate reticulum like epithelium in ameloblastoma only; Altini et al. [19] and Coleman et al. [12] found positive staining in 81.5% cases of unicystic ameloblastomas and 93.5% cases of multicystic ameloblastoma, while Devilliers et al. [3], Sundaragiri et al. [5], and D'Silva et al. [20] found positivity in all cases of ameloblastoma (100%). In all these studies, none of the odontogenic cysts' lining showed positivity, except D'Silva et al. [20] who observed positive staining of the cystic lining epithelium and keratin flakes in the cystic lumen of 40% cases of odontogenic keratocyst. The authors attribute this finding to the aggressive biologic behavior of odontogenic keratocyst similar to a benign neoplasm and its high mitotic activity as compared to other nonneoplastic odontogenic cysts. Also, Piattelli et al. [21] found positivity to calretinin in 8 of 12 parakeratinized keratocysts in the parabasal-intermediate layers of the cyst epithelium. This could point to the aggressive behavior of KCOT and help to explain the differences in the clinical and pathologic behavior of odontogenic keratocysts, in particular the differences found between orthokeratinized keratocysts and parakeratinized keratocysts.

Alaeddini et al. [4] also found that calretinin immunoreactivity was positive only for ameloblastoma when compared to calcifying epithelial odontogenic tumour, adenomatoid odontogenic tumour, ameloblastic fibroma, and odontogenic myxoma, stating that this protein may have a role in the transition of the dental lamina remnants to ameloblastoma. They hypothesized that calretinin may be one of the factors responsible for the differences between this aggressive neoplasm and other odontogenic tumors studied.

Further, in the present study, the distribution pattern of the immunopositive cells was focal in 8 cases (40%) and diffuse in 4 cases (20%). Also, the staining was weak in most of the cases (40%), with 3 cases (15%) showing moderate and only 1 case (5%) intense staining. The staining was not equally distributed throughout the sections with some areas showing intense staining but absolutely no staining in the immediate vicinity. This was in contrast to the earlier studies where most of the cases showed intense staining of the ameloblastic epithelium [3–5, 12, 19, 20].

Altini et al. [19] stated that the better the differentiation of the epithelium was, the lesser the expression of calretinin occurred in their study, where they found little or no immunostaining in those cases of unicystic ameloblastomas that were lined by typical ameloblastic epithelium, while the epithelium which completely lacked ameloblastic features frequently expressed calretinin. Hence they indicated that calretinin expression in some cells varied according to their metabolic activity and may be lost when this activity changes. Later, Coleman et al. [12] observed intense positive staining in both areas of nondescript epithelial lining and areas with typical ameloblastic features in unicystic ameloblastoma, which indicated that although the metaplastic cyst linings may have lost their typical ameloblastic features, the cells have retained their immunophenotypic characteristics resulting in the continued expression of calretinin. Our study can be correlated with the observation of Altini et al. [19] as majority of the unicystic ameloblastoma cases that we observed were lined by typical ameloblastic epithelium, due to which they may not have stained intensely with calretinin.

In a study by Mistry et al. [2] on developing rat molars, calretinin immunoreactivity was present in the inner enamel epithelium and presecretory ameloblasts from the late cap stage onwards. In the cap and late cap stages, many of the specimens were immunopositive for calretinin in the stellate reticulum, and this number increased to >90% for the early and late bell stages. In the present study, the pattern of reactivity of the stellate reticulum observed appeared similar to the late bell stage of normal tooth development. However, in the peripheral layers of the ameloblastic islands, calretinin immunoreactivity was not observed as was the case in normal tooth germs. As enamel organ has been proposed to be one of the possible origins of ameloblastoma [17], this peculiar distribution of calretinin in ameloblastic epithelium is noteworthy and it thus appears that there is no obvious correlation between the staining of normal odontogenic tissues and their neoplastic counterparts [19].

A possible explanation for this dynamic spatial and temporal distribution was that calretinin may be present only in cells that reside directly in the path of calcium in transition on its way to the enamel matrix, acting as a "calcium ferry" [2]. However, Hubbard et al. [22] found that calretinin was primarily expressed during the differentiation stage of enamel formation, and only a faint calretinin band was observed at secretion stage while no such band was detectable during maturation. Based on these findings, the authors suggest retirement of the calcium ferry dogma from enamel biology—in murine models at least.

Gotzos et al. [23, 24] have shown increased expression of calretinin in rapidly proliferating WiDr colon adenocarcinomas cells. Upon being induced to differentiate by treatment with sodium butyrate and hexamethylene bisacetamide, they showed marked reductions in cell proliferation as well as expression of full length calretinin. When treated with oligonucleotides against calretinin synthesis, these cells were blocked in the G1 phase of the cell cycle and subsequently underwent apoptosis. These authors suggested that calretinin may maintain an undifferentiated proliferative state characteristic of neoplastic transformation. Also, calretinin may act as an antiapoptotic factor [25].

The single case of KCOT in our study that showed positivity to calretinin was of a 17-year-old male patient having radiolucency in 24 and 25 region with impacted 23. The hematoxylin and eosin stained sections of the biopsy specimen revealed a highly inflamed odontogenic keratocyst with one bit of tissue depicting stellate reticulum—like epithelium overlying the palisaded basal cell layer. Upon calretinin staining, uniform diffuse immunopositivity of the stellate reticulum like epithelium was observed. This suggests that the previous biopsy may have been misdiagnosed as KCOT on the basis of hematoxylin and eosin staining.

This result can be compared with that of Devilliers et al. [3], wherein they evaluated a tumor from their archives, originally diagnosed as KCOT, which recurred 2 years later. Histologic sections from the tissue biopsied earlier (diagnosed as KCOT) and from the tissue sample of the recurrence (diagnosed as ameloblastoma) were tested with calretinin and both showed positive staining of the neoplastic epithelium, confined to the stellate reticulum.

This finding helps us to understand the importance of calretinin as a differential diagnostic marker for ameloblastoma and how important it is for the pathologist to differentiate both entities, which carry different treatment protocols with potentially serious functional and esthetic consequences for the patient.

Few nonepithelial cells that stained positive for calretinin were also observed in the connective tissue stroma of virtually all cases of ameloblastoma and KCOT in our study. Altini et al. [19] and Coleman et al. [12] also found such darkly stained cells within the tumor or cyst epithelium and in the fibrous connective tissue walls. These were interpreted as being mast cells or Langerhans cells, both of which have been documented as occurring in ameloblastomas and odontogenic cysts.

5. Conclusion

The present study suggests that calretinin may be used as a specific immunohistochemical marker for neoplastic ameloblastic epithelium as calretinin positivity was observed exclusively in ameloblastomas. Hence, it can serve as an important diagnostic adjunct in the differential diagnosis of ameloblastoma and keratocystic odontogenic tumor. The expression of calretinin in these neoplastic lesions might be recapitulating dental ontogeny, as its role during normal tooth development has also been speculated.

Conflict of Interests

The authors declare that there is no conflict of interests regarding the publication of this paper.

Acknowledgment

The authors wish to thank all the members in the Department of Oral and Maxillofacial Pathology for their general support.

References

[1] C. W. Heizmann, "Calcium-binding proteins: basic concepts and clinical implications," *General Physiology and Biophysics*, vol. 11, no. 5, pp. 411–425, 1992.

[2] D. Mistry, M. Altini, H. G. Coleman, H. Ali, and E. Maiorano, "The spatial and temporal expression of calretinin in developing rat molars (*Rattus norvegicus*)," *Archives of Oral Biology*, vol. 46, no. 10, pp. 973–981, 2001.

[3] P. Devilliers, H. Liu, C. Suggs et al., "Calretinin expression in the differential diagnosis of human ameloblastoma and keratocystic odontogenic tumor," *The American Journal of Surgical Pathology*, vol. 32, no. 2, pp. 256–260, 2008.

[4] M. Alaeddini, S. Etemad-Moghadam, and F. Baghaii, "Comparative expression of calretinin in selected odontogenic tumours: a possible relationship to histogenesis," *Histopathology*, vol. 52, no. 3, pp. 299–304, 2008.

[5] S. K. Sundaragiri, J. Chawda, S. Gill, S. Odedra, and G. Parmar, "Calretinin expression in unicystic ameloblastoma: an aid in differential diagnosis," *Journal of Oral Biosciences*, vol. 52, no. 2, pp. 164–169, 2010.

[6] G. V. Sherbet, *Calcium Signalling in Cancer*, Taylor & Francis, Boca Raton, Fla, USA, 2010.

[7] A. Lugli, Y. Forster, P. Haas et al., "Calretinin expression in human normal and neoplastic tissues: a tissue microarray analysis on 5233 tissue samples," *Human Pathology*, vol. 34, no. 10, pp. 994–1000, 2003.

[8] C. Doglioni, A. P. Dei Tos, L. Laurino et al., "Calretinin: a novel immunocytochemical marker for mesothelioma," *The American Journal of Surgical Pathology*, vol. 20, no. 9, pp. 1037–1046, 1996.

[9] L. Barnes, J. W. Eveson, P. Reichart, and D. Sidransky, Eds., *Pathology & Genetics: Head and Neck Tumours*, IARC Press, Lyon, France, 2005.

[10] R. Rajendran and B. Sivapathasundharam, *Shafers Oral Pathology*, Elsevier, New York, NY, USA, 2009.

[11] D. R. Gnepp, *Diagnostic Surgical Pathology of the Head and Neck*, Saunders/Elsevier, Philadelphia, Pa, USA, 2009.

[12] H. Coleman, M. Altini, H. Ali, C. Doglioni, G. Favia, and E. Maiorano, "Use of calretinin in the differential diagnosis of unicystic ameloblastomas," *Histopathology*, vol. 38, no. 4, pp. 312–317, 2001.

[13] A. M. Fernandes, E. C. B. Duarte, F. J. G. S. Pimenta et al., "Odontogenic tumors: a study of 340 cases in a Brazilian population," *Journal of Oral Pathology and Medicine*, vol. 34, no. 10, pp. 583–587, 2005.

[14] R. C. K. Jordan and P. M. Speight, "Current concepts of odontogenic tumours," *Diagnostic Histopathology*, vol. 15, no. 6, pp. 303–310, 2009.

[15] P. A. Reichart, P. Reichart, and H. P. Philipsen, *Odontogenic Tumors and Allied Lesions*, Quintessence, 2004.

[16] M. Shear and P. Speight, *Cysts of the Oral and Maxillofacial Regions*, Wiley, New York, NY, USA, 2008.

[17] B. W. Neville, *Oral and Maxillofacial Pathology*, W.B. Saunders, Philadelphia, Pa, USA, 2002.

[18] H. P. Philipsen and P. A. Reichart, "Unicystic ameloblastoma. A review of 193 cases from the literature," *Oral Oncology*, vol. 34, no. 5, pp. 317–325, 1998.

[19] M. Altini, H. Coleman, C. Doglioni, G. Favia, and E. Maiorano, "Calretinin expression in ameloblastomas," *Histopathology*, vol. 37, no. 1, pp. 27–32, 2000.

[20] S. D'Silva, M. K. Sumathi, N. Balaji et al., "Evaluation of calretinin expression in Ameloblastoma and non-neoplastic odontogenic cysts—an immunohistochemical study," *Journal of International Oral Health*, vol. 5, no. 6, pp. 42–48, 2013.

[21] A. Piattelli, M. Fioroni, G. Iezzi, and C. Rubini, "Calretinin expression in odontogenic cysts," *Journal of Endodontics*, vol. 29, no. 6, pp. 394–396, 2003.

[22] M. J. Hubbard, N. J. McHugh, and J. E. Mangum, "Exclusion of all three calbindins from a calcium-ferry role in rat enamel cells," *European Journal of Oral Sciences*, vol. 119, no. 1, pp. 112–119, 2011.

[23] V. Gotzos, B. Schwaller, N. Hetzel, M. Bustos-Castillo, and M. R. Celio, "Expression of the calcium binding protein calretinin in WiDr cells and its correlation to their cell cycle," *Experimental Cell Research*, vol. 202, no. 2, pp. 292–302, 1992.

[24] V. Gotzos, B. Schwaller, J.-C. Gander, M. Bustos-Castillo, and M. R. Celio, "Heterogeneity of expression of the calcium-binding protein calretinin in human colonie cancer cell lines," *Anticancer Research*, vol. 16, no. 6B, pp. 3491–3498, 1996.

[25] J.-C. Gander, V. Gotzos, B. Fellay, and B. Schwaller, "Inhibition of the proliferative cycle and apoptotic events in WiDr cells after down-regulation of the calcium-binding protein calretinin using antisense oligodeoxynucleotides," *Experimental Cell Research*, vol. 225, no. 2, pp. 399–410, 1996.

16

A Naturally Occurring Feline Model of Head and Neck Squamous Cell Carcinoma

Jackie M. Wypij

Department of Veterinary Clinical Medicine, University of Illinois at Urbana-Champaign, Hazelwood Drive, Urbana, IL 61802, USA

Correspondence should be addressed to Jackie M. Wypij; jwypij@illinois.edu

Academic Editor: R. Montironi

Despite advances in understanding cancer at the molecular level, timely and effective translation to clinical application of novel therapeutics in human cancer patients is lacking. Cancer drug failure is often a result of toxicity or inefficacy not predicted by preclinical models, emphasizing the need for alternative animal tumor models with improved biologic relevancy. Companion animals (dogs and cats) provide an opportunity to capitalize on an underutilized and biologically relevant translational research model which allows spontaneous disease modeling of human cancer. Head and neck squamous cell carcinoma (HNSCC) is a common cancer with a poor prognosis and limited clinical advancements in recent years. One potential novel spontaneous animal tumor model is feline oral squamous cell carcinoma (FOSCC). FOSCC and HNSCC share similar etiopathogenesis (tobacco and papillomavirus exposure) and molecular markers (EGFR, VEGF, and p53). Both human and feline SCCs share similar tumor biology, clinical outcome, treatment, and prognosis. Future clinical trials utilizing FOSCC as a tumor model may facilitate translation of preclinical cancer research for human cancer patients.

1. Introduction

Advances in our understanding of cancer at the molecular level have outpaced clinical application of this information to human patients. It can take more than a decade and $800 million dollars to develop a new drug or diagnostic agent, yet less than 10% of promising drugs achieve FDA-approval [1, 2]. This discouraging drug failure rate is in part due to limited predictive value for drug toxicity and efficacy of accepted preclinical models [2]. The value of pre-clinical models to subsequently predict drug success is inherently based on the relevancy of animal models. Murine models provide crucial opportunities to investigate specific molecular and genetic pathways. These models often incorporate chemically induced cancer or xenografted human cancer cell lines in immunosuppressed animals. Thus, despite their importance these conventional murine models fail to adequately characterize the biologic variations inherent in spontaneously arising human cancer such as long latency period, genomic instability, tumor heterogeneity, and the complexity of the tumor microenvironment. While no single model can provide solutions to all drug-development questions, integration of information from multiple modeling systems can improve the successful translation of a novel drug into human patients. One approach is capitalization on biologically relevant companion animal translational research which allows spontaneous disease modeling with similarities to human cancer that cannot be recreated in induced models [3–6].

Benefits and Limitations of Companion Animal and Murine Models for Cancer Research [3, 4, 4, 5, 5–9]

(1) Cancer-Bearing Pets

(i) Positive Attributes/Similarities to Human HNSCC

- (a) high incidence in native population
- (b) access to normal and cancer-bearing animals
- (c) immune competence
- (d) spontaneous tumor development
- (e) shared environment/diet/risk exposure

(f) similar tumor biology and genetics
(g) similar age, sex
(h) shared molecular targets
(i) proof-of-target analysis
(j) recapitulates tumor microenvironment and cell-stromal interactions
(k) tumor heterogeneity
(l) similar latency period
(m) acquired resistance
(n) spontaneous recurrence and metastasis
(o) similar prognostic factors
(p) similar diagnostics and cancer therapy
(q) multimodality treatment feasible
(r) serial biopsies/biospecimens feasible
(s) increasing species-specific reagents → gene-expression analysis and tumor proteomics
(t) ability to validate biomarkers
(u) not constrained by traditional Phase I/II/III trial design
(v) pet trials similar in caliber yet less costly than human trials
(w) minimally pretreated with good performance scores
(x) good owner/client compliance

(2) Murine Limitations

(i) Positive Attributes

(a) conventional model, well accepted
(b) ability to manipulate gene expression
(c) crucial in evaluating molecular paths

(ii) Limitations

(a) induced disease
(b) tumor homogeneity
(c) inbred population
(d) artificially shortened lifespan
(e) controlled, protected environment.

Traditionally, promising *in vitro* compounds are tested in human-xenografted immunocompromised mice to obtain efficacy and toxicity data in least sentient species. Putative anticancer drugs demonstrating preclinical effectiveness are then tested in primates to assess toxicology, followed by clinical testing in humans. Ethical concerns and recent funding restrictions on nonhuman primate research intensify the need to find alternative animal tumor models. Companion animal models (pets dogs or cats) could provide an essential intermediary safety and efficacy step between artificially induced murine tumor models and human patients. Sixty percent of US households own a pet, with 64% owning ≥2 pets, thus placing approximately 75 million dogs and 85 million cats at risk for cancer [10]. Estimates of age-adjusted overall cancer incidence rates per 100,000 individuals/year at risk are 381 for dogs and 264 for cats [3]. A large number of pets are affected with cancer each year, representing an underutilized resource in translational oncology research. Pet animals have been used in other fields of biomedical research based on similarities in physiology, anatomy, and drug metabolism. Cats in particular have been well studied as models of HIV and viral infections, diabetes mellitus, and obesity [11–14].

Pet owners are motivated to seek cancer treatments to both prolong their pets' lives as well as maintain the quality of life. Pet owners frequently seek out specialized care from board-certified veterinary oncologists, both in private practice and at teaching institutions. Multimodality treatments are consistently available, including surgical oncology, chemotherapy, immunotherapy, and radiation therapy. However, effective "standards of care" do not exist for many types of cancer in companion animals, providing opportunities to implement experimental therapies. Companion animal owners are interesting in pursuing clinical trials to evaluate novel diagnostic and therapeutic modalities, motivated by several potential benefits: for their individual pet, for other pets and pet owners faced with a similar challenge, and translation to benefit human cancer patients. Clinical trials customarily provide financial incentives, which are appealing given the high out-of-pocket expense for conventional treatments given the paucity of health insurance coverage in veterinary medicine. As most clinical trials are designed and administered by veterinary oncologists, they focus on clinical medical applicability and are not terminal studies. All institutional clinical trials are performed under both the auspices of the Institutional Animal Care and Use Committee (IACUC) and the participating veterinary hospital's standard operating procedures. Informed client consent and voluntary participation on part of the pet owner are key aspects. Many veterinary cancers are identified at an advanced stage with limited conventional treatment options, and thus experimental therapies are very acceptable to pet owners, veterinary clinicians, and the public community. Although the timeline for completion of a study in companion animals is longer than in rodents, completion remains rapid compared to human clinical trials as pets with aggressive and/or advanced stage cancer generally die within one year. Compliance is strong compared to human clinical trials, with repeat examination, treatment, and necropsy (autopsy) compliance approaching 90% [3].

2. Head and Neck Squamous Cell Carcinoma (HNSCC) Modeling

2.1. Feline Oral Squamous Cell Carcinoma (FOSCC): A Spontaneous Animal Tumor Model of HNSCC. Feline oral squamous cell carcinoma (FOSCC) has been suggested as a model for human head and neck squamous cell carcinoma (HNSCC), an aggressive cancer with limited advancement in five-year survival rates [7, 15, 16]. Feline models (tumor xenograft, normal cats, and cats with spontaneous disease) can be integrated dynamically with traditional preclinical models to optimize data value in drug testing. By utilizing pet cats that spontaneously develop oral squamous cell carcinoma (SCC), additional information could include drug activity and *in vivo* biomarkers, data in xenografts and clinical cancer patients, toxicity in cancer-bearing cats, PK/PD, drug dose and schedule, combination drug therapy, clinical monitoring, and tumor histology response. Other experimental animal models for human HNSCC include rodent 4NQO models, hamster tongue and check pouch models, and murine transgenic and xenograft models [17, 18]. These models all involve some form of artificial induction, underscoring the need for a relevant spontaneous model.

There have been limited translational and clinical advancements in HNSCC providing a rationale for alternative animal tumor models. Human head and neck cancer is the 8th most common cancer in the US and the 6th most common worldwide, with 40,250 new US cases/year [19]. As a histologic subtype HNSCC comprises approximately 90% of all head and neck cancers. Common initial management strategies include surgery and/or radiation in >65% of patients, with an increasing use of adjuvant chemotherapy [20]. Minimal improvement in overall survival has been made in the last two decades and HNSCC continues to have one of the worst outcomes of all head and neck tumors. For combined stages, the 1-year, 5-year, and 10-year relative survival rates are 84%, 61%, and 50%, respectively [19].

Feline oral squamous cell carcinoma (FOSCC) clinically mimics the disease progression and biologic behavior of HNSCC. Both cancers are locally invasive with metastasis occurring late in disease and most patients succumbing to local disease recurrence. In cats, reported metastases to regional lymph nodes (14.8%–18%) and lungs (12%) occur late in the course of disease and most cats are euthanized due to poor quality of life as a result of primary tumor growth [21, 22]. The incidence in cats is similar to people, with oral cancer accounting for up to 10% of all feline cancers [23]. Squamous cell carcinoma (SCC) is the most common oral tumor in cats (~60%–80%), occurring primarily in geriatric animals (12.5–13.6 years) [23, 24]. Gingiva is the most common intraoral site (51%), followed by lingual/sublingual (34%) [24]. Cats are the only species other than man that frequently develop SCC of the tongue [25]. Oral tumors in cats result in significant morbidity including chronic pain, malaligned dentition, halitosis, oral infection, dysphagia, food aversion, difficulty grooming, and cancer cachexia.

2.2. Comparative Treatment Modalities: HNSCC and FOSCC. The most common initial management strategy for HNSCC includes surgery and/or radiation in >65% of patients [20]. Similar to people, local disease control is the mainstay of therapy in cats with FOSCC. Given the advanced stage at diagnosis in most feline patients, local surgical excision is not considered a curative treatment. The mandible is considered the anatomic region most amenable to surgical resection and when deemed feasible in select cases, mandibulectomy results in median survival times of 5–12 months [26–30]. Given the importance of both functional outcome and primary tumor control, surgical decisions must account for both morbidity and the likelihood of achieving complete excision. In one study, acute and long-term postoperative morbidity were observed in 98% and 76% of the cats, respectively, with 12% of cats never regaining functional ability to eat. Despite curative-intent surgical approaches, 48% of tumor specimens had evidence of residual disease histologically [30]. In one small study, the combination of mandibulectomy and radiation therapy (RT) resulted in a median survival of 14 months, suggesting that for select cases, a better long-term prognosis may be feasible [31].

Radiation therapy is the primary treatment modality for unresectable local disease. Radiation therapy as a single-agent therapy results in overall response rates of 54%–70%, median progression-free intervals of 1.8–3.5 m, and median survival times of 2–5.8 m [22, 32, 33]. Similar to human studies, in cats chemotherapy as a single agent for primary tumor control is considered ineffective [21]. However, adjuvant chemotherapy may have a role in both local tumor control as well as metastatic spread. Cisplatin is routinely used in HNSCC, and a similar protocol using a combination of radiation and carboplatin chemotherapy resulted in a median survival of 5.4 months in cats [34]. Given the hypoxic nature of these tumors, gemcitabine and etanidazole have been investigated in cats as hypoxia/radiosensitizers, with response rates of 75%–100% yet rapid progression with median survival times of approximately 3.7 months [35].

Despite therapy, most cats are euthanized due to local disease progression and the severity of subsequent clinical signs. Overall, median survival times are generally between 2 and 4 months, with a one-year survival of only 10% [27, 29, 33, 36]. While disappointing, these numbers underscore the potential to institute investigational therapies in cats with rapid timelines for study completion.

2.3. Comparative Etiopathogenesis: HNSCC and FOSCC. The etiopathogenesis of HNSCC is multifactorial, with major risk factors including smoking/tobacco consumption, alcohol consumption, betel nut consumption (worldwide), poor oral hygiene, and human papillomavirus infection [37]. Recent studies suggest that human-papillomavirus- (HPV-) associated oropharyngeal cancers are increasing in incidence [19]. In people, oncogenic papillomaviruses alter retinoblastoma protein function, resulting in downstream accumulation of p16CDKN2A protein (p16). This subgroup accounts for ~ 20%–25% of oral cancers and is primarily associated with HPV-16. However, the clinical response and molecular properties of HPV-positive and HPV-negative tumors differ greatly, with HPV-negative HNSCCs having a worse overall survival [38]. In FOSCC, increased p16 immunoreactivity or papillomavirus DNA has been identified in only a small percentage of tissue samples, suggesting a potential role for PV-associated oncogenesis in a subset of FOSCC [39–41]. This suggests that FOSCCs are more similar to HPV-negative HNSCC, with no detectable papillomavirus DNA present in the majority of FOSCC [39–41]. Alternatively, it has been suggested by the "hit-and-run" mechanism of HPV-mediated carcinogenesis in HNSCC that perhaps HPV infection is an early initiating oncogenic event, but not necessary later for tumor progression, and thus HPV DNA may no longer be detectable [38]. However, papillomavirus

DNA is detectable in more than 90% of feline cutaneous SCCs which carries a much better prognosis than FOSCC, similar to the clinical outcome for human cutaneous SCC and HNSCC [42]. Smoking and tobacco consumption are major risk factors for HNSCC. Second-hand tobacco smoke has also been implicated in the pathogenesis of FOSCC, with cats from smoking households at a two- to fourfold increased risk of oral squamous cell carcinoma compared with cats in nonsmoking households [43, 44]. Oral exposure to other chemicals via grooming is also thought to contribute to FOSCC pathogenesis, as cats chronically exposed to flea collars are at an increased risk compared to cats treated with intermittent flea shampoo [43]. In people, an increase in nasopharyngeal cancer has been associated with the consumption of salt-cured meats and fish [37]. Similarly, cats with high canned food intake (particularly tuna) are at increased risk of FOSCC [43]. The significance of this association is not clear and may be related to nutrient content (e.g., protein content) or a relationship between texture of food and oral hygiene.

2.4. Comparative Molecular Aspects: HNSCC and FOSCC

2.4.1. Epidermal Growth Factor Receptor. The epidermal growth factor receptor (EGFR) signaling pathway has been implicated in the oncogenesis of HNSCC. Epidermal growth factor receptor is a transmembrane receptor tyrosine kinase that controls cellular pathways crucial in cancer development, growth, invasion, metastasis, and angiogenesis. Up to 90% of HNSCC exhibit overexpression of EGFR, which is prognostic for overall survival and disease-free interval [37, 45]. EGFR-targeted therapies have been explored, with blocking of EGFR resulting in inhibition of cell proliferation, enhancement of apoptosis, and reduction in the metastatic and angiogenic potential of HNSCC. In addition, monoclonal antibodies (e.g., cetuximab) have been investigated in clinical HNSCC patients with modest results [37].

In cats with FOSCC, EGFR is similarly highly expressed (69%–100%) [46–48]. The significance of EGFR tumor expression is unclear, with two studies demonstrating either high or low EGFR scores associated with better survival [47, 48]. Limitations in comparison of these studies as well as comparison to human studies include the retrospective nature, small sample size, variability in patient treatment, and variability in method of EGFR scoring and cellular localization. *In vitro* in feline cells, EGFR has been associated with proliferation and migration [49]. A population of putative cancer stem cells with enhanced sphere-forming ability, reduced sensitivity to radiation and conventional chemotherapy, and demonstrated resistance to gefitinib (EGFR-targeting drug) has also been demonstrated in FOSCC [50]. Gefitinib results in reduced cell proliferation and migration as well as a change in cell morphology and gene expression suggestive of epithelial to mesenchymal transition [49, 50]. EGFR-targeting with RNAi resulted in reduction in EGFR activity, reversal of acquired gefitinib resistance, and an additive effect on cell killing when combined with radiation [49].

2.4.2. Molecular Markers of Proliferation and Angiogenesis. HNSCC is characterized by tumor-associated angiogenesis, with elevations in the proangiogenic cytokine vascular endothelial growth factor (VEGF) and increased microvessel density (MVD) scores correlated with clinical stage and an overall poor prognosis [51]. In FOSCC, MVD is significantly higher in tumor samples (50.3 ± 23.6), compared with normal feline gingiva (7.6 ± 4.06) with tumor-associated vessels exhibiting morphologic atypia and a thin endothelial lining [52]. There may also be anatomic variability with tongue tumors reported to have the highest MVD [47]. In cats clinically affected with FOSCC, treatment with zoledronate, an aminobisphosphonate used for skeletal malignancies that has putative antiangiogenic properties, rapidly decreases circulating serum VEGF concentrations [16].

Prostaglandins and cyclooxygenase-2 (COX-2) play a critical role in tumor development and growth by regulating numerous biologic processes including tumor angiogenesis. More than 77% of HNSCC express high levels of COX-2 and COX-2 overexpression and higher prostaglandin E2 (PGE2) levels are associated with poor survival and correlated with VEGF expression [53, 54]. In FOSCC, COX-2 expression is variable, with up to 67% of tumors exhibiting COX-2 expression [55–57]. However, COX-2 expression is not reported to be correlated with survival [57]. Although the significance of this is unclear, functional COX-2 enzymatic activity is reported to be dissociated from relative IHC-based COX-2 protein expression in some cell lines including the FOSCC cell line SCCF1 [58]. In HNSCC, lipoxygenase is also overexpressed, and similarly in FOSCC tissue samples there is high-intensity staining of lipoxygenase. Additionally, *in vitro*, the 5-lipoxygenase inhibitor tepoxalin induces apoptosis in feline SCC cells [59].

The tumor suppressor gene p53 is often dysregulated in cancer, with loss of functional p53 protein contributing to disease progression via aberrant cell cycle checkpoint control and regulation of apoptosis. p53 gene mutation associated with allelic loss at 17p is one of the most common genetic abnormalities in HNSCC, and p53 status is an independent predictive factor of response to chemotherapy [60]. In HNSCC HPV-negative tumors, which have a worse overall survival, often have mutated p53, while the HPV-positive HNSCCs have both a better overall survival as well as wild-type p53 [38]. In addition, HPV-positive tumors tend to occur in younger people compared with HPV-negative HNSCC which commonly affects older patients. Similarly, most FOSCCs occur in geriatric cats and are HPV-negative [39, 40]. Aberrant p53 expression has been documented in FOSCC and is associated with tobacco smoke exposure [44, 61].

Ki67 and mitotic index (MI) are markers of proliferation commonly assessed in tumor biopsy samples. Ki67 is a nuclear protein not expressed in senescent cells (G0). In HNSCC, Ki67 expression is related to aberrant p53 expression and is associated with a poor prognosis [62, 63]. In FOSCC, high expression of Ki67 is associated with decreased overall survival [48]. In another study, both Ki 67 and mitotic index exhibited wide variation among tumors, with no correlation between MI and Ki 67 [47].

2.4.3. Malignant Osteolysis. Both HNSCC and FOSCC are highly invasive into surrounding soft tissue structures and frequently characterized by malignant osteolysis of underlying bone. Bone-invasion contributes to clinical morbidity and poorer prognosis for HNSCC patients. In both species, *in vitro* and *in vivo* bone resorption and osteoclastogenesis are associated with high levels of parathyroid hormone-related protein (PTHrP) [15, 24]. PTHrP is known to stimulate osteoclastic bone resorption by increasing the expression of RANKL in osteoblasts. RANKL expression results in differentiation and activation of osteoclasts, ultimately resulting in bone resorption. SCC cells (murine, human, and feline) also express increased receptor activator of nuclear factor kappa-B ligand (RANKL) or an altered RANKL:OPG (osteoprotegerin) ratio [15, 52]. Osteoprotegerin is a decoy receptor for the receptor activator of nuclear factor kappa B ligand (RANKL); binding of RANKL by OPG inhibits nuclear kappa B (NF-κB) downstream signaling. In feline SCC cells, the aminobisphosphonate zoledronate, clinically used in people to inhibit malignant osteolysis, induces a dose-dependent reduction in RANKL expression [16, 52]. In a murine xenograft (feline SCC cells), zoledronate treatment reduced tumor growth and prevented osteolysis [64]. Serum carboxy-terminal collagen crosslink (CTx) is a useful marker of bone resorption and turnover in clinical patients with skeletal malignancies. Cats with naturally occurring bone-invasive SCC have greater serum CTx concentrations in comparison with geriatric, healthy controls and in FOSCC-affected cats treatment with zoledronate rapidly decreased circulating serum CTx levels [16].

3. Conclusions

In conclusion, spontaneous animal tumor models may serve an important role in translating research findings to facilitate clinical improvements in human cancer patients. Spontaneously occurring cancer in pets shares striking molecular and clinical similarities to human malignancies that cannot be reproduced in artificially induced laboratory models. Human HNSCC is one type of cancer that has suffered from limited improvement in effective therapies and outcomes in the last few decades. Given the similarities in clinical progression and therapy as well as tumor biology including EGFR signaling, molecular aspects of cancer progression and angiogenesis, and clinical manifestations of malignant osteolysis, FOSCC is a biologically relevant animal tumor model. Utilization of this naturally occurring cancer may benefit both veterinary and human cancer patients.

References

[1] E. L. Tobinick, "The value of drug repositioning in the current pharmaceutical market," *Drug News and Perspectives*, vol. 22, no. 2, pp. 119–125, 2009.

[2] I. Kola, "The state of innovation in drug development," *Clinical Pharmacology and Therapeutics*, vol. 83, no. 2, pp. 227–230, 2008.

[3] D. M. Vail and D. H. Thamm, "Spontaneous companion animal (pet) cancers," in *Tumor Models in Cancer Research: Cancer Drug Discovery and Development*, B. A. Teicher, Ed., pp. 353–373, Humana Press, New Jersey, NJ, USA, 2nd edition, 2011.

[4] I. K. Gordon and C. Khanna, "Modeling opportunities in comparative oncology for drug development," *ILAR Journal*, vol. 51, no. 3, pp. 214–220, 2010.

[5] M. Paoloni and C. Khanna, "Translation of new cancer treatments from pet dogs to humans," *Nature Reviews Cancer*, vol. 8, no. 2, pp. 147–156, 2008.

[6] K. Hansen and C. Khanna, "Spontaneous and genetically engineered animal models: use in preclinical cancer drug development," *European Journal of Cancer*, vol. 40, no. 6, pp. 858–880, 2004.

[7] S. Tannehill-Gregg, A. Levine, and T. Rosol, "Feline head and neck squamous cell carcinoma: a natural model for the human disease and development of a mouse model," *Veterinary and Comparative Oncology*, vol. 4, no. 2, pp. 84–97, 2006.

[8] C. Khanna, K. Lindblad-Toh, D. Vail et al., "The dog as a cancer model," *Nature Biotechnology*, vol. 24, no. 9, pp. 1065–1066, 2006.

[9] T. Voskoglou-Nomikos, J. L. Pater, and L. Seymour, "Clinical predictive value of the in vitro cell line, human xenograft, and mouse allograft preclinical cancer models," *Clinical Cancer Research*, vol. 9, no. 11, pp. 4227–4239, 2003.

[10] A. J. Shepherd, "Results of the 2006 AVMA survey of companion animal ownership in US pet-owning households," *Journal of the American Veterinary Medical Association*, vol. 232, no. 5, pp. 695–696, 2008.

[11] J. H. Elder, Y. Lin, E. Fink, and C. K. Grant, "Feline immunodeficiency virus (FIV) as a model for study of lentivirus infections: parallels with HIV," *Current HIV Research*, vol. 8, no. 1, pp. 73–80, 2010.

[12] J. C. Kenyon and A. M. L. Lever, "The molecular biology of feline immunodeficiency virus (FIV)," *Viruses*, vol. 3, no. 11, pp. 2192–2213, 2011.

[13] M. S. Henson and T. D. O'Brien, "Feline models of type 2 diabetes mellitus," *ILAR Journal*, vol. 47, no. 3, pp. 234–242, 2006.

[14] M. Hoenig, "The cat as a model for human nutrition and disease," *Current Opinion in Clinical Nutrition and Metabolic Care*, vol. 9, no. 5, pp. 584–588, 2006.

[15] C. K. Martin, W. P. Dirksen, S. T. Shu et al., "Characterization of bone resorption in novel in vitro and in vivo models of oral squamous cell carcinoma," *Oral Oncology*, vol. 48, no. 6, pp. 491–499, 2012.

[16] J. M. Wypij, T. M. Fan, R. L. Fredrickson, A. M. Barger, L. P. De Lorimier, and S. C. Charney, "In vivo and in vitro efficacy of zoledronate for treating oral squamous cell carcinoma in cats," *Journal of Veterinary Internal Medicine*, vol. 22, no. 1, pp. 158–163, 2008.

[17] S. Tannehill-Gregg, E. Kergosien, and T. J. Rosol, "Feline head and neck squamous cell carcinoma cell line: characterization, production of parathyroid hormone-related protein, and regulation by transforming growth factor-β," *In Vitro Cellular and Developmental Biology*, vol. 37, no. 10, pp. 676–683, 2001.

[18] B. Mognetti, F. Di Carlo, and G. N. Berta, "Animal models in oral cancer research," *Oral Oncology*, vol. 42, no. 5, pp. 448–460, 2006.

[19] American Cancer Society, Ed., *Cancer Facts and Figures (2012)*, American Cancer Society, Atlanta, Ga, USA, 2012.

[20] J. S. Cooper, K. Porter, K. Mallin et al., "National cancer database report on cancer of the head and neck: 10-year update," *Head and Neck*, vol. 31, no. 6, pp. 748–758, 2009.

[21] J. J. Marretta, L. D. Garrett, and S. M. Marretta, "Feline oral squamous cell carcinoma: an overview," *Veterinary Medicine*, vol. 102, no. 6, pp. 392–406, 2007.

[22] V. Poirier, B. K. Hotz, D. Vail, and R. Straw, "Efficacy and toxicity of an accelerated hypofractionated radiation therapy protocol in cats with oral squamous cell carcinoma," *Veterinary Radiology Ultrasound*, vol. 54, no. 1, pp. 81–88, 2013.

[23] K. E. Stebbins, C. C. Morse, and M. H. Goldschmidt, "Feline oral neoplasia: a ten-year survey," *Veterinary Pathology*, vol. 26, no. 2, pp. 121–128, 1989.

[24] C. K. Martin, S. H. Tannehill-Gregg, T. D. Wolfe, and T. J. Rosol, "Bone-invasive oral squamous cell carcinoma in cats: pathology and expression of parathyroid hormone-related protein," *Veterinary Pathology*, vol. 48, no. 1, pp. 302–312, 2011.

[25] D. G. Gardner, "Spontaneous squamous cell carcinomas of the oral region in domestic animals: a review and consideration of their relevance to human research," *Oral Diseases*, vol. 2, no. 2, pp. 148–154, 1996.

[26] D. E. Bostock, "The prognosis in cats bearing squamous cell carcinoma," *Journal of Small Animal Practice*, vol. 13, no. 3, pp. 119–125, 1972.

[27] R. L. Bradley, E. G. MacEwen, and A. S. Loar, "Mandibular resection for removal of oral tumors in 30 dogs and 6 cats," *Journal of the American Veterinary Medical Association*, vol. 184, no. 4, pp. 460–463, 1984.

[28] S. K. Salisbury, D. C. Richardson, and G. C. Lantz, "Partial maxillectomy and premaxillectomy in the treatment of oral neoplasia in the dog and cat," *Veterinary Surgery*, vol. 15, no. 1, pp. 16–26, 1986.

[29] N. C. P. Reeves, J. M. Turrel, and S. J. Withrow, "Oral squamous cell carcinoma in the cat," *Journal of the American Animal Hospital Association*, vol. 29, no. 5, pp. 438–441, 1993.

[30] N. C. Northrup, K. A. Selting, K. M. Rassnick et al., "Outcomes of cats with oral tumors treated with mandibulectomy: 42 cases," *Journal of the American Animal Hospital Association*, vol. 42, no. 5, pp. 350–360, 2006.

[31] C. A. Hutson, C. C. Willauer, E. J. Walder, J. L. Stone, and M. K. Klein, "Treatment of mandibular squamous cell carcinoma in cats by use of mandibulectomy and radiotherapy: seven cases (1987–1989)," *Journal of the American Veterinary Medical Association*, vol. 201, no. 5, pp. 777–781, 1992.

[32] C. McDonald, J. Looper, and S. Greene, "Response rate and duration associated with a 4Gy 5 fraction palliative radiation protocol," *Veterinary Radiology Ultrasound*, vol. 53, no. 3, pp. 358–364, 2012.

[33] V. S. Bregazzi, S. M. LaRue, B. E. Powers, M. J. Fettman, G. K. Ogilvie, and S. J. Withrow, "Response of feline oral squamous cell carcinoma to palliative radiation therapy," *Veterinary Radiology and Ultrasound*, vol. 42, no. 1, pp. 77–79, 2001.

[34] J. Fidel, J. Lyons, C. Tripp, R. Houston, B. Wheeler, and A. Ruiz, "Treatment of oral squamous cell carcinoma with accelerated radiation therapy and concomitant carboplatin in cats," *Journal of Veterinary Internal Medicine*, vol. 25, no. 3, pp. 504–510, 2011.

[35] S. M. Evans, F. LaCreta, S. Helfand et al., "Technique, pharmacokinetics, toxicity, and efficacy of intratumoral etanidazole and radiotherapy for treatment of spontaneous feline oral squamous cell carcinoma," *International Journal of Radiation Oncology Biology Physics*, vol. 20, no. 4, pp. 703–708, 1991.

[36] A. M. Hayes, V. J. Adams, T. J. Scase, and S. Murphy, "Survival of 54 cats with oral squamous cell carcinoma in United Kingdom general practice," *Journal of Small Animal Practice*, vol. 48, no. 7, pp. 394–399, 2007.

[37] L. G. Marcu and E. Yeoh, "A review of risk factors and genetic alterations in head and neck carcinogenesis and implications for current and future approaches to treatment," *Journal of Cancer Research and Clinical Oncology*, vol. 135, no. 10, pp. 1303–1314, 2009.

[38] J. Rautava and S. Syrjanen, "Biology of human papillomavirus infections in head and neck carcinogenesis," *Head and Neck Pathology*, vol. 6, supplement 1, pp. S3–S15, 2012.

[39] J. S. Munday, L. Howe, A. French, R. A. Squires, and H. Sugiarto, "Detection of papillomaviral DNA sequences in a feline oral squamous cell carcinoma," *Research in Veterinary Science*, vol. 86, no. 2, pp. 359–361, 2009.

[40] S. H. O'Neill, K. M. Newkirk, E. A. Anis, R. Brahmbhatt, L. A. Frank, and S. A. Kania, "Detection of human papillomavirus DNA in feline premalignant and invasive squamous cell carcinoma," *Veterinary Dermatology*, vol. 22, no. 1, pp. 68–74, 2011.

[41] J. S. Munday, C. G. Knight, and A. F. French, "Evaluation of feline oral squamous cell carcinomas for p16CDKN2A protein immunoreactivity and the presence of papillomaviral DNA," *Research in Veterinary Science*, vol. 90, no. 2, pp. 280–283, 2011.

[42] J. S. Munday, M. Kiupel, A. F. French, and L. Howe, "Amplification of papillomaviral DNA sequences from a high proportion of feline cutaneous in situ and invasive squamous cell carcinomas using a nested polymerase chain reaction," *Veterinary Dermatology*, vol. 19, no. 5, pp. 259–263, 2008.

[43] E. R. Bertone, L. A. Snyder, and A. S. Moore, "Environmental and lifestyle risk factors for oral squamous cell carcinoma in domestic cats," *Journal of Veterinary Internal Medicine*, vol. 17, no. 4, pp. 557–562, 2003.

[44] L. A. Snyder, E. R. Bertone, R. M. Jakowski, M. S. Dooner, J. Jennings-Ritchie, and A. S. Moore, "p53 expression and environmental tobacco smoke exposure in feline oral squamous cell carcinoma," *Veterinary Pathology*, vol. 41, no. 3, pp. 209–214, 2004.

[45] S. Kalyankrishna and J. R. Grandis, "Epidermal growth factor receptor biology in head and neck cancer," *Journal of Clinical Oncology*, vol. 24, no. 17, pp. 2666–2672, 2006.

[46] J. Looper, D. Malarkey, D. Ruslander, D. Proulx, and D. Thrall, "Epidermal growth factor receptor expression in feline oral squamous cell carcinomas," *Veterinary and Comparative Oncology*, vol. 4, no. 1, pp. 33–40, 2006.

[47] H. Yoshikawa, E. J. Ehrhart, J. Charles, D. Thamm, and S. Larue, "Immunohistochemical characterization of feline oral squamous cell carcinoma," *American Journal of Veterinary Research*, vol. 73, no. 11, pp. 1801–1806, 2012.

[48] G. T. Bergkvist, D. J. Argyle, L. Morrison, N. Macintyre, A. Hayes, and D. A. Yool, "Expression of epidermal growth factor receptor (EGFR) and Ki67 in feline oral squamous cell carcinomas (FOSCC)," *Veterinary and Comparative Oncology*, vol. 9, no. 2, pp. 106–117, 2011.

[49] G. T. Bergkvist, D. J. Argyle, L. Y. Pang, R. Muirhead, and D. A. Yool, "Studies on the inhibition of feline EGFR in squamous cell carcinoma: enhancement of radiosensitivity and rescue of resistance to small molecule inhibitors," *Cancer Biology and Therapy*, vol. 11, no. 11, pp. 927–937, 2011.

[50] L. Y. Pang, G. T. Bergkvist, A. C. Arias, D. A. Yool, R. Muirhead, and D. J. Argyle, "Identification of tumour initiating cells in feline head and neck squamous cell carcinoma and evidence for gefitinib induced epithelial to mesenchymal transition," *The Veterinary Journal*, vol. 193, no. 1, pp. 46–52, 2012.

[51] P. A. Kyzas, I. W. Cunha, and J. P. A. Ioannidis, "Prognostic significance of vascular endothelial growth factor immunohistochemical expression in head and neck squamous cell carcinoma: a meta-analysis," *Clinical Cancer Research*, vol. 11, no. 4, pp. 1434–1440, 2005.

[52] J. M. Wypij, *Anti-neoplastic effects of zoledronate in feline oral squamous cell carcinoma [Masters]*, University of Illinois at Urbana-Champaign, Urbana, Ill, USA, 2009.

[53] O. Gallo, E. Masini, B. Bianchi, L. Bruschini, M. Paglierani, and A. Franchi, "Prognostic significance of cyclooxygenase-2 pathway and angiogenesis in head and neck squamous cell carcinoma," *Human Pathology*, vol. 33, no. 7, pp. 708–714, 2002.

[54] G. Pannone, P. Bufo, M. F. Caiaffa et al., "Cyclooxygenase-2 expression in oral squamous cell carcinoma," *International Journal of Immunopathology and Pharmacology*, vol. 17, no. 3, pp. 273–282, 2004.

[55] S. L. Beam, K. M. Rassnick, A. S. Moore, and S. P. McDonough, "An immunohistochemical study of cyclooxygenase-2 expression in various feline neoplasms," *Veterinary Pathology*, vol. 40, no. 5, pp. 496–500, 2003.

[56] L. DiBernardi, M. Doré, J. A. Davis et al., "Study of feline oral squamous cell carcinoma: potential target for cyclooxygenase inhibitor treatment," *Prostaglandins Leukotrienes and Essential Fatty Acids*, vol. 76, no. 4, pp. 245–250, 2007.

[57] A. Hayes, T. Scase, J. Miller, S. Murphy, A. Sparkes, and V. Adams, "COX 2 expression in feline oral squamous cell carcinoma (FOSCC)—an immunohistochemical study and analysis of survival," *Veterinary and Comparative Oncology*, vol. 3, no. 1, pp. 44–45, 2005.

[58] D. A. Heller, C. A. Clifford, M. H. Goldschmidt, D. E. Holt, M. J. Manfredi, and K. U. Sorenmo, "Assessment of cyclooxygenase-2 expression in canine hemangiosarcoma, histiocytic sarcoma, and mast cell tumor," *Veterinary Pathology*, vol. 42, no. 3, pp. 350–353, 2005.

[59] J. J. Wakshlag, J. Peters-Kennedy, J. J. Bushey, and J. P. Loftus, "5-lipoxygenase expression and tepoxalin-induced cell death in squamous cell carcinomas in cats," *American Journal of Veterinary Research*, vol. 72, no. 10, pp. 1369–1377, 2011.

[60] A. Cabelguenne, H. Blons, I. De Waziers et al., "p53 alterations predict tumor response to neoadjuvant chemotherapy in head and neck squamous cell carcinoma: a prospective series," *Journal of Clinical Oncology*, vol. 18, no. 7, pp. 1465–1473, 2000.

[61] J. P. Teifke and C. V. Lohr, "Immunohistochemical detection of P53 overexpression in paraffin wax-embedded squamous cell carcinomas of cattle, horses, cats and dogs," *Journal of Comparative Pathology*, vol. 114, no. 2, pp. 205–210, 1996.

[62] P. J. Slootweg, R. Koole, and G. J. Hordijk, "The presence of p53 protein in relation to Ki-67 as cellular proliferation marker in head and neck squamous cell carcinoma and adjacent dysplastic mucosa," *European Journal of Cancer B*, vol. 30, no. 2, pp. 138–141, 1994.

[63] S. D. Silva, M. Agostini, I. N. Nishimoto et al., "Expression of fatty acid synthase, ErbB2 and Ki-67 in head and neck squamous cell carcinoma. A clinicopathological study," *Oral Oncology*, vol. 40, no. 7, pp. 688–696, 2004.

[64] C. K. Martin, J. L. Werbeck, N. K. Thudi et al., "Zoledronic acid reduces bone loss and tumor growth in an orthotopic xenograft model of osteolytic oral squamous cell carcinoma," *Cancer Research*, vol. 70, no. 21, pp. 8607–8616, 2010.

17

FAP Associated Papillary Thyroid Carcinoma: A Peculiar Subtype of Familial Nonmedullary Thyroid Cancer

Francesco Cetta

IRCCS MultiMedica, Viale Fantoli 16/15, 20138 Milan, Italy

Correspondence should be addressed to Francesco Cetta; cetta_francesco@libero.it

Academic Editor: Hanlin L. Wang

Familial Nonmedullary Thyroid Carcinoma (FNMTC) makes up to 5–10% of all thyroid cancers, also including those FNMTC occurring as a minor component of familial cancer syndromes, such as Familial Adenomatous Polyposis (FAP). We give evidence that this extracolonic manifestation of FAP is determined by the same germline mutation of the APC gene responsible for colonic polyps and cancer but also shows some unusual features (F : M ratio = 80 : 1, absence of LOH for APC in the thyroid tumoral tissue, and indolent biological behaviour, despite frequent multicentricity and lymph nodal involvement), suggesting that the APC gene confers only a generic susceptibility to thyroid cancer, but perhaps other factors, namely, modifier genes, sex-related factors, or environmental factors, are also required for its phenotypic expression. This great variability is against the possibility of classifying all FNMTC as a single entity, not only with a unique or prevalent causative genetic factor, but also with a unique or common biological behavior and a commonly dismal prognosis. A new paradigm is also suggested that could be useful (1) for a proper classification of FAP associated PTC within the larger group of FNMTC and (2) for making inferences to sporadic carcinogenesis, based on the lesson from FAP.

1. Introduction

Familial Nonmedullary Thyroid Carcinoma (FNMTC) is a nonmedullary thyroid cancer occurring in a subject with germline mutation for a gene responsible for an inherited multitumoral syndrome, including thyroid carcinoma as a part of the syndrome (or in more than 3 members of the same kindred, even in the absence of a known mutation in a putative gene). FNMTC makes up to 5–10% of all thyroid cancers, also including those FNMTC occurring as a minor component of familial cancer syndromes, such as Gardner's syndrome, Cowden's disease, Carney complex type-1, Werner's syndrome, McCune Albright syndrome, or Familial Adenomatous Polyposis (FAP) [1, 2]. In particular, a recent review outlines that "FNTMC is associated with more aggressive disease than sporadic cases, with higher rates of multicentric tumours, lymph node metastasis, extrathyroidal invasion, and shorter disease-free survival" [1].

In addition, it has been suggested that "the genetic inheritance of FNMTC, (in patients in whom it is the predominant feature), remains 'unknown...'", but "it has been observed an increased percentage of male patients with FNMTC compared to those with sporadic NMTC" [1].

We have collected the largest world series of patients with FAP (Familial Adenomatous Polyposis) associated FNMTC (n = 18, all females) and were the first to show a significant genotype-phenotype correlation, suggesting that most of APC (Adenomatous Polyposis Coli) germline mutations in patients with FAP associated FNMTC are located in a well defined genomic area, that is, $5'$ to codon 1200 [3–17].

FAP is inherited in an autosomal dominant fashion and is characterized by multiple adenomatous polyps in the colon and rectum and a near certainty of developing colorectal cancer unless a risk-reducing prophylactic colectomy is performed. Therefore, early identification and intervention in FAP patients is of paramount importance. FAP is also associated with several extracolonic malignancies, including malignancies of the upper gastrointestinal tract, hepatobiliary tract, central nervous system, and endocrine system (thyroid, adrenal) [3–10].

While many individuals are diagnosed with FAP due to the discovery of colonic polyps, the identification of CMV (cribriform-morular variant) histology in patients with PTC provides clinicians with a unique opportunity to diagnose occult cases of FAP [18–25].

During the last decade we have continued (1) to recruit FAP associated FNMTC, (2) to follow up those previously collected, and (3) to collect all available data from the literature [11–17, 26].

2. Female Prevalence

In our review of the various series (often including just 1 or 2 cases) we could document that whereas in our first report on FAP associated FNMTC, the prevalence for females was 17 : 1, after 2000, there was a striking increase (female to male ratio = 80 : 1 versus 2.5–3.1) in sporadic tumors [11–17, 26].

3. Age at Diagnosis of PTC and/or Colonic Polyps

More than 80% of FAP associated FNPTC were diagnosed between 18 and 35 years of age. In particular, in our 18 patients, diagnosis was concomitant in 6 (1/3), whereas in 6 (1/3) FAP preceded and in 6 (1/3) PTC preceded. This is very important, because the early occurrence of PTC can facilitate diagnosis in some kindred with undetected FAP [5, 16].

4. Long-Term Prognosis

In an overall series of 200 cases reported in the literature (112 before 2000 and 90 after that year), there were very few recurrences and only 1 death, possibly related to FAP associated PTC [16, 17, 26]. In particular, there was no recurrence in 9 of our patients, with a follow-up longer than 15 years (180 months) in every subject [26].

5. Prevalence of PTC in FAP Patients

Concerning the actual prevalence of PTC in FAP patients, it has been reported as 0.4% to 2% in various retrospective series. More recently, results of prospective registry screening programs for PTC in patients with FAP have reported prevalences of 2.6% [27] to 11.8% [28]. This is an increased value in comparison with the previously reported data (1.2%) [23]. We deem that a 3 to 5% prevalence of PTC in FAP patients could be a more realistic value in the present era of improved early diagnosis [26]; even if recent intensive screening protocols in patients belong to FAP registries, the prevalence was 6.1% overall and 11.1% in women [29, 30].

The main criticism that can be raised in the interpretation of the findings of the last series, in which all FAP patients underwent intensive screening, concerns the significance of observed data. In fact, in some cases thyroid nodules resulted positive at FNAB, even in males and after age 60. This observation contrasts with previous observations, suggesting that these tumors are likely to be different from those currently associated with FAP, occurring in females aged less than 35.

6. Age of Patients

In our first report the mean age of patients was 24.8 years, in a series of 15 female patients [5], but it was also 24.8 years in a series of 97 patients collected from the literature. The mean age has been similar in the 81 patients reported in the literature after 2000 [26].

7. Histologic Variants of PTC

Harach et al. [19] reported 4 cases of thyroid carcinoma in FAP patients and noted the following unusual features: multifocality (differing from sporadic PTC) multifocality-tumors encapsulated, and unusual histologic patterns: cribriform, solid, spindling, and whorls. They concluded that FAP associated thyroid carcinomas were likely related to PTC but were sufficiently different.

Cameselle-Teijeiro and Chan [20] described 4 cases with similar or identical morphology, apparently occurring in patients without FAP. These findings were also observed by others [21]. These tumors have been termed the "cribriform morular" variant of PTC (CMV PTC). The cribriform areas are composed of anastomosing bars and arches of cells without intervening stroma with the follicular spaces devoid of colloid. The morulas are composed of spindled cells with "peculiar nuclear clearing." These clear nuclei differ from both the optically clear nuclei and intranuclear pseudoinclusions more typically seen in PTC and consist of accumulation of biotin [20–22].

Harach et al. [19] speculated that the morphology of this variant could be related to the involvement of the APC gene in the pathogenesis. However, we never found balletic inactivation in the thyroid tumoral tissue (that was found in the colonic tumoral tissue); Soravia et al. [25] in 9 samples from 4 patients found somatic APC mutations in 1 sample. These findings suggest that although somatic mutations of APC may be seen in a few cases of FAP associated thyroid carcinoma, it is not a required step in the pathogenesis of these neoplasms. On the contrary, we were the first to show a very high incidence of ret/PTC oncogene activation, which is known to be an early molecular event in papillary thyroid carcinoma oncogenesis [7]. These findings support the concept that FAP associated thyroid tumors are variant of PTC [7]. In a subset of CMV of PTC Xu et al. [22] have demonstrated that aberrant nuclear accumulation of mutant beta-catenin may substitute for APC mutations. It is thought that these sporadic cases are due to a somatic mutation in exon 3 of the beta-catenin gene (CTNNB1), further highlighting the analogous role to the APC-beta-catenin pathway. In fact, not only sporadic CMV PTC but also FAP associated PTC usually, but not always, show nuclear and cytoplasmatic expression of beta-catenin [12, 16, 26].

On the contrary, the most common genetic abnormality in papillary thyroid carcinoma BRAF mutation appears to be absent in FAP associated thyroid cancer, suggesting that BRAF and APC RET/PTC mutations are mutually exclusive of each other in the occurrence of different types of PTC [16, 17, 26].

However, there are some clinical, demographic, and prognostic differences between sporadic CMV-PTCs, which may occur in males (instead of exclusively in females) and in old age, and many reports show an aggressive behavior with distant metastasis [20, 21, 29] and the typical indolent behavior of FAP associated PTC, occurring almost always in females and showing an indolent behavior [5, 26]. There was only 1 death because of thyroid related complications out of 200 FAP associated PTCs [26].

Therefore, we suggest caution before stating that, despite similar features and the possibility of diagnosing CMV PTC preoperatively by FNAB, these tumors (sporadic and FAP associated) should be considered as a single entity [16, 17].

Interestingly, whereas tumors in the colon rectum occur invariably in almost 100% of subjects with APC germline mutations, with no prevalence for any sex and with the same incidence in males and in females (and in most colorectal polyps or cancers, there is a complete loss of the APC function documented by the high rate of LOH for APC in the tumoral tissue), FAP associated FNMTC occurs in a minority of affected siblings, in the absence of LOH for APC [6] and almost invariably in the female sex [26]. This is opposite to what has been reported for FNMTC as a homogeneous entity [1], since these authors observed a relative prevalence of males in comparison to the usual F : M ratio = 3 : 1 in sporadic tumors.

In particular, this is a very unusual finding in an inherited multitumoral syndrome. There is no doubt that FAP associated FNMTC is part of the multitumoral syndrome due to germline mutations of a tumor suppressor gene as APC. In fact, there is a frequent association of FNMTC in siblings with the same germline mutation (all the 23 siblings with FAP associated FNMPC were female).

There is a statistically significant association between FNMTC and the site of germline mutations (almost all mutations are located in the proximal portion of the gene, 5′ to codon 1220) [5].

However, the absence of complete inactivation of the gene [6] suggests that the germline mutation of the APC gene confers only a generic susceptibility to thyroid cancer [5–11], but perhaps other factors, namely, modifier genes, sex-related factors (hormonal, but also dietary, metabolic, and immunological), or environmental factors [31], are also required for the phenotypic expression.

It is likely that FAP associated FNMTC represents a veritable example of cooperation between purely inherited factors (APC germline mutation) and epigenetic or environmental factors, namely, those strictly connected with the female sex, as the striking female to male ratio of 80 : 1 strongly suggests [26].

These peculiar features have been documented in detail only for FAP associated FNMTC, with the striking female preponderance.

In FNMTC associated with Werner syndrome, a relative male prevalence has been suggested by some authors [1]; as well in other FNMTC associated with other inherited multitumoral syndromes there could be other associations with epigenetic or environmental factors [1].

We suggest that a similar multifactorial cooperation could also occur for the most frequent variant of FNMTC that is not associated with a germline mutation of a known tumor suppressor gene. We suspect that the 5–10% of FNMTC do not include just a few rare manifestations of 3-4 inherited multitumoral syndromes (such as those quoted in a recent review) [1], whereas the remaining patients belong to a unique disease, for which (in addition to a common prognosis or similar biological behavior) also a single predisposing gene or a common molecular or pathophysiologic mechanism should be envisaged. This is an oversimplification of a complex entity.

Actually, Navas-Carrillo et al. [1] report (1) on the American family with 5 members affected by PTC, one by colon cancer and 2 by papillary renal neoplasm, with a possible susceptibility gene (PTC/PRN), located at 1q21 [32], (2) on the susceptibility locus (NMTC1) on chromosome 2q21, firstly identified in a large Tasmanian pedigree with recurrence of PTC [33], and (3) on the susceptibility locus to chromosome 8p23.1-p22 in a large Portuguese family with 11 cases of benign thyroid disease and 5 cases of thyroid cancer [34]. In particular, patients with these genetic alterations may partially overlap with, or be completely different from, those showing genetic anticipation (i.e., diagnosis at an earlier age in patients of the second generation) [35].

Anyway all these patients are smaller in number than the 200 homogeneous patients with FAP associated NMPTC, with documented association with an inherited germline mutation, for whom we have shown a biological behavior (striking female prevalence and little tumor aggressiveness) different from that suggested by Navas-Carrillo et al. [1] for the total amount of FNMTC.

On the basis of these cumulative data, it is more likely that there is a galaxy, a wide multiplicity, of potential germline mutations, each of which can confer an increased susceptibility, but other genes or factors, namely, environmental factors (maybe playing a greater role than congenital predisposition), are also required for PTC manifestation.

This great variability of germline predisposing factors and of epigenetic and environmental factors is against the possibility of classifying all FNMTC as a single entity, not only with a unique or prevalent causative genetic factor, but also with a unique or common biological behavior, such as "higher rates of metastases, extrathyroidal invasion, and shorter disease free survival."

The only common characteristic (in addition to the possibility of earlier diagnosis, because of a previous affected sibling in the same kindred) is the frequent multicentricity. But, also in this respect, it must be outlined that we had no recurrence in the contralateral lobe (after a minimum follow-up of 180 months for all patients), in 5 out of 5 subjects with FAP associated FNMTC, who had hemithyroidectomy, because they refused total thyroidectomy, in association with total colectomy and other concomitant invasive operations at a young age, which are usually required in FAP subjects [16, 17, 26].

In particular, there is no single genetic alteration predisposing specifically to FNMTC in all cases. On the contrary, there are various syndromes, also including some familial cancer syndromes, that have multiple siblings with FNMTC as a part of the syndrome.

Therefore, if FNMTC is a very heterogeneous syndrome, to try to select common features as well as a uniform prognosis or the same biological behavior can be misleading.

Furthermore, the lesson from the galaxy of heterogeneous FNMTC, if correctly interpreted, could contribute to open new avenues for a deeper knowledge of pathogenic factors determining the occurrence of all "common" or most frequent types of cancers.

From a more general point of view, concerning inherited predisposition of tumors, we hypothesize that, concerning genetic predisposition, in the vast majority of "common cancers" (such as lung, breast, cancer, pancreas, and liver, also including thyroid cancer), there is an individual way to cancer occurrence; that is, there is a single gene or an oligogenic alteration, that is, one or more germline mutations occurring in some cancer facilitating or controlling genes, but also in genes controlling immune response or other functions, which predisposes to cancer. This cancer predisposition that is not due to a single germline mutation in a tumor suppressor gene (such as in the rare inherited multitumoral syndromes), but due to a combination of genes, could segregate more frequently in siblings, facilitating the familial occurrence of some cancers [36].

In particular, our recent studies on oligogenic germline mutations in nonsmoker-discordant siblings with lung adenocarcinoma (1) confirmed, as a "proof of concept," the hypothesis of an oligogenic combination for cancer susceptibility, (2) further support a model of "private genetic epidemiology" for a better understanding of the genetic effects in families with common cancers, and (3) suggest the possibility that each individual may have his/her personal way to cancer. These findings could have important implications for personalized medicine [36]. It is noteworthy that, for thyroid cancer, the common exposure to radiation [31] or other environmental factors to which siblings living in the same site could be exposed, in association with inherited predisposition from a wide range of susceptibility genes, should also be taken into account [26].

8. Conclusion and Lesson from FAP Associated PTC to Familial and Sporadic Carcinogenesis

(1) Concerning FNMTC, the preliminary knowledge of the familial aggregation of a given cancer could be a useful tool for early tumor detection. But this should not be used to conclude that FNMTC should be considered as a single entity, a unique disease, with a common pathogenic mechanism.

(2) We must recognize that, on the basis of present data, we are unable to answer uniformly to the question as to whether FNMTC is more or less aggressive than its sporadic counterpart. The correct answer could be "in some cases yes, in others no." It depends on inherited genetic alterations facilitating cancer susceptibility, but also on the individual tumor of a given subject.

(3) We suggest that time has come that, on the basis of current clinical evidence, we must challenge and also try to confute the "old scientific paradigm" and to provide a "new paradigm" that is more in accordance with actual genetic, pathologic, and clinical evidence. After the "genetic revolution" following DNA discovery and human genome sequencing, together with the observation that a single base change in a single gene (as a germline mutation) could be responsible for the occurrence of a given cancer in 100% of affected subjects (such as in FAP), the utopian dream has been cultivated that "targeted genetic engineering" could cure clinically evident cancer. Unfortunately, this is not the case. Analogously, clinical evidence and long-term follow-up (as in FAP associated FNMTC or in MEN 2A associated endocrine tumors) have shown that it is not true that a tumor belonging to an inherited multitumoral syndrome (even if frequently multifocal) has a more aggressive behavior and a worse prognosis than its sporadic counterpart.

(4) Not only many multitumoral syndromes (such as FAP), but also nontumoral diseases (Alport syndrome, etc.), instead of being determined by a single germline mutation in a single gene, may be determined not only by mutually exclusive mutations in different genes (APC and MYH) [37], but also by concomitant mutations in multiple genes, so determining digenic diseases (with at least 2 pathogenic germline mutations in at least 2 of the 3 genes COL4A3, COL4A4, and COL4A5, responsible for Alport syndrome) [38] or even by somatic mosaicism [39]. In summary, things and tumors have a greater complexity than what was initially hypothesized. Better classification and grouping of similar diseases can be useful, but incorrect grouping (mixing apples and oranges) can be misleading [36].

(5) The new paradigm can be the following. A single genetic mutation, but also, and perhaps more frequently, an oligogenic group of germline mutations (in some cancer related genes, but also in other genes) sometimes overlapping among individuals, but often differing from one individual to another, can be responsible for cancer (or common diseases) predisposition, together with a wide range of epigenetic or environmental factors (the "weight" of which can also be greater than that of congenital predisposition), or necessary for its full phenotypic manifestation. In addition, biological behavior, aggressiveness of the tumor, and also susceptibility to tumor occurrence, do not depend only on the quantity or the "potential danger" of the "offending agent," but also on the resistance of the subject, not only at the level of the targeted cell or tissue, but also as "host resistance" as an entire "indivisible" organism [36].

(6) The true challenge of the near future is that available data from the literature can be used and interpreted according to the "old paradigm," considering FNMTC as a single entity, with a common biological

behavior, or according to the "new paradigm" as "a galaxy of different diseases," each one with its peculiar combination between congenital predisposing factors, also facilitating familial aggregation, and environmental factors, determining in every patient a "unique type of cancer." This new paradigm fits more and is more in accordance with the so-called "personalized medicine" [36].

Conflict of Interests

The author declares that there is no conflict of interests regarding the publication of this paper.

References

[1] D. Navas-Carrillo, A. Ríos, J. M. Rodríguez, P. Parrilla, and E. Orenes-Piñero, "Familial nonmedullary thyroid cancer: screening, clinical, molecular and genetic findings," *Biochimica et Biophysica Acta—Reviews on Cancer*, vol. 1846, no. 2, pp. 468–476, 2014.

[2] F. Cetta, "Familial nonmedullary thyroid carcinomas: a heterogeneous syndrome with different natural history and variable long-term prognosis," *Journal of Clinical Endocrinology and Metabolism*, vol. 82, no. 12, pp. 4274–4275, 1997.

[3] F. Cetta, P. Toti, M. Petracci et al., "Thyroid carcinoma associated with familial adenomatous polyposis," *Histopathology*, vol. 31, no. 3, pp. 231–236, 1997.

[4] F. Cetta, S. Olschwang, M. Petracci et al., "Genetic alterations in thyroid carcinoma associated with familial adenomatous polyposis: clinical implications and suggestions for early detection," *World Journal of Surgery*, vol. 22, no. 12, pp. 1231–1236, 1998.

[5] F. Cetta, G. Montalto, M. Gori, M. C. Curia, A. Cama, and S. Olschwang, "Germline mutations of the APC gene in patients with familial adenomatous polyposis—associated thyroid carcinoma: results from a European cooperative study," *Journal of Clinical Endocrinology and Metabolism*, vol. 85, no. 1, pp. 286–292, 2000.

[6] F. Cetta, M. C. Curia, G. Montalto et al., "Thyroid carcinoma usually occurs in patients with familial adenomatous polyposis in the absence of biallelic inactivation of the adenomatous polyposis coli gene," *Journal of Clinical Endocrinology and Metabolism*, vol. 86, no. 1, pp. 427–432, 2001.

[7] F. Cetta, G. Chiappetta, R. M. Melillo et al., "The ret/ptcl oncogene is activated in familial adenomatous polyposis-associated thyroid papillary carcinomas," *The Journal of Clinical Endocrinology & Metabolism*, vol. 83, no. 3, pp. 1003–1006, 1998.

[8] G. Chiappetta, P. Toti, F. Cetta et al., "The RET/PTC oncogene is frequently activated in oncocytic thyroid tumors (Hurthle cell adenomas and carcinomas), but not in oncocytic hyperplastic lesions," *Journal of Clinical Endocrinology and Metabolism*, vol. 87, no. 1, pp. 364–369, 2002.

[9] F. Cetta, M. Gori, C. Baldi, N. Raffaelli, M. Zuckermann, and G. Montalto, "The relationships between phenotipic expression in patients with familial adenomatous polyposis (FAP) and the site of mutations in the adenomatous polyposic coli (APC) gene," *Annals of Surgery*, vol. 229, pp. 445–446, 1999.

[10] F. Cetta, M. R. Pelizzo, M. C. Curia, and A. Barbarisi, "Genetics and clinicopathological findings in thyroid carcinomas associated with familial adenomatous polyposis," *American Journal of Pathology*, vol. 155, no. 1, pp. 7–9, 1999.

[11] C. Francesco, M. L. Brandi, F. Tonelli, M. Zuckermann, and A. Cariati, "Papillary thyroid carcinoma," *The American Journal of Surgical Pathology*, vol. 27, no. 8, pp. 1176–1177, 2003.

[12] F. Cetta, A. Dhamo, G. Malagnino, and L. Barellini, "Germ-line and somatic mutations of the APC gene and/or β catenin gene in the occurrence of FAP associated thyroid carcinoma," *World Journal of Surgery*, vol. 31, no. 6, pp. 1366–1367, 2007.

[13] F. Cetta and A. Dhamo, "Inherited multitumoral syndromes including colorectal carcinoma," *Surgical Oncology*, vol. 16, pp. S17–S23, 2007.

[14] F. Cetta, A. Dhamo, A. Azzarà, and L. Moltoni, "The role of inherited predisposition and environmental factors in the occurrence of multiple different solid tumors in the same individual. The experience of the University Hospital of Siena," in *Multiple Primary Malignancies*, A. Renda, Ed., pp. 157–178, Springer, Milan, Italy, 2009.

[15] F. Cetta, A. Dhamo, S. Civitelli, and R. Zangari, "Comment on 'extra-intestinal manifestations of familial adenomatous polyposis'," *Annals of Surgical Oncology*, vol. 15, pp. 1446–1448, 2008.

[16] F. Cetta, G. Ugolini, L. Barellini, S. Civitelli, and M. Carmellini, "FAP associated cribriform morular variant of PTC: striking female prevalence and indolent course," *Endocrine Journal*, vol. 58, no. 9, pp. 817–818, 2011.

[17] F. Cetta, L. Moltoni, L. Barellini, M. Monti, and G. Gotti, "Familial adenomatous polyposis-associated papillary thyroid carcinoma shows an indolent course and usually, but not always, belongs to the cribriform-morular variant of papillary thyroid carcinoma," *Acta Cytologica*, vol. 56, no. 1, pp. 107–108, 2012.

[18] R. O. Plail, H. J. R. Bussey, G. Glazer, and J. P. S. Thomson, "Adenomatous polyposis: an association with carcinoma of the thyroid," *British Journal of Surgery*, vol. 74, no. 5, pp. 377–380, 1987.

[19] H. R. Harach, G. T. Williams, and E. D. Williams, "Familial adenomatous polyposis associated thyroid carcinoma: a distinct type of follicular cell neoplasm," *Histopathology*, vol. 25, no. 6, pp. 549–561, 1994.

[20] J. Cameselle-Teijeiro and J. K. C. Chan, "Cribriform-morular variant of papillary carcinoma: a distinctive variant representing the sporadic counterpart of familial adenomatous polyposis-associated thyroid carcinoma?" *Modern Pathology*, vol. 12, no. 4, pp. 400–411, 1999.

[21] S. B. Ng, K. Sittampalam, Y. H. Goh, and K. W. Eu, "Cribriform-morular variant of papillary carcinoma: the sporadic counterpart of familial adenomatous polyposis-associated thyroid carcinoma. A case report with clinical and molecular genetic correlation," *Pathology*, vol. 35, no. 1, pp. 42–46, 2003.

[22] B. Xu, K. Yoshimoto, A. Miyauchi et al., "Cribriform-morular variant of papillary thyroid carcinoma: a pathological and molecular genetic study with evidence of frequent somatic mutations in exon 3 of the β-catenin gene," *Journal of Pathology*, vol. 199, no. 1, pp. 58–67, 2003.

[23] C. Tomoda, A. Miyauchi, T. Uruno et al., "Cribriform-morular variant of papillary thyroid carcinoma: clue to early detection of familial adenomatous polyposis-associated colon cancer," *World Journal of Surgery*, vol. 28, no. 9, pp. 886–889, 2004.

[24] N. D. Perrier, J. A. Van Heerden, J. R. Goellner et al., "Thyroid cancer in patients with familial adenomatous polyposis," *World Journal of Surgery*, vol. 22, no. 7, pp. 738–743, 1998.

[25] C. Soravia, S. L. Sugg, T. Berk et al., "Familial adenomatous polyposis-associated thyroid cancer. A clinical, pathological,

and molecular genetics study," *The American Journal of Pathology*, vol. 154, no. 1, pp. 127–135, 1999.

[26] F. Cetta, G. Ugolini, J. Martellucci, and G. Gotti, "Screening for thyroid cancer in patients with familial adenomatous polyposis," *Annals of Surgery*, vol. 261, pp. e13–e14, 2015.

[27] A. M. Jarrar, M. Milas, J. Mitchell et al., "Screening for thyroid cancer in patients with familial adenomatous polyposis," *Annals of Surgery*, vol. 253, no. 3, pp. 515–521, 2011.

[28] M. Herraiz, G. Barbesino, W. Faquin et al., "Prevalence of thyroid cancer in familial adenomatous polyposis syndrome and the role of screening ultrasound examinations," *Clinical Gastroenterology and Hepatology*, vol. 5, no. 3, pp. 367–373, 2007.

[29] E. Steinhagen, J. G. Guillem, G. Chang et al., "The prevalence of thyroid cancer and benign thyroid disease in patients with familial adenomatous polyposis may be higher than previously recognized," *Clinical Colorectal Cancer*, vol. 11, no. 4, pp. 304–308, 2012.

[30] E. Steinhagen, V. W. Hui, R. A. Levy et al., "Results of a prospective thyroid ultrasound screening program in adenomatous polyposis patients," *The American Journal of Surgery*, vol. 208, no. 5, pp. 764–769, 2014.

[31] F. Cetta, G. Montalto, M. Petracci, and A. Fusco, "Thyroid cancer and the Chernobyl accident. Are long-term and long distance side effects of fall-out radiation greater than estimated?" *The Journal of Clinical Endocrinology and Metabolism*, vol. 82, no. 6, pp. 2015–2017, 1997.

[32] J. R. Burgess, A. Duffield, S. J. Wilkinson et al., "Two families with an autosomal dominant inheritance pattern for papillary carcinoma of the thyroid," *Journal of Clinical Endocrinology and Metabolism*, vol. 82, no. 2, pp. 345–348, 1997.

[33] J. D. McKay, D. Thompson, F. Lesueur et al., "Evidence for interaction between the TCO and NMTC1 loci in familial nonmedullary thyroid cancer," *Journal of Medical Genetics*, vol. 41, no. 6, pp. 407–412, 2004.

[34] B. M. Cavaco, P. F. Batista, L. G. Sobrinho, and V. Leite, "Mapping a new familial thyroid epithelial neoplasia susceptibility locus to chromosome 8p23.1-p22 by high-density single-nucleotide polymorphism genome-wide linkage analysis," *Journal of Clinical Endocrinology and Metabolism*, vol. 93, no. 11, pp. 4426–4430, 2008.

[35] M. Capezzone, S. Marchisotta, S. Cantara et al., "Familial non-medullary thyroid carcinoma displays the features of clinical anticipation suggestive of a distinct biological entity," *Endocrine-Related Cancer*, vol. 15, no. 4, pp. 1075–1081, 2008.

[36] A. Renieri, M. A. Mencarelli, F. Cetta et al., "Oligogenic germline mutations identified in early non-smokers lung adenocarcinoma patients," *Lung Cancer*, vol. 85, no. 2, pp. 168–174, 2014.

[37] G. Aceto, M. C. Curia, S. Veschi et al., "Mutations of APC and MYH in unrelated Italian patients with adenomatous polyposis coli," *Human Mutation*, vol. 26, no. 4, article 394, 2005.

[38] M. A. Mencarelli, L. Heidet, H. Storey et al., "Evidence of digenic inheritance in Alport syndrome," *Journal of Medical Genetics*, vol. 52, no. 3, pp. 163–174, 2015.

[39] S. Amitrano, A. Marozza, S. Somma et al., "Next generation sequencing in sporadic retinoblastoma patients reveals somatic mosaicism," *European Journal of Human Genetics*, vol. 23, no. 11, pp. 1523–1530, 2015.

18

Trypanosoma vivax Adhesion to Red Blood Cells in Experimentally Infected Sheep

Alpidio A. Boada-Sucre,[1] Marcello Salvatore Rossi Spadafora,[2,3] Lucinda M. Tavares-Marques,[4] Héctor J. Finol,[5] and Armando Reyna-Bello[4,6]

[1]*Laboratorio de Microscopía Electrónica, Centro de Estudios Biomédicos y Veterinarios, Instituto de Estudios Científicos y Tecnológicos, Universidad Nacional Experimental Simón Rodríguez, Caracas, Venezuela*
[2]*Unidad de Toxoplasmosis y Protozoosis, Departamento de Parasitología, Centro Nacional de Microbiología, Instituto de Salud Carlos III, Calle Alejandro Casona 7, Piso 6D, 28035 Madrid, Spain*
[3]*Sección de Inmunohistoquímica y Microscopía Electrónica, Instituto Anatomopatológico "José A. O'Daly", Facultad de Medicina, Universidad Central de Venezuela, Caracas, Venezuela*
[4]*Grupo de Inmunobiología, Centro de Estudios Biomédicos y Veterinarios, Instituto de Estudios Científicos y Tecnológicos, Universidad Nacional Experimental Simón Rodríguez, Caracas, Venezuela*
[5]*Centro de Microscopía Electrónica "Mitsuo Ogura", Facultad de Ciencias, Universidad Central de Venezuela, Caracas, Venezuela*
[6]*Investigador Prometeo, Universidad de Las Fuerzas Armadas ESPE, Departamento de Ciencias de la Vida, Grupo de Investigación de Sanidad Animal y Humana (GISAH), Sangolquí, Ecuador*

Correspondence should be addressed to Marcello Salvatore Rossi Spadafora; rossimarcell@gmail.com

Academic Editor: Piero Tosi

Trypanosomosis, a globally occurring parasitic disease, poses as a major obstacle to livestock production in tropical and subtropical regions resulting in tangible economic losses. In Latin America including Venezuela, trypanosomosis of ruminants is mainly caused by *Trypanosoma vivax*. Biologically active substances produced from trypanosomes, as well as host-trypanosome cellular interactions, contribute to the pathogenesis of anemia in an infection. The aim of this study was to examine with a scanning electron microscope the cellular interactions and alterations in ovine red blood cells (RBC) experimentally infected with *T. vivax*. Ovine infection resulted in changes of RBC shape as well as the formation of surface holes or vesicles. A frequent observation was the adhesion to the ovine RBC by the trypanosome's free flagellum, cell body, or attached flagellum in a process mediated by the filopodia emission from the trypanosome surface. The observed RBC alterations are caused by mechanical and biochemical damage from host-parasite interactions occurring in the bloodstream. The altered erythrocytes are prone to mononuclear phagocytic removal contributing to the hematocrit decrease during infection.

1. Introduction

In Venezuela, trypanosomosis, a globally occurring parasitic disease, in animals is mainly caused by *Trypanosoma vivax*. Trypanosomosis is responsible for tangible economic losses due to impaired livestock production. The detrimental effects produced by *T. vivax* in livestock include growth retardation, loss of body weight, low production of animal proteins (meat and milk) [1, 2], and diminished fertility [3]. These effects are responsible for increasing production costs through an increased need for treatment and veterinary care [4–6]. The economic implications of trypanosomosis in developing subtropical regions underscore the value in research covering the pathogenesis of *T. vivax*.

Animal trypanosomosis is characterized by periodic fevers, parasitemia, and anemia, changes in blood chemistry, body mass loss, and often death. The anemia developed by animals is considered the most characteristic symptom [7]. It seems that the anemia is hemolytic in nature, intravascular in the early stages of the disease, and extravascular in the chronic phase [6, 8].

Current experimental and clinical evidence on animal trypanosomosis suggests that the main pathogenetic mechanisms of anemia include hemolysis, red blood cells (RBC) sequestration, hemodilution, platelet aggregation, lipid peroxidation, bleeding, and bone marrow dysfunction [9, 10]. However, insufficient research has been done to associate the structural and biochemical changes in RBCs as consequences of the interaction between RBC and trypanosomes. For example, existing reports list the following as possible mechanisms responsible for RBC injury: mechanical damage produced by the interaction of trypanosomes with RBC [11], adhesion and membrane fusion mediated filopodia [12], immune complexes adsorbed to erythrocytes [13], and biologically active substances released by live or dead trypanosomes which produce erythrocyte injury [14–17].

In Venezuela, *T. vivax* is the causative agent of trypanosomosis in ruminants. The pathogenesis, characterized by anemia and fever, seriously compromises the animal's health [1, 6, 18]. The aim of this study was to examine, with a scanning electron microscope (SEM), the cellular interactions and alterations in ovine RBCs experimentally infected with a Venezuelan *T. vivax* isolate.

2. Material and Methods

2.1. Experimental Animals. A total of nine (9) crossbreed male sheep in reproductive age (30–35 kg body weight) were used in the study. Two of them were used as control and seven as the experimental group. Sheep in the experimental group were randomly selected and inoculated simultaneously with strain LIEM-176 of *T. vivax*. Both groups were housed in separate corrals covered with antimosquito nets to prevent contact with blood sucking flies and disease vectors. All the animals were fed concentrated food (Purina®, 500 g/animal/day), hay, and water *ad libitum*.

Both groups were clinically, parasitologically, and PCR examined one week before starting the study (preinfection period) in order to confirm the negativity to *T. vivax* and other hemoparasites. All tests were conducted at the Instituto de Estudios Científicos y Tecnológicos under veterinary supervision.

2.2. Trypanosomes. The strain LIEM-176 of *T. vivax* used in this work was previously morphometric and molecularly characterized [19–21], isolated from naturally infected cattle in the Trujillo State (Venezuela), and kindly provided by Drs. Glenda Moreno and Laura Moron of Universidad de Los Andes and expanded by inoculation into sheep.

2.3. Experimental Infection of Sheep. One mL of blood containing approximately 1×10^6 blood trypomastigotes of *T. vivax* was inoculated intravenously in the jugular vein of each sheep of the experimental group. Control animals were inoculated with 1 mL of isotonic saline solution. Once inoculated, experimental and control groups were clinically and parasitologically examined every 4 days for 45 days. Values collected as indicators of *T. vivax* infection included the temperature, hematocrit, total plasma proteins, hemoglobin, and parasitemia by the Brener method [22].

During experimental infection, all animals were maintained under veterinary supervision to safeguard health and minimize animal suffering. Protocols used were approved by the Ethical Committee for Laboratory Animal Use under number 013-11 according to the Ethics Chart of animal experimentation.

2.4. Scanning Electron Microscopy (SEM). Aliquots of blood from sheep experimentally infected with *T. vivax* taken every 4 days from the jugular vein (Vacutainer System®) and prefixed with Karnovsky fixative solution (2.5% glutaraldehyde and 4% *p*-formaldehyde in Millonig's phosphate buffer 0.10 M, pH 7.4) were contained in vacuum-glass tubes of 5 mL. The blood fixation process was done following the technique described by Boada-Sucre et al. [23]. Briefly, fixation began at the time of blood sampling for 1 hour at 4°C. Finally, 100 μL of prefixed blood was spotted on to coverslips pretreated with poly-L-lysine 0.1% v/v in order to promote the adhesion of blood cells. The excess of glutaraldehyde was removed by washing with Millonig's phosphate buffer and the postfixation was performed with 1% m/v osmium tetroxide (OsO_4) for 1 hour at 4°C. Osmium excess was removed by washing with deionized water and samples were dehydrated in increasing concentrations of ethanol at 4°C. The biological material adsorbed to the coverslips was dried by evaporation on a critical point dryer (Hitachi HCP-2) using carbon dioxide (CO_2) as liquid transition fluid. Then, samples were mounted on the sample holder and covered with platinum ion (Electron Microscopy Science EMS-350). Observations and micrographic records were performed on a field emission scanning electron microscope (FE Hitachi S-4500) with an accelerating voltage of 5 keV.

2.5. Transmission Electron Microscopy (TEM). The liver samples were processed for TEM using the standard methods described by Boada-Sucre et al., 1999 [23]. Pieces of liver were fixed at 2 mm in diameter with glutaraldehyde 2.5% and OsO_4 1% (Millonig-buffered solutions pH 7.4; 300 mOsm), dehydrated in increasing ethanol concentrations, and embedded in Epon 812. Sections were cut with a diamond knife in a RMC Ultramicrotome MT 7.000, and stained with uranyl acetate and lead citrate. Sections were observed with a Hitachi H-7100 transmission electron microscope (75 kV accelerating voltage).

2.6. Statistical Analysis. Each SEM preparation was examined 15, 30, or 45 days after infection. For each SEM preparation, one hundred trypomastigotes were counted and the proportion of observed parasite-RBC adhesion was quantified. For the adhered trypomastigotes, the method of adhesion was counted; the proportion of cell body adhesion, free flagellum adhesion, and attached flagellum adhesion was calculated. The proportions of *T. vivax* adhesion and the cell body structures involved in the attachment were compared using a two-tailed Fisher's Exact Test at a 95% confidence level. Differences between observations were considered statistically significant when $p < 0.05$.

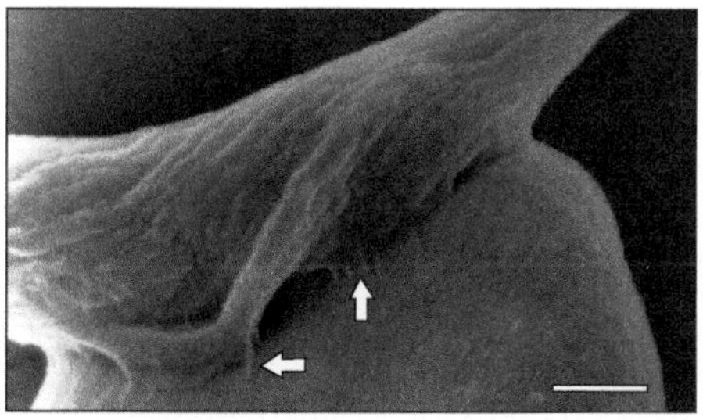

FIGURE 1: Scanning electron micrograph showing a large area (⇒) of *T. vivax* in close contact to sheep erythrocytes at 30 days after infection. Bar = 1.2 μm.

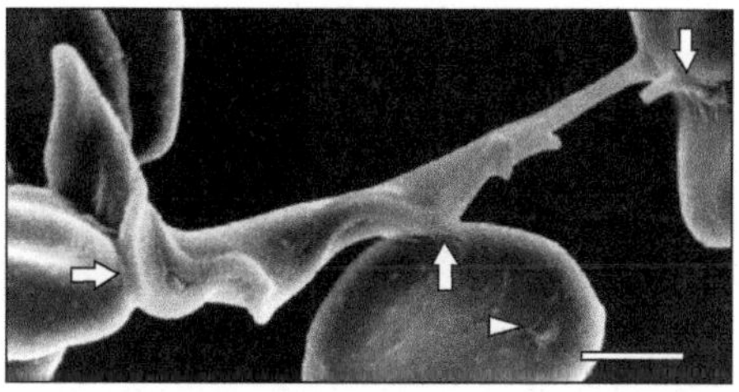

FIGURE 2: Adhesion of *T. vivax* to three RBCs through its body and flagellum (⇒). Note the presence of a vesicle (△) in one RBC at 15 days after infection. Bar = 1.4 μm.

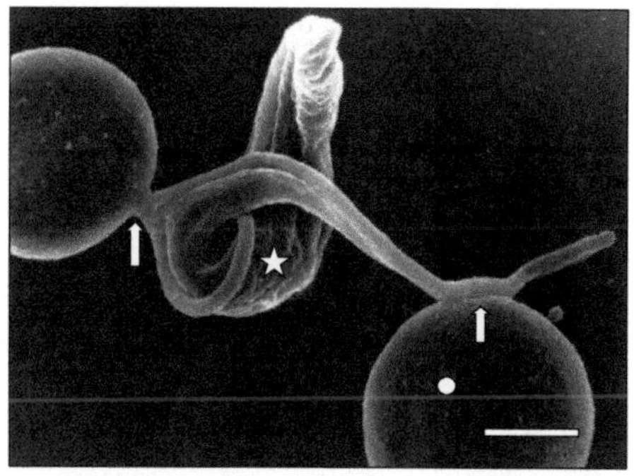

FIGURE 3: Attached (⇒) trypanosome (☆) to two sheep RBCs (○) at 30 days of infection. Bar = 1.4 μm.

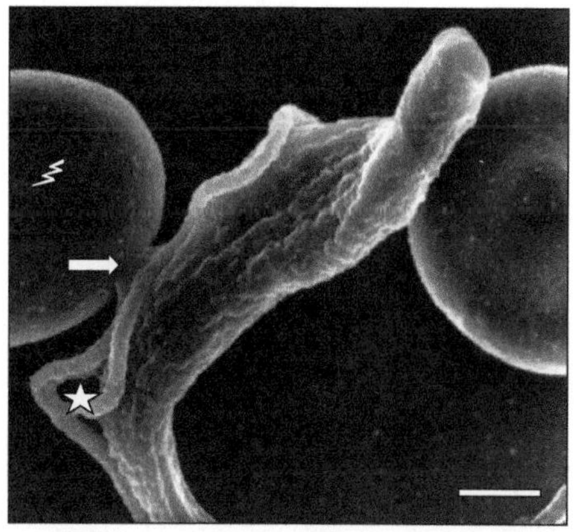

FIGURE 4: High resolution of a parasite in division process (☆) and contact (⇒) with an erythrocyte sheep at 45 days of infection. Note the holes in RBC (↯). Bar = 2.0 μm.

3. Results

Scanning electron microscopy showed the interaction of *T. vivax* with sheep RBCs. The interactions of *T. vivax* trypomastigotes with RBCs from experimentally infected sheep can be observed in the scanning electron micrographs of Figures 1–11. As it can be observed, the interaction was achieved through the establishment of a very narrow cell contact and the subsequent development of RBC clusters. This adhesion was favored by the emission of filamentous and membranous projections through the trypanosome cell body (Figure 1). Figures 2–6 show RBC adhesion mediated by the attached *T. vivax* flagellum. Free flagellum participation is observed in Figures 3 and 7–9, while the direct involvement of *T. vivax* cell body is shown in Figures 1, 2, and 9–11. This interaction between *T. vivax* and RBCs was measured as the proportion of *T. vivax* adhered at 15, 30, or 45 days after infection and is summarized in Table 1.

The proportion of adhered trypomastigotes at 15 days after infection is significantly higher than the proportion at 30 and 45 days after infection according to Fisher's Exact Test ($p < 0.001$). There was no significant difference between 30 and 45 days after infection (Table 1). Moreover, the parasite segments (cell body, free flagellum, and attached flagellum) adhered to the RBCs were quantified and the proportions were examined 15, 30, and 45 days after infection (Table 2).

Trypomastigotes adhered to sheep RBCs through the free flagellum at any time after infection are significantly higher ($p < 0.0001$) than the cell body and attached flagellum. Furthermore, the proportion of trypanosomes adhered to RBC through the attached flagellum is significantly lower ($p < 0.0001$) than the proportion of parasites adhered through the cell body.

The proportion of trypanosomes adhered to sheep RBC through the flagellum was very significant at day 15 when it was compared with the adhesion observed at days 30 and 45 ($p < 0.0001$). In addition, trypanosomes adhered through the cell body was significantly higher ($p < 0.0001$) at 15 and 45 days after infection, while the proportion of parasites adhered through the attached flagellum was significantly lower ($p < 0.0001$) at days 15 and 45 after infection.

Additionally, SEM images depict the emission of filopodia by *T. vivax* during the experimental infection process (Figure 10). The interaction of bloodstream trypanosomes with RBCs induces vesicle formation (Figure 2). Moreover, SEM images show pore formation on the erythrocyte surface during experimental infection (Figures 4, 9, and 12). Other common findings were morphological alterations in RBC (Figures 13 and 14), activated white blood cells (WBC) (Figure 15), WBC in contact with RBC (Figures 14 and 16), microspherocytosis (results not showed), and erythrophagocytosis process extravascularly (Figure 17) and intravascularly in liver sinusoid (Figure 18).

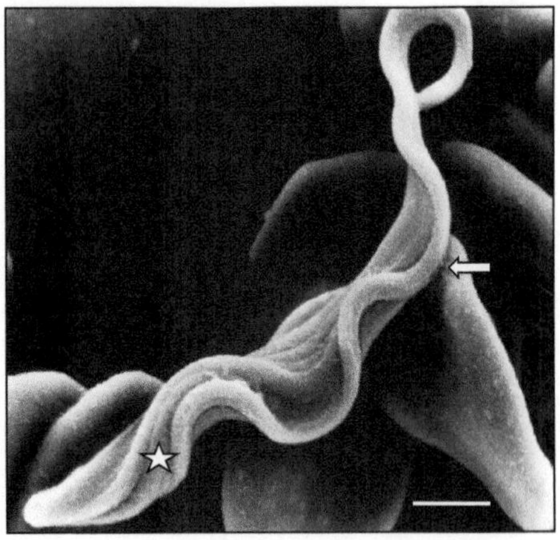

Figure 5: Scanning electron microscopy of adhesion (⇒) from one parasite in division (☆) to sheep erythrocyte at 45 days of infection. Bar = 2.0 μm.

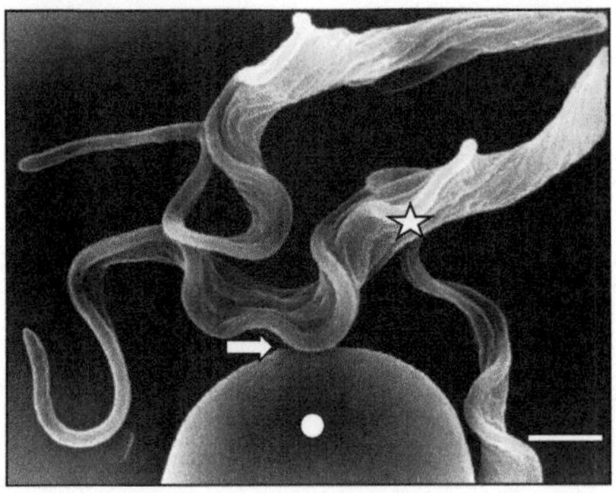

Figure 6: Electron microscopy of adhesion (⇒) of *T. vivax in division* (☆) to a sheep RBC (◯) through the attached flagellum at 30 days of infection. Bar = 2.0 μm.

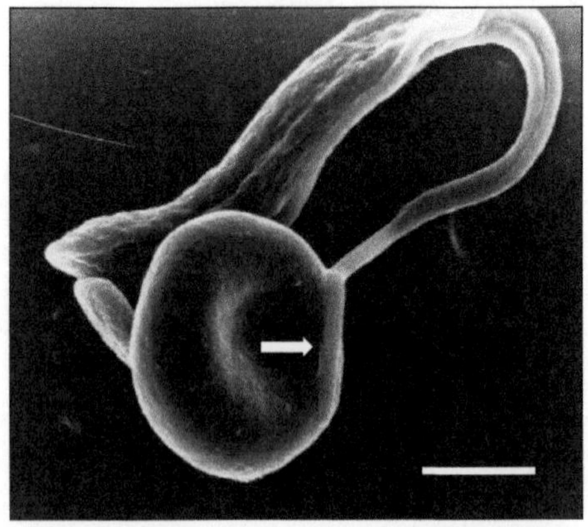

Figure 7: *T. vivax* flagellum contact (⇒) with a RBC at 15 days of inoculation. Bar = 1.7 μm.

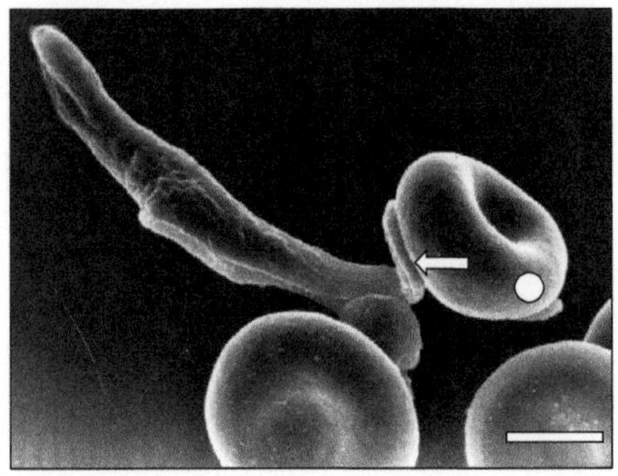

Figure 8: Scanning electron micrographs showing a large area of *T. vivax* flagellum in close adhesion (⇒) to a sheep erythrocyte (◯) at 30 days after infection. Bar = 1.6 μm.

Table 1: Percentage (%) of trypanosomes adhered to RBC or free, during infection process.

Days after infection	% of *T. vivax* adhered to RBC	% of *T. vivax* nonadhered to RBC
15	40	60
30	38	62
45	38	62

Table 2: Percentage (%) of trypanosomes adhered to RBC through cell body, flagellum, and attached flagellum during infection process.

Days after infection	Cell body	Free flagellum	Attached flagellum
15	12	20	8
30	11	18	9
45	12	18	8

4. Discussion

In the RBC-*Trypanosoma* adhesion observed by SEM, morphological changes in the RBCs are found to be a contributing factor in the pathophysiology of anemia in sheep trypanosomosis by *T. vivax*.

In this paper, we have described the adhesion between *T. vivax* and sheep RBC mediated by the parasite's cell body, attached flagellum, and free flagellum. Free flagellum adhesion appears to be favored by the emission of filopodia and filamentous material of parasitic origin. Similar observations were reported between *T. brucei* and *T. evansi* to murine RBC [12, 13].

This adhesion of *T. vivax* to sheep RBC led to notable observations. First, Table 1 shows higher adhesion during the early stage of the disease compared to the latest stage, suggesting that the adhesion of *T. vivax* to RBC is inhibited by the sheep's antibodies against the parasite membrane. As it was described as a capping effect in *T. evansi*, mediated by antibodies [24].

Next, Table 2 shows higher adhesion of *T. vivax* to RBC through free flagellum than cell bodies or attached flagellum. This difference is remarkable since it may be due to the free flagellum's continuous whiplash movement.

The emission of filopodia by the African trypanosomes has been described by several researchers since the 1970s in infections caused by *T. b. brucei* and *T. b. rhodesiense* [25] and African isolates of *T. vivax* [26] and *T. venezuelense* (*T. evansi*)

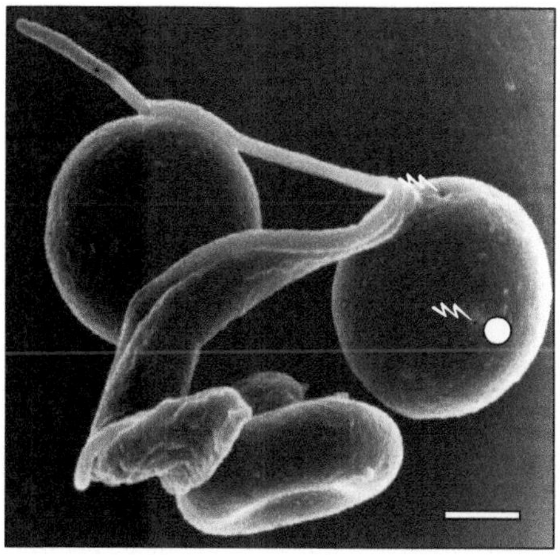

FIGURE 9: Scanning electron micrograph showing the adhesion of a *T. vivax* bloodstream trypomastigote to two sheep RBCs (○) with holes (⚡) at 45 days of infection. The adhesion was through free flagellum and cell body. Bar = 2.0 μm.

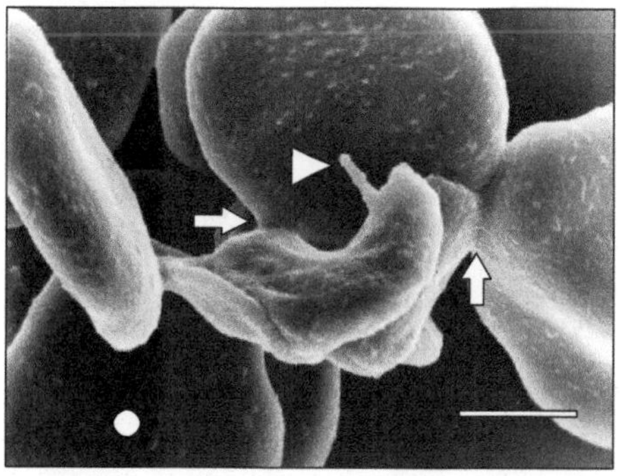

FIGURE 10: Trypomastigote in a close contact to a RBC cluster (○) at 15 days after infection. Notice the emission of a pseudopod prolongation from *T. vivax* (△) and the adhesion of *T. vivax* trypomastigote to RBCs (⇒). Bar = 1.4 μm.

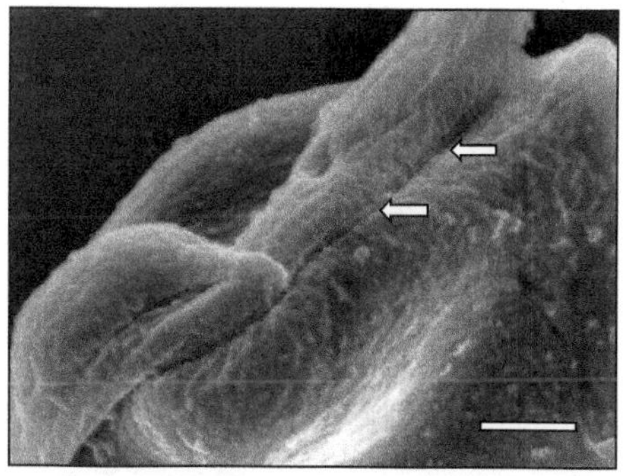

FIGURE 11: Scanning electron micrograph showing a large area (⇒) of *T. vivax* in close contact to an erythrocyte at 30 days after infection. Bar = 0.8 μm.

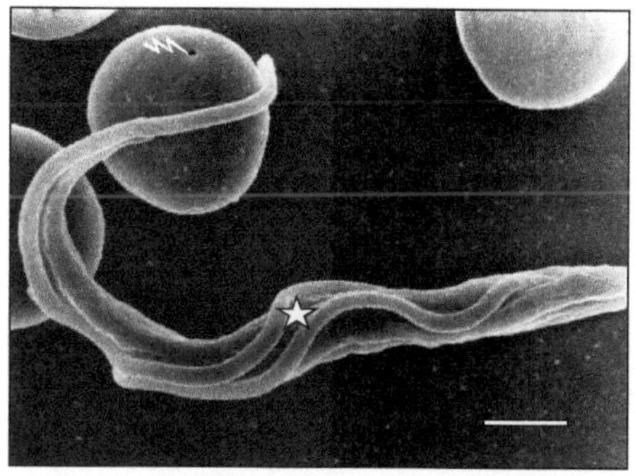

FIGURE 12: Scanning electron micrograph of a *T. vivax* trypomastigote in division process (☆) at 45 days of infection. Note the presence of holes on the RBC surface (⚡) and its round-morphology. Bar = 2.0 μm.

[27]. Furthermore, their involvement in the adhesion of *T. vivax* to the proboscide of Tsetse fly (*Glossina fuscipes*) has been documented [28]. The emission of these filamentous material and filopodia of parasitic origin has been described in phagocytes of cattle infected with *T. vivax* [29] and in the adhesion of *T. congolense* to endothelial cells from bovine aorta [30].

According to Rossi [13], filopodia and filamentous material help the trypanosome-RBC interaction in a process that is mediated by receptors on the erythrocyte surface. Additionally, the filamentous material could act by promoting the establishment of zip-type connections or hemidesmosome formations as it has been described in the adhesion of *T. congolense* to bovine endothelial cells [30]. Similarly, *T. vivax* is capable of developing this zip-type connection (Figure 12) and filopodia (Figure 3).

The close contact between trypanosomes and RBC via sialic acid receptors causes injuries to erythrocyte membranes at the point of contact [11]. In addition to the aforementioned RBC injuries, the apparent membrane fusion, changes in the oligosaccharide composition of the surface of RBC, and mechanical damage "pinching out" caused by the motility of the trypanosomes in the bloodstream [13, 17, 31] induce ultrastructural, biochemical, and antigenic alterations of the RBC, which increases erythrophagocytosis, as shown in Figure 16.

At the level of the RBC plasma membrane, the modification of its composition by trypanosomal antigens, such as neuraminidases [13], activates effector mechanisms of the immune system leading to the formation and adsorption of antigen-antibody complexes and complements on the surface [32]. This mechanism could explain the occurrence of holes in the RBC surface as is observed in Figures 15, 16, and 17. Those holes may facilitate erythrolysis and/or recognition and removal of RBC by mononuclear phagocytic system. A similar response to this erythrophagocytosis is the autoimmune mechanism observed in alterations of horse muscles naturally infected with *T. evansi* [33].

Furthermore, the action of biologically active substances secreted [34] or derived from live or dead trypanosomes [35–37], particularly sialidase secreted/excreted from *T. vivax*, in the bloodstream [18, 37, 38] contributes to the intravascular erythrophagocytosis [12, 38] described in this paper (Figures 17 and 18). In contrast, changes in the glycocalyx of RBCs

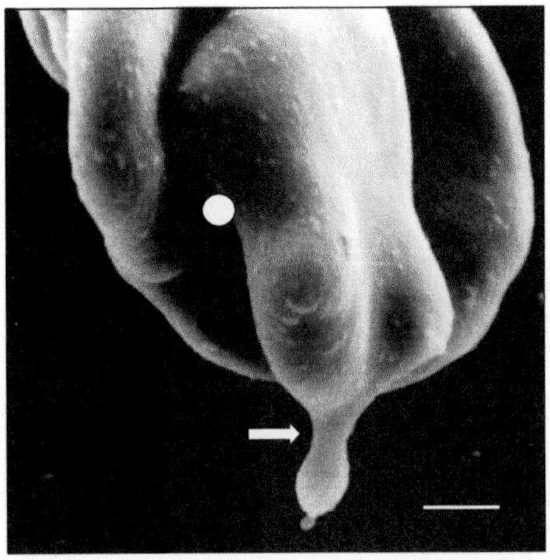

Figure 13: High resolution micrograph of a sheep RBC cluster showing a deformed RBC (○) with small vesicles and emission of a pseudopod (⇒) at 15 days of infection. Bar = 1.3 *μ*m.

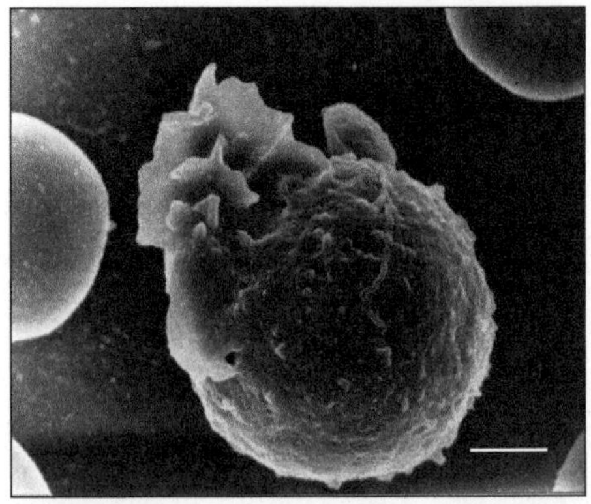

Figure 15: Electron micrograph showing an activated WBC in peripheral blood of a sheep at 15 days after infection with *T. vivax*. Bar = 2.5 *μ*m.

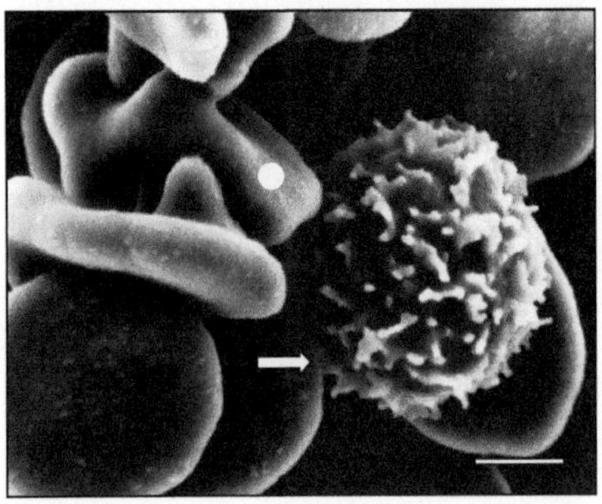

Figure 14: Adhesion (⇒) of one WBC to a deformed RBC (○) in the peripheral blood of sheep at 15 days of infection with *T. vivax*. Bar = 1.0 *μ*m.

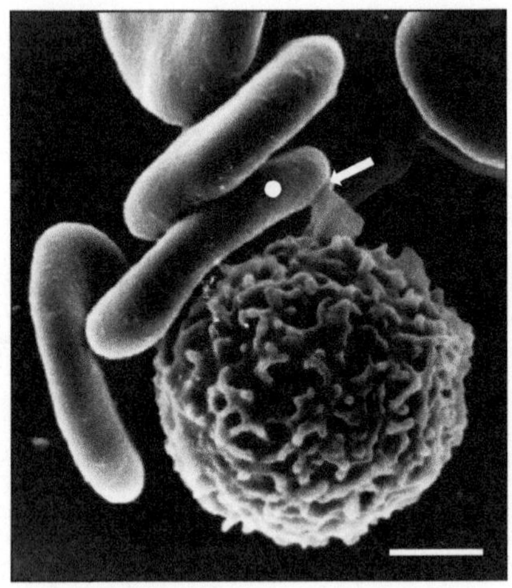

Figure 16: Adhesion (⇒) of WBC to RBC cluster (○) in sheep peripheral blood at 15 days of infection with *T. vivax*. Bar = 2.0 *μ*m.

induce extravascular erythrophagocytosis mediated by the mononuclear phagocyte system [10, 12, 39–41].

Sialidases secreted/excreted by trypanosomes have the ability to remove sialic acid residues from the RBC glycocalyx, enabling glycoconjugate degradation and elimination of fatty acids from cell membranes by other biologically active substances such as proteases, glycosidases, and phospholipases [15, 42, 43]. In this sense, Guegan et al. [18] characterized a multigenic family of transsialidases in *T. vivax* Y486, some of which are released and able to induce erythrophagocytosis by desialylating the glycophorins.

Cluster formations of thrombi composed of RBC and leukocytes (Figures 14 and 15) have also been described in infections caused by *T. brucei* and *T. evansi* and may complicate the pathophysiology of the ovine trypanosomosis caused by *T. vivax*. The systemic complications triggered by anemia together with microthrombi of parasitic origin not only compromise the normal gas and metabolites exchange between blood and host tissues by way of the occlusion of the vascular lumen of capillary, but also contribute to the cell

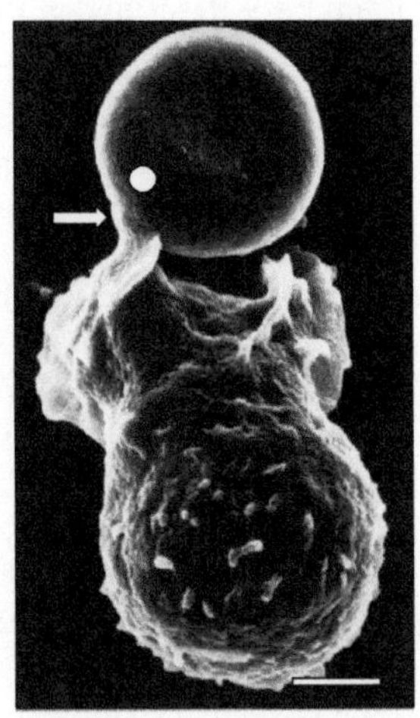

Figure 17: Phagocytosis (⇒) of a RBC (○) by an activated WBC in peripheral blood of a sheep at 15 days of infection with *T. vivax*. Bar = 3.0 *μ*m.

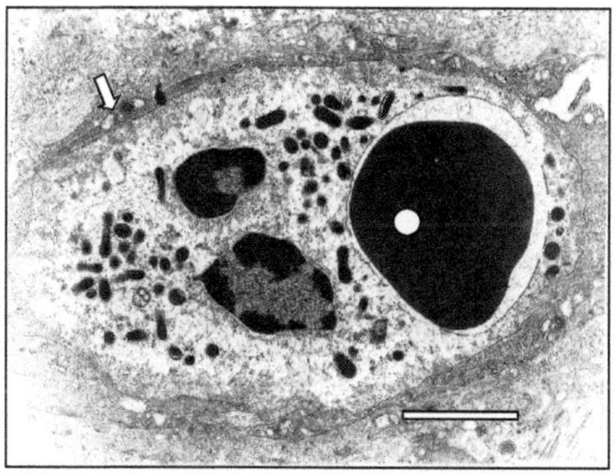

FIGURE 18: Transmission electron microscopy of a RBC phagocytosed (◯) by a polymorphonuclear cell-neutrophil (⇒) in the liver of a sheep infected with *T. vivax* at 15 days. Notice the RBC inside a phagocytic vacuole surrounded by lysosomes. Bar = 1.5 μm.

necrosis aggravated by endothelial alterations that occur in the disease [12, 13, 41, 44, 45].

Forty-five years ago, Goodwin [31] pointed out that abnormalities of the RBC in trypanosomosis are a consequence of changes that occur in the small blood vessels. With the Venezuelan strain of *T. evansi*, this alteration in vessels was observed by Finol et al. [45]. Moreover, these authors concluded that the observed alterations on vessels contribute to modifications of the RBC morphological and cytoskeletal structure. The proteolytic lysosomal enzymes released into the circulation system from trypanosomes cleave sialic acid fractions [46] resulting in the vascular endothelium adopting a tortuous shape [47]. While observing the SEM images of sheep tissue experimentally infected with *T. vivax*, we found occurrences of the aforementioned endothelium damage in small vessels.

In experimental infection of mice with *T. evansi*, changes such as thickening of the basement membrane, proliferation, and vacuolization of endothelial cells and mechanical damage for action of trypanosome flagella and bodies also contribute in the modification of the erythrocyte cytoskeleton structure and morphology [13, 44, 47].

Furthermore, as it has been described in the infections of *Camelus dromedarius* [48] and rats with *T. evansi* [49], the infection of sheep with *T. vivax* could generate an oxidative stress with the generation of free radicals and superoxide reactive species that attack the proteins and lipid membranes with osmotic fragility. The peroxidation of lipids determines the degradation of polyunsaturated fatty acids with the interruption of the plasma membrane and a concomitant loss of its basic functions and features, as was described by a different author [15, 50, 51].

The RBC alterations described in this study, like emission of filopodia, vesicles, roughness, and holes on the erythrocyte surface are similar compared to those reported in *T. brucei* [12] and *T. evansi* infections [13].

5. Conclusion

The adhesion of *Trypanosoma vivax* (LIEM-176) to sheep erythrocytes described in this study is the first evidence for *T. vivax* infection. Moreover, the presence of holes and vesicles caused by the adhesion to RBC is an important factor to be considered in parasite-host interactions and contributes to anemia during trypanosomosis.

Competing Interests

The authors (Alpidio A. Boada-Sucre, Marcello Salvatore Rossi Spadafora, Lucinda M. Tavares-Marques, Héctor J. Finol, and Armando Reyna-Bello) declare that there are no competing interests regarding the publication of this paper.

Acknowledgments

This research was supported by Project G-98003462-Fondo Nacional de Ciencia, Tecnología e Innovación (FONACIT), Caracas, Venezuela, and the Instituto de Estudios Científicos y Tecnológicos from Universidad Nacional Experimental Simón Rodríguez. The authors thank Beatriz Cajade for critical reading of this paper.

References

[1] M. I. Gonzatti, B. González-Baradat, P. M. Aso, and A. Reyna-Bello, "*Trypanosoma* (*Duttonella*) *vivax* and typanosomosis in Latin America: secadera/huequera/cacho hueco," in *Trypanosomes and Trypanosomiasis*, S. Magez and M. Radwanska, Eds., pp. 261–285, Springer, 2014.

[2] M. Desquesnes, *Livestock Trypanosomoses and Their Vectors in Latin America*, OIE, Paris, France, 4th edition, 2004.

[3] E. Elhassan, B. O. Ikede, and O. Adeyemo, "Trypanosomosis and reproduction: I. Effect of *Trypanosoma vivax* infection on the oestrous cycle and fertility in the ewe," *Tropical Animal Health and Production*, vol. 26, no. 4, pp. 213–218, 1994.

[4] B. J. S. Batista, C. M. F. Rodrigues, H. A. García et al., "Association of *Trypanosoma vivax* in intracellular sites with central nervous system lesions and changes in cerebrospinal fluid in experimentally infected goats," *Veterinary Research*, vol. 42, no. 63, pp. 1–7, 2011.

[5] J. S. Batista, F. Riet-Correa, M. M. G. Teixeira, C. R. Madruga, S. D. V. Simões, and T. F. Maia, "Trypanosomiasis by *Trypanosoma vivax* in cattle in the Brazilian semiarid: description of an outbreak and lesions in the nervous system," *Veterinary Parasitology*, vol. 143, no. 2, pp. 174–181, 2007.

[6] G. J. N. Galiza, H. A. García, A. C. O. Assis et al., "High mortality and lesions of the central nervous system in trypanosomosis by *Trypanosoma vivax* in Brazilian hair sheep," *Veterinary Parasitology*, vol. 182, no. 2–4, pp. 359–363, 2011.

[7] T. M. Silva, R. G. Olinda, C. M. Rodrigues et al., "Pathogenesis of reproductive failure induced by *Trypanosoma vivax* in experimentally infected pregnant ewes," *Veterinary Research*, vol. 44, article 1, 2013.

[8] T. S. G. A. M. Van den Ingh, D. Zwart, A. S. J. P. A. M. Van Miert, and A. J. H. Schotman, "Clinico-pathological and pathomorphological observations in *Trypanosoma vivax* infection cattle," *Veterinary Parasitology*, vol. 2, no. 3, pp. 237–250, 1976.

[9] K. A. N. Esievo and D. I. Saror, "Immunochemistry and immunopathology of animal trypanosomiasis," *Veterinary Bulletin*, vol. 61, pp. 755–777, 1991.

[10] V. O. Anosa, "Haematological and biochemical changes in human and animal trypanosomiasis Part I," *Revue D'élevage et de Médecine Vétérinaire des Pays Tropicaux*, vol. 41, no. 1, pp. 65–78, 1988.

[11] A. Mbaya, H. Kumshe, and C. Okwudiri-Nwosu, "The mechanism of anaemia in trypanosomosis: a review," in *Anemia*, D. Silverberg, Ed., pp. 269–282, In Tech, 2012.

[12] V. O. Anosa and J. J. Kaneko, "Pathogenesis of *Trypanosoma brucei* infection in deer mice (*Peromyscus maniculatus*): hematologic, erythrocyte biochemical, and iron metabolic aspects," *American Journal of Veterinary Research*, vol. 44, no. 4, pp. 639–644, 1983.

[13] S. M. S. Rossi, *Trypanosoma evansi: estudios parasitológicos, ultraestructurales y quimioterapéuticos en la infección experimental del ratón [Ph.D. thesis]*, Facultad de Ciencias, Universidad Central de Venezuela, Caracas, Venezuela, 2009.

[14] G. C. Jenkins, "Effects of trypanosomes on the haemopoietic system," *Transactions of the Royal Society of Tropical Medicine and Hygiene*, vol. 74, no. 2, pp. 268–270, 1980.

[15] I. O. Igbokwe, "Mechanism of cellular injury in African trypanosomiasis," *Veterinary Bulletin*, vol. 64, pp. 611–620, 1994.

[16] J. Naessens, H. Kitani, Y. Yagi, K. Sekikawa, and F. Iraqqi, "TNF-α mediates the development of anaemia in a murine *Trypanosoma bruceirhodesiense* infection, but not the anaemia associated with a murine *T. congolense* infection," *Clinical & Experimental Immunology*, vol. 139, no. 3, pp. 403–410, 2005.

[17] L. E. J. Huson, E. Authié, A. F. Boulangé, J. P. D. Goldring, and T. H. T. Coetzer, "Modulation of the immunogenicity of the *Trypanosoma congolense* cysteine protease, congopain, through complexation with α2-macroglobulin," *Veterinary Research*, vol. 40, article 52, 2009.

[18] F. Guegan, N. Plazolles, T. Baltz, and V. Coustou, "Erythrophagocytosis of desialylated red blood cells is responsible for anaemia during *Trypanosoma vivax* infection," *Cellular Microbiology*, vol. 15, no. 8, pp. 1285–1303, 2013.

[19] L. E. González, J. A. García, C. Núñez et al., "*Trypanosoma vivax*: a novel method for purification from experimentally infected sheep blood," *Experimental Parasitology*, vol. 111, no. 2, pp. 126–129, 2005.

[20] G. Greif, M. P. de Leon, G. Lamolle et al., "Transcriptome analysis of the bloodstream stage from the parasite *Trypanosoma vivax*," *BMC Genomics*, vol. 14, article 149, 2013.

[21] E. Gómez-Piñeres, A. A. Boada-Sucre, A. Bretaña, M. Contreras-Bretaña, F. García, and A. Reyna-Bello, "Comparative morfometric of five Venezuelan *Trypanosoma vivax* isolates," *Revista de la Facultad de Ciencias Veterinarias de la Universidad Central de Venezuela*, vol. 55, no. 1, pp. 25–33, 2014.

[22] Z. Brener, "Therapeutic activity and criterion of cure on mice experimentally infected with *Trypanosoma cruzi*," *Revista do Instituto de Medicina Tropical de São Paulo*, vol. 4, pp. 389–396, 1962.

[23] A. A. Boada-Sucre, H. De Stefano, B. González, H. Soto, S. Godoy, and A. Bretaña, "Microscopía electrónica de barrido de las alteraciones presentes en los espermatozoides de toros mestizos Siboney," *Revista Cientifica FCV-LUZ*, vol. 9, no. 3, pp. 235–242, 1999.

[24] M. Mendoza, G. L. Uzcanga, R. Pacheco et al., "Anti-VSG antibodies induce an increase in *Trypanosoma evansi* intracellular Ca^{2+} concentration," *Parasitology*, vol. 135, no. 11, pp. 1303–1315, 2008.

[25] R. F. Macadam and W. J. Herbert, "Fine structural demonstration of cytoplasmic protrusions (Filopodia) in Trypanosomes," *Experimental Parasitology*, vol. 27, no. 1, pp. 1–8, 1970.

[26] K. Vickerman, "The mode of attachment of *Trypanosoma vivax* in the proboscis of the tsetse fly *Glossina fuscipes*: an ultrastructural study of the epimastigote stage of the trypanosome," *Journal of Protozoology*, vol. 20, no. 3, pp. 394–404, 1973.

[27] R. Hernández-Páez, "Consideraciones ultraestructurales sobre el *Trypanosoma venezuelense*, Mesnil 1910; Aspecto morfológico normal del *Trypanosoma venezuelense*," *Revista Facultad de Ciencias Veterinarias, UCV*, vol. 28, pp. 83–106, 1980.

[28] C. Hoare, *The Trypanosomes of Mammals. A Zoological Monograph*, Blackwell Scientific Publications, Oxford, UK, 1972.

[29] D. J. Williams, L. L. Logan-Henfrey, E. Authie, C. Seely, and F. McOdimba, "Experimental infection with a haemorrhage-causing *Trypanosoma vivax* in n'dama and boran cattle," *Scandinavian Journal of Immunology*, vol. 36, supplement 1, pp. 34–36, 1992.

[30] A. Hemphill and C. A. Ross, "Flagellum-mediated adhesion of *Trypanosoma congolense* to bovine aorta endothelial cells," *Parasitology Research*, vol. 81, no. 5, pp. 412–420, 1995.

[31] L. G. Goodwin, "The pathology of African trypanosomiasis," *Transactions of the Royal Society of Tropical Medicine and Hygiene*, vol. 64, pp. 797–812, 1970.

[32] D. Bratosin, J. Mazurier, J. P. Tissier et al., "Cellular and molecular mechanisms of senescent erythrocyte phagocytosis by macrophages. A review," *Biochimie*, vol. 80, no. 2, pp. 173–195, 1998.

[33] M. E. Quiñones-Mateu, H. J. Finol, L. E. Sucre, and S. H. Torres, "Muscular changes in Venezuelan wild horses naturally infected with *Trypanosoma evansi*," *Journal of Comparative Pathology*, vol. 110, no. 1, pp. 79–89, 1994.

[34] M. Rossi, A. Bremo, M. Gonzatti, and S. Giardina, "*Trypanosoma evansi* secretes proteins to the extracelular medium," in *Proceedings of the XXV Convención Anual de AsoVAC*, Universidad Simón Bolívar, Caracas, Venezuela, November 1995.

[35] G. Knowles, G. Abebe, and S. J. Black, "Peptidase in the plasma of mice infected with *Trypanosoma brucei brucei*," *Parasitology*, vol. 95, pp. 291–300, 1987.

[36] D. M. Okenu, K. N. Opara, R. I. Nwuba, and M. Nwagwu, "Purification and characterization of an extracellular release protease of *Trypanosoma brucei*," *Parasitology Research*, vol. 85, no. 5, pp. 424–428, 1999.

[37] K. A. N. Esievo, "*In vitro* production of neuraminidase (sialidase) by *Trypanosoma vivax*," in *Proceedings of the OAU/STRC International Council for Trypanosomiasis Research and Control*, pp. 205–210, Yaounde, Cameroum, 1979.

[38] B. A. Kimeto, G. M. Mugera, and P. N. Nyaga, "Haemorrhagic pancarditis in cattle infected with *Trypanosoma vivax*," *Veterinary Parasitology*, vol. 34, no. 4, pp. 295–301, 1990.

[39] K. A. N. Esievo and D. I. Saror, "Leukocyte response in experimental *Trypanosoma vivax* infection in cattle," *Journal of Comparative Pathology*, vol. 93, no. 2, pp. 165–169, 1983.

[40] V. O. Anosa, L. L. Logan-Henfrey, and M. K. Shaw, "A light and electron microscopic study of changes in blood and bone marrow in acute hemorrhagic *Trypanosoma vivax* infection in calves," *Veterinary Pathology*, vol. 29, no. 1, pp. 33–45, 1992.

[41] S. M. S. Rossi, A. A. Boada-Sucre, G. Hernández et al., "Ultrastructural analysis of liver in mice experimentally infected with a Venezuelan isolated of *Trypanosoma evansi* (Kinetoplastida:

Trypanosomatidae)," *Acta Microscópica*, vol. 17, no. 2, pp. 5–12, 2008.

[42] A. Samad, B. Licht, M. E. Stalmach, and A. Mellors, "Metabolism of phospholipids and lysophospholipids by *Trypanosoma brucei*," *Molecular and Biochemical Parasitology*, vol. 29, no. 2-3, pp. 159–169, 1988.

[43] M. Engstler and R. Schauer, "Sialidases from African *Trypanosomes*," *Parasitology Today*, vol. 9, no. 6, pp. 222–225, 1993.

[44] M. Rossi, A. Boada-Sucre, H. J. Finol et al., "Ultrastructural alterations in the adrenal gland cortex of mice experimentally infected with a Venezuelan isolate of *Trypanosoma evansi*," *Journal of Submicroscopic Cytology and Pathology*, vol. 31, no. 4, pp. 509–513, 1999.

[45] H. J. Finol, A. A. Boada-Sucre, M. Rossi, and F. Tejero, "Skeletal muscle ultrastructural pathology in mice infected with *Trypanosoma evansi*," *Journal of Submicroscopic Cytology and Pathology*, vol. 33, no. 1-2, pp. 65–71, 2001.

[46] G. M. W. Cook, D. H. Heard, and G. V. F. Seaman, "A sialomucopeptide liberated by trypsin from the human erythrocyte," *Nature*, vol. 188, no. 4755, pp. 1011–1012, 1960.

[47] A. A. Boada-Sucre, *Histopatología y patología ultraestructural de la glándula adrenal, el hígado y el testículo de ovinos infectados experimentalmente con Trypanosoma vivax [Ph.D. thesis]*, Facultad de Ciencias. Universidad Central de Venezuela, Caracas, Venezuela, 2009.

[48] M. A. Saleh, M. B. Al-Salahy, and S. A. Sanousi, "Oxidative stress in blood of camels (*Camelus dromedaries*) naturally infected with *Trypanosoma evansi*," *Veterinary Parasitology*, vol. 162, no. 3-4, pp. 192–199, 2009.

[49] A. Mijares, J. Vivas, C. Abad et al., "*Trypanosoma evansi*: effect of experimental infection on the osmotic fragility, lipid peroxidation and calcium-ATPase activity of rat red blood cells," *Experimental Parasitology*, vol. 124, no. 3, pp. 301–305, 2010.

[50] B. A. Freeman and J. D. Crapo, "Biology of disease: free radicals and tissue injury," *Laboratory Investigation*, vol. 47, no. 5, pp. 412–426, 1982.

[51] I. A. Umar, E. Ogengy, D. Okodaso et al., "Amelioration of anaemia and organ damage by combined intraperitoneal administration of vitamin A and C to *Trypanosoma brucei* brucei infected rats," *African Journal of Biotechnology*, vol. 6, no. 18, pp. 2083–2086, 2007.

19

Morphological and Chemical Study of Pathological Deposits in Human Aortic and Mitral Valve Stenosis: A Biomineralogical Contribution

Valentina Cottignoli,[1] Elena Cavarretta,[2] Loris Salvador,[3] Carlo Valfré,[3] and Adriana Maras[1]

[1]Department of Earth Sciences, Sapienza University of Rome, Piazzale Aldo Moro 5, 00185 Rome, Italy
[2]Department of Medical-Surgical Sciences and Biotechnologies, Sapienza University of Rome, Corso della Repubblica 79, 04100 Latina, Italy
[3]Division of Cardiac Surgery, San Bortolo Hospital, Viale Rodolfi 37, 36100 Vicenza, Italy

Correspondence should be addressed to Adriana Maras; adriana.maras@uniroma1.it

Academic Editor: Elizabeth Wiley

Aim of this study was to investigate heart valve calcification process by different biomineralogical techniques to provide morphological and chemical features of the ectopic deposit extracted from patients with severe mitral and aortic valve stenosis, to better evaluate this pathological process. Polarized light microscopy and scanning electron microscopy analyses brought to light the presence of nodular and massive mineralization forms characterized by different levels of calcification, as well as the presence of submicrometric calcified globular cluster, micrometric cavities containing disorganized tissue structures, and submillimeter pockets formed by organic fibers very similar to amyloid formations. Electron microprobe analyses showed variable concentrations of Ca and P within each deposit and the highest content of Ca and P within calcified tricuspid aortic valves, while powder X-ray diffraction analyses indicated in the nanometer range the dimension of the pathological bioapatite crystals. These findings indicated the presence of highly heterogeneous deposits within heart valve tissues and suggested a progressive maturation process with continuous changes in the composition of the valvular tissue, similar to the multistep formation process of bone tissue. Moreover the micrometric cavities represent structural stages of the valve tissue that immediately precedes the formation of heavily mineralized deposits such as bone-like nodules.

1. Introduction

Several physiological and pathological mineralized deposits are present in the human body. The major mineralized products (enamel, dentin, and bone) are formed by well-controlled processes of mineralization [1, 2]. Other deposits (e.g., dental calculus, urinary stones, arthritic cartilage, and heart valve calcification) are produced by pathologic mineralization. Calcific aortic valve stenosis is a major health problem facing our aging society and, after hypertension and coronary artery disease, is the third most common cardiovascular disorder and the most common indication for surgical valve replacement in the United States [3]. Despite the fact that ectopic deposits within heart valve tissues are intensively investigated, their formation mechanism is still unclear, and currently there are no effective medical treatments to delay valve calcification course progression.

The calcified deposits are composed of mineral and organic components and represent inorganic phases produced by the activity of living organisms, better known as biominerals [4]. Most pathologic biomineral deposits, generically termed calcifications or ectopic calcifications, are composed of a mixture of calcium phosphate phases. The formation of each phase depends on the combination of pH, temperature, and solution composition [5–8], and the characteristics of these deposits are different from normal mineralized tissues and from their inorganically produced counterparts. As the formation of biominerals is associated

TABLE 1: Patients characteristics, experimental analyses performed (SEM-EDS, scanning electron microscopy with energy dispersive spectrometry; PXRD, powder X-ray diffraction; EMP, electron microprobe analysis; PLM, polarized light microscopy), and average content of calcium (Ca) and phosphorus (P) in different types of calcified valve. Ca and P contents are expressed as oxide-weight percent values and as atomic Ca : P ratio. Values are mean ± SD.

Characteristic	Overall $N = 36$	Tricuspid aortic valve $N = 29$	Bicuspid aortic valve $N = 3$	Mitral valve $N = 4$
Age, y	72.4 ± 10	74.5 ± 7.8	55 ± 15	69 ± 9
Males	25 (69.4%)	20 (69%)	3 (100%)	2 (50%)
SEM-EDS	20 (55.5%)	13 (45%)	3 (100%)	4 (100%)
PXRD	27 (75%)	23 (79%)	2 (66%)	2 (50%)
EMP	5 (14%)	2 (7%)	2 (66%)	1 (25%)
PLM	5 (14%)	2 (7%)	2 (66%)	1 (25%)
CaO	40 ± 5.7	44.3 ± 4.3	35.3 ± 8.2	40.7 ± 3.4
P_2O_5	28.1 ± 4.2	30.85 ± 3.3	25 ± 6	28.85 ± 2.3
Ca : P	1.8 ± 0.08	1.82 ± 0.05	1.8 ± 0.105	1.78 ± 0.09

with different processes involving complex physicochemical and biological mechanisms, we sought to better comprehend this pathological process by conducting an interdisciplinary study focusing on the biomineralogical features of the ectopic deposits in heart valves and to present a novel biomineralogical approach that may provide important insights into the growth mechanisms of pathological events.

2. Materials and Methods

2.1. Valve Samples. Calcified aortic valves (tricuspid type, $n = 29$; bicuspid type, $n = 3$) and mitral valves ($n = 4$) were obtained from Caucasian patients of both sexes and different ages (41–90 years old) (Table 1). Samples were collected as resection materials from patients undergoing valve replacement due to severe aortic valve and mitral stenosis. All surgical interventions were performed at the Department of Cardiac Surgery, Treviso Regional Hospital, Italy. An institutional committee approved the study, and the patients gave written informed consent. Calcified valves without any sign of inflammation were included in this study. For a mineralogical preparation of the samples, after extraction tissues were preserved and dehydrated in absolute alcohol, then to sterilize the biological material, samples were exposed to UV radiation for almost 72 hours.

2.2. Preparation of Polished Thin Sections. As the dehydration treatment of the samples gave to the calcified valves the consistency of a soft rock (Figure 1) the same procedure used for rock samples was applied for the preparation of polished thin sections (PTS) of calcified deposits. Only samples with an extensive calcification were chosen for PTS, because the preparation method requires a significant amount of calcification to obtain good-quality PTS. The epoxy mounting method was used to prepare PTS with 30 μm thicknesses [9, 10].

2.3. Polarized Light Microscopy and Electron Microprobe Analyses. PTS were studied with an Olympus BX60 microscope with transmitted- and reflected-polarized light (PLM). Cross

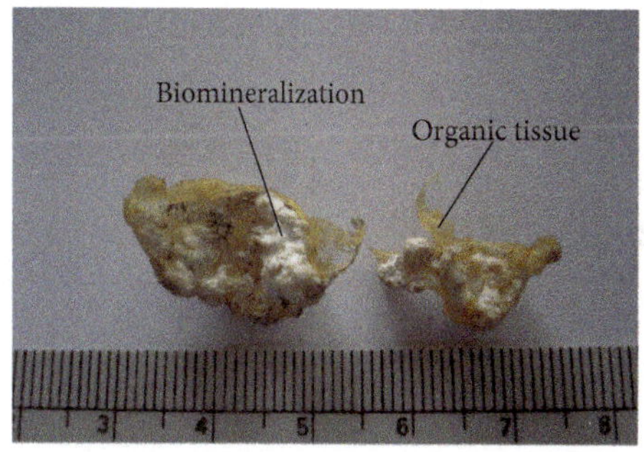

FIGURE 1: Macroscopic images of a large mineralized deposit on a valve leaflet after the mineralogical preparation (dehydration in absolute alcohol and exposure to UV radiation) of the sample. The white deposit represents the biomineral formation grown within the organic tissue (in yellow) of the human heart valve.

polarized light was used to test birefringence of samples. PTS were then coated with a thin layer of graphite, sputter-coated with an Edwards E306A High Vacuum System, and analyzed with a Cameca SX 50 EMP equipped with four wavelength dispersive spectrometers (WDS) and one energy dispersive spectrometer (EDS), at a beam current of 15.0 nA and an accelerating voltage of 15 kV. The samples were investigated using a defocused beam, as described by Ballirano et al. [11]. Standards used for the quantitative chemical analyses were all synthetic, apart from the natural fluorapatite from Durango (Mexico) used for phosphorus (P). The synthetic standards used were barite for sulfur (S), periclase for magnesium (Mg), wollastonite for calcium (Ca), magnetite for iron (Fe), and jadeite for sodium (Na). Electron microprobe (EMP) was used to obtain quantitative chemical analysis of micron-sized crystallites and backscattered electron images, very helpful to find high-resolution spatial variations in the chemical composition of the samples. They were used in conjunction with spot probe analyses, either EDS or WDS methods. At least 16 to 30 points were analyzed for each specimen.

2.4. Scanning Electron Microscopy. A FEI Quanta 400 MK2 scanning electron microscope (SEM) was used for morphological investigations. Samples were fixed on a graphite stub with double-faced tape and investigated in high- and low-vacuum modes. In order to monitor that no artifacts associated with sputter coating were formed, morphological investigations were conducted on coated and uncoated samples. Samples were coated with a thin layer of graphite, as for the PTS, only for high-vacuum mode analysis. To investigate the internal structure of pathological mineralized deposits, some samples were fractured to allow analysis of freshly broken surfaces. X-ray microanalysis was carried out with an EDS Genesis XM2, manufactured by EDAX, and several measurements were taken for each sample. Four PTS were investigated by SEM as well, and X-ray maps of individual chemical elements were acquired at a beam energy of 15 kV using the Kα lines of Ca, P, Na, Mg, and S, with a collection time of 2 hours.

2.5. Powder X-Ray Diffraction Analyses. Powder X-ray diffraction (PXRD) patterns were collected on a parallel X-ray beam Bruker AXS D8 FOCUS automated diffractometer, equipped with the parabolically shaped Göbel Mirror, using the Cu Kα_1 radiation (1.54051 Å) at 40 kV and 40 mA and operating in θ-2θ geometry. Data were collected in the 5–90° 2θ range with a step size of 0.02° and a counting time of 10 s at each step. Measurements were collected at room temperature in rotating 0.5 mm capillary tube. The samples were ground in an agate mortar into a fine powder. Two sets of diffractograms were collected: one on untreated powders and another on powders which have undergone deproteination treatment made to remove the organic component of the samples from the powders which significantly reduces the quality of the collected data. The deproteination treatment was performed through an enzymatic attack using trypsin in basic pH conditions. The cards from the International Center for Diffraction Data were used for phase identification.

The crystallite size as expression of mean diameter of the coherent-scattering domains (D) was determined with indirect measurements using diffraction peak broadening analysis. This was estimated using the Scherrer equation $D = (k\lambda)/(\beta \cos\theta)$ assuming (i) the line width/shape dominated only by particle-size effects, (ii) the Scherrer constant (K) as 0.9, and (iii) the peak broadening as Full Width Half Maximum (FWHM). The physical broadening of different diffraction lines, between ~25° and ~50° 2θ, was used after computer fit using the Gaussian line shape to determine the FWHM.

2.6. Statistical Analysis. Computations were performed with SPSS 19 (IBM, Armonk, NY, USA). Continuous variables are reported as mean ± standard deviation and categorical variables as n (%). Comparative analyses could not be performed due to the differences among groups.

3. Results

3.1. Polarized Light Microscopy Analyses. Under PLM, the ectopic deposit within heart valve tissue appeared as nodules of variable dimensions from 500 μm to 2-3 mm completely embedded within valve tissue and made up of a mishmash of amorphous material and mineral (Figures 2(a) and 2(c)). Under cross polarized light (XPL) the latter had the typical first-order gray interference color of apatite (Figures 2(b) and 2(d)). Anomalous interference colors were sometimes seen at the sample interface, probably due to reaction between organic material and the epoxy resin used for polished thin section preparation.

3.2. Backscattered Electron Images and Scanning Electron Microscopy. Backscattered electron (BSE) images on PTS, obtained by either EMP or SEM-EDS analyses, confirmed the presence of millimeter nodular formations completely embedded in the heart valve tissue that instead appeared to be not mineralized. Within the millimeter nodules we observed areas with different brightness showing a grayscale range indicative of differences in mean atomic number (Figure 3(a)): a massive mineral formation with a lower brightness and micrometric nodules with higher brightness embedded within the massive mineral matrix. The presence of grayscale range allowed us to infer a nonuniform chemical composition of the mineralized tissue. Both micrometric nodules and the massive formation had the same chemical elemental composition, as indicated by energy dispersive spectrometry (EDS) spectra (Figures 3(b) and 3(c)), even if we noted a different amount of carbon (C) independently of the carbon coating and sulphur (S) between the light grey and the grey minerals in Figure 3(a). In particular the areas having lower brightness (lowest mean atomic number) were always associated with high content of C and S (Figure 4) indicating a greater amount of organic extracellular matrix (ECM).

Elemental mapping confirmed the presence of high concentrations of Ca and P within the brightest zones of Figure 3(a) and the presence of high concentration of S only in association with the ECM surrounding the pathological deposit. In contrast, the concentrations of Na and Mg were very low and probably below the detection limit of the instrument (Figure 5).

Investigations on PTS brought to light also the presence of circular cavities (Figure 6) of variable size similar to vugs found within rocks, filled with fragments of disorganized and mineralized collagen (Figures 6(b) and 6(c)). Very large pockets filled with organic fibers formed by C, Na, and S without any trace of biomineralization, similar to amyloid-like fibrils [12, 13], were also observed (Figure 7).

At high magnifications SEM analyses revealed the presence of coalescent spherical particles (Figure 8). The latter were variably sized and had a diameter from few micrometers up to nanometer range (Figure 8(d)). They were present in all the types of valves studied (bicuspid aortic valve, tricuspid aortic valve, and mitral valve), but in some samples they presented with a different degree of agglomeration.

High-resolution images also revealed a strict relationship between fine collagen fibers and spherical particles (Figure 8(b)). SEM analyses conducted on coated and uncoated samples confirmed the same results.

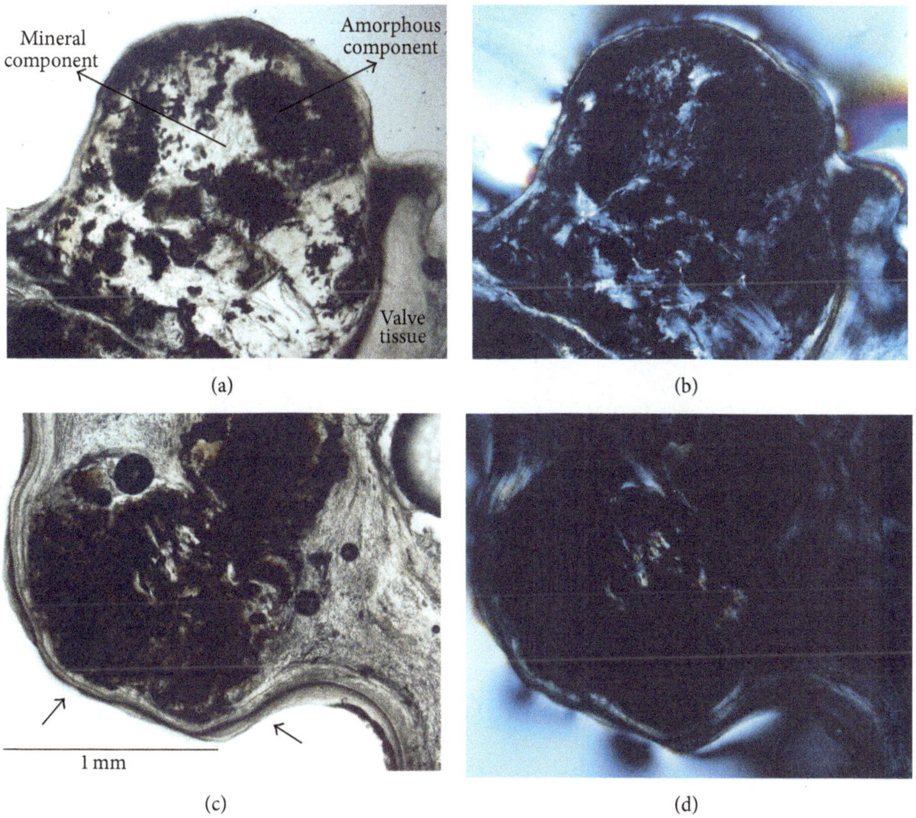

FIGURE 2: PLM analysis of valve nodules. Appearance of nodules of variable dimensions embedded in the valve tissue of a mineralized bicuspid aortic valve (Tv20ab) under transmitted PLM (a, c). (b, d) Under XPL the presence of extinguished zones is indicative of amorphous component. Zones having the typical first-order gray interference color are suggestive for apatite within the nodule. Contact between organic tissue and the epoxy resin was characterized by the presence of anomalous colors due to reaction between the two (b).

3.3. Electron Microprobe Analyses. EMP data indicated that the chemical variability of each sample was great; Ca and P concentrations, as well as the atomic Ca : P ratio, changed significantly from point to point. In addition, there was substantial chemical variability also in the different types of heart valve studied. Calcified tricuspid aortic valves had the highest and most uniformly distributed Ca and P concentrations and a high Ca : P ratio; bicuspid aortic valves had the lowest Ca and P concentrations, with less uniform distribution of Ca and P within the calcified deposits; the mitral valve analyzed presented Ca and P concentrations similar to those in tricuspid aortic valves. The chemical variability of Ca and P is given in Figure 9, whereas their average content and the mean Ca : P ratio are given in Table 1. Moreover the comparison between the two different types of aortic calcified valves showed a greater content of Ca and P within the tricuspid aortic valve than bicuspid aortic valve (Figure 10).

Despite the variable concentrations of Ca and P in each sample, the atomic Ca : P ratio for each calcified valve was relatively uniform (Table 1). The calculated mean Ca : P values fell in the so-called "AB-type carbonated apatite" range, which corresponds to the presence of carbonate (CO_3^{2-}) in the apatite lattice [14]. Thus, the chemical variability of each sample seems to be strictly regulated by its carbonate content. This is not detectable by EMP, but we have well documented its presence with Raman and infrared spectroscopy published elsewhere [15].

3.4. Powder X-Ray Diffraction Analyses. X-ray diffraction patterns of the untreated powders showed a diffuse background due to organic component (Figure 11(a)); however the enzymatic attack cleaned successfully the powders from the organic matter and revealed how this is extended in the samples (Figure 11(b)). PXRD patterns confirmed the lattice structure to be consistent with that of standard hydroxylapatite, although the latter is significantly more crystalline. However the calcification appears to have a good crystallinity degree as indicated by the resolved diffraction peaks. All samples showed the same diffraction pattern and broadening of the diffraction peaks indicating very small crystallite size. According to Scherrer equation, all samples appear to be in the nanometer range with average crystallite domains size between 20 and 24 nm (see Supplementary Tables 1 and 2 in Supplementary Material available online at http://dx.doi.org/10.1155/2015/342984).

3.5. Feasibility. Several difficulties arise when studying the mineral component of calcified tissue and its organic matrix through purely mineralogical techniques. The main difficulties are linked to (1) the application of complementary

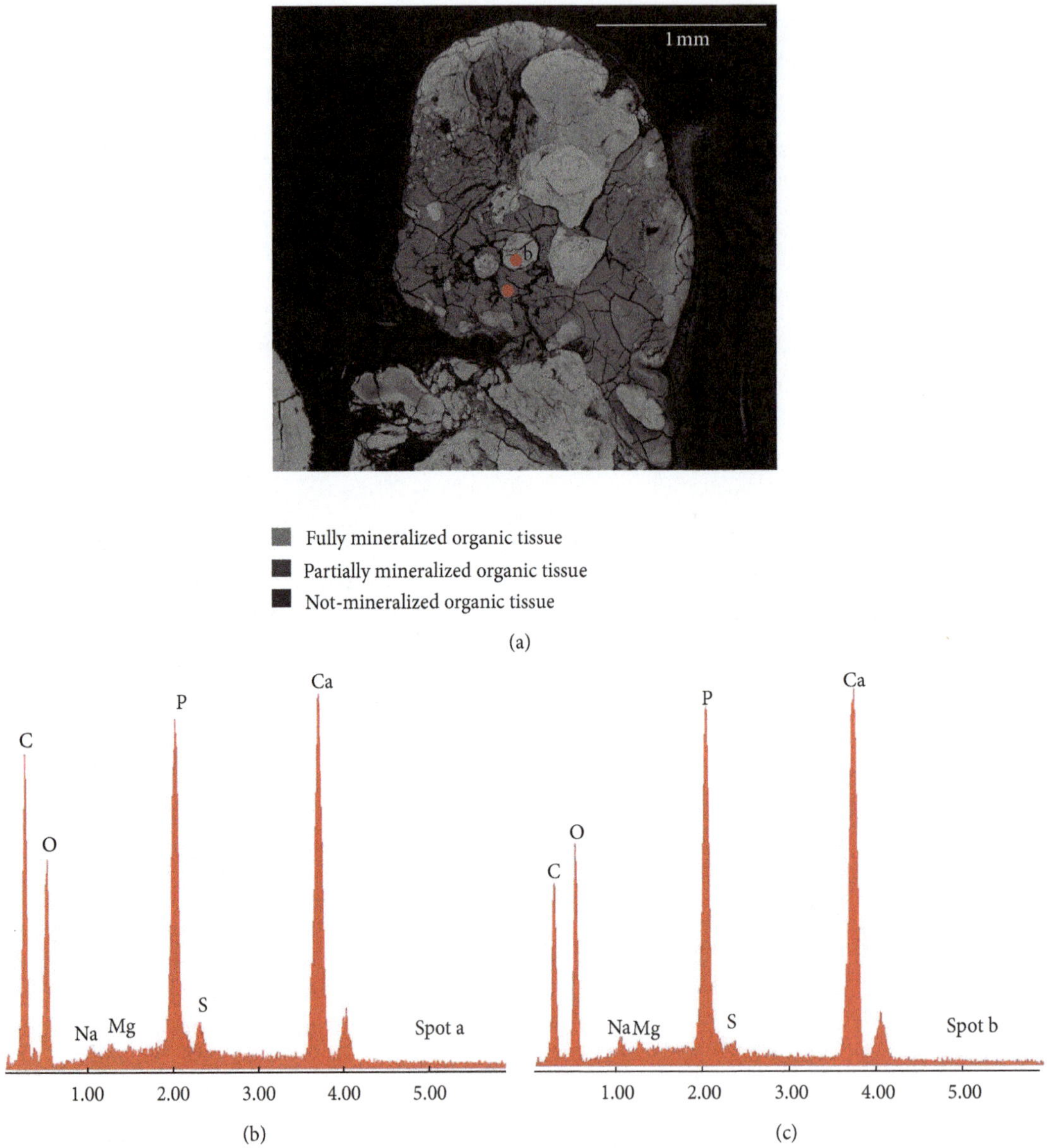

FIGURE 3: BSE image and EDS analyses of PTS (sample Tv20ab). (a) Millimeter nodule embedded in the heart valve tissue. The nodule appears to be formed by a massive mineral formation with a low brightness in which smaller nodules with higher brightness are visible. The EDS spectra of these zones with different brightness are given in panels (b) and (c); these show that Ca, P, and O are the main chemical elements that made up the heart valve mineralized tissues, confirming their calcium phosphate nature. Mg, Na, and S were also detected; the massive mineral formation characterized by a lower brightness (spot a) than micrometric nodules (spot b) had a greater content of carbon (C) and sulphur (S) and represents a partially mineralized tissue while the micrometric nodules represent fully mineralized areas. The darkest zones represent the organic matrix not mineralized (lowest mean atomic number), while the black zones represent voids in the embedding material.

experimental techniques to obtain reliable and interpretable results, (2) the very small amount of material, not allowing application of all experimental techniques, (3) the sample preparation procedures, and (4) the specific features of the pathological deposit under investigation; indeed calcium phosphate biominerals possess peculiar characteristics that make them very difficult to be analyzed. For example, these are soft and beam-sensitive materials and can be subjected to phase instability and artifacts formation. Therefore an accurate biomineralogical study such as this work is not easy.

To date application of EMP for studying standard geological materials such as inorganic crystals formed in abiotic systems is a routine analytical procedure; thus for calcium phosphate phases of geological environment recommended protocols and various operating conditions are indicated in the literature. Conversely, analytical protocols and sample preparation procedures for EMP analysis of specific biominerals are not still well defined. Therefore we made an accurate samples selection to evaluate the more suitable samples for each type of experimental analysis and then

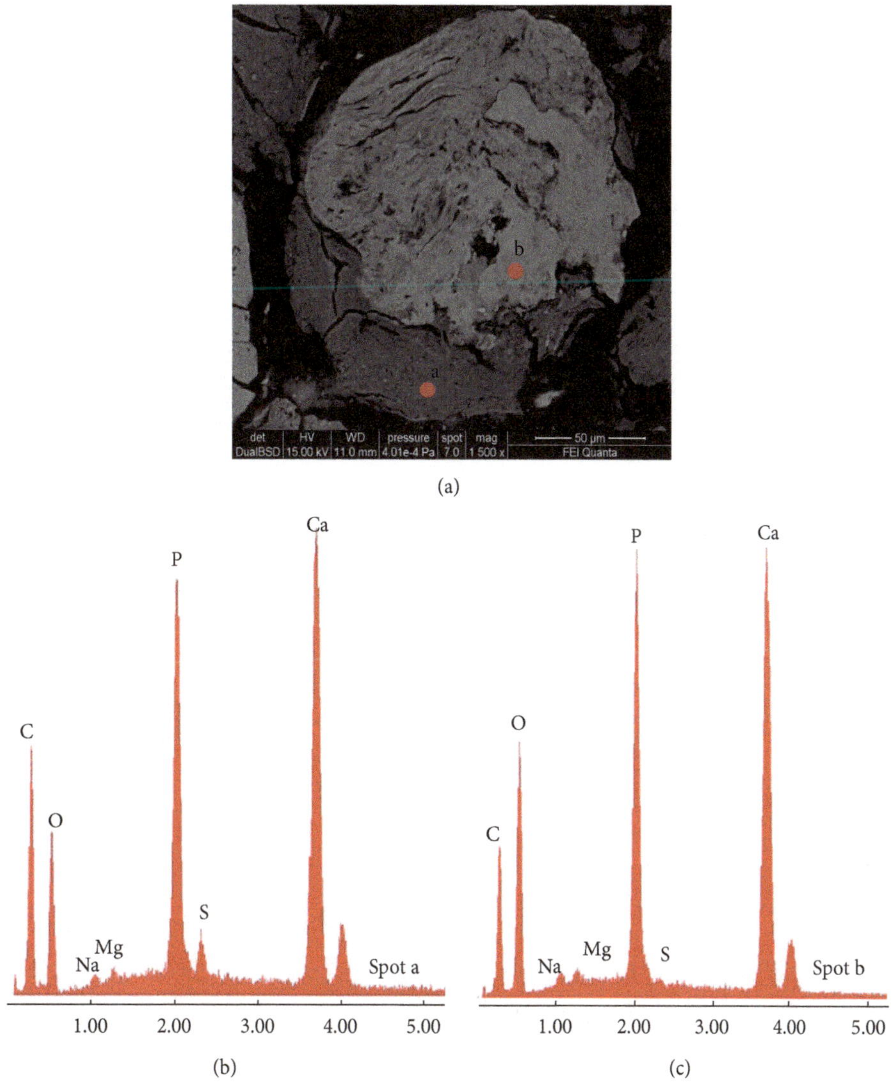

FIGURE 4: BSE-SEM analyses of PTS (sample Tv20ab). (a) High magnification image of a micrometric nodule formed by two different stages of mineralization. The lower zone of the nodule having lower brightness had greater content of C and S (spot a) (b) than the upper zone of the nodule (spot b) (c). This indicates a partially mineralized organic matrix for the lower zone of the nodule and a fully mineralized tissue for the upper zone.

an evaluation of the optimal analytical conditions to obtain correct information. We used the same criterion for SEM analyses; moreover as the preparation of organic material for SEM investigations can introduce a variety of damage and artifacts, we made several morphological investigations, as described in the text, to monitor the formation of artifacts associated with the organic component of the samples.

4. Discussion

The first detailed report of aortic valve calcification was published by Moenckeburg in 1904, who proposed two different mechanisms to explain this phenomenon: (1) degeneration of the valve leaflet layers, originating near the sinuses of Valsalva and propagating toward the tips of the cusps, and (2) a sclerotic process of the aortic wall involving the cusps. Since then, a growing scientific body of evidence has been collected on the cellular and molecular mechanisms underlying calcification [16, 17]. Currently valve calcification is not considered a simple, passive, degenerative deposition of calcium phosphate complexes on the injured valve leaflet surface. Several mechanisms potentially promoting the cusps dystrophic calcification have been proposed, ranging from mechanical stress, inflammation, Ca/P homeostasis, focal energy dissipation, immune response, and metabolic changes to upregulation of osteogenic genotype. Progression of calcification seems to be mediated primarily by valve interstitial cells (VICs) [18, 19]. In particular, changes in VIC phenotype seem to have an important role in the pathogenesis of valve calcification [20, 21], as well as in the ECM maladaptations occurring with disease [22]. The calcifying osteoblast phenotype is considered the final common pathway of the heart

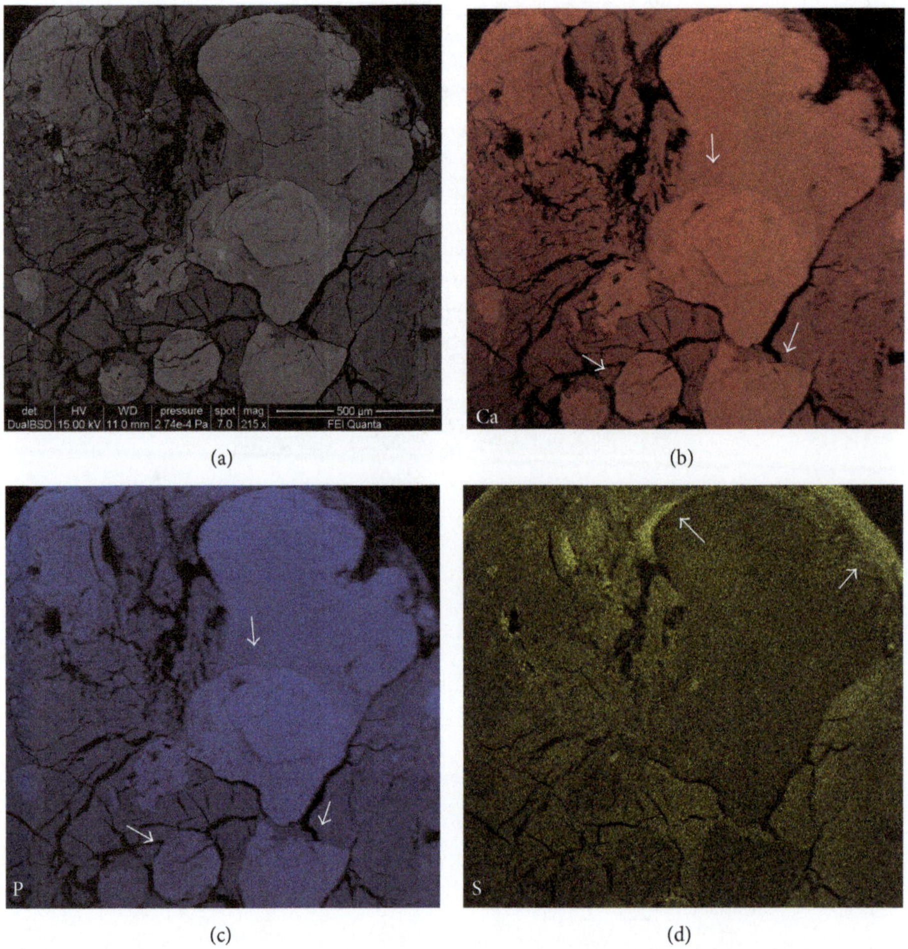

FIGURE 5: Elemental maps (sample Tv20ab). (a) BSE-SEM image of the area used to generate elemental maps. (b) Distribution of Ca. (c) Distribution of P. (d) Distribution of S. The arrows in panels (b) and (c) indicate completely mineralized areas characterized by very high concentrations of Ca and P. The arrows in panel (d) indicate high concentrations of S associated only with the extracellular organic matrix surrounding the pathological deposit.

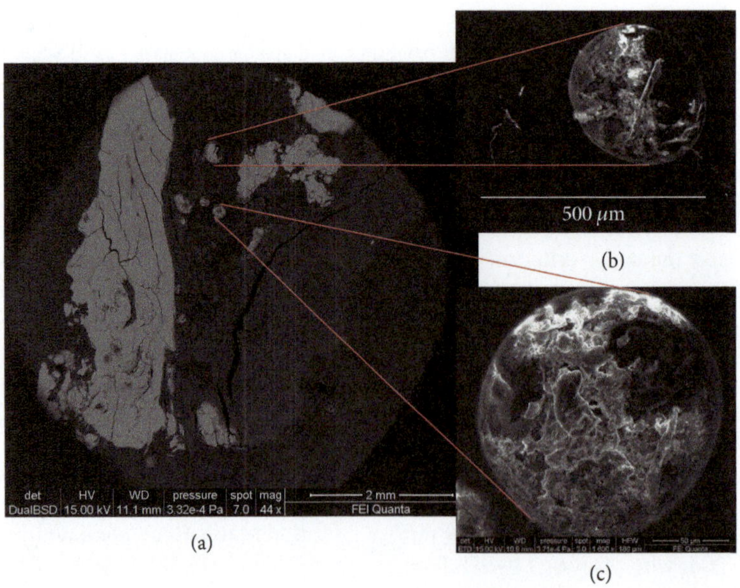

FIGURE 6: BSE-SEM analysis of circular cavities (sample Tv16 m). (a) Low magnification image of a PTS. The brightest areas represent fully mineralized zones. On the left, a massive and homogeneous deposit is visible, while in the center micrometric circular cavities are visible. (b, c) Magnified view of the small cavities indicated in panel (a); fragments of disorganized and mineralized collagen are visible within the cavities.

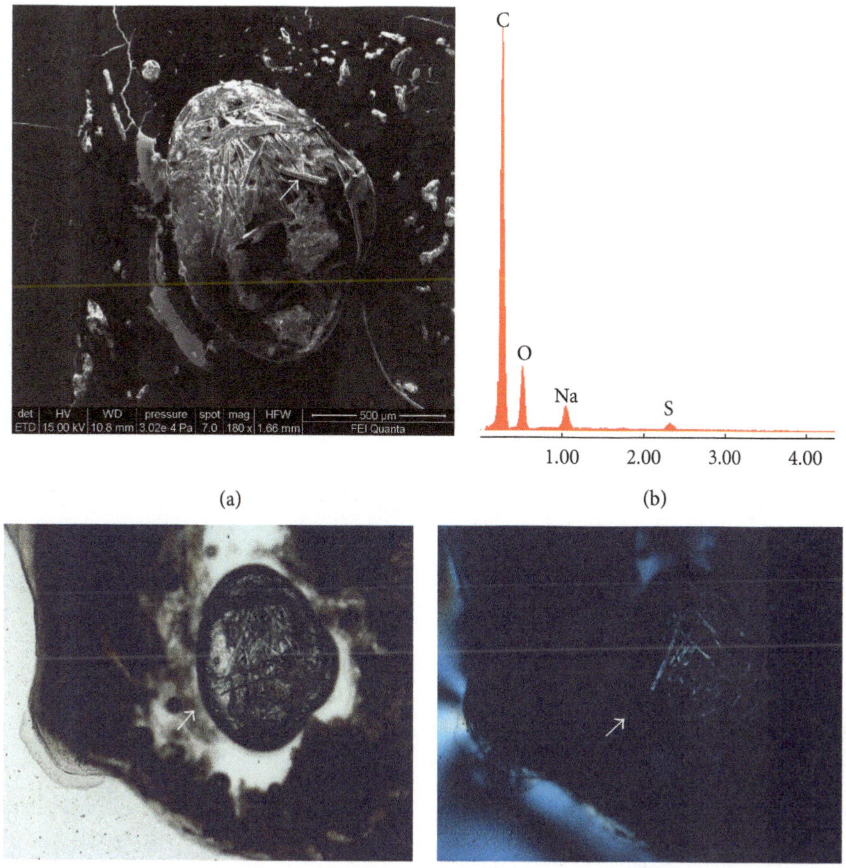

(a) (b)

(c) (d)

FIGURE 7: (a) SEM image (sample Tvl2a) of a pocket filled only with proteins, *oxidized lipids*, and collagen fibers, formed by carbon (C), oxygen (O), sodium (Na), and sulphur (S) as indicated by the spectrum EDS in panel (b); the absence of P and Ca in the spectrum demonstrates the nonmineralized nature of the fibers. Images of the pocket under PLM (c) and XPL (d). The birefringent of the organic fibers within the pocket is clearly visible as well as their morphology very similar to amyloid fibrils.

valve calcification process [23], and the identification of osteoblast-specific transcripts supports the hypothesis that degenerative aortic valve stenosis can be considered the result of an active, multifactorial, highly regulated process similar to skeletal bone formation, although the regulation of these processes is fundamentally different [24].

One mechanism involved in the pathogenesis of valve calcification seems to be based on the activation of normally quiescent VICs in response to different environmental stimuli and on their differentiation into osteoblastic VICs [25]. Moreover, microRNAs are small noncoding RNAs implicated in several cardiovascular pathologies [26], including calcific aortic stenosis, where miR-26a, miR-195, and miR-30b were found reduced [27]; in particular, miR-30b attenuates bone morphogenetic protein 2-induced osteoblast differentiation by targeting Runx2, Smadl, and caspase-3 [28]. miR-30b has been proposed as a regulator of human aortic valvular calcification and apoptosis, regulating the osteoblastic VICs, but the exact link with the inorganic phase remains to be established. Recent findings demonstrated that cells from an extracardiac origin, such as circulating hematopoietic stem cells, may contribute to vascular and valvular calcification, by driving the differentiation processes. The presence of bone marrow-derived hematopoietic stem cells has been documented in adult valves, even if the function of these cells in valvular pathogenesis has not been defined [29]. Although much progress has been made in understanding the cellular mechanisms involved in the calcification process of human heart valves, it is not clear which signaling pathways are responsible for initiation and progression of this complex process. Despite the different biological mechanisms described in valve calcification, the inorganic phase has been less systematically analyzed. We aimed to apply the mineralogical point of view to heart valve calcification, to analyze the content of Ca and P and the physicochemical features of the biominerals included in the valve calcifications. Therefore, we report in detail the morphological and chemical features of the calcified deposits found on valve tissue. Chemically, these deposits are constituted by calcium phosphate with an apatite crystal structure very similar to hydroxylapatite. This is in agreement with the phase indicated in previous reports on human heart calcification [30–37].

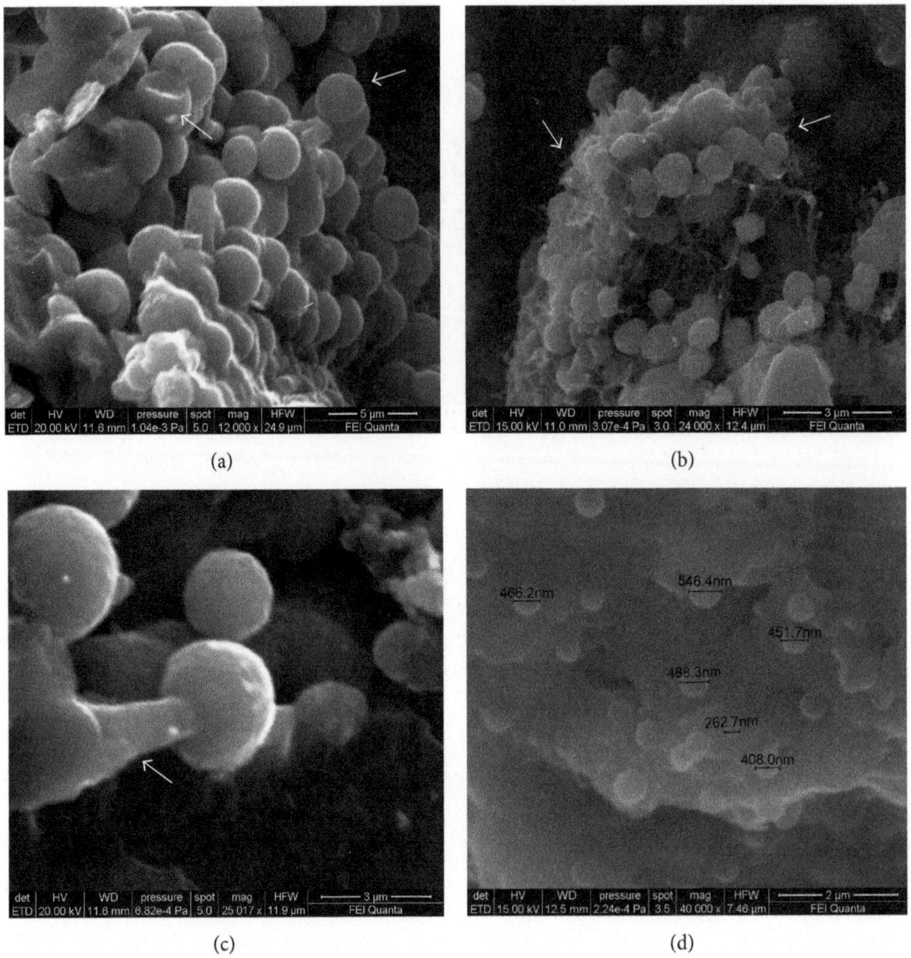

FIGURE 8: SEM analysis of pathological biomineralization morphology. (a) Agglomeration of variably sized (micrometer range) calcified nanoparticles, indicated by the arrows (12000x, mitral valve sample). (b) Agglomeration of spherical calcified nanoparticles in a framework of organic filaments (bicuspid aortic valve sample), formed by extracellular matrix proteins. (c) Magnified view (25000x) of individual spherical nanoparticle along a mineralized filament, indicated by the arrow (mitral valve sample). (d) Agglomeration of spherical calcified nanoparticles in the nanometer range at 40000x; the smallest measured nanoparticle was 262.7 nm in diameter (bicuspid aortic valve sample).

Our elemental maps clearly show that the composition of the pathological phase is restricted to Ca and P, with a high content of CO_3^{2-}, very similar to the carbonate content of normal mineralized tissues, such as bone [15].

BSE images revealed the presence of different levels of calcification. We observed a heavily mineralized tissue, characterized by nodular formations, inside a mineral-deficient tissue in which the organic component was still dominant. The areas around the nodule formations represented this type of calcification. We consider these different levels of calcification as the expression of two different stages of the calcification process. In this sense, the mineral-deficient tissue appears to be in an initial stage of calcification and is indicative of an ongoing maturation process. We hypothesize that pathological mineral formation on valve tissue is a continuous process, similar to the multistep formation process of bone tissue [38–40]: as the organic part of the valve is lost, the mineral component increases. The brightest zones such as nodules were ascribed to the final bioapatite deposit, while the mineral-deficient tissue with minor brightness was ascribed to the initial stage of the process.

We also identified the presence of small cavities in the calcifications. High magnification images revealed the presence of disorganized tissue and in some cases of calcified and fragmented fibers, within these cavities. We consider these cavities of particular interest because they clearly show in three dimensions the degradation and abnormal remodeling of the ECM involved in the calcification process. We suggest that these localized zones, which are characterized by a disorganized matrix, represent a stage immediately preceding the formation of a heavily mineralized formation, such as bone-like nodule formations [29], and after the activation and transition of VIC phenotype.

Calcification appears to be morphologically organized in globular clusters of spherical particles. To date, the nature and mechanisms of nucleation and growth of spherical calcium

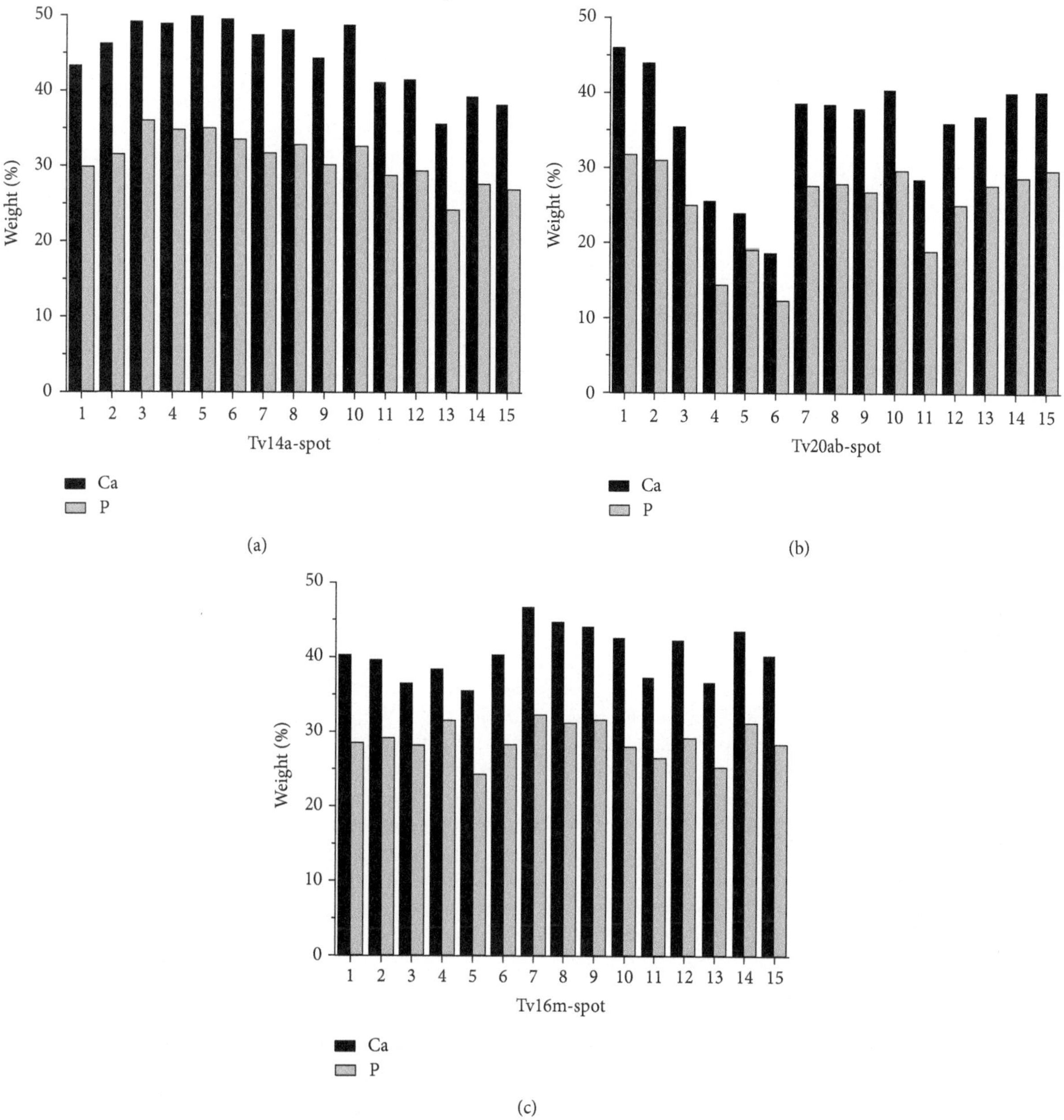

FIGURE 9: Chemical variability of Ca and P for three different calcified valves. The concentrations of Ca and P indicated in the histograms represent the concentrations determined in oxide-weight percent (CaO, P_2O_5) for fifteen punctual analyses (indicated as spot) taken within the same calcified deposit. Histograms showed that bicuspid aortic valves (b) were characterized by a lower content of Ca and P and by greater variations in Ca : P concentrations. In contrast, mitral (c) and tricuspid aortic valves (a) were characterized by a higher content of Ca and P and less variation in Ca and P concentration.

phosphate particles in pathologic states are still unclear. It is still uncertain if these spherical particles are self-replicating life forms or if they derive from a physicochemical phenomenon without any relation to living organisms. *The so-called nanobacteria (or nanobacteria-like particles, nanobes, and calcifying nanoparticles)* have been considered *by mistake* for many years the pathogenic agents involved in the calcification processes, and this bacteriomorphic hypothesis was very diffuse [41–50]. However, it has been documented that *the nanoparticles observed in pathological calcification lack RNAs and metabolic activity* [50] but are associated with mineraloprotein *complexes as albumin and fetuin-A* [51, 52], also called calciprotein particles (CPPs) [52]. The estimated values obtained from powder X-ray diffraction analyses are in agreement with values of literature reported for similar "pathological" deposits [53] and are indicative of anisotropic crystallites longer in the *c*-direction than in the *a*- or *b*-direction, suggesting a preferential growth orientation and

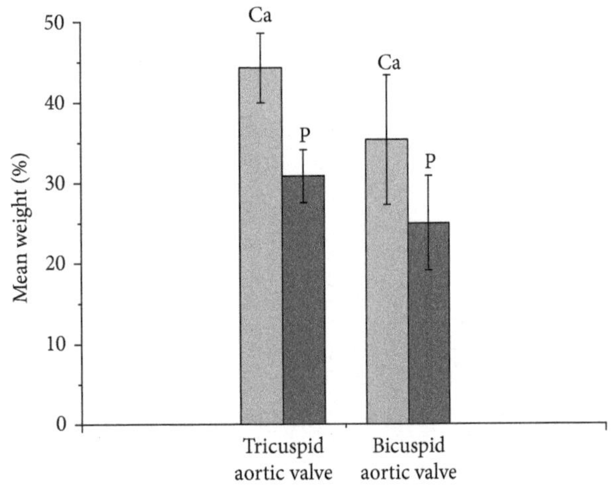

FIGURE 10: Comparison between two different types of calcified aortic valve. Histograms showed that the tricuspid aortic valve had a major content of Ca and P (expressed as mean weight %) compared to bicuspid aortic valve. The mean value was calculated on thirty spots taken within each valve. The vertical bars represent the standard deviation.

elongated shapes such as rod- or needle-like. In particular the measurements based on the peak linked to 002 reflection that is considered the most reliable peak for quantitative purposes, because of being well resolved and without overlapping with other peaks, are in agreement with the values estimated by Rusu et al. [54] for fully formed hydroxylapatite. We consider these spherical aggregates the morphological manifestation of calcifying nanoparticles of mineralo-protein and mineralo oxidized lipids that provide structural scaffolds for carbonate apatite crystals [55, 56] associated with a self-assembly process between organic and inorganic components [54]. In fact, the smallest spherical particle we measured was about 263 nm, whereas the mean size of crystallites calculated from PXRD was about 21 nm (see Supplementary Tables). Therefore, we propose that these biological aggregations are tiny bioapatite nanoparticles with crystals growing with the support of proteins as albumin, fetuin-A, and apolipoprotein A1, even if these types of nanoparticles simply adsorb any available protein from their surrounding environment [56]. At the same time, these spherical morphologies can be ascribed to extracellular vesicles- (EVs-) like particles [57, 58]. Their presence in calcified human heart valve supports the role of an active extracellular vesicular compartment in the formation of ectopic deposits within soft tissues.

However, complementary microanalytical techniques applied to harder minerals, such as focused ion beam, transmission electron microscopy, and laser ablation [59], are needed in order to obtain more information on these bioapatite nanoparticles. We plan to apply these techniques in further studies.

To the best of our knowledge, this is the first study to highlight the quantitative difference in Ca and P tissue concentrations between tricuspid and bicuspid aortic valves. The bicuspid aortic valve (BAV) is the most common congenital valve anomaly, with a prevalence of 2% in the general population and a male preponderance ratio of 2 : 1 [60]. The Ca and P content of tricuspid aortic valve (TAV) and mitral valve were similar, but the magnitude and the distribution of Ca and P were less in bicuspid valves (Figure 10). On the contrary, macroscopically, the congenital deformity of the BAV is associated with accelerated degeneration and heavier calcification than tricuspid, with a histoarchitecture of a rock-like mass of poorly mobile valve tissue. The Ca content of sinus, cusps, and arterial walls are similar in normal mammalian native semilunar valves [61] and the regional variation in normal semilunar valve tissue Ca concentrations is not predictive of later dystrophic calcification. The difference concentrations in calcified BAV are intriguing, as these valves are more subject to dystrophic calcification not only in the cusps, but also in the sinus and aortic wall. Impact of the asymmetrical hydraulic stress, inflammation, endothelial dysfunction, and neoangiogenesis probably affects more intensively the ECM when compared to tricuspid valves. It has been demonstrated that genetic factors affect the different behavior of aortic aneurisms in BAV and TAV cases [62], as in BAV there is a reduction in endothelial nitric oxide (NO) tissue endothelium levels, lower NO production, and increased release of MMP-2 and -9, determining endothelial dysfunction, activation of stretch and stress pathways, increased hypertension, increased apoptosis of smooth muscle cells, and weakening ECM. The molecular, cellular, and genetic differences between BAV and TAV affect also the Ca and P content, but further studies are needed to validate the biomineralogical difference of both types of aortic valve.

Understanding the features of pathological crystals is important if we are to obtain new insight into the mechanisms involved in valve calcification. This is fundamental for the development of therapies targeting the biomineralization process in order to improve the durability of surgically and transcatheter-implanted bioprosthetic valves. Invasive and costly surgical intervention and transcatheter implantation are today the only effective treatments of calcific valve stenosis.

5. Limitations

We are aware of the fact that a small sample size is the major limitation of this study. As described above this limitation is strictly linked to the methods of sample preparation for specific mineralogical techniques that require a very big amount of calcification, first of all to obtain accurate experimental results and to make reproducible analyses in order to verify their reliability when specific analytical protocols are missing. However, the large number of different and accurate analyses performed and the magnitude of the results are of relevance. Moreover, to our knowledge, this is the first report using pure mineralogical techniques applied to the study of soft bioapatite in humans. Studies comparing data from ultrastructural analyses, inflammatory markers, and

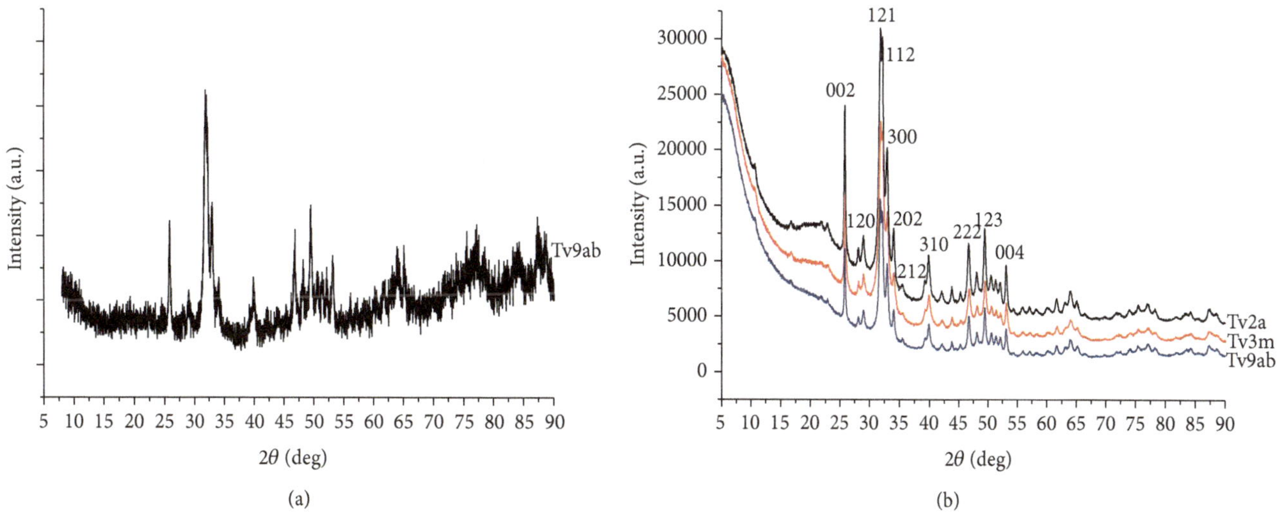

FIGURE 11: Experimental XRD patterns relative to three different types of mineralized human cardiac valves. (a) X-ray diffraction pattern of the untreated powders. (b) X-ray powder diffraction pattern of the biomineralization after the enzymatic attack. The main characteristic peaks match the hydroxylapatite pattern numbers 9–432 from the ICDS. The broadening of the peaks indicates a small crystal size within the nanometer range. a = aortic valve, ab = bicuspid aortic valve, and m = mitral valve.

biomineralogical data are ongoing and will be the object of future publications.

Abbreviations

BAV: Bicuspid aortic valve
BSE: Backscattered electron microscopy
ECM: Extracellular matrix
EDS: Energy dispersive spectrometer/spectrometry
EMP: Electron microprobe
PLM: Polarized light microscope/microscopy
PTS: Polished thin sections
PXRD: Powder X-ray diffraction
TAV: Tricuspid aortic valve
SE: Secondary electron
SEM: Scanning electron microscope/microscopy
VICs: Valve interstitial cells
WDS: Wavelength dispersive spectrometer/spectrometry
XPL: Cross polarized light.

Conflict of Interests

The authors declare no conflict of interests.

Acknowledgments

The authors wish to thank the cardiac surgery staff of Treviso Regional Hospital (Italy) for assistance during the surgical interventions and preserving valves for this study. They are grateful to technical staff of CNR-IGAG, La Sapienza section, for assistance with EMP and SEM. This work was supported by the University of Rome La Sapienza (Project C26A14258W), the Research Project of National Interest (PRIN 2010-2011) "Minerals-Biosphere Interaction: Environmental and Health Consequences," and "Gli Amici del Cuore" Association, Vicenza, Italy.

References

[1] J. C. Elliott, "Calcium phosphate biominerals," *Reviews in Mineralogy and Geochemistry*, vol. 48, no. 1, pp. 427–453, 2002.

[2] H. C. W. Skinner, "Mineralogy of bone," in *Essentials of Medical Geology: Impacts of the Natural Environment on Public Health*, pp. 667–693, Elsevier/Academic Press, New York, NY, USA, 2005.

[3] L. G. Svensson, D. H. Adams, R. O. Bonow et al., "Aortic valve and ascending aorta guidelines for management and quality measures: executive summary," *The Annals of Thoracic Surgery*, vol. 95, no. 4, pp. 1491–1505, 2013.

[4] S. Weiner and P. M. Dove, "An overview of biomineralization processes and the problem of the vital effect," *Reviews in Mineralogy and Geochemistry*, vol. 54, no. 1, pp. 1–29, 2003.

[5] R. Z. LeGeros, "Formation and transformation of calcium phosphates: relevance to vascular calcification," *Zeitschrift für Kardiologie*, vol. 90, no. 3, pp. 116–124, 2001.

[6] R. Z. LeGeros and J. P. LeGeros, "Phosphate minerals in human tissue," in *Phosphate Minerals*, pp. 351–385, Springer, Berlin, Germany, 1984.

[7] S. Shimoda, T. Aoba, E. C. Moreno, and Y. Miake, "Effect of solution composition on morphological and structural features of carbonated calcium apatites," *Journal of Dental Research*, vol. 69, no. 11, pp. 1731–1740, 1990.

[8] S. Liao, F. Watari, G. Xu, M. Ngiam, S. Ramakrishna, and C. K. Chan, "Morphological effects of variant carbonates in biomimetic hydroxyapatite," *Materials Letters*, vol. 61, no. 17, pp. 3624–3628, 2007.

[9] J. Sinkankas, "High pressure epoxy impregnation of porous materials for thin-section and microprobe analysis," *American Mineralogist*, vol. 53, pp. 339–342, 1968.

[10] J. L. Woodbury and T. A. Vogel, "A rapid, economical method for polishing thin sections for microprobe and petrographic analyses," *American Mineralogist*, vol. 55, pp. 2095–2102, 1970.

[11] P. Ballirano, A. Maras, and P. R. Buseck, "Crystal chemistry and IR spectroscopy of Cl- and SO_4-bearing cancrinite-like minerals," *American Mineralogist*, vol. 81, no. 7-8, pp. 1003–1012, 1996.

[12] A. Audet, N. Côté, C. Couture et al., "Amyloid substance within stenotic aortic valves promotes mineralization," *Histopathology*, vol. 61, no. 4, pp. 610–619, 2012.

[13] L. Millucci, L. Ghezzi, E. Paccagnini et al., "Amyloidosis, inflammation, and oxidative stress in the heart of an alkaptonuric patient," *Mediators of Inflammation*, vol. 2014, Article ID 258471, 12 pages, 2014.

[14] B. Wopenka and J. D. Pasteris, "A mineralogical perspective on the apatite in bone," *Materials Science and Engineering: C*, vol. 25, no. 2, pp. 131–143, 2005.

[15] S. Mangialardo, V. Cottignoli, E. Cavarretta, L. Salvador, P. Postorino, and A. Maras, "Pathological biominerals: raman and infrared studies of bioapatite deposits in human heart valves," *Applied Spectroscopy*, vol. 66, no. 10, pp. 1121–1127, 2012.

[16] J. A. Leopold, "Cellular mechanisms of aortic valve calcification," *Circulation: Cardiovascular Interventions*, vol. 5, no. 4, pp. 605–614, 2012.

[17] A. H. Chester, "Molecular and cellular mechanisms of valve calcification," *Aswan Heart Centre Science & Practice Series*, vol. 2011, no. 1, p. 4, 2011.

[18] C. Y. Y. Yip, J.-H. Chen, R. Zhao, and C. A. Simmons, "Calcification by valve interstitial cells is regulated by the stiffness of the extracellular matrix," *Arteriosclerosis, Thrombosis, and Vascular Biology*, vol. 29, no. 6, pp. 936–942, 2009.

[19] A. C. Liu, V. R. Joag, and A. I. Gotlieb, "The emerging role of valve interstitial cell phenotypes in regulating heart valve pathobiology," *The American Journal of Pathology*, vol. 171, no. 5, pp. 1407–1418, 2007.

[20] E. R. Mohler III, M. K. Chawla, A. W. Chang et al., "Identification and characterization of calcifying valve cells from human and canine aortic valves," *The Journal of Heart Valve Disease*, vol. 8, no. 3, pp. 254–260, 1999.

[21] J.-H. Chen and C. A. Simmons, "Cell-matrix interactions in the pathobiology of calcific aortic valve disease: critical roles for matricellular, matricrine, and matrix mechanics cues," *Circulation Research*, vol. 108, no. 12, pp. 1510–1524, 2011.

[22] N. M. Rajamannan, "Calcific aortic stenosis. Lessons learned from experimental and clinical studies," *Arteriosclerosis, Thrombosis, and Vascular Biology*, vol. 29, no. 2, pp. 162–168, 2009.

[23] N. M. Rajamannan, M. Subramaniam, D. Rickard et al., "Human aortic valve calcification is associated with an osteoblast phenotype," *Circulation*, vol. 107, no. 17, pp. 2181–2184, 2003.

[24] M. R. Dweck, N. A. Boon, and D. E. Newby, "Calcific aortic stenosis: a disease of the valve and the myocardium," *Journal of the American College of Cardiology*, vol. 60, no. 19, pp. 1854–1863, 2012.

[25] M. D. Combs and K. E. Yutzey, "Heart valve development: regulatory networks in development and disease," *Circulation Research*, vol. 105, no. 5, pp. 408–421, 2009.

[26] G. Condorelli, M. V. G. Latronico, and E. Cavarretta, "MicroRNAs in cardiovascular diseases: current knowledge and the road ahead," *Journal of the American College of Cardiology*, vol. 63, no. 21, pp. 2177–2187, 2014.

[27] V. Nigam, H. H. Sievers, B. C. Jensen et al., "Altered microRNAs in bicuspid aortic valve: a comparison between stenotic and insufficient valves," *The Journal of Heart Valve Disease*, vol. 19, no. 4, pp. 459–465, 2010.

[28] M. Zhang, X. Liu, X. Zhang et al., "MicroRNA-30b is a multifunctional regulator of aortic valve interstitial cells," *Journal of Thoracic and Cardiovascular Surgery*, vol. 147, no. 3, pp. 1073–e2, 2014.

[29] R. P. Visconti, Y. Ebihara, A. C. LaRue et al., "An in vivo analysis of hematopoietic stem cell potential: hematopoietic origin of cardiac valve interstitial cells," *Circulation Research*, vol. 98, no. 5, pp. 690–696, 2006.

[30] L. G. Gilinskaya, T. N. Grigorieva, G. N. Okuneva, and Y. A. Vlasov, "Investigation of pathogenic mineralization on human heart valves. I. Chemical and phase composition," *Journal of Structural Chemistry*, vol. 44, no. 4, pp. 622–631, 2003.

[31] B. B. Tomazic, "Physicochemical principles of cardiovascular calcification," *Zeitschrift für Kardiologie*, vol. 90, no. 3, supplement, pp. 68–80, 2001.

[32] D. W. Foreman and P. K. Fulkerson, "Crystallochemical characteristics of the inorganic phase of human calcific aortic valvar stenosis," *Cardiovascular Research*, vol. 21, no. 10, pp. 761–765, 1987.

[33] L. Stork, P. Müller, R. Dronskowski, and J. R. Ortlepp, "Chemical analyses and X-ray diffraction investigations of human hydroxyapatite minerals from aortic valve stenoses," *Zeitschrift für Kristallographie*, vol. 220, no. 2-3, pp. 201–205, 2005.

[34] J. Kapolos, D. Mavrilas, Y. Missirlis, and P. G. Koutsoukos, "Model experimental system for investigation of heart valve calcification in vitro," *Journal of Biomedical Materials Research*, vol. 38, no. 3, pp. 183–190, 1997.

[35] S. P. Marra, C. P. Daghlian, M. F. Fillinger, and F. E. Kennedy, "Elemental composition, morphology and mechanical properties of calcified deposits obtained from abdominal aortic aneurysms," *Acta Biomaterialia*, vol. 2, no. 5, pp. 515–520, 2006.

[36] D. Mikroulis, D. Mavrilas, J. Kapolos, P. G. Koutsoukos, and C. Lolas, "Physicochemical and microscopical study of calcific deposits from natural and bioprosthetic heart valves. Comparison and implications for mineralization mechanism," *Journal of Materials Science: Materials in Medicine*, vol. 13, no. 9, pp. 885–889, 2002.

[37] G. Boivin and P. J. Meunier, "Methodological considerations in measurement of bone mineral content," *Osteoporosis International*, vol. 14, no. 5, supplement, pp. S22–S27, 2003.

[38] C. Lukas, P. Kollmannsberger, D. Ruffoni, P. Roschger, P. Fratzl, and R. Weinkamer, "The heterogeneous mineral content of bone using stochastic arguments and simulations to overcome experimental limitations," *Journal of Statistical Physics*, vol. 144, no. 2, pp. 316–331, 2011.

[39] P. Roschger, E. P. Paschalis, P. Fratzl, and K. Klaushofer, "Bone mineralization density distribution in health and disease," *Bone*, vol. 42, no. 3, pp. 456–466, 2008.

[40] L. G. Gilinskaya, N. A. Rudina, G. N. Okuneva, and Y. A. Vlasov, "Pathogenic mineralization on human heart valves. III. Electron microscopy," *Journal of Structural Chemistry*, vol. 44, no. 6, pp. 1038–1045, 2003.

[41] L. G. Gilinskaya, Y. N. Zanin, and N. A. Rudina, "Bacterial genesis of calcium phosphates in human organism and nature," *Lithology and Mineral Resources*, vol. 42, no. 1, pp. 56–67, 2007.

[42] E. O. Kajander and N. Çiftçioglu, "Nanobacteria: an alternative mechanism for pathogenic intra- and extracellular calcification

and stone formation," *Proceedings of the National Academy of Sciences of the United States of America*, vol. 95, no. 14, pp. 8274–8279, 1998.

[43] V. M. Miller, G. Rodgers, J. A. Charlesworth et al., "Evidence of nanobacterial-like structures in calcified human arteries and cardiac valves," *American Journal of Physiology—Heart and Circulatory Physiology*, vol. 287, no. 3, pp. H1115–H1124, 2004.

[44] N. Çiftçioğlu, K. Vejdani, O. Lee et al., "Association between Randall's plaque and calcifying nanoparticles," *International Journal of Nanomedicine*, vol. 3, no. 1, pp. 105–115, 2008.

[45] N. Ciftcioglu, D. S. McKay, G. Mathew, and E. O. Kajander, "Nanobacteria: fact or fiction? Characteristics, detection, and medical importance of novel self-replicating, calcifying nanoparticles," *Journal of Investigative Medicine*, vol. 54, no. 7, pp. 385–394, 2006.

[46] L. G. Puskás, L. Tiszlavicz, Z. Rázga, L. L. Torday, T. Krenács, and J. G. Y. Papp, "Detection of nanobacteria-like particles in human atherosclerotic plaques," *Acta Biologica Hungarica*, vol. 56, no. 3-4, pp. 233–245, 2005.

[47] Y. R. Hu, Y. Zhao, Y. W. Sun et al., "Detection of nanobacteria-like material from calcified cardiac valves with rheumatic heart disease," *Cardiovascular Pathology*, vol. 19, no. 5, pp. 286–292, 2010.

[48] T. M. Jelic, H.-H. Chang, R. Roque, A. M. Malas, S. G. Warren, and A. P. Sommer, "Nanobacteria-associated calcific aortic valve stenosis," *The Journal of Heart Valve Disease*, vol. 16, no. 1, pp. 101–105, 2007.

[49] K. Benzerara, V. M. Miller, G. Barell et al., "Search for microbial signatures within human and microbial calcifications using soft x-ray spectromicroscopy," *Journal of Investigative Medicine*, vol. 54, no. 7, pp. 367–379, 2006.

[50] I. Barba, E. Villacorta, M.-A. Bratos-Perez et al., "Aortic valve-derived calcifyng nanoparticles: no evidence of life," *Revista Espanola de Cardiologia*, vol. 65, no. 9, pp. 813–818, 2012.

[51] J. D. Young, J. Martel, D. Young et al., "Characterization of granulations of calcium and apatite in serum as pleomorphic mineralo-protein complexes and as precursors of putative nanobacteria," *PLoS ONE*, vol. 4, no. 5, Article ID e5421, 2009.

[52] G. Schlieper, T. Krüger, A. Heiss, and W. Jahnen-Dechent, "A red herring in vascular calcification: 'nanobacteria' are protein-mineral complexes involved in biomineralization," *Nephrology Dialysis Transplantation*, vol. 26, no. 11, pp. 3436–3439, 2011.

[53] A. Becker, M. Epple, K. M. Müller, and I. Schmitz, "A comparative study of clinically well-characterized human atherosclerotic plaques with histological, chemical, and ultrastructural methods," *Journal of Inorganic Biochemistry*, vol. 98, no. 12, pp. 2032–2038, 2004.

[54] V. M. Rusu, C. H. Ng, M. Wilke, B. Tiersch, P. Fratzl, and M. G. Peter, "Size-controlled hydroxyapatite nanoparticles as self-organized organic-inorganic composite materials," *Biomaterials*, vol. 26, no. 26, pp. 5414–5426, 2005.

[55] A. P. Sommer and T. Tsurumoto, "Vascular cemeteries formed by biological nanoparticles," *Journal of Nanoparticle Research*, vol. 15, no. 4, article 1506, 2013.

[56] H. Kumon, E. Matsuura, N. Nagaoka et al., "Ectopic calcification: importance of common nanoparticle scaffolds containing oxidized acidic lipids," *Nanomedicine: Nanotechnology, Biology, and Medicine*, vol. 10, no. 2, pp. 441–450, 2014.

[57] B. György, T. G. Szabó, M. Pásztói et al., "Membrane vesicles, current state-of-the-art: emerging role of extracellular vesicles," *Cellular and Molecular Life Sciences*, vol. 68, no. 16, pp. 2667–2688, 2011.

[58] E. E. Golub, "Biomineralization and matrix vesicles in biology and pathology," *Seminars in Immunopathology*, vol. 33, no. 5, pp. 409–417, 2011.

[59] D. Bleiner, M. Macrì, P. Gasser, V. Sautter, and A. Maras, "FIB, TEM and LA-ICPMS investigations on melt inclusions in Martian meteorites—analytical capabilities and geochemical insights," *Talanta*, vol. 68, no. 5, pp. 1623–1631, 2006.

[60] W. C. Roberts and J. M. Ko, "Frequency by decades of unicuspid, bicuspid, and tricuspid aortic valves in adults having isolated aortic valve replacement for aortic stenosis, with or without associated aortic regurgitation," *Circulation*, vol. 111, no. 7, pp. 920–925, 2005.

[61] G. Acharya, M. Armstrong, C. McFall et al., "Calcium and phosphorus concentrations in native and decellularized semilunar valve tissues," *Journal of Heart Valve Disease*, vol. 23, no. 3, pp. 259–270, 2014.

[62] C. R. Balistreri, C. Pisano, G. Candore, E. Maresi, M. Codispoti, and G. Ruvolo, "Focus on the unique mechanisms involved in thoracic aortic aneurysm formation in bicuspid aortic valve versus tricuspid aortic valve patients: clinical implications of a pilot study," *European Journal of Cardio-thoracic Surgery*, vol. 43, no. 6, pp. e180–e186, 2013.

20

Mycobacterium genavense Infections in a Tertiary Hospital and Reviewed Cases in Non-HIV Patients

M. Santos,[1] A. Gil-Brusola,[2] A. Escandell,[3] M. Blanes,[3] and M. Gobernado[1]

[1] *Arevalo Baca Street 3, 46010 Valencia, Spain*
[2] *Department of Microbiology, University Hospital La Fe, Avenida Campanar 21, 46009 Valencia, Spain*
[3] *Infectious Diseases Unit, University Hospital La Fe, 46009 Valencia, Spain*

Correspondence should be addressed to A. Gil-Brusola; agilbru@hotmail.com

Academic Editor: Maria M. Picken

Mycobacterium genavense is a relatively new species of nontuberculous mycobacterium reported to cause disseminated infections in patients with AIDS and later on in non-HIV immunosuppressed patients. We describe clinical and laboratory features and response to therapy in 7 patients, three of them with HIV infection and four non-HIV—three organ transplant recipients and one with hyper-IgE syndrome—in Valencia, Spain, in a ten years period. We then summarize the published cases of *M. avium complex* infection, with invasion of peripheral blood, liver, spleen, bone marrow, lymph nodes, and lungs. In clinical samples a large number of acid-fast bacilli were observed. *M. genavense* grew only from liquid media and after a prolonged incubation period. Its identification was accomplished through molecular methods. Patients were treated with prolonged combinations of antimicrobial agents. There was clinical favourable outcome in 4 patients.

1. Introduction

Mycobacterium genavense is a nontuberculous mycobacterium (NTM), first described in 1990 [1], proposed as a new species in 1992 [2, 3], and characterized in 1993 [4]. It is a slowly growing fastidious mycobacterium that has been found in tap water [5], animals (birds, rabbits, cats, ferrets, and rabbits) [6–9], and intestinal tract of healthy humans [10]. No human to human transmission has been demonstrated. It can cause infection in birds—it is the most frequently isolated mycobacterium in parrots and parakeets [11, 12]—and humans [13–16]. In the latter, symptoms vary from nonspecific in otherwise healthy patients to disseminated symptomatology in immunosuppressed ones. These are similar to those observed in *Mycobacterium avium complex* (MAC) infection and can include fever, abdominal pain, diarrhea, weight loss, lymphadenitis, hepatosplenomegaly, and progressive anemia, being the bowel the most affected organ [17]. Other less frequently involved organs are the lungs [18], central nervous system [19], skin and soft tissues [20, 21], and genital tract [22]. Its tendency to colonize the small intestine suggests that the digestive tract could act as a reservoir and that transmission could be oral or intestinal [10].

Most reports of *M. genavense* infection are from the pre-HAART era, in AIDS patients from Europe [14, 16, 23, 24], America [3, 13, 25], Asia [26], and Australia [27, 28]. Since 1997, few cases in non-HIV patients have been reported, mainly in immunosuppressed patients, including solid organ transplant recipients [23, 29], and patients with lymphoproliferative malignancies [30] or other immunosuppressive therapy [31, 32].

M. genavense is a fastidious NTM that needs liquid media, acid pH, higher than usual temperature (45°C), mycobactin J as supplement, and at least 3 months of incubation to grow [3, 15, 17, 33]. Molecular methods are needed for its definitive identification to a species level [2, 17, 24, 34]. Nevertheless, these are also difficult since this species is related, from a phylogenetic point of view, to *M. simiae* and *M. malmoense* [35, 36]. Susceptibility testing of *M. genavense* is also arduous, not only due to its problematical isolation, but also due to the large incubation period required for its growth [4, 15, 17]. Several studies inform that it is resistant to isoniazid with variable results with ethambutol and susceptible to streptomycin, rifampicin, clarithromycin, amikacin, fluoroquinolones, and pyrazinamide [17, 37]. Even though its optimal treatment is not set, combinations of at least three active drugs are used, similarly to other NTM infections.

We hereon present a retrospective analysis of the clinical and microbiological aspects of the cases of *M. genavense* infection diagnosed in a tertiary hospital in Valencia, Spain, between 2003 and 2013, and also review the published cases from non-HIV patients in order to describe the clinical profile of this type of infection.

2. Materials and Methods

Retrospective search through the database of the Microbiology Department of the University Hospital La Fe in Valencia, Spain, of all isolates identified *M. genavense* between 2003 and 2013. This hospital has around 1000 beds with a catchment area of 360,000 inhabitants including 20 primary care centres. Data recovered included type of samples, culture and identification methods, and susceptibility results. The medical records of all patients with *M. genavense* isolation in any clinical sample were reviewed. Data collected included age, sex, underlying diseases, immune status with CD4 lymphocyte count, radiological, radioscopic and histological findings, treatment received, and outcome.

Microbiologic processing followed the standard protocol of the laboratory. Samples from nonsterile sites were decontaminated using the N-acetyl-L-cysteine-sodium hydroxide treatment. Staining with Ziehl-Neelsen method was always done. The samples were cultured in two Löwenstein-Jensen (LJ) solid media and liquid media: either BACTEC 12B Mycobacteria Medium which contains 4 mL of Middlebrook 7H12 to be periodically measured in the BACTEC 460TB radiometric instrument until 2008 or the BBL Mycobacteria Growth Indicator Tube (MGIT) with 7 mL modified Middlebrook 7H9 with the BD MGIT 960 automated fluorometric system, from that year onwards. Blood samples and bone marrow were directly inoculated in 13A radiometric medium until the year 2008 and later into BACTEC MYCO/F Lytic medium designed for use with the BACTEC 9050 automated system. Incubation was routinely done at 37°C for at least 6 weeks, extended to 3 or even 4 months when this mycobacterium was suspected. Processing of positive cultures included Ziehl-Neelsen stain, subculturing to a LJ with and without pyruvate, chocolate, Sabouraud dextrose, and blood agar plates incubated at both 37°C and 42°C. Identification was partially accomplished through biochemical methods but was then definitively made through DNA probes (GenoType HAIN Lifescience) or 16S rRNA gene sequencing. Antibiotic susceptibility testing in liquid media (BACTEC 12B Mycobacteria Medium or BD MGIT) included isoniazid, rifampicin, streptomycin, ethambutol, and pyrazinamide drugs.

To assess lung infection caused by *M. genavense* we used the American Thoracic Society (ATS) 2007 criteria [37], and for the intestinal infection we considered intestinal isolates in several successive samples in patients with prolonged symptoms. Disseminated infection was considered as the presence of signs or symptoms involving two or more organs or systems and/or isolation of *M. genavense* in blood, bone marrow, or other organs.

For the review of non-HIV cases published in literature, information from Medline databases (PubMed and Ovid) was used.

3. Results

In the period of study, 7 cases of *M. genavense* infection were identified, three HIV positive and four non-HIV. Table 1 shows demographic data of the patients, together with information concerning their underlying diseases, main symptoms, radiological findings, antibiotic treatment, and final outcome. Pathologic findings from biopsies (jejunal, duodenal lymph nodes, lung, and spleen) showed inflammatory changes, granulomas, and a large amount of intracytoplasmatic AFB, compatible with atypical mycobacteriosis. The three AIDS patients were receiving antiretroviral treatment and cotrimoxazole prophylaxis for *Pneumocystis jirovecii*, the three transplant recipients were on immunosuppressive drugs, and the child had no immunosuppressive therapy. The interval between start of immunosuppression and the *M. genavense* diagnosis was of 4 years in case 4, 1 year in case 5, and 6 years in case 6. In the rest of patients, initiation of immunosuppression is difficult to determine since they were attended at our hospital in a late stage of HIV infection. All patients had disseminated infection, five of them with symptoms and/or radiological images compatible with pulmonary infection, three (cases 2, 6 and 7) according to ATS criteria [37] and isolation of *M. genavense*.

Table 2 collects year of isolation, microbiological aspects such as type and number of samples cultured, whether AFB were observed in the initial stain, culture medium where it grew, in which samples was the mycobacterium isolated or was DNA detected, and *in vitro* drug susceptibility results. Culturing in liquid broth was always successful, being not the case of the solid LJ medium, in which *M. genavense* did not grow neither from the original samples nor from the subcultures. The identification at species level, in order to exclude *M. tuberculosis* and other NTM, was always done by conventional and molecular methods. All strains of *M. genavense* were urease producers.

Table 3 shows the cumulative cases of *M. genavense* infection in non-HIV patients published in the scientific literature from 1997 to present, including four of this study.

4. Discussion

All documented infections by *M. genavense* have been in immunocompromised hosts, mainly AIDS patients with CD4 count below 50/μL in the pre-HAART era, except for one reported case of lymphadenitis in a healthy human [44]. The incidence of *M. genavense* infection in the Swiss HIV cohort study was found to be 12.8% of all NTM cases, making it the second most frequent NTM, after MAC [14].

Table 1: Clinical characteristics, treatment, and outcome of the patients.

P	Age/sex	Underlying conditions	Signs and symptoms	Radiologic findings	Treatment	Outcome
1	38/M	Terminal HIV; CD4: 7/μL	Fever, abdominal pain, diarrhea	CT: retroperitoneal adenopathies	CL + RIF + ETM	Death (1 month)
2	38/F	HIV (2 months); CD4: 9/μL; Wilson's disease	Fever, productive cough; abdominal pain, lower limb xerosis	CXR: bilateral interstitial pattern, LUL condensation; AXR: right echogenic image	INH + RIF + PRZ	Recovery
3	35/M	HIV (<1 m); CD4: 9/μL	Fever, cough, abdominal pain, enlarged cervical lymph nodes	CT: retroperitoneal and mesenteric adenopathies; mesenteric edema	AZ + ETM + AK	Recovery
4	66/M	Kidney Tx (2004); CD4: 85/μL	Fever, productive cough; abdominal pain, anemia, bilateral tibiomaleolar oedema	CXR: blunting of right costophrenic angle; ARX: left echogenic image; colonoscopy: multiple adenomatous polyps	CL + ETM + LEV	Recovery
5	28/F	AML (UCBT, 2009)	Fever, anemia, abdominal pain, diarrhea, ankle and leg oedema	CXR: RUL micronodule; CT: pericardial effusion, pleural thickening; endoscopy: duodenal villous hypertrophy	First ETM + AK + LIN; then CL + RIB + ETM	Death (6 months)
6	52/F	Heart Tx (2004)	Fever, diarrhea, abdominal pain, ankle and leg oedema; lower limb petechiae	Abdominal Echo: hepatosplenomegaly, intra- and retroperitoneal lymphadenopathy; CXR: multiple bilateral infiltrates	RIF + ETM + PRZ + LEV	Death (5 months)
7	7/F	Hiper-IgE Syndrome	Fever, diarrhea, abdominal pain	CT: RLL bronchiectasies	CL + RIF + ETM + LEV	Recovery

P: patient; M: male; F: female; Tx: transplantation; AML: acute myeloid leukaemia; CT: computed tomography scan; UCBT: umbilical cord blood transplantation; CXR: chest X-ray; AXR: abdominal X-ray; LUL: left upper lobe; RLL: right lower lobe; CL: clarithromycin; INH: isoniazid; RIF: rifampicin; RIB: rifabutin; ETM: ethambutol; PRZ: pyrazinamide; AZ: azithromycin; AK: amikacin; LEV: levofloxacin; LIN: linezolid.

TABLE 2: Year, samples and microbiological characteristics of the study.

P	Year	Samples studied	ZN	Culture media growth	Samples with growth/DNA	Identification	Susceptibility testing (INH/RIF/STR/ETM/PRZ)
1	2003	Retroperitoneal adenopathy*	+	Bactec 12B and 13A	Retroperitoneal adenopathy	CONV and MB	R/S/S/I/—
2	2007	Blood (2), BAL	−	Bactec 12B and 13A	Blood and BAL	CONV and MB	R/S/S/S/—
3	2007	Retroperitoneal biopsy*, blood, faeces*, sputum	+	Bactec 12B and 13A	Retroperitoneal biopsy, blood, faeces	CONV and MB	R/S/S/S/—
4	2008	Faeces* (3), blood (4), urine (3), BM, sputum	+	Bactec 12B	Faeces	CONV and MB	R/S/S/I/—
5	2010	Faeces* (10), BM*, blood, sputum	+	MGIT and MYCO/F	Faeces, BM, blood	CONV and MB	Not done
6	2010	Faeces* (4), blood, BM*, BAS, spleen*	+	MGIT and MYCO/F	Faeces**, blood, BM**, BAS**, Spleen**	CONV and MB	R/S/S/R/S
7	2011	Faeces* (7) blood, lung biopsy*	+	MYCO/F	Faeces**, blood	CONV and MB	Not done

P: patient; BAL: bronchoalveolar lavage; BM: bone marrow; BAS: bronchoaspirate; ZN: Ziehl-Neelsen staining method; LJ: Löwenstein-Jensen; CONV: convencional; MB: molecular biology; INH: isoniazid; RIF: rifampicin; STR: streptomycin; ETM: ethambutol; PRZ: pyrazinamide; R: resistant; S: susceptible; I: intermediate.

*Samples with acid-fast bacilli.

**Samples in which DNA was detected.

TABLE 3: Cumulative cases of *M. genavense* infection in non-HIV patients.

Patient	Age/sex	Underlying condition	Disseminated disease	Outcome	Reference/year
1	47/F	Immunological disorder	Yes	Died	[20] 1997
2	38/F	Sarcoidosis chronic lymphopenia	Iliac abscess	Recovery	[21] 2000
3	80/F	CLL	Yes	Recovery	[30] 2000
4	67/F	Renal Tx	Yes	Died	[38] 2007
5	38/M	SLE	Yes	Improve	[39] 2008
6	56/M	Steam cell Tx	Duodenitis	Recovery	[27] 2009
7	55/F	SLE	Yes	Recovery	[31] 2009
8	39/M	Myasthenia gravis thymectomy	Enteritis	Recovery	[28] 2009
9	72/M	Sarcoidosis	Yes	Died	[32] 2009, [24] 2013
10	58/M	Sarcoidosis	Yes	Died	[32] 2009
11	44/M	Renal Tx	Yes	Recovery	[18] 2011
12	41/F	Renal Tx	Yes	Recovery	[23] 2011
13	63/M	Liver Tx	Yes	Died	[23] 2011
14	37/M	Heart Tx	Yes	Recovery	[40] 2008, [23] 2011
15	64/M	Renal Tx	Yes	Recovery	[29] 2011
16	43/M	Innate IL-12 deficiency	Yes	Improve*	[41] 2012, [24] 2013
17	43/F	Lung Tx	Yes	Died	[42] 2012
18	55/M	Possible RA	Pulmonar	Recovery	[24] 2013
19	57/M	Sarcoidosis	Pulmonar	Improve	[24] 2013
20	63/M	NHL	Yes	Improve*	[24] 2013
21	73/F	Renal Tx	Yes	Died	[24] 2013
22	54/F	Liver Tx	Yes	Improve*	[24] 2013
23	57/M	Interstitial nephritis	Yes	Died	[24] 2013
24	42/M	Idiopathic CD4+ lymphocytopenia	Yes	Improve*	[24] 2013
25	35/F	Autoimmune hepatitis IL-12 deficiency	Yes	Recovery	[43] 2013
26	66/M	Renal Tx	Yes	Recovery	Present study
27	28/F	AML umbilical cord Tx	Yes	Died	Present study
28	52/F	Heart Tx	Yes	Died	Present study
29	7/F	Hiper-IgE syndrome	Enteritis	Recovery	Present study

Tx: transplantation; CLL: chronic lymphocytic leukaemia; SLE: systemic lupus erythematosus; AML: acute mieloide leukaemia; RA: rheumatoid arthritis; NHL: non-Hodgkin lymphoma. *Chronic treatment.

However, data concerning the frequency of infection caused by this mycobacterium is few and disperse, probably due to its difficult clinical suspicion and microbiological isolation, so the disease might be underdiagnosed. In our series, the 7 patients had a diminished immune system: 3 HIV positive, 3 transplant recipients, and one child with hyper-IgE syndrome. In the different studies more cases of infection were found in adults [14, 16, 23], being less frequent in children [44–46] and with no discrimination concerning sex.

The majority of reported cases are disseminated, so clinicians should suspect this disease when a patient presents symptoms similar to those of disseminated MAC infection. *M. genavense* often affects the bowel and has less frequently been related to pleuropulmonary involvement [18, 20, 29, 47]. Other less commonly reported localizations are cutaneous, cerebral as a solitary lesion, and genital tract [19, 20, 22]. It sometimes appears associated with other opportunistic infections, making its diagnosis even more difficult. In our series, all patients had disseminated infections with intestinal tract invasion. Pulmonary infection was proofed with isolation of the mycobacterium in three cases, even though five patients had fever and productive cough and four had altered chest X ray.

Clinical presentation in affected patients usually includes fever, diarrhea, weight loss, abdominal pain, swelling of lymph nodes, hepatosplenomegaly, progressive anemia, low CD4 lymphocyte count, and sometimes hyperammonemia [38]. All these signs and symptoms are difficult to differentiate from disseminated MAC infection, except for the abdominal pain, present in the seven cases in our series, which is more frequent in *M. genavense* infection [17].

Pathologic findings from spontaneous samples and biopsies show inflammatory changes, granulomas, and a large amount of intracytoplasmatic AFB, all indistinguishable from MAC infection [15, 23, 48], in accordance with our results.

Microbiological findings are also similar to those of MAC infection. Samples like faeces and biopsies show a large amount of AFB. These are small, thin coccobacilli and appear disperse in direct staining from samples and accumulated when cultured. In our series, we observed these same facts in all stools and biopsies (retroperitoneal, duodenal, lung, and spleen).

Culture in liquid broth is preferred, BACTEC 13A medium as a good classic option [3]. Subculture in solid media is accomplished after adjusting pH, supplementing Mycobactin J, better on Middlebrook 7H11 agar than in LJ, in microaerophilic conditions, and incubation temperature of 37–45°C [3, 4, 49]. It is important to suspect *M. genavense* and incubate the samples for a longer period of time, even up to 4 months if AFB were observed in the direct staining of the sample. Our strains grew only in liquid medium after a 3-4-month period of incubation, since we do not use supplemented solid media. Neither an enriched CO_2 atmosphere nor a higher temperature facilitated the growth of the mycobacterium. It is important to consider a prolonged incubation period, especially when using automated machines with closed protocols. Blood and bone marrow, biopsies, and stools were samples that showed good microbiological results—the first ones probably due to their direct inoculation in the liquid media without previous processing and the stools because of their abundant AFB load.

During the period of study, there were some samples with acid-fast coccobacilli similar to *M. genavense*, which neither grew nor were identified. These could have been *M. genavense* but also other subspecies of MAC that have similar clinical presentation and are also difficult to grow and mycobactin J dependent [3].

Biochemical identification to species level is problematic, being urease slowly positive. Chromatography and commercial DNA probes relate this species to *M. simiae* and *M. malmoense*, so 16S rRNA sequencing is actually needed for its identification [3, 15, 24]. We had good results using the GenoType HAIN Lifescience probes that do not discriminate it from *M. triplex* although the latter grows on solid media.

In vitro susceptibility testing is not standardized due to its difficult growth, the need of an acid pH, and its requirement of a longer time of incubation than other mycobacteria [17]. We could do it in 5 cases. All our strains, in concordance to the scientific literature [17], were resistant to isoniazid, susceptible to rifampicin and streptomycin, and with variable susceptibility to ethambutol.

In general, according to our experience and other authors', differences between infection by *M. genavense* and MAC are as follows. The first is more frequently associated with abdominal pain, with more AFB found in faeces; growth in solid medium is poor in *M. genavense* and good in MAC; *M. genavense* needs a more acid pH to grow (optimal pH 5.5), as well as a longer incubation period and addition of supplements; MAC is more resistant to standard anti-TB drugs [17].

No optimal treatment protocols for *M. genavense* disease have been reported [37], but animal models found an important reduction in AFB after 15–30 days of treatment with clarithromycin and rifabutin, after 30 days of amikacin and ethambutol, and no effect with ciprofloxacin [50]. Antimycobacterial therapy should be similar to that used in MAC infection, during several months, and must be prolonged until one year of negative culture. A combination of antibiotics should be used, among them clarithromycin, although some studies discuss the *in vitro* susceptibility of this drug [51], rifampicin, ethambutol, amikacin, moxifloxacin, and others [17]. In addition to antibiotics, immunosuppressants should be minimized. Standardized antituberculous treatment is not useful in these cases. During treatment and also similar to MAC infection, patients may develop immune reconstitution syndrome (IRIS), requiring gamma interferon [23, 52].

Outcome is poor, mainly because most patients have an underlying deep immunodeficiency. Nevertheless, survival has improved over the years—in the pre-HAART era it was around 10% in AIDS patients, while as in 2011, data of 53% survival rate at 5 years follow-up was recorded [23]. Four of our patients had good evolution, including the child who required retreatment for partial lack of compliment. The other three died during the treatment—case 1, after a month secondary to terminal AIDS; case 5, with good initial evolution, but final multiorganic failure after 8 months of treatment; and case 6, after 3 months of therapy, by pulmonary complication with respiratory insufficiency. Due to the complexity of the underlying diseases of the patients, it is difficult to determine whether any of the deaths was attributable to *M. genavense*.

In the review of non-HIV patients published from 1997 until now, we have found 29 cases of infection with *M. genavense*, mainly collected in recent years (Table 3). The prototype patient is one who, due to an underlying disease, either innate or acquired, or secondary to immunosuppressive treatments, has reached a chronic immunosuppressant situation. All were adults except a child. Nearly half of the cases [13/29] were transplant recipients and the remaining had either hematological or immunological disorders, connective diseases, or others. Most patients had disseminated infection with serious mortality [8/21], focusing on the group of transplant recipients [6/10].

In summary, *M. genavense* is an emerging opportunistic pathogen with increasingly frequency in varied immunocompromised patients. The disease mimics that of other disseminated NTM, being very similar to MAC infection, but with more abdominal involvement. There is therefore a need to obtain biopsies of enlarged lymph nodes and do a systematic analysis of stool samples, to search for AFB or nucleic acid of *M. genavense*, for early diagnosis and treatment of infection. The slow and special culture requirements are useful to confirm the diagnosis. Susceptibility testing is difficult and not always accomplished. However, treatment, although long and complex, can lead to recovery. Nevertheless, mortality remains serious.

Conflict of Interests

The authors declare that there is no conflict of interests regarding the publication of this paper.

References

[1] B. Hirschel, H. R. Chang, N. Mach et al., "Fatal infection with a novel, unidentified mycobacterium in a man with the acquired immunodeficiency syndrome," *The New England Journal of Medicine*, vol. 323, no. 2, pp. 109–113, 1990.

[2] E. C. Bottger, A. Teske, P. Kirschner et al., "Disseminated "Mycobacterium genavense" infection in patients with AIDS," *The Lancet*, vol. 340, no. 8811, pp. 76–80, 1992.

[3] M. B. Coyle, L. D. C. Carlson, C. K. Wallis et al., "Laboratory aspects of "Mycobacterium genavense" a proposed species isolated from AIDS patients," *Journal of Clinical Microbiology*, vol. 30, no. 12, pp. 3206–3212, 1992.

[4] E. C. Bottger, B. Hirschel, and M. B. Coyle, "*Mycobacterium genavense* sp. Nov," *International Journal of Systematic Bacteriology*, vol. 43, no. 4, pp. 841–843, 1993.

[5] M. E. Hillebrand-Haverkort, A. H. J. Kolk, L. F. F. Kox, J. J. A. M. Ten Velden, and J. H. Ten Veen, "Generalized mycobacterium genavense infection in HIV-infected patients: detection of the mycobacterium in hospital tap water," *Scandinavian Journal of Infectious Diseases*, vol. 31, no. 1, pp. 63–68, 1999.

[6] T. E. Kiehn, H. Hoefer, E. C. Bottger et al., "Mycobacterium genavense infections in pet animals," *Journal of Clinical Microbiology*, vol. 34, no. 7, pp. 1840–1842, 1996.

[7] M. S. Hughes, N. W. Ball, D. N. Love et al., "Disseminated *Mycobacterium genavense* infection in a FIV-positive cat," *Journal of Feline Medicine and Surgery*, vol. 1, no. 1, pp. 23–29, 1999.

[8] J. Lucas, A. Lucas, H. Furber et al., "Mycobacterium genavense infection in two aged ferrets with conjunctival lesions," *Australian Veterinary Journal*, vol. 78, no. 10, pp. 685–689, 2000.

[9] E. Ludwig, U. Reischl, D. Janik, and W. Hermanns, "Granulomatous pneumonia caused by mycobacterium genavense in a dwarf rabbit (*Oryctolagus cuniculus*)," *Veterinary Pathology*, vol. 46, no. 5, pp. 1000–1002, 2009.

[10] J.-M. Dumonceau, P.-A. Fonteyne, L. Realini, A. Van Gossum, J. P. Van Vooren, and F. Portaels, "Species-specific *Mycobacterium genavense* DNA in intestinal tissues of individuals not infected with human immunodeficiency virus," *Journal of Clinical Microbiology*, vol. 33, no. 9, pp. 2514–2515, 1995.

[11] R. K. Hoop, E. C. Bottger, P. Ossent, and M. Salfinger, "Mycobacteriosis due to *Mycobacterium genavense* in six pet birds," *Journal of Clinical Microbiology*, vol. 31, no. 4, pp. 990–993, 1993.

[12] F. Portaels, L. Realini, L. Bauwens, B. Hirschel, W. M. Meyers, and W. De Meurichy, "Mycobacteriosis caused by *Mycobacterium genavense* in birds kept in a zoo: 11-Year survey," *Journal of Clinical Microbiology*, vol. 34, no. 2, pp. 319–323, 1996.

[13] M. T. Bessesen, J. Shlay, B. Stone-Venohr, D. L. Cohn, and R. R. Reves, "Disseminated *Mycobacterium genavense* infection: clinical and microbiological features and response to therapy," *AIDS*, vol. 7, no. 10, pp. 1357–1361, 1993.

[14] M. Pechere, M. Opravil, A. Wald et al., "Clinical and epidemiologic features of infection with *Mycobacterium genavense*," *Archives of Internal Medicine*, vol. 155, no. 4, pp. 400–404, 1995.

[15] P. Rodríguez, F. March, M. Garrigó et al., "Disseminated *Mycobacterium genavense* infection in patients with HIV infection. Description of 5 cases and review of the literature," *Enfermedades Infecciosas y Microbiología Clínica*, vol. 14, pp. 220–226, 1996.

[16] E. Tortoli, F. Brunello, A. E. Cagni et al., "Mycobacterium genavense in AIDS patients, report of 24 cases in Italy and review of the literature," *European Journal of Epidemiology*, vol. 14, no. 3, pp. 219–224, 1998.

[17] V. Ø. Thomsen, U. B. Dragsted, J. Bauer, K. Fuursted, and J. Lundgren, "Disseminated infection with *Mycobacterium genavense*: a challenge to physicians and mycobacteriologists," *Journal of Clinical Microbiology*, vol. 37, no. 12, pp. 3901–3905, 1999.

[18] B. Rammaert, L.-J. Couderc, E. Rivaud et al., "Mycobacterium genavense as a cause of subacute pneumonia in patients with severe cellular immunodeficiency," *BMC Infectious Diseases*, vol. 11, article 311, 2011.

[19] S. M. Berman, R. C. Kim, D. Haghighat, M. E. Mulligan, J. Fierer, and F. C. Wyle, "Mycobacterium genavense infection presenting as a solitary brain mass in a patient with AIDS: Case report and review," *Clinical Infectious Diseases*, vol. 19, no. 6, pp. 1152–1154, 1994.

[20] C. Bogdan, P. Kern, E. Richter et al., "Systemic infection with *Mycobacterium genavense* following immunosuppressive therapy in a patient who was seronegative for human immunodeficiency virus," *Clinical Infectious Diseases*, vol. 24, no. 6, pp. 1245–1247, 1997.

[21] S. Léautez, D. Boutoille, P. Bemer-Melchior, T. Ponge, and F. Raffi, "Localized *Mycobacterium genavense* soft tissue infection in an immunodeficient HIV-negative patient," *European Journal of Clinical Microbiology and Infectious Diseases*, vol. 19, no. 1, pp. 51–52, 2000.

[22] M. Vergnaud, C. Dauga, A. Dompmartin, B. Malbruny, C. Bazin, and P. A. D. Grimont, "Genital infection due to *Mycobacterium genavense* in a patient with AIDS," *Clinical Infectious Diseases*, vol. 27, no. 6, p. 1531, 1998.

[23] P. Charles, O. Lortholary, A. Dechartres et al., "Mycobacterium genavense infections: a retrospective multicenter study in France, 1996–2007," *Medicine*, vol. 90, no. 4, pp. 223–230, 2011.

[24] W. Hoefsloot, J. van Ingen, E. J. G. Peters et al., "Mycobacterium genavense in the Netherlands: an opportunistic pathogen in HIV and non-HIV immunocompromised patients. An observational study in 14 cases," *Clinical Microbiology and Infection*, vol. 19, no. 5, pp. 432–437, 2013.

[25] D. J. Hadad, S. C. Smole, C. C. Martins et al., "Disseminated *Mycobacterium genavense* in an HIV-infected patient from South America," *International Journal of Tuberculosis and Lung Disease*, vol. 7, no. 5, pp. 502–503, 2003.

[26] J.-J. Yan, W.-C. Ko, H.-M. Tsai, Y.-T. Jin, and I.-J. Su, "Disseminated mycobacterium genavense infection in a patient with acquired immunodeficiency syndrome: first case report in Taiwan," *Journal of the Formosan Medical Association*, vol. 98, no. 1, pp. 62–65, 1999.

[27] K. J. Lu, A. Grigg, D. Leslie, M. Finlay, and J. Sasadeusz, "Mycobacterium genavense duodenitis following allogeneic peripheral blood stem cell transplantation: case report," *Transplant Infectious Disease*, vol. 11, no. 6, pp. 534–536, 2009.

[28] A. Sharifian, J. Humphris, R. W. L. Leong, and D. B. Jones, "Gastrointestinal: *Mycobacterium genavense* enteritis in an immunosuppressed patient," *Journal of Gastroenterology and Hepatology*, vol. 24, no. 8, p. 1474, 2009.

[29] J. S. Doggett and L. Strasfeld, "Disseminated *Mycobacterium genavense* with pulmonary nodules in a kidney transplant recipient: case report and review of the literature," *Transplant Infectious Disease*, vol. 13, no. 1, pp. 38–43, 2011.

[30] T. Krebs, S. Zimmerli, T. Bodmer, and B. Lämmle, "Mycobacterium genavense infection in a patient with long-standing chronic lymphocytic leukaemia," *Journal of Internal Medicine*, vol. 248, no. 4, pp. 343–348, 2000.

[31] J. Lorenzen, D. Meyer-Olson, M. Haubitz et al., "Infection with *Mycobacterium genavense* in a patient with systemic lupus erythematosus," *Clinical Rheumatology*, vol. 28, no. 1, pp. S39–S41, 2009.

[32] H. Dumouchel-Champagne, C. Charlier-Woerther, A. Boibieux et al., "Disseminated nontuberculous infections with *Mycobacterium genavense* during sarcoidosis," *European Respiratory Review*, vol. 18, no. 114, pp. 299–301, 2009.

[33] E. C. Böttger, "*Mycobacterium genavense*: an emerging pathogen," *European Journal of Clinical Microbiology & Infectious Diseases*, vol. 13, pp. 932–936, 1994.

[34] O. Esparcia, M. Español, M. Garrigo et al., "Utilización de diferentes técnicas de biología molecular integradas en un algoritmo de identificación de micobacterias no tuberculosas," *Enfermedades Infecciosas y Microbiología Clínica*, vol. 30, pp. 3–10, 2012.

[35] A. Roth, M. Fischer, M. E. Hamid, S. Michalke, W. Ludwig, and H. Mauch, "Differentiation of phylogenetically related slowly growing mycobacteria based on 16S-23S rRNA gene internal transcribed spacer sequences," *Journal of Clinical Microbiology*, vol. 36, no. 1, pp. 139–147, 1998.

[36] E. Tortoli, "Phylogeny of the genus *Mycobacterium*: many doubts, few certainties," *Infection, Genetics and Evolution*, vol. 12, no. 4, pp. 827–831, 2012.

[37] D. E. Griffith, T. Aksamit, B. A. Brown-Elliott et al., "An official ATS/IDSA statement: diagnosis, treatment, and prevention of nontuberculous mycobacterial diseases," *American Journal of Respiratory and Critical Care Medicine*, vol. 175, no. 4, pp. 367–416, 2007.

[38] S. Nurmohamed, A. Weenink, H. Moeniralam, C. Visser, and F. Bemelman, "Hyperammonemia in generalized *Mycobacterium genavense* infection after renal transplantation," *American Journal of Transplantation*, vol. 7, no. 3, pp. 722–723, 2007.

[39] S. Daum, V. Moos, C. Loddenkemper et al., "Immunrekonstitutionssyndrom des Dünndarms bei einer immunsupprimierten Patientin mit systemischem Lupus erythematodes und nicht-tuberkulöser Mykobakteriose," *Z Rheumatol*, vol. 67, pp. 277–283, 2008.

[40] V. de Lastours, R. Guillemain, J.-L. Mainardi et al., "Early diagnosis of disseminated mycobacterium genavense infection," *Emerging Infectious Diseases*, vol. 14, no. 2, pp. 346–347, 2008.

[41] J. Potjewijd, R. A. de Paus, A. van Wengen, J. Damoiseaux, A. Verbon, and E. van de Vosse, "Disseminated *Mycobacterium genavense* infection in a patient with a novel partial interleukin-12 receptor $\beta 1$ deficiency," *Clinical Immunology*, vol. 144, pp. 83–86, 2012.

[42] E. Lhuillier, O. Brugière, N. Veziris et al., "Relapsing *Mycobacterium genavense* infection as a cause of late death in a lung transplant recipient: case report and review of the literature," *Experimental and Clinical Transplantation*, vol. 10, pp. 618–620, 2012.

[43] L. Tassone, A. C. Carvalho, A. Calabresi, E. Tortoli, A. Apostoli, and O. Scomodon, "Disseminated Mycobacterium genavense infection after immunosuppressive therapy shows underlying new composite heterozygous mutations of b 1 subunit of IL-12 receptor gene," *Journal of Allergy and Clinical Immunology*, vol. 131, pp. 607–610, 2013.

[44] V. Liberek, C. Soravia, B. Ninet, B. Hirschel, and C.-A. Siegrist, "Cervical lymphadenitis caused by *Mycobacterium genavense* in a healthy child," *Pediatric Infectious Disease Journal*, vol. 15, no. 3, pp. 269–270, 1996.

[45] D. Nadal, R. Caduff, R. Kraft et al., "Invasive infection with *Mycobacterium genavense* in three children with the acquired immunodeficiency syndrome," *European Journal of Clinical Microbiology & Infectious Diseases*, vol. 12, no. 1, pp. 37–43, 1993.

[46] D. Reymond, P. Birrer, and U. B. Schaad, "Mycobacterium genavense invasive infection in two children with AIDS: long-term followup," *European Journal of Pediatrics, Supplement*, vol. 154, no. 4, pp. S74–S76, 1995.

[47] C. D. Gaynor, R. A. Clark, F. P. Koontz, S. Emler, B. Hirschel, and L. S. Schlesinger, "Disseminated *Mycobacterium genavense* infection in two patients with AIDS," *Clinical Infectious Diseases*, vol. 18, no. 3, pp. 455–457, 1994.

[48] M. Wilson, K. Seilstad, M. Bessesen, D. Cohn, and S. Winter, "Pathologic findings in disseminated *Mycobacterium genavense* infection," *American Society for Microbiology*, vol. 93, article 185, 1993.

[49] L. Realini, K. De Ridder, J.-C. Palomino, B. Hirschel, and F. Portaels, "Microaerophilic conditions promote growth of *Mycobacterium genavense*," *Journal of Clinical Microbiology*, vol. 36, no. 9, pp. 2565–2570, 1998.

[50] G. Vrioni, C. Nauciel, G. Kerharo, and P. Matsiota-Bernard, "Treatment of disseminated *Mycobacterium genavense* infection in a murine model with ciprofloxacin, amikacin, ethambutol, clarithromycin and rifabutin," *Journal of Antimicrobial Chemotherapy*, vol. 42, no. 4, pp. 483–487, 1998.

[51] N. Rastogi and K. S. G. Khye Seng Goh, "Effect of pH on radiometric MICs of clarithromycin against 18 species of mycobacteria," *Antimicrobial Agents and Chemotherapy*, vol. 36, no. 12, pp. 2841–2842, 1992.

[52] S. Ehlers and E. Richter, "Gamma interferon is essential for clearing *Mycobacterium genavense* infection," *Infection and Immunity*, vol. 68, no. 6, pp. 3720–3723, 2000.

21

Pathologic and Radiologic Correlation of Adult Cystic Lung Disease: A Comprehensive Review

Prajwal Boddu,[1] Vamsi Parimi,[2] Michale Taddonio,[3] Joshua Robert Kane,[4] and Anjana Yeldandi[5]

[1] *Department of Internal Medicine, Advocate Illinois Masonic Medical Center, 836 West Wellington Avenue, Chicago, IL 60657, USA*
[2] *Department of Pathology, Loyola University Medical Center, 2160 S. 1st Avenue, Maywood, IL 60153, USA*
[3] *Department of Radiology, UC San Diego, 200 West Arbor Drive, San Diego, CA 92103, USA*
[4] *Department of Anatomic Pathology, Feinberg School of Medicine, Northwestern University, 303 E. Chicago Ave., Chicago, IL 60611, USA*
[5] *Northwestern University, Chicago, IL, USA*

Correspondence should be addressed to Prajwal Boddu; bprajwalc@gmail.com

Academic Editor: Piero Tosi

The presence of pulmonary parenchymal cysts on computed tomography (CT) imaging presents a significant diagnostic challenge. The diverse range of possible etiologies can usually be differentiated based on the clinical setting and radiologic features. In fact, the advent of high-resolution CT has facilitated making a diagnosis solely on analysis of CT image patterns, thus averting the need for a biopsy. While it is possible to make a fairly specific diagnosis during early stages of disease evolution by its characteristic radiological presentation, distinct features may progress to temporally converge into relatively nonspecific radiologic presentations sometimes necessitating histological examination to make a diagnosis. The aim of this review study is to provide both the pathologist and the radiologist with an overview of the diseases most commonly associated with cystic lung lesions primarily in adults by illustration and description of pathologic and radiologic features of each entity. Brief descriptions and characteristic radiologic features of the various disease entities are included and illustrative examples are provided for the common majority of them. In this article, we also classify pulmonary cystic disease with an emphasis on the pathophysiology behind cyst formation in an attempt to elucidate the characteristics of similar cystic appearances seen in various disease entities.

1. Introduction

Cystic air spaces represent sustained, unresolved insults to the pulmonary airways and parenchyma. Reversibility of these cysts depends on the stage in the natural history of a particular disease entity and on their response to resolution of the inciting insult [1]. Radiological classifications of lung cysts have suffered from standardization due to a lack of a uniform definition. Nomenclature has undergone periodic revisions, and the most recent glossary of definitions has been based on the radiological anatomy descriptions, as recommended by the third Fleischer Society committee meeting. These definitions have helped categorize cystic lung disease broadly into "true cystic," "cavitary," and "cystic mimics." For the purpose of this discussion, we will include and study cavitary lung disease and cystic disease mimickers under the broad umbrella of cystic lung disease.

As per the third Fleischer Society committee meeting criteria, a cyst may be defined as any low-attenuating circumscribed space, containing gas or liquid that is enclosed by an epithelial or fibrous wall and has a well-defined interface with the normal lung tissue [2]. A cavity, on the other hand, is a gas-filled space within a pulmonary consolidation or mass that is characterized by markedly thicker walls [2]. A lung cyst is usually less than 4 mm in wall thickness. By contrast, cavities have walls greater than 4 mm in thickness [3]. Diseases characterized by true cysts are relatively uncommon and are usually distinguishable from their mimicking entities like bullae, honeycombing, and bronchiectasis [4]. Bullae are sharply demarcated areas of emphysema with a wall thickness of less than 1 millimeter [2, 3, 5]. Pneumatoceles are thin-walled, gas-filled spaces occurring in association with acute infections and after trauma [2, 3]. Bullae can grow to larger volumes and occupy up to an entire lobe, while pneumatoceles tend to resolve with the improvement of the underlying infection [6]. Bullae and pneumatoceles are considered subcategories of cysts [2, 3]. Other important mimics include honeycombing, bronchiectasis, and loculated parapneumonic effusions [3, 7, 8]. Honeycombing refers to a patterning of irregular, thick-walled air spaces [2]. This condition is a sign of end stage pulmonary fibrosis. Although several disease processes present with similar pathologic and radiologic features, honeycombing is considered specific to usual interstitial pneumonia (UIP) [6, 9]. Honeycombing on CT allows distinction of UIP from other idiopathic interstitial pneumonias [7]. On the other hand, emphysema is characterized by abnormal air spaces distal to the terminal bronchiole with destruction of the alveolar walls. Emphysematous bullae may be differentiated from cysts on CT by their indefinable walls and decreased vascularity [3]. Bronchiectatic air spaces, when viewed "en face," may carry a similar appearance to cysts creating significant diagnostic confusion. However, the presence of bronchovascular bundles adjacent to air spaces can help differentiate bronchiectasis from true cysts.

One of the most important factors of cyst causation is the presence of interstitial abnormality upstream to the site of cyst formation, creating a ball valve effect. These check valves prevent egress of air on exhalation while allowing air to enter on inspiration. The coexistence of interstitial abnormalities in a small airway disease may be required for cyst formation. This supposition is supported by the lack of cystic air spaces as a pathologic or HRCT finding in pure bronchiolitic disorders without peribronchiolar infiltration [4]. Other mechanisms of cyst formation include traction bronchiectasis/bronchioloectasis, alveolar wall dissolution and conflation, and local emphysema from collateral air drifts into collapsed acini distal to obstructed bronchioles [1, 10].

2. Cystic Lung Disease

We classified cystic lung diseases based on their dominant mechanism of cyst formation (as in Table 1). This mechanistic classification is an attempt to offer better insights into the association between histopathology and radiologic characteristics. It is important to keep in mind that such mechanisms are neither exhaustive nor mutually exclusive in causation and more than one mechanism may contribute at any specific phase to disease evolution. It must also be noted, from Table 1, that some of the disease entities (e.g., lung micrometastasis) may present with atypical radiologic manifestations consequent to cystic mechanisms less frequently operating in that disease entity. These atypical presentations will be discussed further under individual disease entities.

We have subdivided cystic lung disease entities based on underlying cystic mechanism into (1) cystic dilation of lung structures: (a) ball valve effects, (b) traction bronchiectasis/alveolar ectasia, and (c) cystic suppurative/necrotic bronchiectasis; (2) parenchymal necrosis: (a) suppurative, (b) caseous, (c) ischemic, and (d) intratumoral; (3) alveolar rupture and air space conflation; (4) cyst expansion with lung displacement: (a) infectious, (b) congenital, and (5) miscellaneous.

2.1. Cystic Dilation of Lung Structures

2.1.1. Ball Valve Effects

(i) Lymphangioleiomyomatosis (LAM). LAM is an uncommon interstitial lung disease that affects women in the reproductive age group [3, 11, 12]. It may occur sporadically or in association with tuberous sclerosis caused by mutations in one of the two genes, TSC1 and TSC2 [3]. The clinicoradiologic picture is characterized by progressive pulmonary cystic changes and chylous pleural effusions [12]. Morphology is characterized by the presence of nodules, composed of two dimorphic populations of abnormally proliferating cells [3]. Proliferation of smooth muscle cells along the peribronchiolar lymphatics leads to bronchiolar obstruction and formation of lung cysts [11] (see Figure 1). Proliferation of smooth muscle cells of the lymphovascular structures results in blocking of the axial lymphatics by lymphangiomyoma which leads to chylous effusions and ascites. Centrilobular nodules on the CT correspond to type 2 pneumocyte hyperplasia. The smooth muscle proliferation represents focal ground-glass opacities; the lymphatic obstruction is seen as septal thickening [3, 11]. The characteristic CT findings in LAM are randomly distributed, diffuse thin-walled cysts, ranging from 0.5 to 2 cm in diameter, surrounded by normal lung parenchyma [12] (see Figure 2). The cyst size may vary proportionately with the severity of the disease. These LAM cells have partial melanocytic differentiation and stain positive for HMB-45 (a glycoprotein occurring in the premelanosomes in the cytoplasm). In contrast to PLCH, cysts in LAM are evenly distributed throughout the parenchyma and are more regular in shape and more uniform in size [11]. Nodules are characteristically absent in LAM and, if rarely present, are not larger than 10 millimeters in size [13, 14]. A combination of random cyst distribution and absence of ground-glass distribution helps distinguish LAM from other disease entities. In fact, the diagnosis can be arrived at with a reasonably high degree of accuracy without requiring a biopsy [14].

(ii) Respiratory Bronchiolitis-Interstitial Lung Disease (RB-ILD) and Desquamative Interstitial Pneumonia (DIP). Interstitial lung disorders (ILD) are a heterogeneous group of entities with similar clinical, radiologic, physiologic, and pathologic features. Pulmonary Langerhans cell histiocytosis (PLCH), RB-ILD, and DIP are a group of smoking related interstitial lung disorders characterized by cysts. RB-ILD and DIP share clinical and histological similarities and represent different manifestations of the same disease

TABLE 1: Cysts and cyst-like lesions based on the mechanism of cyst formation^.

Mechanism of cyst formation	Principal pathophysiology	Associated diseases	Other features
Cystic dilatation of lung structures	Ball valve effect due to proximal obstruction by peribronchiolar infiltration	*LAM* [11] *Lymphoid Interstitial pneumonia* [17, 19, 20] *PLCH* [29]* *RB-ILD* [7, 16] *DIP* [25] *P. jirovecii* [26] Primary neoplasms Endobronchial neoplasms Metastasis or micrometastases Lymphoma [25]****	Generally thin-walled (<4 mm)[3], uniform in size, and rounded in shape. May change size depending on phase of respiration due to communication with airways [5]; infiltration/nodules may be observed either radiologically or histopathologically proximal to cysts. May be diffuse (as in LAM, PLCH, and LIP) [6, 17] or focal (as in solitary neoplasms) [18, 56].
Cystic dilatation of lung structures	Traction bronchiolectasis or alveolar ectasia due to retraction from surrounding interstitial fibrosis	*Honeycombing UIP/IPF* [7] *Collagen vascular disorders, asbestosis, hypersensitive pneumonitis*, and *drug induced fibrosis* [56] *PLCH* [29]* *Viral bronchiolitis* [5] *Follicular bronchiolitis* [17] Lymphoma [25]****	Air spaces are clustered to resemble a honeycomb. Cysts are associated with other features indicating fibrosis including architectural distortion, interstitial thickening, and traction bronchiectasis. Granuloma induced fibrosis in PLCH results in irregular shaped cysts when compared to the more uniform shaped cysts as in LAM.
Cystic dilatation of lung structures	Cystic bronchiectatic air spaces formed due to fibrosing dilatation of the bronchi as a result of suppurative and/or necrotizing inflammation	*Chronic infections, immunodeficiency disorders, genetic syndromes*, and *cystic fibrosis* [5, 31]	Air spaces can be confused for cysts when viewed "en face." The bronchi have thick walls and do not taper when followed to the periphery. Cysts are more central than bullae and may contain fluid and change size with phase of respiration due to communication with airways [5].
Parenchymal necrosis	Suppurative necrosis	*Abscesses (bacterial and amoebic)* [45] *Fungal infections, nontuberculous mycobacterial infections* [52] *Postinfectious pneumatoceles* [46]	Thick-walled (>4 mm) with irregular margins seen as low areas of attenuation within an area of pulmonary consolidation or nodule on CT[3]. Air fluid levels present due to superimposed infection. May be thin-walled in resolved consolidations as seen in pneumatoceles [46].
Parenchymal necrosis	Caseous necrosis	*Tuberculosis, cryptococcosis, coccidioidomycosis*, and *histoplasmosis* [51]	Thick-walled cavitations with irregular margins predominantly in upper lobes; NTM cavitations more thin-walled and commonly associated with bronchiectasis [40, 52, 80].
Parenchymal necrosis	Ischemic necrosis	*Pulmonary infarcts* *Vasculitides* [54] *Amyloidosis* [33]** *Rheumatic disorders* [53] PLCH*	Multiple or solitary thick-walled cavitations depending on the extent of involvement.

Table 1: Continued.

Mechanism of cyst formation	Principal pathophysiology	Associated diseases	Other features
Parenchymal necrosis	Desquamation of tumor tissue with subsequent liquefaction	*Malignancies* *Primary**** *Squamous cell carcinoma* [56], *adenocarcinoma* [18, 81] *Secondary pulmonary lymphoma, AIDS lymphoma* [17] *Metastasis Mesenchymal sarcomas* [58, 59], *epithelial carcinomas* [60, 82], and *airway papillomatosis* [61]	Cavities are typically thick-walled and are usually found in an area of mass or nodule, multifocal or solitary. Very rarely thin-walled indicating formation by other mechanisms and can present as a diagnostic pitfall [83].
Alveolar rupture and/or confluence of air spaces	Alveolar dissolution from ischemia or alveolar rupture and further conflation resulting in large air spaces	*Emphysematous bullae* *COPD, connective tissue syndromes (e.g., EDS* [69]*)*Later stages of MCLD including PLCH, *amyloidosis* *BHD syndrome* [68]	Blebs and bullae have imperceptible walls (<1 mm). Tend to be peripheral and do not communicate with airways [5]. Bizarre large cysts are seen in later stages due to confluence of cystic air spaces [29].
Cystic expansion with lung displacement	Parasitic cysts	*Parasitic cysts* *Echinococcosis* [42] *Paragonimiasis* [43]	See description in Sections 2 and 3.
Cystic expansion with lung displacement	Congenital cyst formations manifesting in adults	*CPAM* *Bronchogenic cyst* [75] *Sequestration* [73]	Cysts may present very similar to acquired cystic lesions.
Miscellaneous	Iatrogenic herniation of the bowel into the thorax	*Lucite plombage* [5] *Traumatic diaphragmatic rupture* [84] *Bochdalek hernia* [85]	Apical distribution, in resistant tuberculosis. Herniation of abdominal structures into the thorax, with a cystic appearance on CT.

^Diseases whose cystic formation is predominated by the particular mechanism are written in italics. *Different mechanisms involved in cyst formation including bronchiolectasis and cavitary necrosis of nodules in early stages with confluence of air spaces in end stages of disease. **Various mechanisms proposed for cysts in amyloidosis including air trapping, ischemia by amyloid deposits on vascular walls, and bronchiolectasis. ***Majority of the solitary/multifocal neoplastic cavitations are due to squamous cell neoplasms and rarely due to adenocarcinomas. ****Rarely reported in adult lymphomas from check valve and traction fibrosis.

MCLD: multiple cystic lung disorder; IPF: idiopathic pulmonary fibrosis; LIP: lymphocytic interstitial pneumonia; LAM: lymphangioleiomyomatosis; PLCH: pulmonary Langerhans cell histiocytosis; HRCT: high-resolution CT scan; DIP: desquamative interstitial pneumonia; RB-ILD: respiratory bronchiolitis interstitial lung disorder; OP: organizing pneumonia.

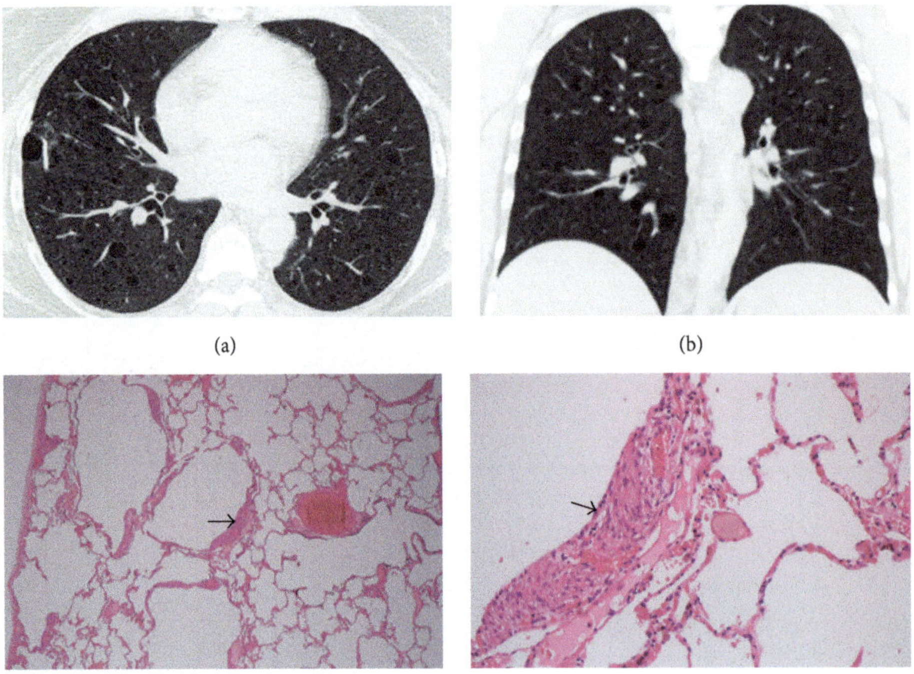

(a) (b) (c) (d)

FIGURE 1: Lymphangioleiomyomatosis (LAM). High-resolution CT scan in axial (a) and coronal (b) views demonstrating numerous well-defined, thin-walled lung cysts varying in size from 2 to 18 mm. There is diffuse involvement of all lung fields, and the lung parenchyma between the cysts is normal. (c) Thin-walled cystic air spaces interspersed between uninvolved lung parenchymata (magnification ×40). (d) Focal cyst wall thickening from smooth muscle proliferation (arrow) (magnification ×100).

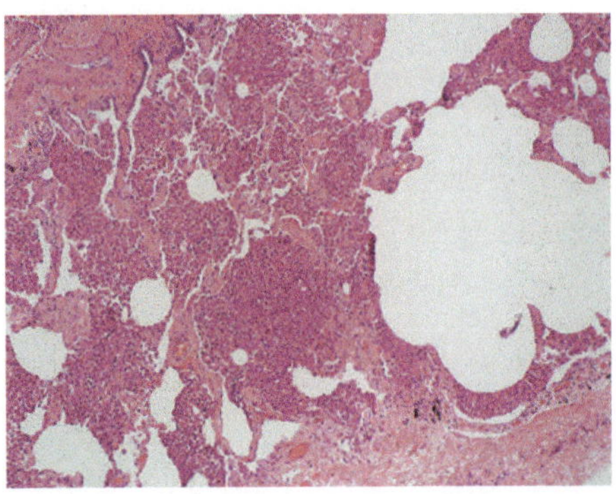

FIGURE 2: Histopathology image of a RB-ILD specimen demonstrates diffuse accumulation of macrophages in the peribronchiolar, bronchiolar regions. Interspersed among the macrophage collections are alveolar septae with a large cystic air space on the right (magnification ×100).

continuum. RB-ILD/DIP is characterized by accumulation by pigmented macrophages around the terminal airways with mild interstitial inflammatory changes which are confined to peribronchiolar parenchyma in case of RB-ILD and diffusely involve parenchyma in case of DIP [7]. RB-ILD predominantly involves the peripheral lower lobe and is typified by the occasional presence of centrilobular nodules and areas of patchy ground-glass opacities (due to alveolar inflammation and accumulation of intra-alveolar macrophages) [14, 15]. DIP is a more diffuse parenchymal reaction and is characterized by basally predominant ground-glass opacities (corresponding to intra-alveolar macrophages and minimal fibrosis) (Figure 2) [7]. Cysts are not a predominant feature of either disease and usually arise late in presentation as result of the ball valve effect from bronchiolar stenosis. On the other hand, cystic changes seen are generally emphysematous areas as a direct result of smoking. These hardly perceptible, thin-walled cysts arising in areas of ground-glass attenuation are features that characterize RB-ILD/DIP and they help differentiate this entity from the pathophysiologically related emphysema, where cysts are not surrounded by ground-glass attenuation [14]. The cysts are reversible in nature and may resolve with time unlike in the case of UIP [16].

(iii) Pulmonary Lymphoproliferative Disorders. Lymphoproliferative disorders comprise a range of disease entities and are classified into reactive or neoplastic on the basis of cellular morphology and presence of clonality [17].

Lymphocytic Interstitial Pneumonia (LIP). Benign reactive pulmonary lymphoproliferative diseases comprise three disease entities: follicular bronchiolitis, nodular lymphoid hyperplasia, and LIP [18]. LIP can be idiopathic or can occur in association with autoimmune disorders (Sjögren's syndrome), infections (*P. jiroveci*, HIV, hepatitis B, and

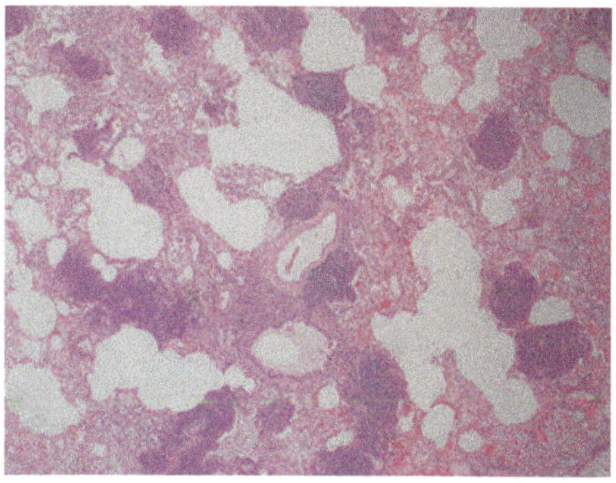

FIGURE 3: Pathology of lung biopsy specimen from a patient with lymphoid interstitial pneumonia. (a) Low power view showing peribronchiolar and interstitial lymphocytic follicular aggregates alongside dilated cystic air spaces (magnification ×40). (b) Low power view of another LIP specimen with diffuse lymphocytic follicular aggregates infiltrating the interstitium (magnification ×40).

Epstein-Barr virus), collagen vascular diseases, and immunodeficiency states (AIDS, SCID), among others [3, 11, 19, 20]. LIP is characterized microscopically by a polymorphous inflammatory infiltrate of lymphocytes, plasma cells, and histiocytes that diffusely expand the alveolar septa (Figure 3) [3, 20]. Lymphocyte predominant areas involving the bronchovascular bundles, interlobular septae, and subpleural areas are affected. The characteristic HRCT findings consist of small-sized centrilobular nodules (<10 mm), ground-glass opacities, and scattered, randomly distributed, thin-walled cysts [14, 20]. Cysts are seen in more than half the cases of LIP and are generally distributed randomly without clustering [21]. GGOs are due to the diffuse interstitial inflammation while centrilobular branching nodules are due to peribronchiolar cellular infiltration. The cysts are formed due to partial bronchial obstruction due to peribronchiolar infiltration [19]. The cysts are reversible on resolution of disease. They are typically few in number, measuring less than 3 cm in diameter. The presence of cysts and the absence of consolidation and effusion rule in favor of LIP when compared to a lymphoma [17]. In contrast to the perilymphatic distribution of LIP, follicular bronchiolitis involvement is limited to the airways with minimal peribronchial disease and lack of cysts on CT [11, 17]. CT findings are frequented by interlobular septal and bronchovascular thickening, which in combination with random cystic distributions help distinguish and differentiate LIP from other disease entities.

Lymphoma. Malignant lymphoproliferative disease may be primary or secondary in nature. The most common primary pulmonary malignant lymphoproliferative disorder is MALToma [17]. MALT lymphoma can present similarly to LIP histopathologically and radiologically, posing diagnostic difficulty. However, the presence of cysts is far more common in LIP and helps in its differentiation [17]. Most importantly, it is imperative to recognize and differentiate lymphoma from LIP as the treatment and prognosis are markedly different. Honda et al. [22] reported characteristic findings on CT which help differentiate LIP from lymphoma, cysts being characteristic of LIP and presence of consolidations with large nodules and pleural effusions being characteristic of lymphoma. It must be kept in mind that radiologic findings vary depending on the histological subtype of lymphoma. More aggressive high grade lymphomas occurring in immunosuppressed patients have more nodular presentations [23]. It is worthwhile to note that lymphomas can also cavitate and present with similar radiologic findings as solitary bronchogenic carcinomas [3, 17].

Secondary pulmonary lymphomas, including Hodgkin's and non-Hodgkin's lymphomas, can less frequently involve the lung parenchyma with varied and nonspecific imaging features, ranging from solitary nodules to parenchymal lymphangitic involvement [17]. A study by Filly et al. [24] analyzing the incidence of intraparenchymal involvement in HL and NHL revealed nodules and cysts in only 11.6% of Hodgkin's disease patients and an even lower percent in the NHL population.

Sakashita et al. [25] described a case of acute T-cell lymphoma in which there was an alloy wheel appearance with a large cyst in the center of the ground-glass opacities surrounded peripherally by smaller clustered cysts from a combination of check valve effect and traction bronchiolectasis.

(iv) Pneumocystis jiroveci Associated Multiple Cystic Lung Disease. Pneumocystis jiroveci has emerged as an important opportunistic pathogen in immunocompromised patients. The typical pulmonary features of *P. jiroveci* infection consist of diffuse pulmonary ground-glass and reticular opacities usually without pleural effusion and lymphadenopathy. However, the radiological features of *P. jiroveci* pneumonia have changed since the epidemic of AIDS from a classic CT pattern of extensive ground-glass attenuation [6] to lung cysts with an upper lobe distribution of parenchymal opacities. The formation of cystic lesions is attributed to long-standing low grade inflammation before a clinical diagnosis of PCP is made [26]. The latter radiological picture has become less common, due to early intervention with antiretroviral and PJP prophylaxis therapy [27]. Pathologically, the extensive ground-glass opacities in PJP correspond to accumulation of intra-alveolar fibrin, necrotic debris, and organisms. In patients without HIV infection, the extent of ground-glass opacity tends to be greater, reflecting pulmonary damage by an active host inflammatory immune response. The cystic lesions (Figure 4) disappear or reduce in size following treatment (as in pneumatoceles of another infectious origin). The presence of extensive GGOs with apically predominant cysts is indicative of PCP in AIDS patients. Of note, PCP lesions may infrequently manifest as cavitary infiltrates making a diagnosis extremely difficult [28].

2.1.2. Traction Bronchiolectasis/Alveolar Ectasia

(i) Interstitial Lung Disorders

Pulmonary Langerhans Cell Histiocytosis (PLCH). Pulmonary Langerhans cell histiocytosis (PLCH) is an isolated form of LCH involving the lung. The most characteristic radiological

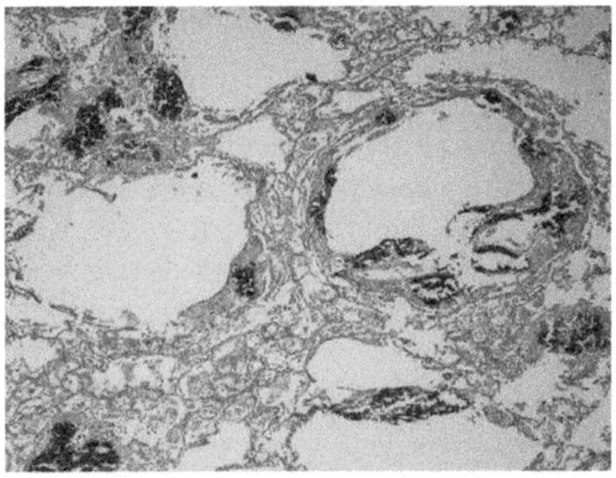

FIGURE 4: A patient with *Pneumocystis jirovecii* pneumonia. Low power view showing thin-walled cystic air spaces lined by inflammatory cells and necrotic debris with dystrophic calcification; inflammatory exudate in the interstitium and alveolar septae (magnification ×40).

presentation is the presence of apical nodules and cysts in young adult smokers [29]. Morphology is characterized by peribronchiolar Langerhans cell infiltrates forming stellate nodules (see Figure 5(b)). The nodular lesions may cavitate to form thick-walled cysts [11]. Some of these cystic nodules enlarge with increasing degrees of cicatrization, resulting in irregular thin- or thick-walled cysts [14] (see Figures 5(a), 5(c), and 5(d)). The cellular infiltrates disappear, leaving behind fibrotic scars surrounded by distorted and enlarged air spaces, typically 2 mm to 2 cm in diameter [29]. Bronchiolocentric cellular nodules correspond to the radiographic nodules on the CT and the fibrous cavitations correspond to the cysts [3]. The cysts enlarge and coalesce to form bizarre shaped cystic air spaces [3, 30]. Cystic air spaces in PLCH may be distinguished from the round cysts in LAM and LIP by their distorted shapes as well as by their characteristic apical location [29]. Cyst configurations in PLCH are more frequently lobulated than in other diseases. Centrilobular emphysema may be distinguished from PLCH by the lack of a perceptible wall and the central location of vascular structures in the former [6, 11]. PLCH shares it cystic pathogenesis with usual interstitial pneumonia which is distinguished by clustered distribution of its cysts preponderant in the lower lung zones [14].

2.1.3. Cystic Suppurative/Necrotic Bronchiectatic Air Spaces

(i) Bronchiectasis. Bronchiectasis is irreversible localized or diffuse bronchial dilatation, usually resulting from chronic infection, proximal airway obstruction, or congenital bronchial abnormalities [1]. HRCT criteria include the signet ring sign, lack of normal tapering of the bronchi towards the periphery such that bronchi are seen within a centimeter of the pleural surface [9, 31]. The signet ring appearance corresponds to a cross section of dilated bronchus adjacent to its accompanying pulmonary artery [9]. Tree-in-bud pattern and grape-like clusters in the peripheral airways are other signs of bronchiectasis seen on CT. The tree-in-bud appearance is due to mucous debris within the airways and the grape-like clusters are due to the resultant air trapping [6, 31]. Bronchial wall thickening, despite being frequent, is not necessarily diagnostic with thin-walled spaces occurring in congenital forms of bronchiectasis [32]. Bronchiectasis is caused by a vicious cycle of inflammation and an altered response to infection [33]. Normal mucosal and muscular layers fail to heal because of repeated infectious insults. Transmural inflammation occurs, not only destroying important supportive mural tissues such as smooth muscle and cartilage causing bronchomalacia, but also resulting in scarring of the wall, leading to both airway thickening and dilatation of the airways up to the periphery of the lung [34] (Figure 6). Bronchomalacia can make bronchi excessively collapsible and further air trapping [35]. CT is the gold standard for diagnosis and grading of disease severity in bronchiectasis. Disease severity is graded on the basis of the severity of bronchial dilatation, as cylindrical or tubular, a mild form; varicoid, a moderate form; and cystic or saccular, a severe form [9, 31]. Bronchiectasis can be distinguished from pulmonary cysts by following the dilated airways on multiple sequential CT slices [36]. Cystic bronchiectasis may be differentiated from bullae by the difference in the inspiration and expiration CT. Cystic bronchiectatic spaces communicate with the airways and show an increase on the inspiration CT and reduction on expiration CT whereas bullae remain largely unchanged regardless of the phase of respiration [36]. The underlying causes of bronchiectasis, for example, due to infectious or fibrosing disease, may be diagnosed in the appropriate clinical context by their zonal cystic distributions and ancillary pulmonary radiologic findings [37]. Another disorder associated with cavities is bronchiolitis obliterans organizing pneumonia, an organizing pneumonic process triggered by a variety of insults including drugs, toxins, autoimmune disease, and viral pathogens [38]. Cavitations occur in a small minority of cases and are nonspecific, thus warranting a lung biopsy for diagnosis [39].

2.2. Parenchymal Necrosis

2.2.1. Suppurative. Infectious cavities may occur during or subsequent to a necrotizing pneumonic process *(Staphylococcus aureus or Streptococcus pneumonia)*, postprimary tuberculosis (upper lobe preference) [3, 30, 40], or chronic fungal infections like *Mucor* [3] (Figure 12). Pulmonary actinomycosis, which can mimic a bronchogenic carcinoma [30], may present as a persistent pulmonary mass or consolidation with cavitations [41]. Atypical causes of cavities that are not frequently seen outside endemic areas include paragonimiasis and echinococcosis and should be considered depending on the clinical setting [3, 42, 43]. Unlike in purely cystic lung disease, pathogenic causes of cavitary lesions are not easily predicted by radiographic algorithms and require supplementary microbiological and pathological evaluations [44].

(i) Lung Abscess. A lung abscess is defined as a lesion formed by pulmonary tissue necrosis with cavity formation from expulsion of necrotic debris. Lung abscesses are recognized by their round or oval configuration, presence of air-fluid

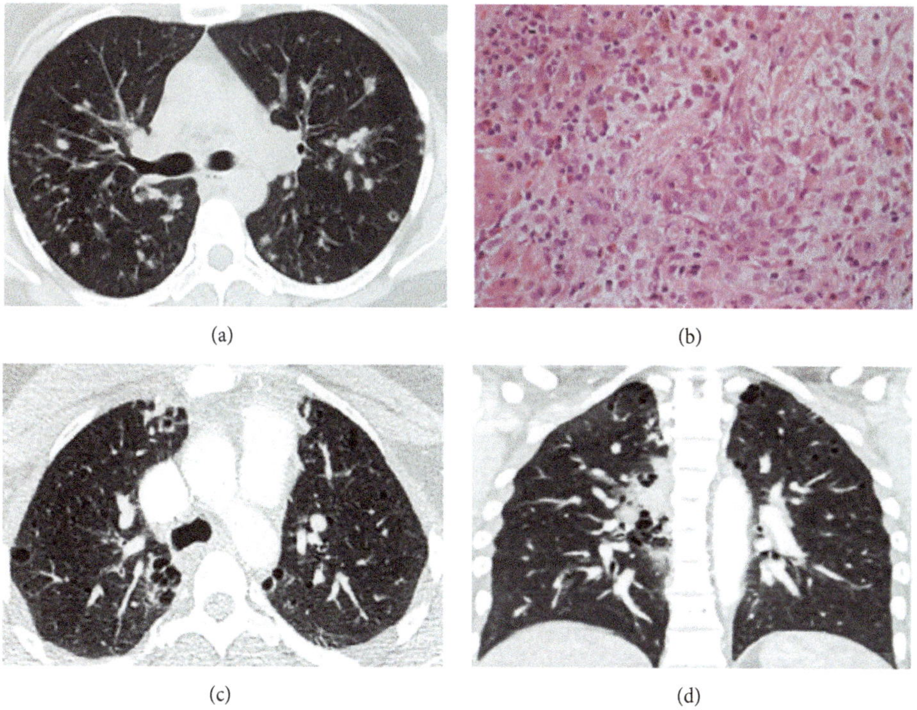

FIGURE 5: Pulmonary Langerhans cell histiocytosis. HRCT axial view (a) demonstrating a nodular phase of PLCH with multiple bronchiolocentric variable-sized nodules. The nodules correspond to granulomas on histology (b) showing high power view of Langerhans histiocytic cell aggregates surrounded by lymphocytes, eosinophils, and plasma cells (magnification ×400). Nodular phase eventually evolves to a cystic phase. Axial (c) and coronal (d) views demonstrating multiple subcentimeter lung cysts with thickened and irregular walls. Coronal view shows predominance of these lesions in the upper lobes, with relative sparing of the lung bases.

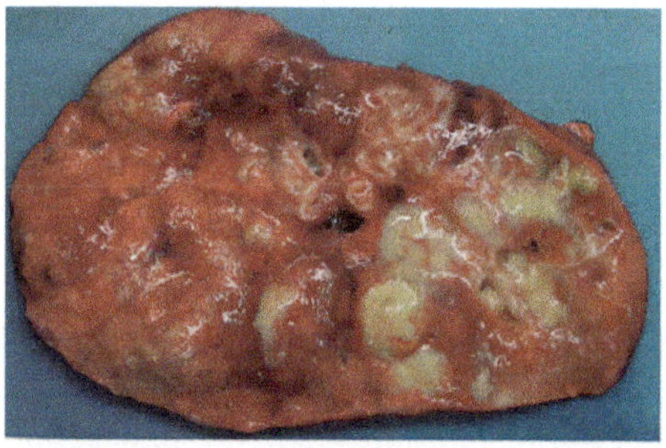

FIGURE 6: Gross specimen of resected lung from a patient with cystic fibrosis. Extensive cystic bronchiectasis with pus filled bronchial air spaces, dilated bronchi extending into the periphery.

levels, and thick walls. Pneumonia complicated by the formation of multiple, small (less than 2 cm) abscesses is referred to as necrotizing pneumonia. Abscesses may be classified as either primary or secondary depending on the presence of a preexisting condition. A primary abscess is caused by infection in an otherwise healthy host. A secondary abscess may be secondary to postobstructive pneumonia, bronchiectasis (Figure 10), or extrapulmonary or hematogenous spread of infection, among others. Aspiration is the most common cause of pulmonary abscesses, making the superior segment of the right lower lobe the most common site for infection. CT is the most sensitive and specific imaging modality to diagnose a lung abscess. Acute abscesses, over time, develop a chronic inflammatory layer of lymphocytes, plasma cells, histiocytes, and fibrosis around the pyogenic membrane creating better defined margins [45]. The typical appearance is that of a cavity containing an air-fluid level corresponding to necrotic debris and infected fluid, surrounded by a thick wall corresponding to a layer of fibrosis formed from chronic inflammation. CT distinction may be difficult between true abscesses and their radiologic mimickers, including cavitary neoplasms (see below). This may be resolved with the administration of contrast which helps identify abscess margins from the surrounding consolidation. Cavities are a very rare feature of emboli/infarcts and their presence in a case of suspected pulmonary infarct indicates septic embolization [5].

(ii) Pneumatocele. Pneumatoceles are usually transient cysts resulting from an inflammatory process that causes central necrosis with subsequent retraction by surrounding pulmonary tissue. The mechanism is primarily a combination of parenchymal necrosis and check valve obstruction [9]. The most common cause is infectious, often in patients with a localized bacterial pneumonia. Pneumatoceles differ in appearance from abscesses by way of their air-filled cavities and thin, regular walls. The cyst is frequently larger than the preceding cavitation due to resulting expansion from

elastic recoil by surrounding lung. Infectious pneumatoceles are most commonly seen in staphylococcal and streptococcal infections but have also been seen in pneumococcus and Gram negative infections [3, 5, 46]. Pneumatoceles may also be seen in immunocompromised patients due to *Pneumocystis jiroveci* infection (see above). Infectious cysts that persist despite resolution of primary infection should raise suspicion of less common infections like *Pneumocystis* or *Echinococcus*. Pneumatoceles may also occur as a complication of blunt trauma [47, 48] or aspiration of hydrocarbon fluid [5, 49].

(iii) Aspergillus. Cavitations secondary to tuberculosis and other chronic infections can provide a nidus for fungus balls, visible as intracavitary soft tissue lesions with an air meniscus on CT [6]. Although there is a significant overlap in the appearances of aspergilloma and malignancy, dependent location, adjacent bronchiectasis, and nonenhancement of the mass on contrast favor aspergilloma [50]. Other forms of *Aspergillus* infections include allergic bronchopulmonary aspergillosis (ABPA) in patients with chronic airway disease and invasive and semi-invasive pulmonary aspergillosis seen in immunocompromised patients. ABPA may cause proximal central bronchiectasis, due to bronchial damage. In invasive pulmonary aspergillosis, air crescents on CT result from cavitary necrosis of infected tissue presenting with a characteristic halo sign and indicate immune system recovery [6]. The soft tissue density in invasive aspergillosis represents necrotic tissue and is not freely movable as in the case of an aspergilloma. Chronic necrotizing pulmonary aspergillosis is another form that is associated with cavitary infiltrates that occur in patients with chronic lung disease and immunosuppressive conditions such as alcoholism and diabetes [30].

2.2.2. Caseous

(i) Tuberculosis. Tuberculomas are granulomas usually less than 3 cm in diameter, frequently seen in an upper lobe [40]. These lesions are characterized by a lack of temporal progression and evidence of dystrophic calcification. Long-standing tuberculomas undergo caseous necrosis resulting in expulsion of necrotic debris into the bronchial airways. Caseous necrosis has also been described in other fungal infections like cryptococcosis, coccidioidomycosis, and histoplasmosis [51]. The walls of an untreated tuberculous cavity are usually thick and irregular [5]. Calcified hilar lymphadenopathy supports the diagnosis. Nontuberculous mycobacterial (NTM) infections are also known to cause cysts which are more thin-walled and surrounded by less dense consolidation when compared with tuberculous lesions [5]. The presence of cavitation in association with right middle lobe and lingular bronchiectasis and nodules often suggests nontuberculous mycobacterial disease. Cystic lesions and bronchiectasis are more characteristic CT findings in NTM infections and help in differentiation [52].

A mimicker of tuberculomas is actinomycosis which typically manifests as an area of persistent consolidation or a mass, either of which may contain cavitation [41]. Chest wall invasion may occur. Bronchogenic carcinoma must also be considered as it may present as a cavitary lesion (see below).

2.2.3. Ischemic

(i) Autoimmune/Rheumatologic Diseases. Among the autoimmune disorders, Wegener's granulomatosis with angiitis and rheumatoid disease is most commonly associated with cavitations [5, 30]. Lung involvement in rheumatoid arthritis is not uncommon and may present as necrobiotic nodules which are characteristically multiple, peripheral, and thick-walled, resolving with treatment [53] (Figure 13). Wegener's granulomatosis with angiitis is a clinicopathological entity characterized by necrotizing granulomas involving the upper and lower respiratory tract causing cavitations in up to half the cases of lung involvement [54]. Cavitations occasionally occur within nodules distributed along the bronchovascular bundles, interlobular septa, major fissures, and subpleural regions in pulmonary sarcoidosis [34]. Cavities are less frequently encountered in other autoimmune diseases and are more likely to be infectious in origin from immunosuppressive use [44].

(ii) Amyloidosis. AL is generally found in primary amyloidosis in association with monoclonal plasma cell proliferation such as multiple myeloma, whereas protein AA is the major component of secondary amyloidosis, a feature of chronic inflammatory disorders [33]. Amyloidosis can present in the lung in three forms: nodular, diffuse parenchymal, and tracheobronchial. The formation of cysts is a late and relatively rare manifestation and they occur most commonly in localized amyloidosis in association with Sjögren's syndrome, resulting from peribronchiolar deposition of amyloid [11]. However, cysts in Sjögren's syndrome may also present secondary to LIP (see section on LIP) [55]. It must be remembered that Sjögren's syndrome can present with a wide range of interstitial patterns including nonspecific interstitial pneumonia, lymphocytic interstitial pneumonia, usual interstitial pneumonia, and organizing pneumonia. Pulmonary amyloidosis accompanying Sjögren's syndrome and lymphoproliferative disease generally manifests as multiple, large, thin-walled cysts and nodules in areas of lymphocyte predominance which include the interlobular septae, bronchovascular interstitium, and subpleural areas; honeycombing and traction bronchiectasis may also be seen [11, 55]. Such cases may be differentiated from bronchiectasis in which the cysts have thicker walls and are more centrally located [33]. Calcified nodules on CT are a fairly characteristic finding in amyloidosis.

2.2.4. Intratumoral

(i) Neoplasms. A study by Woodring et al. [12] showed that it is possible to make a specific diagnosis of benignancy or malignancy based on the measurement of the thickest part of the cavity wall, with lesions with less than 4 mm of

wall thickness considered as benign and greater than 15 mm of wall thickness considered as malignant. Chronic cavities (greater than 1 month in duration) are more likely to be malignant, congenital, or a result of chronic inflammatory disorders; acute cavities (less than 1 month from onset) are often infectious, inflammatory, septic embolic, or traumatic in origin [3].

Cavitary neoplasms are formed by central necrosis with expulsion of the necrotic tumor debris into the communicating airways. Other mechanisms for cyst formation in both primary and metastatic lung tumors include check valve effects (formed by neoplastic stenosis) and destruction of the alveolar sacs. Uniformly distended progressively enlarging cysts on serial CT scans suggest check valve effects from micrometastastic tumor lesions. Also, tumors in the lung can masquerade as abscesses or other forms of benign cysts [18]. A tumor may very rarely present as benign looking thin-walled cyst [56]. Hence, early and complete resection of benign lung cysts is advisable [18]. Alternatively, a high degree of suspicion is required and careful detection of the changes in clinical and radiologic findings over time is important to avoid missing the diagnosis [56]. Cavitary tumor lesions in the lung are usually from squamous cell carcinomas [5] (Figure 9). Lung adenocarcinoma can rarely present with cystic lesions and should be suspected in patients with mediastinal masses and diffuse cystic lesions in the lung [53] (Figure 10). Endobronchial neoplasms may also cause a solitary cyst via a check valve mechanism. Cysts may also develop as a postchemotherapy effect due to cavitary necrosis of solid tumor masses [57].

Cystic metastases have been described in endometrial, pancreatic, and colon cancers. Cystic lung metastases occur more frequently in tumors of epithelial origin and less frequently in tumors of mesenchymal and hematopoietic origin. Nevertheless, cystic lesions have been described in metastatic osteosarcoma [58], leiomyosarcoma [59], synovial sarcoma [59], and epithelioid sarcoma [60], among others.

(ii) Airway Papillomatosis. Squamous cell papillomata are benign proliferation of squamous mucosa. Papillomata are the most common benign tumors in the laryngotracheal region [61]. Lesions are often limited to the nasopharynx but can descend to involve the tracheobronchial tree and lung by microaspiration or a multicentric origin, causing small solid or cavitary lesions (Figure 11). Cysts may result either from obstructive emphysema or from cavitatory necrosis of the papillomatous lesions [5].

2.3. Alveolar Rupture and Air Space Confluence

(i) Emphysema. Emphysema is characterized by permanently enlarged air spaces distal to the terminal bronchiole with destruction of the alveolar walls [9]. Emphysema may be classified into various types, based on the pattern of lung parenchyma destruction with respect to the secondary pulmonary lobule: proximal acinus in centriacinar (centrilobular) emphysema and distal in paraseptal and whole acinus in panacinar (panlobular) emphysema. Centrilobular type is more often found in upper lung zones (i.e., the posterior and apical segments of the upper lobes or the superior segments of the lower lobes) and is commonly associated with cigarette smoking [62]. The emphysematous centriacinar air spaces over time may conflate into large air spaces with bizarre shapes. Typical findings by CT include irregular, small, round, or confluent areas of low attenuation interspersed within normal lung, often in proximity to the center of a secondary pulmonary artery. The cysts in the centrilobular form of emphysema have central nodularity due to the presence of intralobular pulmonary artery allowing differentiation from the cysts seen in PLCH and LAM [6]. Centriacinar emphysema, unlike panacinar emphysema, is recognizable by its easily discernible contrast from the surrounding normal lung [63]. Other differentiating radiologic features from panlobular emphysema include upper lobe predominance, greater degree of lung inflation, and less frequent bullous formation [64, 65]. Bullous emphysema can occur either in centrilobular or in panlobular emphysema and does not refer to any specific pathological entity. It is simply a more advanced form of emphysema characterized by the presence of blebs/bullae conflated by ruptured pulmonary alveoli. These giant blebs may grow to achieve significantly large volumes occupying an entire lobe with the potential to rupture and complicate as pneumothorax [10, 66] (Figure 7). Bullous emphysema is the most common attributable cause of lung cyst formation [5].

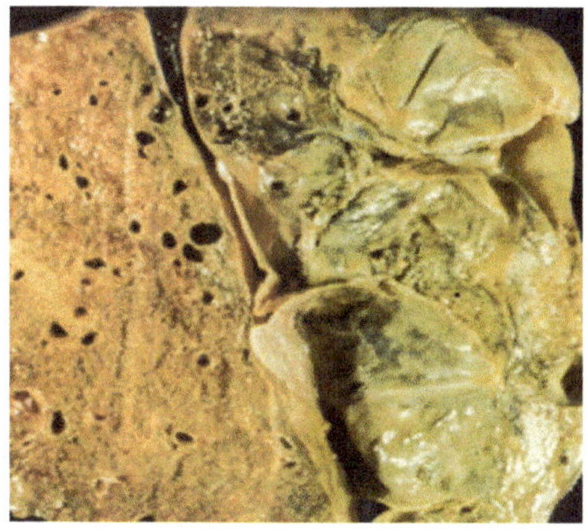

Figure 7: Gross specimen showing lung tissue with scattered thin-walled bullae. Large bullous cavity resulting from expansion of one of the bullous air spaces.

(ii) Syndromes

Birt-Hogg-Dubé (BHD) Syndrome. Birt-Hogg-Dubé (BHD) syndrome is an autosomal dominant condition characterized by cutaneous papular skin lesions, multiple lung cysts that may cause pneumothorax, and an increased risk of renal tumors [67]. The syndrome is caused by a deletion of the FLCN gene on chromosome 17 which encodes the protein folliculin. The lung cysts are elongated and oval, closely associated with the peripheral interlobular septum, visceral pleura, or septal-pleural junctional region; the rupture of these cysts may result in pneumothoraces (Figure 8). These cysts are lined by a layer of alveolar epithelium. Several

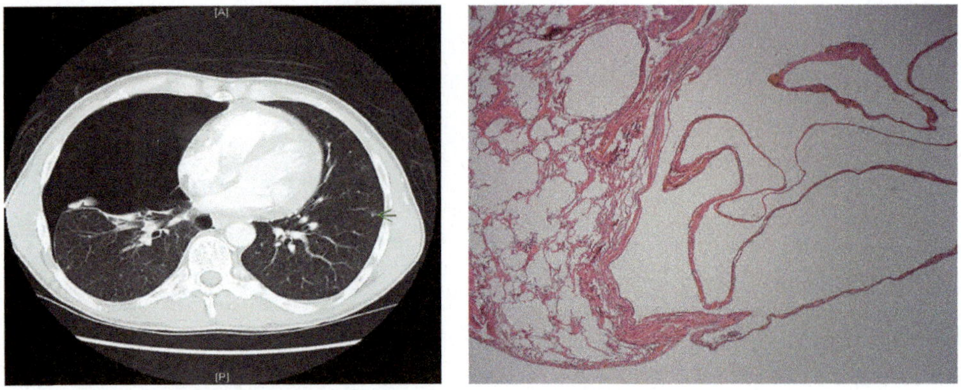

(a) (b)

FIGURE 8: (a) HRCT of the lung showing pneumothorax on the right. Pneumothoraces tend to arise from the rupture of peripherally located cysts as pointed out on the left of the image (green arrow). (b) A low power view (×40) showing the ruptured cyst lined by a thin-walled alveolar epithelium.

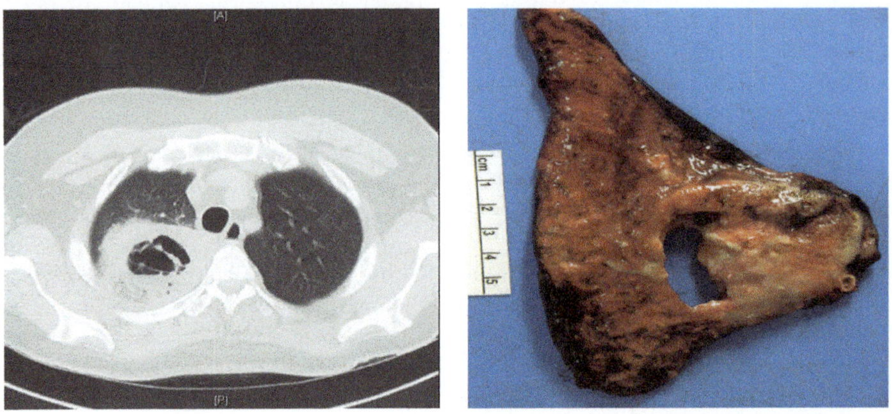

(a) (b)

FIGURE 9: Squamous cell carcinoma. (a) HRCT of the right lung demonstrating a large thick-walled solitary cavitation with internal septations. (b) Gross specimen demonstrating a large area of cavitation with thick surrounding walls from malignant infiltration.

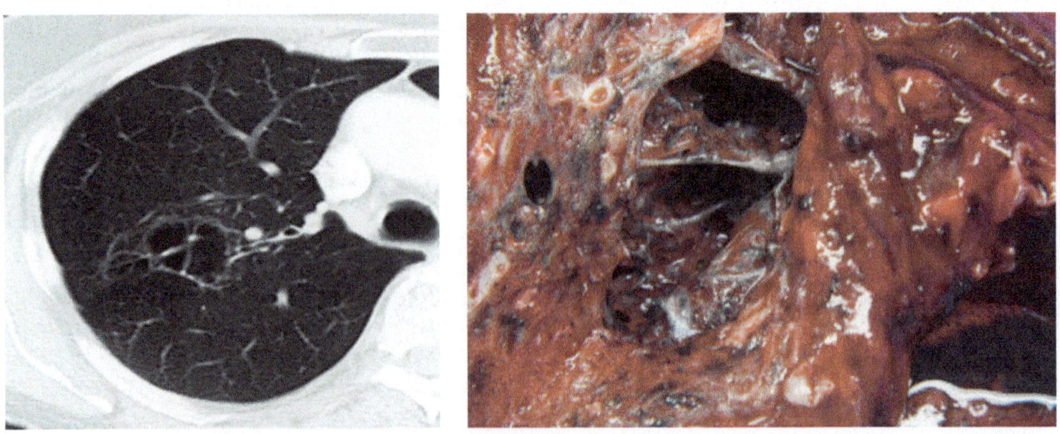

(a) (b)

FIGURE 10: Adenocarcinoma with cystic change. (a) Gross surgical specimen of resected lung tissue showing the cystic mass, with thin-walled septations. (b) High-resolution CT scan of the right lung demonstrates a large, thick-walled cavitary mass in the upper lobe. Multiple thin septations are present within the mass.

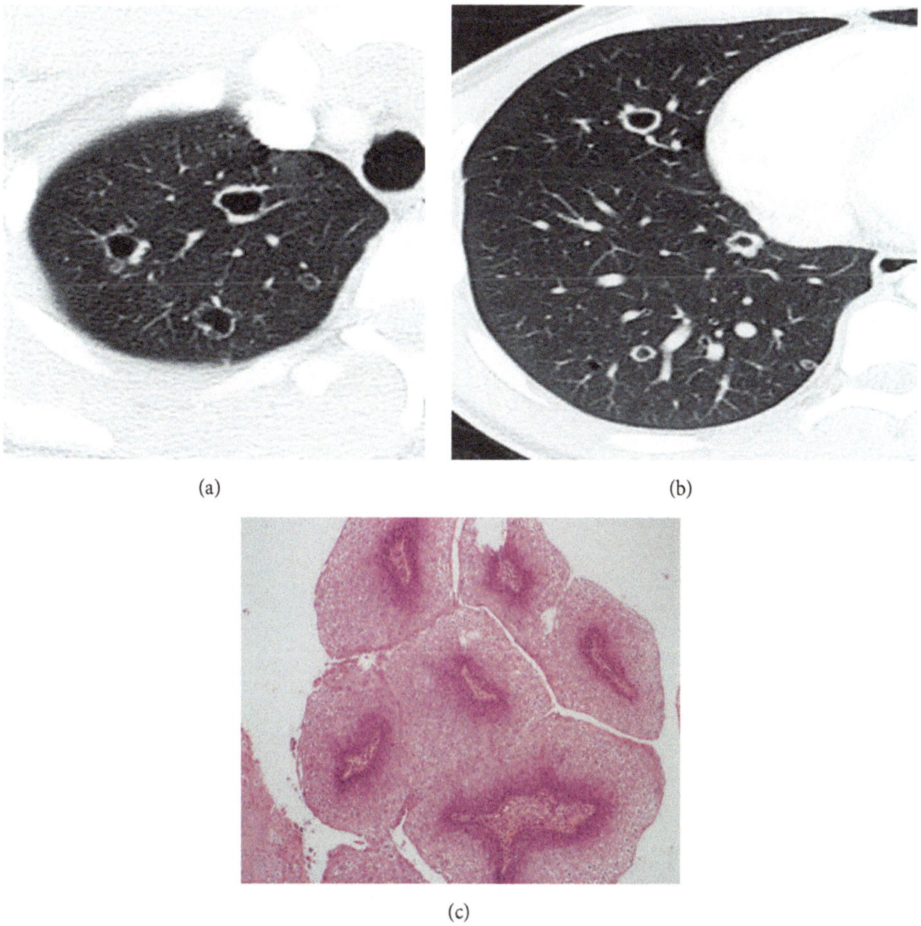

FIGURE 11: Airway papillomatosis. (a and b) HRCT of the right lung at descending levels reveals multiple pulmonary nodules, many of which have undergone cavitation to form irregular thin-walled cysts. (c) High power view showing papillomata with central fibrovascular core surrounded by benign squamous epithelium with evidence of hyperkeratosis and parakeratosis (magnification ×100).

mechanisms have been proposed for the mechanism of formation of the lung cysts in BHD including inflammation and growth failure (secondary to haploinsufficiency of folliculin leading to deranged alveolar development) [68]. Both BHD and lymphangioleiomyomatosis may be seen in middle-aged women. However, unlike the cysts of LAM, those seen in BHD are larger and nonprogressive and are predominant in the lower and medial zones of the lung [68].

Ehlers-Danlos Syndrome (EDS). Ehlers-Danlos syndrome (EDS) is an inherited disorder of connective tissue with multiple thoracic manifestations. One of the thoracic manifestations of EDS is the presence of parenchymal cysts. The cysts are due to formation of hematomas with subsequent cavitation which may result in hemoptysis following communication with the tracheobronchial tree [69]. Repair by osseous metaplasia results in the formation of fibroosseous nodules, a rather unusual thoracic manifestation [69].

(iii) Traumatic. Posttraumatic pneumatoceles (traumatic pulmonary pseudocysts) following blunt thoracic trauma are not frequently observed [37, 47]. Pulmonary contusion is the usual pattern of lung injury following blunt chest trauma. The mechanism of cyst formation appears to be due to inciting trauma with subsequent elastic recoil of the normal surrounding parenchyma creating clefts between the normal and injured parenchymata [37]. These clefts may be alveolar or interstitial. Pneumatoceles may also form secondary to increased intrapulmonary pressure due to positive pressure ventilation. These are typically transient and resolve with time.

2.4. Cystic Expansion of Structures with Lung Displacement

2.4.1. Infectious

Parasitic Cysts

Hydatid Cyst. Hydatid cysts primarily involve the liver. In the case of pulmonary involvement, a simple hydatid cyst is most common in the right lower lobe [42], though it may arise anywhere including the upper lobes. Cysts in the lung are commonly multiple with wall thickness from 0.2 to 1 cm. CT and radiography are the diagnostic methods of choice, considering high false positive results with serodiagnosis

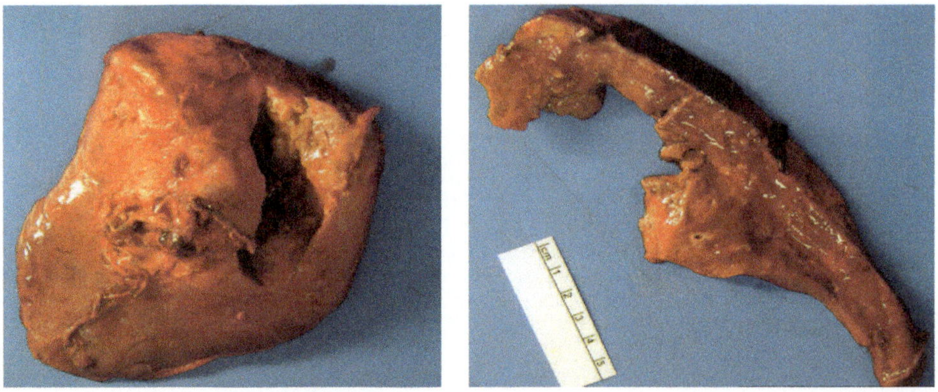

(a) (b)

FIGURE 12: (a) Gross surgical specimen of lung demonstrating a necrotic fungal cavity; (b) cut section of the lung showing an irregular contoured necrotic wall.

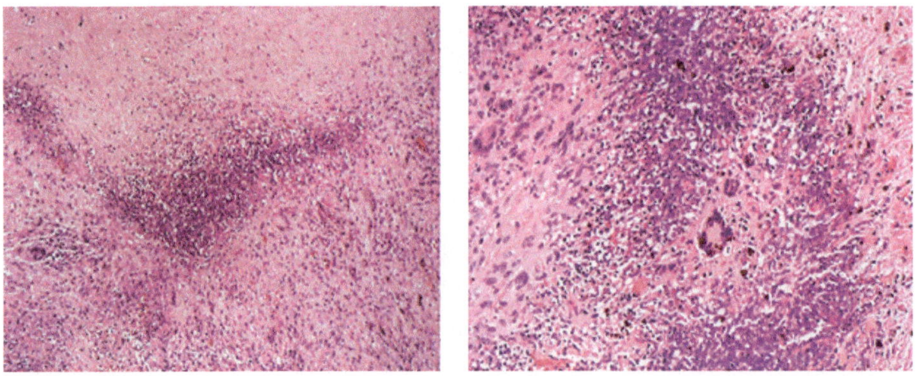

(a) (b)

FIGURE 13: Left: (a) high power view showing coagulative necrosis (upper center) surrounded by multinucleated giant cells in a poorly formed granuloma surrounded by palisading histiocytes (magnification ×100). Right: (b) a higher power view demonstrating necrobiotic granuloma comprising multinucleated giant cells (center of the image), surrounded by palisading histiocytes (magnification ×200).

[42]. Bronchiolar erosion into the pericyst may introduce air between the pericyst and the laminated membrane. These air collections appear as radiolucent crescents in the upper part of the cyst and are known as the crescent sign. Demonstration of air bubbles (formed by air dissecting between the pericyst and the parasitic membrane) with ring enhancement is a strong indicator of infected hydatid cysts [42].

Paragonimiasis. Paragonimiasis is an infection caused by lung flukes of the genus *Paragonimus*. In Asia, *P. westermani* infections are relatively common where diets include raw or salted crustaceans. Mammals acquire the infection when they ingest raw or undercooked crustaceans [70]. Features seen on CT include linear opacities (due to worm migration tracks or focal atelectasis due to obstruction of the airway lumina); focal air space consolidation (due to hemorrhagic pneumonia, as the parasite travels through the parenchyma); and cysts due to the infarction by blocking of the arteriole or vein by the expansion of the parasite in the lung tissue [43]. Clinicians should consider the diagnosis of paragonimiasis in all patients with cough, fever, and pleural effusion with peripheral eosinophilia [70].

2.4.2. Congenital/Hamartomatous. Congenital cystic lesions typically present during childhood but may rarely manifest in adults. These lesions must be distinguished from other acquired adult cystic diseases. A brief discussion on the more common congenital cystic diseases is included.

(i) Congenital Pulmonary Airway Malformation (CPAM), Formally Congenital Cystic Adenomatoid Malformation (CCAM). CPAM is rare in adults and can be a frequently underdiagnosed entity. Bronchoalveolar dysgenesis during the first trimester results in adenomatoid hamartomatous proliferation of terminal bronchiolar units (hence its former name). Histologically, the CPAM lesions are characterized by bronchiolar proliferation and columnar or cuboidal epithelium lined micro- and macrocysts [71]. CPAM was originally classified into 3 types, by Stocker, and was later revised to include Type 0 and Type 4 [72, 73]. Type 1 is the most

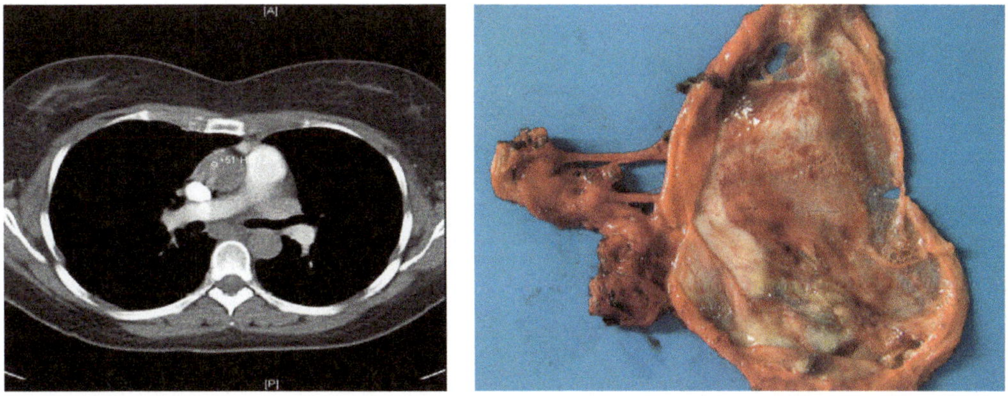

(a) (b)

FIGURE 14: (a) Bronchogenic cyst. High-resolution CT scan reveals a 5.0 × 7.0 cm, well-circumscribed, thin-walled cystic mass of fluid density (+51 Hounsfield units) arising within the right lung and abutting the posterior aspect of the heart. There is no communication with the bronchus. (b) Gross specimen of a bronchogenic cyst bisected to reveal a smooth inner surface with punctate hemorrhagic foci and mucoid material and interrupted by trabeculations.

common form with large cysts ranging from 2 to 10 cm in diameter. Type 1 CPAM is a known precursor for mucinous adenocarcinoma [74]. Type 4 CPAM can present as a solitary cyst typically involving a single lobe [73]. These lesions, unlike bronchogenic cysts, have a connection with the central airways. Lack of reliable differentiating characteristics, due to shared pathogenesis, sometimes necessitates histologic exam in order to rule out the latter. Additionally, histological diagnosis may be difficult to make due to architectural distortions from prior infections [71].

(ii) Bronchogenic Cysts. Bronchogenic cysts (BC) represent congenital abnormalities resulting from abnormal budding of the developing tracheobronchial tree. While they typically appear as intraparenchymal masses, they may also manifest as cystic cavities, usually within the lower lobes [30]. As alluded to, they do not communicate with the tracheobronchial tree. However, supervening infection may establish a communication with airways allowing the cysts to enlarge rapidly [3].

The high attenuation of bronchogenic cysts on CT scans is caused by hemorrhage, mucoid proteinaceous fluid, or calcium oxalate [73, 75] (see Figure 14). These cysts may be intrapulmonary or mediastinal in location [75]. These cysts are frequently superinfected further complicating the clinical picture. Sometimes, definitive diagnosis is only possible by coupled histopathological examination. Along these lines, the most reliable criterion for the diagnosis of intrapulmonary BC is considered as the presence of cartilage in the cyst wall.

(iii) Sequestration. Bronchopulmonary sequestration refers to the isolation of a portion of the lung with development under its own arterial supply. Sequestration is a rare phenomenon in adults [76, 77]. Two variants exist based on whether visceral pleura encompasses the isolated segment along with (intralobar sequestration) or distinctly from (extralobar sequestration) the main [30, 73]; 75% of sequestrations are intralobar with the majority of them occurring in the basilar segment of the left and right lower lobes [78]. Intralobar sequestrations are complicated by recurrent infections and bronchial obstruction. As in intralobar sequestration, extralobar sequestration occurs most often on the left, is often peripheral, and presents as a wedge-shaped density associated with the left diaphragm in almost 90% of cases [3]. A definitive diagnosis can be made by demonstrating the aberrant systemic arterial blood supply as a linearly enhancing structure adjacent to the aorta on contrast CT [79]. Diagnosis requires maintaining a high degree of clinical suspicion in young and middle-aged patients with left lower lobe cystic lesions.

3. Conclusions

In this review, we provided an overview of the diseases most commonly associated with cystic lung lesions in adults, by illustration and description of pathologic and radiologic features of each entity. We also classified pulmonary cystic disease with an emphasis on pathophysiology behind cyst formation in an attempt to explain the characteristics of similar cystic appearances seen in various disease entities. It is possible to make a fairly specific diagnosis during early stages of disease evolution by its relatively distinct radiological presentation which is very well appreciated on high-resolution CT scans. Distinct pathologic presentations caused by a variety of insults to the lung, over time, progress to converge into relatively nonspecific chronic injury patterns characterized by cysts among other features. Although specificities of HRCTs are much improved with resultant decrease for the need of surgical biopsies, microscopic analysis may provide the only method of diagnosis during the later stages of lung injury where gross pathologic and radiologic manifestations tend to be relatively nonspecific. Some of these diseases may manifest rarely with atypical and unusual presentations, requiring a multidisciplinary approach to arrive at an accurate diagnosis.

Competing Interests

The authors certify that they have no affiliations with or involvement in any organization or entity with any financial interest or nonfinancial interest in the subject matter or materials discussed in this manuscript.

Authors' Contributions

All the authors had a role in writing this manuscript.

References

[1] G. P. Genereux, "The end stage lung. Pathogenesis, pathology, and radiology," *Radiology*, vol. 116, no. 2, pp. 279–289, 1975.

[2] W. J. Tuddenham, "Glossary of terms for thoracic radiology: recommendations of the nomenclature committee of the Fleischner society," *American Journal of Roentgenology*, vol. 143, no. 3, pp. 509–517, 1984.

[3] G. P. Cosgrove, S. K. Frankel, and K. K. Brown, "Challenges in pulmonary fibrosis. 3: cystic lung disease," *Thorax*, vol. 62, no. 9, pp. 820–829, 2007.

[4] C. Rowan, D. M. Hansell, E. Renzoni et al., "Diffuse cystic lung disease of unexplained cause with coexistent small airway disease: a possible causal relationship?" *American Journal of Surgical Pathology*, vol. 36, no. 2, pp. 228–234, 2012.

[5] J. D. Godwin, W. R. Webb, C. J. Savoca, G. Gamsu, and P. C. Goodman, "Multiple, thin-walled cystic lesions of the lung," *American Journal of Roentgenology*, vol. 135, no. 3, pp. 593–604, 1980.

[6] J. Collins, "CT signs and patterns of lung disease," *Radiologic Clinics of North America*, vol. 39, no. 6, pp. 1115–1135, 2001.

[7] A. K. Attili, E. A. Kazerooni, B. H. Gross, K. R. Flaherty, J. L. Myers, and F. J. Martinez, "Smoking-related interstitial lung disease: radiologic-clinical-pathologic correlation," *Radiographics*, vol. 28, no. 5, pp. 1383–1396, 2009.

[8] P. J. Friedman and C. A. G. Hellekant, "Radiologic recognition of bronchopleural fistula," *Radiology*, vol. 124, no. 2, pp. 289–295, 1977.

[9] D. M. Hansell, A. A. Bankier, H. MacMahon, T. C. McLoud, N. L. Müller, and J. Remy, "Fleischner society: glossary of terms for thoracic imaging," *Radiology*, vol. 246, no. 3, pp. 697–722, 2008.

[10] D. Geddes, M. Davies, H. Koyama et al., "Effect of lung-volume-reduction surgery in patients with severe emphysema," *The New England Journal of Medicine*, vol. 343, no. 4, pp. 239–245, 2000.

[11] D. M. Seaman, C. A. Meyer, M. D. Gilman, and F. X. McCormack, "Diffuse cystic lung disease at high-resolution CT," *American Journal of Roentgenology*, vol. 196, no. 6, pp. 1305–1311, 2011.

[12] J. H. Woodring, A. M. Fried, and V. P. Chuang, "Solitary cavities of the lung: diagnostic implications of cavity wall thickness," *American Journal of Roentgenology*, vol. 135, no. 6, pp. 1269–1271, 1980.

[13] F. S. Bonelli, T. E. Hartman, S. J. Swensen, and A. Sherrick, "Accuracy of high-resolution CT in diagnosing lung diseases," *American Journal of Roentgenology*, vol. 170, no. 6, pp. 1507–1512, 1998.

[14] M. Koyama, T. Johkoh, O. Honda et al., "Chronic cystic lung disease: diagnostic accuracy of high-resolution CT in 92 patients," *American Journal of Roentgenology*, vol. 180, no. 3, pp. 827–835, 2003.

[15] J. S. Park, K. K. Brown, R. M. Tuder, V. A. E. Hale, T. E. King Jr., and D. A. Lynch, "Respiratory bronchiolitis-associated interstitial lung disease: radiologic features with clinical and pathologic correlation," *Journal of Computer Assisted Tomography*, vol. 26, no. 1, pp. 13–20, 2002.

[16] M. Akira, S. Yamamoto, H. Hara, M. Sakatani, and E. Ueda, "Serial computed tomographic evaluation in desquamative interstitial pneumonia," *Thorax*, vol. 52, no. 4, pp. 333–337, 1997.

[17] S. S. Hare, C. A. Souza, G. Bain, J. M. Seely, M. M. Gomes, and M. Quigley, "The radiological spectrum of pulmonary lymphoproliferative disease," *British Journal of Radiology*, vol. 85, no. 1015, pp. 848–864, 2012.

[18] D. Cabibi, A. Sciuto, G. Geraci, C. Lo Nigro, G. Modica, and M. Cajozzo, "Cystic mucinous adenocarcinoma of the lung: a case report," *Journal of Cardiothoracic Surgery*, vol. 6, no. 1, article 128, 2011.

[19] Y. Ichikawa, M. Kinoshita, T. Koga, K. Oizumi, K. Fujimoto, and N. Hayabuchi, "Lung cyst formation in lymphocytic interstitial pneumonia: Ct features," *Journal of Computer Assisted Tomography*, vol. 18, no. 5, pp. 745–748, 1994.

[20] C. I. S. Silva, J. D. Flint, R. D. Levy, and N. L. Müller, "Diffuse lung cysts in lymphoid interstitial pneumonia: high-resolution CT and pathologic findings," *Journal of Thoracic Imaging*, vol. 21, no. 3, pp. 241–244, 2006.

[21] T. Johkoh, N. L. Müller, H. A. Pickford et al., "Lymphocytic interstitial pneumonia: thin-section CT findings in 22 patients," *Radiology*, vol. 212, no. 2, pp. 567–572, 1999.

[22] O. Honda, T. Johkoh, K. Ichikado et al., "Differential diagnosis of lymphocytic interstitial pneumonia and malignant lymphoma on high-resolution CT," *American Journal of Roentgenology*, vol. 173, no. 1, pp. 71–74, 1999.

[23] M. Corti, M. F. Villafañe, N. Trione, R. Schtirbu, and M. Narbaitz, "Primary pulmonary AIDS-related lymphoma," *Revista do Instituto de Medicina Tropical de São Paulo*, vol. 47, no. 4, pp. 231–234, 2005.

[24] R. Filly, N. Blank, and R. A. Castellino, "Radiographic distribution of intrathoracic disease in previously untreated patients with Hodgkin's disease and non Hodgkin's lymphoma," *Radiology*, vol. 120, no. 2, pp. 277–281, 1976.

[25] A. Sakashita, K. Ashizawa, K. Minami et al., "Localized ground glass opacities with multiple pulmonary small cysts in adult T-cell leukemia or lymphoma: an "alloy wheel" appearance," *Journal of Thoracic Imaging*, vol. 24, no. 4, pp. 321–324, 2009.

[26] E. Hardak, O. Brook, and M. Yigla, "Radiological features of pneumocystis jirovecii pneumonia in immunocompromised patients with and without AIDS," *Lung*, vol. 188, no. 2, pp. 159–163, 2010.

[27] J. P. Kanne, D. R. Yandow, and C. A. Meyer, "*Pneumocystis jiroveci* pneumonia: high-resolution CT findings in patients with and without HIV infection," *American Journal of Roentgenology*, vol. 198, no. 6, pp. W555–W561, 2012.

[28] C. Ferre, F. Baguena, D. Podzamczer et al., "Lung cavitation associated with Pneumocystis carinii infection in the acquired immunodeficiency syndrome: a report of six cases and review of the literature," *European Respiratory Journal*, vol. 7, no. 1, pp. 134–139, 1994.

[29] A. C. Greiwe, K. Miller, C. Farver, and C. T. Lau, "AIRP best cases in radiologic-pathologic correlation: pulmonary langerhans cell histiocytosis," *Radiographics*, vol. 32, no. 4, pp. 987–990, 2012.

[30] J. H. Ryu and S. J. Swensen, "Cystic and cavitary lung diseases: focal and diffuse," *Mayo Clinic Proceedings*, vol. 78, no. 6, pp. 744–752, 2003.

[31] B. C. Moulton and A. F. Barker, "Pathogenesis of bronchiectasis," *Clinics in Chest Medicine*, vol. 33, no. 2, pp. 211–217, 2012.

[32] K. B. Newman and W. R. Beam, "Congenital bronchiectasis in an adult," *The American Journal of Medicine*, vol. 91, no. 2, pp. 198–201, 1991.

[33] S. Ohdama, S. Akagawa, O. Matsubara, and Y. Yoshizawa, "Primary diffuse alveolar septal amyloidosis with multiple cysts and calcification," *European Respiratory Journal*, vol. 9, no. 7, pp. 1569–1571, 1996.

[34] N. L. Muller, P. Kullnig, and R. R. Miller, "The CT findings of pulmonary sarcoidosis: analysis of 25 patients," *American Journal of Roentgenology*, vol. 152, no. 6, pp. 1179–1182, 1989.

[35] M. Nishino, B. Siewert, D. H. Roberts et al., "Excessive collapsibility of bronchi in bronchiectasis: evaluation on volumetric expiratory high-resolution CT," *Journal of Computer Assisted Tomography*, vol. 30, no. 3, pp. 474–478, 2006.

[36] L. Marti-Bonmati, F. J. Catala, and F. R. Perales, "Computed tomography differentiation between cystic bronchiectasis and bullae," *Journal of Thoracic Imaging*, vol. 7, no. 1, pp. 83–85, 1991.

[37] B. Milliron, T. S. Henry, S. Veeraraghavan, and B. P. Little, "Bronchiectasis: mechanisms and imaging clues of associated common and uncommon diseases," *Radiographics*, vol. 35, no. 4, pp. 1011–1030, 2015.

[38] J. Murphy, P. Schnyder, C. Herold, and C. Flower, "Bronchiolitis obliterans organising pneumonia simulating bronchial carcinoma," *European Radiology*, vol. 8, no. 7, pp. 1165–1169, 1998.

[39] Kyung Soo Lee, P. Kullnig, T. E. Hartman, and N. L. Muller, "Cryptogenic organizing pneumonia: CT findings in 43 patients," *American Journal of Roentgenology*, vol. 162, no. 3, pp. 543–546, 1994.

[40] J. M. Goo and J.-G. Im, "CT of tuberculosis and nontuberculous mycobacterial infections," *Radiologic Clinics of North America*, vol. 40, no. 1, pp. 73–87, 2002.

[41] R. A. Smego Jr. and G. Foglia, "Actinomycosis," *Clinical Infectious Diseases*, vol. 26, no. 6, pp. 1255–1261, 1998.

[42] D. Biswas, A. Dey, S. Biswas, and M. Chakraborty, "It's easy to miss complicated hydatid cyst of lung," *Lung India*, vol. 27, no. 3, pp. 164–166, 2010.

[43] J. G. Im, Y. Kong, Y. M. Shin et al., "Pulmonary paragonimiasis: clinical and experimental studies," *Radiographics : a review publication of the Radiological Society of North America, Inc*, vol. 13, no. 3, pp. 575–586, 1993.

[44] L. B. Gadkowski and J. E. Stout, "Cavitary pulmonary disease," *Clinical Microbiology Reviews*, vol. 21, no. 2, pp. 305–333, 2008.

[45] I. Kuhajda, K. Zarogoulidis, K. Tsirgogianni et al., "Lung abscess-etiology, diagnostic and treatment options," *Annals of Translational Medicine*, vol. 3, no. 13, p. 183, 2015.

[46] S. Al-Saleh, H. Grasemann, and P. Cox, "Necrotizing pneumonia complicated by early and late pneumatoceles," *Canadian Respiratory Journal*, vol. 15, no. 3, pp. 129–132, 2008.

[47] K. Kaira, T. Ishizuka, N. Yanagitani, N. Sunaga, T. Hisada, and M. Mori, "Pulmonary traumatic pneumatocele and hematoma," *Japanese Journal of Radiology*, vol. 27, no. 2, pp. 100–102, 2009.

[48] T. C. Yang, C. Huang, J. Yu, F. Hsieh, and Y. Huang, "Traumatic pneumatocele," *Pediatrics & Neonatology*, vol. 51, no. 2, pp. 135–138, 2010.

[49] V. J. Harris and R. Brown, "Pneumatoceles as a complication of chemical pneumonia after hydrocarbon ingestion," *"The American Journal of Roentgenology, Radium Therapy, and Nuclear Medicine*, vol. 125, no. 3, pp. 531–537, 1975.

[50] Y. Park, T. S. Kim, C. A. Yi, E. Y. Cho, H. Kim, and Y. S. Choi, "Pulmonary cavitary mass containing a mural nodule: differential diagnosis between intracavitary aspergilloma and cavitating lung cancer on contrast-enhanced computed tomography," *Clinical Radiology*, vol. 62, no. 3, pp. 227–232, 2007.

[51] E. Sada Diaz, N. Hernandez, and J. Perez Roman, "Pulmonary histoplasmosis. Experience at the National Institute of Respiratory Diseases," *Revista de Investigación Clínica*, vol. 40, no. 4, pp. 333–339, 1988.

[52] M.-K. Yuan, C.-Y. Chang, P.-H. Tsai, Y.-M. Lee, J.-W. Huang, and S.-C. Chang, "Comparative chest computed tomography findings of non-tuberculous mycobacterial lung diseases and pulmonary tuberculosis in patients with acid fast bacilli smear-positive sputum," *BMC Pulmonary Medicine*, vol. 14, article 65, 2014.

[53] F. G. Burrows, "Pulmonary nodules in rheumatoid disease: a report of two cases," *British Journal of Radiology*, vol. 40, no. 472, pp. 256–261, 1967.

[54] A. S. Fauci and S. M. Wolff, "Wegener's granulomatosis: studies in eighteen patients and a review of the literature," *Medicine*, vol. 52, no. 6, pp. 535–561, 1973.

[55] Y. J. Jeong, K. S. Lee, M. P. Chung et al., "Amyloidosis and Lymphoproliferative disease in Sjögren syndrome: thin-section computed tomography findings and histopathologic comparisons," *Journal of Computer Assisted Tomography*, vol. 28, no. 6, pp. 776–781, 2004.

[56] T. Iwata, N. Nishiyama, K. Nagano et al., "Squamous cell carcinoma presenting as a solitary growing cyst in lung: a diagnostic pitfall in daily clinical practice," *Annals of Thoracic and Cardiovascular Surgery*, vol. 15, no. 3, pp. 174–177, 2009.

[57] J. B. Hoag, M. Sherman, Q. Fasihuddin, and M. E. Lund, "A comprehensive review of spontaneous pneumothorax complicating sarcoma," *Chest*, vol. 138, no. 3, pp. 510–518, 2010.

[58] N. Songür, A. Karakaş, M. Arikan, S. Demir, A. Bozkurt, and A. Uçaner, "Multiple cystic pulmonary metastases from osteosarcoma," *Respiration*, vol. 72, no. 4, article no. 418, 2005.

[59] S. T. Traweek, A. J. Rotter, W. Swartz, and N. Azumi, "Cystic pulmonary metastatic sarcoma," *Cancer*, vol. 65, no. 8, pp. 1805–1811, 1990.

[60] J. K. C. Chan, W. Y. W. Tsang, M. Y. Pau, M. C. Tang, S. W. Pang, and C. D. M. Fletcher, "Lymphangiomyomatosis and angiomyolipoma: closely related entities characterized by hamartomatous proliferation of HMB-45-positive smooth muscle," *Histopathology*, vol. 22, no. 5, pp. 445–455, 1993.

[61] L. Zawadzka-Głos, A. Jakubowska, M. Chmielik, A. Bielicka, and M. Brzewski, "Lower airway papillomatosis in children," *International Journal of Pediatric Otorhinolaryngology*, vol. 67, no. 10, pp. 1117–1121, 2003.

[62] A. Choromańska and K. J. Macura, "Role of computed tomography in quantitative assessment of emphysema," *Polish Journal of Radiology*, vol. 77, no. 1, pp. 28–36, 2012.

[63] E. J. Stern and M. S. Frank, "CT of the lung in patients with pulmonary emphysema: diagnosis, quantification, and correlation with pathologic and physiologic findings," *American Journal of Roentgenology*, vol. 162, no. 4, pp. 791–798, 1994.

[64] W. M. Thurlbeck, "The incidence of pulmonary emphysema, with observations on the relative incidence and spatial distribution of various types of emphysema," *The American Review of Respiratory Disease*, vol. 87, pp. 206–215, 1963.

[65] R. S. Mitchell, G. W. Silvers, N. Goodman, G. Dart, and J. C. Maisel, "Are centrilobular emphysema and panlobular emphysema two different diseases?" *Human Pathology*, vol. 1, no. 3, pp. 433–441, 1970.

[66] W. Mitlehner, M. Friedrich, and W. Dissmann, "Value of computer tomography in the detection of bullae and blebs in patients with primary spontaneous pneumothorax," *Respiration*, vol. 59, no. 4, pp. 221–227, 1992.

[67] A. Garg and B. R. Herts, "Birt-Hogg-Dube syndrome," *Journal of Urology*, vol. 188, no. 4, pp. 1343–1344, 2012.

[68] K. Tobino, T. Hirai, T. Johkoh et al., "Differentiation between Birt-Hogg-Dubé syndrome and lymphangioleiomyomatosis: quantitative analysis of pulmonary cysts on computed tomography of the chest in 66 females," *European Journal of Radiology*, vol. 81, no. 6, pp. 1340–1346, 2012.

[69] R. A. Murray, T. B. Poulton, M. G. Saltarelli et al., "Rare pulmonary manifestation of ehlers-danlos syndrome," *Journal of Thoracic Imaging*, vol. 10, no. 2, pp. 138–141, 1995.

[70] M. A. Lane, L. A. Marcos, N. F. Onen et al., "Paragonimus kellicotti Fluke infections in Missouri, USA," *Emerging Infectious Diseases*, vol. 18, no. 8, pp. 1263–1267, 2012.

[71] G. Vicidomini, M. Santini, A. Baldi, T. Cesarano, M. P. Di Marino, and F. Baldi, "Cystic adenomatoid malformation of the lung in an adult," *Minerva Chirurgica*, vol. 52, no. 4, pp. 469–473, 1997.

[72] J. T. Stocker, J. E. Madewell, and R. M. Drake, "Congenital cystic adenomatoid malformation of the lung. Classification and morphologic spectrum," *Human Pathology*, vol. 8, no. 2, pp. 155–171, 1977.

[73] F. Watarai, M. Takahashi, T. Hosoya, and K. Murata, "Congenital lung abnormalities: a pictorial review of imaging findings," *Japanese Journal of Radiology*, vol. 30, no. 10, pp. 787–797, 2012.

[74] R. J. Summers, B. M. Shehata, J. C. Bleacher, C. Stockwell, and L. Rapkin, "Mucinous adenocarcinoma of the lung in association with congenital pulmonary airway malformation," *Journal of Pediatric Surgery*, vol. 45, no. 11, pp. 2256–2259, 2010.

[75] A. Kosar, C. Tezel, A. Orki, H. Kiral, and B. Arman, "Bronchogenic cysts of the lung: report of 29 cases," *Heart Lung and Circulation*, vol. 18, no. 3, pp. 214–218, 2009.

[76] J.-H. Lee and M.-J. Kim, "Intradiaphragmatic extralobar pulmonary sequestration in adult," *Journal of Cardiothoracic Surgery*, vol. 9, no. 1, article no. 112, 2014.

[77] C. Hertzenberg, E. Daon, and J. Kramer, "Intralobar pulmonary sequestration in adults: three case reports," *Journal of Thoracic Disease*, vol. 4, no. 5, pp. 516–519, 2012.

[78] B. Savic, F. J. Birtel, W. Tholen, H. D. Funke, and R. Knoche, "Lung sequestration: report of seven cases and review of 540 published cases," *Thorax*, vol. 34, no. 1, pp. 96–101, 1979.

[79] J. Ikezoe, S. Murayama, J. D. Godwin, S. L. Done, and J. A. Verschakelen, "Bronchopulmonary sequestration: CT assessment," *Radiology*, vol. 176, no. 2, pp. 375–379, 1990.

[80] S. M. Albelda, J. A. Kern, D. L. Marinelli, and W. T. Miller, "Expanding spectrum of pulmonary disease caused by nontuberculous mycobacteria," *Radiology*, vol. 157, no. 2, pp. 289–296, 1985.

[81] J. Zhang, Y.-L. Zhao, M.-X. Ye et al., "Rapidly progressive diffuse cystic lesions as a radiological hallmark of lung adenocarcinoma," *Journal of Thoracic Oncology*, vol. 7, no. 2, pp. 457–458, 2012.

[82] D. P. N. Chan, J. F. Griffith, T.-W. Lee, L. T. C. Chow, and A. P. C. Yim, "Cystic pulmonary metastases from epithelioid cell sarcoma," *Annals of Thoracic Surgery*, vol. 75, no. 5, pp. 1652–1654, 2003.

[83] H. J. Anderson and J. W. Pierce, "Carcinoma of the bronchus presenting as thin-walled cysts," *Thorax*, vol. 9, no. 2, pp. 100–105, 1954.

[84] L. A. Christiansen, P. Stage, E. Bille Brahe, and S. Bertelsen, "Rupture of the diaphragm," *Thorax*, vol. 29, no. 5, pp. 559–563, 1974.

[85] K. S. Hamid, S. S. Rai, and J. A. Rodriguez, "Symptomatic bochdalek hernia in an adult," *Journal of the Society of Laparoendoscopic Surgeons*, vol. 14, no. 2, pp. 279–281, 2010.

22

Plasmin Activation of Glial Cells through Protease-Activated Receptor 1

André R. Greenidge,[1] Kiana R. Hall,[1] Ian R. Hambleton,[1] Richelle Thomas,[1] Dougald M. Monroe,[2] and R. Clive Landis[1]

[1] *Edmund Cohen Laboratory For Vascular Research, Chronic Disease Research Centre, University of the West Indies, Cave Hill, Barbados*
[2] *Division of Hematology/Oncology, School of Medicine, University of North Carolina, Chapel Hill, NC, USA*

Correspondence should be addressed to R. Clive Landis; clive.landis@cavehill.uwi.edu

Academic Editor: Piero Tosi

The objective of this study was to determine whether plasmin could induce morphological changes in human glial cells via PAR1. Human glioblastoma A172 cells were cultured in the presence of plasmin or the PAR1 specific activating hexapeptide, SFLLRN. Cells were monitored by flow cytometry to detect proteolytic activation of PAR1 receptor. Morphological changes were recorded by photomicroscopy and apoptosis was measured by annexinV staining. Plasmin cleaved the PAR1 receptor on glial cells at 5 minutes ($P = 0.02$). After 30 minutes, cellular processes had begun to retract from the basal substratum and by 4 hours glial cells had become detached. Similar results were obtained by generating plasmin de novo from plasminogen. Morphological transformation was blocked by plasmin inhibitors aprotinin or epsilon-aminocaproic acid ($P = 0.03$). Cell viability was unimpaired during early morphological changes, but by 24 hours following plasmin treatment 22% of glial cells were apoptotic. PAR1 activating peptide SFLLRN (but not inactive isomer FSLLRN) promoted analogous glial cell detachment ($P = 0.03$), proving the role for PAR1 in this process. This study has identified a plasmin/PAR1 axis of glial cell activation, linked to changes in glial cell morophology. This adds to our understanding of pathophysiological disease mechanisms of plasmin and the plasminogen system in neuroinjury.

1. Introduction

Plasmin is a serine protease best known for its thrombolytic properties in the coagulation system. However, it can also act on cells that bear receptors belonging to the protease-activated receptor (PAR) family to cause secretion of inflammatory cytokines, oxidative radicals, matrix metalloproteinases, proliferation, cell migration, and platelet aggregation [1–6]. PARs are widely expressed in the central nervous system [7].

Plasmin is generated from plasminogen, by proteolytic cleavage with either tissue-type plasminogen activator (tPA), urinary plasminogen activator (uPA), or bacterial streptokinase. It catalyzes the breakdown of fibrin into D-dimers, hence acting as a brake on coagulation. Antifibrinolytics are in clinical use to limit bleeding in cardiac surgery and intracranial bleeding in traumatic brain injury [8, 9]. Antifibrinolytics fall into two categories: lysine analogues that prevent plasmin generation from plasminogen, (e.g., ε-aminocaproic acid), or active site inhibitors (e.g., serine protease inhibitor aprotinin [10]).

A pathophysiological role has been recognized for the plasminogen-activating system in exacerbating intracranial bleeding, excitotoxicity and cell death in neurons or white matter, ischemia reperfusion injury, and increased permeability of the blood-brain barrier (BBB) [11–17]. Alterations in BBB permeability were accompanied by profound changes in cell shape to astroglial cell lines or primary glial cells, via an incompletely understood receptor mechanism [15]. This phenomenon has been confirmed in cardiac surgery patients with clinical evidence for glial cell injury [18].

PAR receptors share a common activation mechanism, whereby proteolytic cleavage unmasks a hexapeptide ligand sequence in the exodomain of the receptor, which can

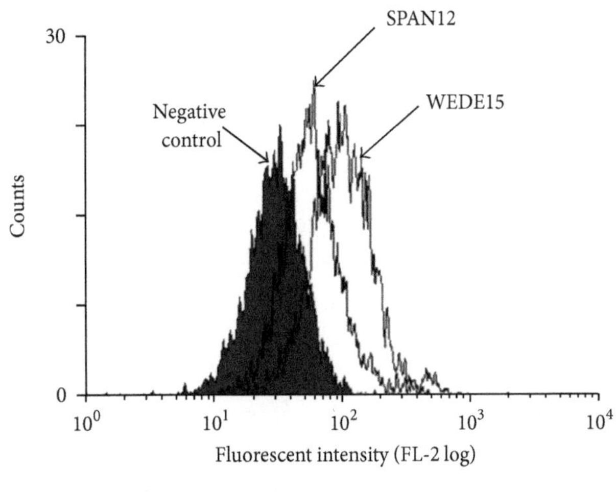

FIGURE 1: Expression of PAR1 epitopes. Flow cytometric histogram depicting expression of WEDE15 (a pan-receptor antibody) and SPAN12 (an activation-dependent antibody) on human A172 glioma cells. The filled histogram represents background staining with control antibody of the same isotype (IgG_1).

then dock intramolecularly and transmit G-protein-coupled signals into the cell [19]. PAR1 is activated by any serine protease that cuts specifically at arginine^{41}-serine^{42} of the receptor generating the hexapeptide serine^{42}-phenylalanine-leucine-leucine-arginine-asparagine^{47} (SFLLRN) at the new N-terminus. PAR1 activating proteases include thrombin, plasmin, and trypsin [20–22].

Although plasmin and PAR1 have independently been implicated in pathways of cerebral injury, a plasmin/PAR1 axis remains to be identified in cells of the central nervous system. In mice, genetic deletion of the PAR1 homolog or deletion of tPA confers neuroprotection in a model of transient cerebral ischemia [16, 22, 23]. Although plasmin has not been studied in this context, other PAR1 agonists trigger excitotoxicity, cell invasion, and apoptosis in neurons, astrocytes, and microglia [13, 16, 22, 24–28]. Hence, we investigated the ability of plasmin to activate central nervous system glial cells via PAR1 in an effort to identify key cellular events and highlight potential therapeutic targets.

2. Methods

2.1. Materials. Plasmin, plasminogen, streptokinase, aprotinin, and ε-aminocaproic acid were purchased from Sigma-Aldrich (St. Louis, MO). Phycoerythrin (PE) conjugated antibodies WEDE15(PE) and SPAN12(PE) were purchased from Beckman-Coulter (Caguas, PR). Phycoerythrin conjugated control antibody of the same isotype (IgG1-PE) was also purchased from Beckman-Coulter. PAR1 receptor activating hexapeptide (SFLLRN) and inactive scramble peptide (FSLLRN) were generated in house (University of North Carolina, Chapel Hill, NC) using an Applied Biosystems 432A Peptide Synthesizer (Life Technologies Corporation, Foster City, CA) and purified by reverse phase HPLC.

2.2. Cell Culture. The human glioma cell line A172 was purchased from the American Type Culture Collection (ATCC; Manassas, VA). Cells were maintained in Dulbecco's Modified Eagle's Medium (DMEM) enriched with 10% fetal calf serum, 2 mmoles/L L-glutamine, 100 U/mL penicillin, and 100 μg/mL streptomycin (all Sigma-Aldrich) at 37°C in a humidified environment with 5% CO_2. At confluence cells were detached using cell dissociation medium (Sigma Aldrich), a trypsin-free detachment step that avoids possible PAR1 activation by trypsin [20, 29]. For plasmin activation, cells were cultured to confluence in Corning Costar 24-well tissue culture plates (Sigma-Aldrich). Purified plasmin (Sigma-Aldrich) was used at 5 U/mL. Plasmin was also generated in situ from plasminogen and streptokinase (Sigma-Aldrich), monitoring plasmin generation spectrophotometrically with Spectrozyme colour reagent (American Diagnostica, Stanford, CT) at 405 nm using a Multimode Detector (Dynex Technologies, Chantilly, VA). Where indicated, aprotinin was used at 200 KIU/mL and ε-aminocaproic acid at 10 mmoles/L. SFLLRN or FSLLRN peptides were used at a concentration of 25 μmoles/L.

2.3. PAR1 Expression and Cleavage. PAR1 receptor expression and cleavage was carried out by flow cytometry as previously described [29]. Briefly, total receptor expression was assessed using the pan-reactive anti-PAR1 antibody WEDE15, whereas receptor activation due to plasmin cleavage was monitored using antibody SPAN12. SPAN12 detects only the intact (i.e., unactivated) PAR1 receptor; therefore, loss of SPAN12 staining provides a linear measure of receptor activation [30]. Staining was carried out on freshly passaged cells in suspension following stimulation with plasmin for 5 minutes at 37°C. Staining with WEDE15, SPAN12, or class-matched (IgG_1) control antibody was carried out at 20 μg/mL for 15 minutes on ice, followed by three washes in ice-cold PBS. Flow cytometric analysis was performed using an EPICS XL flow cytometer (Beckman Coulter). WEDE-15 or SPAN12 staining was expressed in units of relative fluorescent intensity (RFI), a ratio of the mean fluorescent staining intensity obtained with detection antibody versus the staining intensity of a class-matched control antibody (i.e., an RFI of 1.00 is equivalent to no detectable expression). Results were expressed as median ± IQR (RFI units).

2.4. Morphological Changes. Cells were observed and photographed at 0 min, 30 min, 4 h, and 24 h using a Leica DM IL inverted microscope (Leica Microsystems, Wetzlar, Germany) at ×40 or ×100 magnification. Morphological changes were scored on a 6-point ordinal scale according to the scheme: 1 = fully confluent lawn of cells; 2 = cellular pseudopodia have started to retract from one area; 3 = cell processes has started to retract from multiple areas; 4 = cell lawns show visible detachment from well substrata and flapping; 5 = cells have completely detached from well substrata to form a floating island; 6 = floating island of cells with shrivelled appearance.

2.5. Apoptosis. Apoptosis of A172 cells was monitored flow cytometrically by staining with Annexin V FITC Apoptosis Detection Kit according to the manufacturer's instructions (Sigma-Aldrich). The percentage of apoptosis was calculated

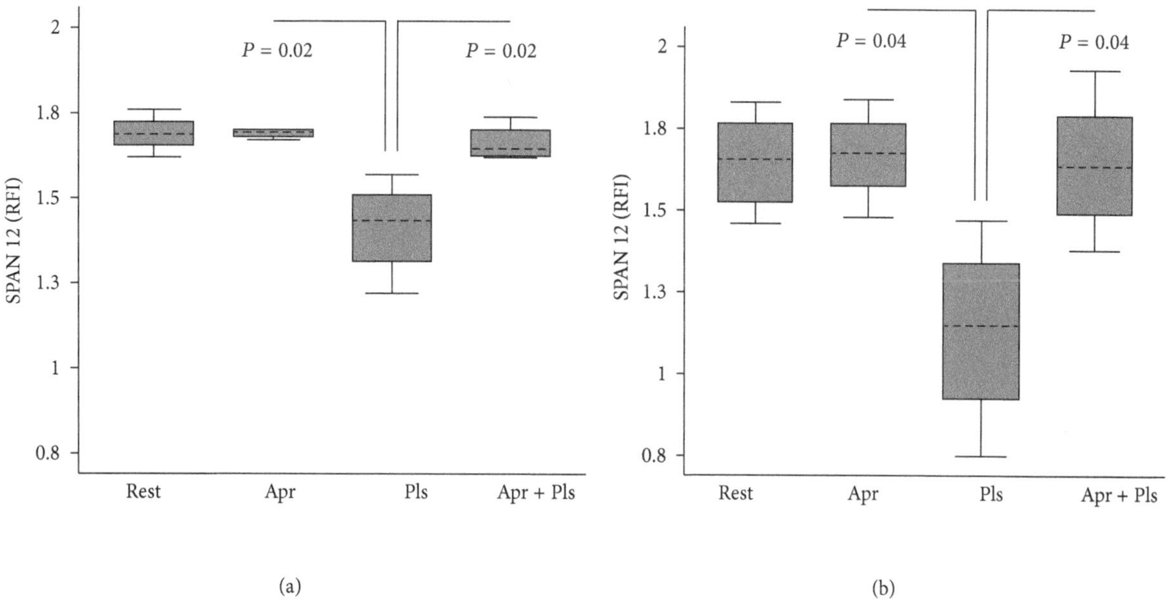

FIGURE 2: Effect of plasmin on PAR1 receptor activation. Proteolytic activation of PAR1 at 5 minutes was monitored flow cytometrically using antibody SPAN12 to detect intact (i.e., unactivated) receptor. Results were expressed in units of relative fluorescent intensity (RFI), calculated by dividing the mean fluorescent staining intensity obtained with SPAN12 antibody by the staining intensity obtained with a class matched (IgG_1) control antibody. Results were expressed as the median ± interquartile range (IQR) from $n = 4$ experiments. (a) Preformed plasmin (5 U/mL). (b) Plasmin generated *in situ* from plasminogen. Rest = resting; Pls = plasmin; Apr = aprotinin 200 KIU/mL.

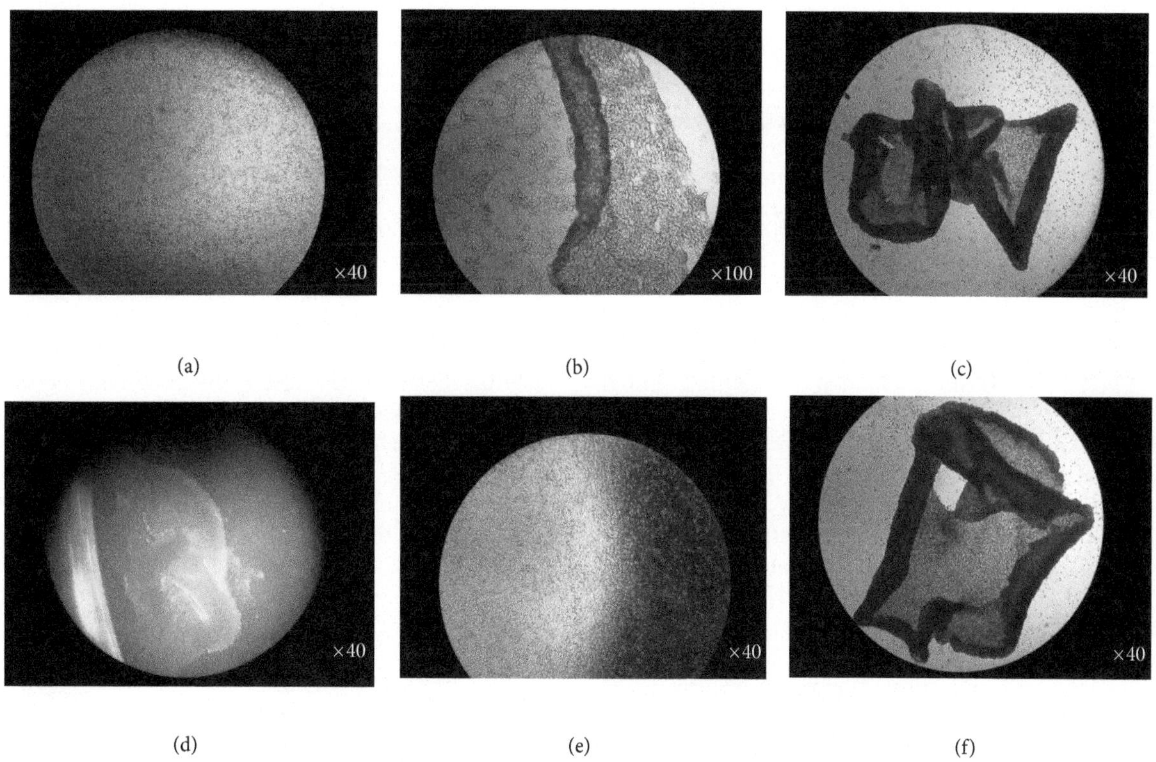

FIGURE 3: Effect of plasmin on cell morphology. (a) Time 0: confluent lawn of resting A172 glial cells. (b) 30 minutes after addition of plasmin: cell processes have started retracting from basal substrata, and flaps of detached cells were observed, although cell-to-cell contacts were maintained. (c) 4 hours: A172 cells fully detached into a floating island. (d) 24 hours: shrivelled floating cell mass. (e) 24 hours: aprotinin (200 KIU/mL) preserved the confluent monolayer of A172 cells in the face of plasmin activation. (f) 24 hours: a PAR1 agonist peptide SFLLRN (25 μmoles/L) triggered analogous glial cell detachment as observed for plasmin in (d). Control peptide FSLLRN did not trigger any morphological changes (not shown). The magnification is indicated at the bottom right of each panel. Representative photomicrographs from $n = 3$–5 experiments are shown.

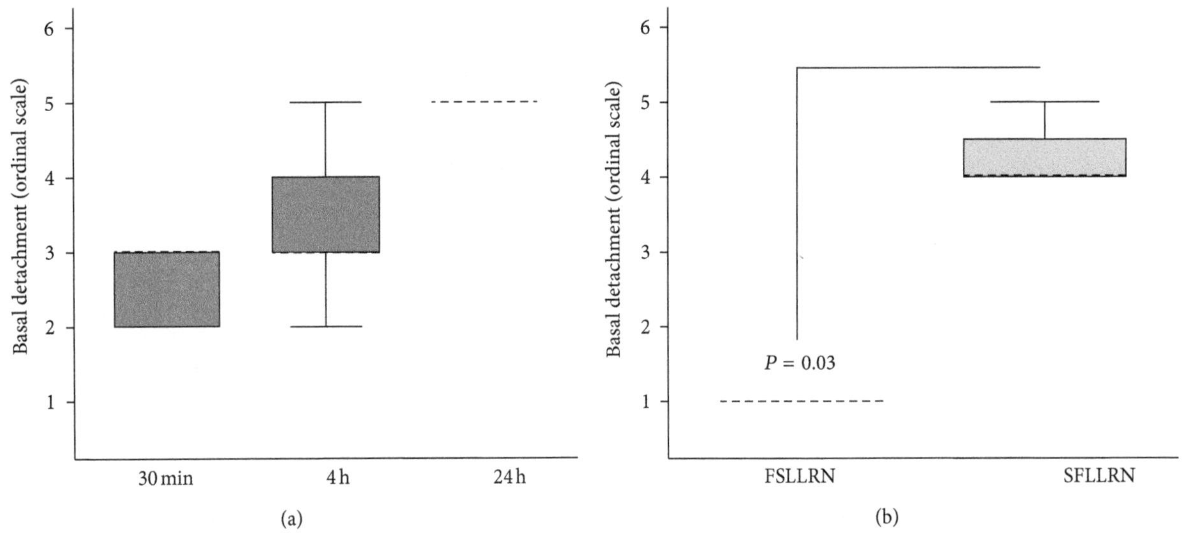

FIGURE 4: Effect of plasmin or PAR1 agonist peptide on glial cell detachment. (a) A172 cells were stimulated with plasmin (5 U/mL) for the length of time indicated, and cell detachment was quantified as defined in the Materials and Methods. (b) Effect of PAR1 specific activating peptide SFLLRN or inactive control peptide FSLLRN (both 25 μmoles/L) on cell detachment at 24 hours. Results were expressed as the median $\pm$ interquartile range (IQR) from $n = 4$ experiments.

by determining the area under the histogram greater than background staining in resting cells. Serum starvation was used as a positive control for apoptosis.

2.6. Statistics. Relative flourescent intensity and the morphological change scale were summarised using robust measures: median and interquartile range. Group differences were plotted using boxplots and assessed formally using the Wilcoxon-Mann-Whitney test for two-group comparisons. Statistical analyses used exact algorithms performed in Stata 10 (Stata Corp., College Station, TX).

3. Results

3.1. PAR1 Receptor Cleavage Induced by Plasmin. Initial experiments examined whether PAR1 was expressed on resting A172 glioma cells. A representative flow cytometric histogram illustrates expression of PAR1 detected with a pan-receptor antibody WEDE15 (Figure 1). WEDE15 staining from pooled samples ($n = 8$) demonstrated expression at an intensity of 2.31 $\pm$ 0.33 (median $\pm$ interquartile range (IQR)) relative fluorescent intensity units (RFI units) at the cell surface. Proteolytic activation of PAR1 due to plasmin was monitored using a different antibody, SPAN12, specific to only the intact (i.e., unactivated) receptor (Figures 1 and 2). This antibody was expressed at a fluorescent intensity of 1.69 $\pm$ 0.05 RFI units (median $\pm$ IQR.) on resting cells ($n = 8$). Activation with a purified plasmin preparation caused a statistically significant loss of SPAN12 expression at 5 minutes (1.69 $\pm$ 0.07 resting cells versus 1.43 $\pm$ 0.20 plasmin activated; $P = 0.02$; Figure 2(a)). To demonstrate whether this was due to proteolytic cleavage of the receptor by plasmin, experiments were repeated in the presence of the serine protease inhibitor aprotinin: this showed complete restoration of SPAN12 expression (1.65 $\pm$ 0.08; $P = 0.02$ versus plasmin alone). Analogous results were obtained when plasmin was generated *in situ* from plasminogen (Figure 2(b)).

3.2. Morphological Changes Induced by Plasmin. A time-course of photomicrographs taken at 30 minutes, 4 hours and 24 hours after plasmin activation illustrates remarkable morphological transformation of A172 glioma cells (Figures 3 and 4(a)). At 30 minutes cell processes could be observed retracting from the basal substratum, and flap formation was seen at the edges of cell lawns (Figure 3(b)). By 4 hours the cell lawn had completely detached from the well into a floating island, apparently preserving cell-to-cell contacts (Figure 3(c)). Video microscopy showing cell detachment in real time illustrated the release of individual tethers from the end of cell processes (http://youtube/FkSUdWKfoxE). The morphological changes were abrogated by 200 KIU/mL aprotinin, indicating they were dependent on serine proteolytic activity of plasmin (Figure 3(e)). To demonstrate a specific role for PAR1 in this process, a PAR1 specific activating peptide SFLLRN (25 μmoles/L) was examined. This revealed exactly analagous morphological changes triggered through SFLLRN, but not through an inert scramble peptide FSLLRN even when used at high concentrations up to 250 μmoles/L (Figures 3(f) and 4(b)). Morphological changes up to 4 hours following plasmin treatment were not accompanied by any detectable apoptosis as assessed with Annexin V staining by flow cytometry (Figure 5). However, at 24 hours the floating mass of glial cells had a shrivelled appearance (Figure 3(d)) and flow cytometric analysis indicated 22% of cells were apoptotic (Figure 5).

3.3. Effect of Antifibrinolytics. The effect of antifibrinolytics on glial cell morphology was determined in cultures in which plasmin was generated *in situ* from plasminogen.

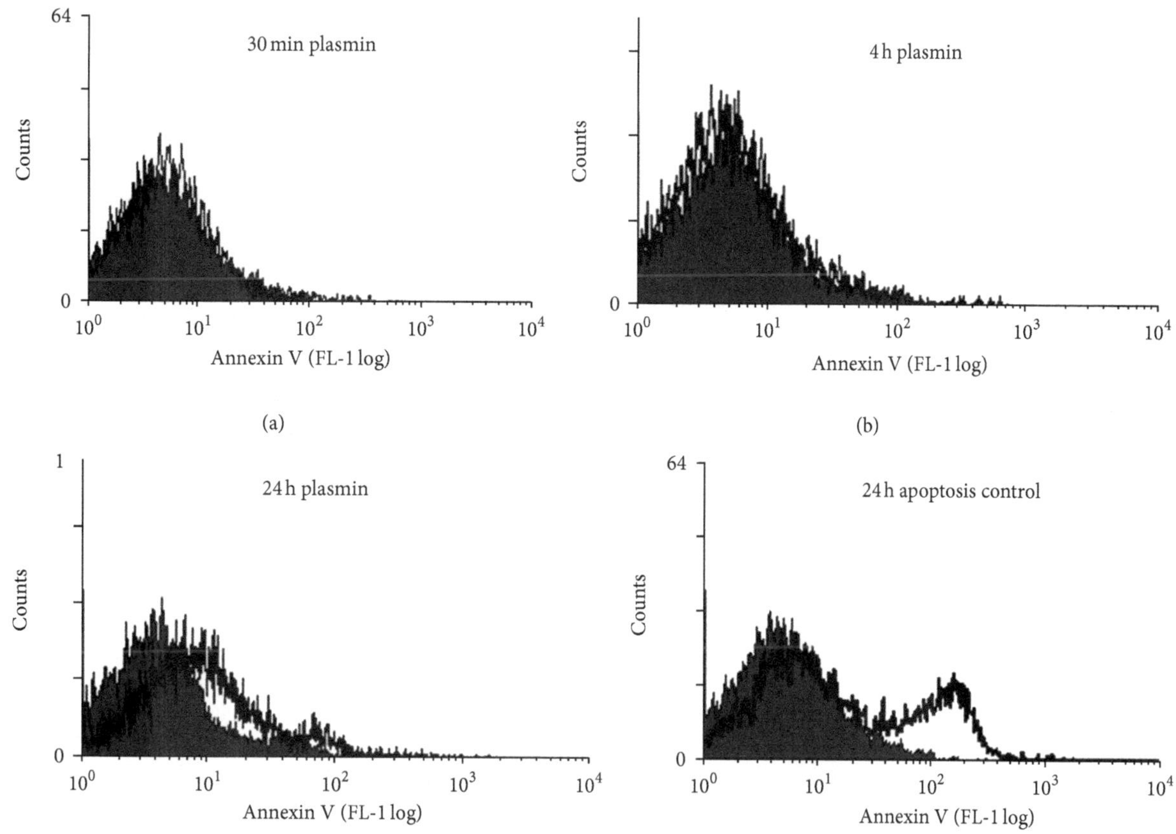

FIGURE 5: Effect of plasmin on glial cell apoptosis. A172 cells were stimulated with plasmin (5 U/mL) for the length of time indicated and monitored flow cytometrically for apoptosis (programmed cell death) by staining with Annexin V. Representative flow cytometric histograms depict the effect of plasmin (open histogram) versus resting cells (filled histogram) on Annexin V expression. Serum starvation was used as a positive control for apoptosis.

The antiplasmin(ogen) agents aprotinin (200 KIU/mL) and ε-aminocaproic acid (10 mmoles/L), used at concentrations equivalent to their clinical usage, statistically significantly inhibited glial cell detachment due to plasmin (each $P = 0.03$; Figure 6). Biochemical assays for plasmin activity in cell cultures confirmed that each of the antifibrinolytics had abrogated plasmin activity at the concentrations employed (data not shown).

4. Discussion

The present study has proven the principle that plasmin can activate human glial cells via proteolytic cleavage of PAR1. The type of cell-lawn detachment observed was similar to that previously described in A172 cells treated with an integrin antagonist, that also caused separation from basal substratum and accumulation of cells into floating spheroids [31]. Although immediate cytotoxicity due to plasmin was ruled out in apoptosis assays, gradual expression of annexin V occurred in our culture system after 24 hours following plasmin activation. The fact that SFLLRN (but not the inactive scramble peptide FSLLRN) could recapitulate the morphological changes in A172 cells proved the role of PAR1 in this process.

These findings add to a growing literature that morphological transformation of astroglial cells can take place in a pathway involving the plasminogen activating system and components of the focal cell adhesion machinery [15, 31, 32]. An important recent study showed that tPA was capable of eliciting morphological changes and increased BBB permeability in mouse astroglial cells, through alterations to the Rho kinase (ROCK) pathway regulating focal adhesion contacts with extracellular matrix proteins [15]. A two-receptor mechanism was postulated in that study, one of which remained unknown. The unknown receptor was a receptor for plasminogen, as shown by antagonism with the antifibrinolytic agents aprotinin or tranexamic acid. The plasmin/PAR1 axis described by us was similarly antagonized by aprotinin or a lysine analog and may therefore present a plausible alternative receptor pathway.

Most studies investigating the effect of serine proteases on neuronal PAR1 have focused on thrombin, which can either be neuroprotective or, conversely, induce apoptosis in neurons, depending on concentration and length of exposure to thrombin [7, 24, 25, 28, 33]. Initial studies using our

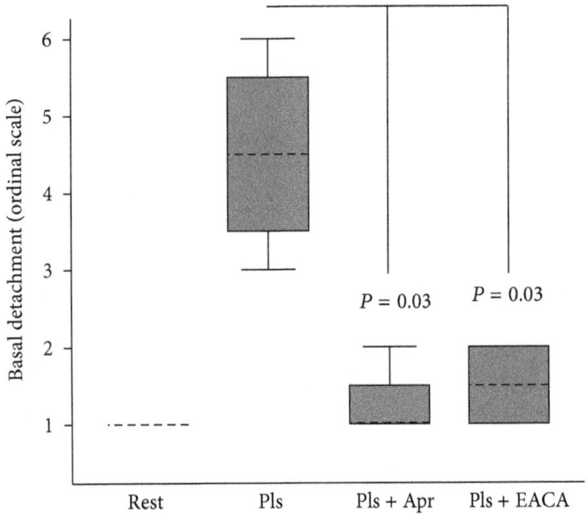

FIGURE 6: Effect of antifibrinolytics on plasmin induced glial cell detachment. A172 cells were stimulated with plasmin generated *in situ* from plasminogen (5 U/mL) and streptokinase (50 KU/mL) in the presence of aprotinin or ε-aminocaproic acid. Cell detachment was expressed in arbitrary units defined in Section 2. Results were expressed as the median ± interquartile range (IQR) from n = 4 experiments. Rest = Resting; Pls = plasmin; Apr = aprotinin (200 KIU/mL); EACA = ε-aminocaproic acid (10 mmoles/L).

culture system indicated that alpha-thrombin did not activate PAR1 on A172 glial cells within a physiological concentration range, but that plasmin activated PAR1 efficiently [34]. The plasmin/PAR1 axis of glial activation identified here may synergise to cause neurodegeneration with pathways of excitotoxic potentiation of N-methyl D-aspartate responses in neurons, also mediated via PAR1 activation with plasmin or thrombin [27, 35].

Cell lawn detachment may represent a manifestation of natural morphological processes, such as cell migration or astrocyte stellation. Reversal of the stellate phenotype by thrombin or changes in astrocyte morphology described for tPA may utilize the same cellular pathway, since both are regulated by ROCK [15, 36]. Local restructuring of focal adhesion contacts and cell detachment may emulate important physiological functions linked to cell migration, wound healing, proliferation, glial scarring, and neurite formation [17, 37–40]. Video microscopy of the cell detachment process appeared to indicate the release of individual pseudopod tethers, similar to what had been described for release or thinning of astrocyte cell processes induced by thrombin agonist [38, 41].

The morphological changes described here may be most relevant in the setting of neurotrauma or neuroinjury secondary to BBB breakdown, when zymogens such as plasmin that are normally confined to the systemic circulation can enter the brain [42]. A common surgical insult that compromises BBB function is cardiopulmonary bypass: this is linked to changes in glial cell morphology, neurocognitive deficits and stroke [18, 43–46]. The demonstration that glial cells are activated via plasmin/PAR1 expands our understanding of neurodegenerative mechanisms and focuses attention on PAR1 as a possible drug target for neuroprotection. While PAR1 deficient mice are protected in various models of ischemia, it is simplistic to consider PAR1 antagonism as a treatment option to block astroglial pathways of neuroinjury, since a clinical trial with the oral PAR1 antagonist vorapaxar for treatment of acute coronary syndromes was associated with significantly higher rates of intracerebral hemorrhage [22, 47, 48]. A desirable outcome would be to combine thrombolytic properties without hemorrhage or compromise of BBB permeability; however, this outcome remains elusive. However, plasmin inhibitors are neuroprotective, and the plasmin/PAR1 axis identified here may be explored further as a therapeutic target [17, 49–51].

There are some limitations to this study. The cell culture system may fail adequately to model the homeostatic environment of the brain, which is endowed not only with serine proteases and their zymogens but also naturally occurring serine protease inhibitors (serpins) [52, 53]. Furthermore, the *in vitro* cell culture model may not faithfully replicate *in vivo* pathways of glial injury caused by plasmin nor the three-dimensional cell-cell and cell-substrate interaction that arises from the precise cellular organization that exists within the brain. However, a reductionist cell culture approach as employed here is well suited to prove unequivocally that glial cells can be activated through proteolytic cleavage of PAR1 due to plasmin.

In conclusion, we have identified a PAR1 axis of glial cell activation triggered by plasmin or the plasminogen system. This may be especially relevant under conditions of BBB breakdown or intracranial hemorrhage when serine proteases gain access to the neurovascular unit.

Acknowledgments

R. C. Landis discloses unrestricted research grants from the Barbados Diabetes Foundation and Bayer Pharmaceuticals Inc. which supported this work. The authors declare that they have no conflict of interests.

References

[1] I. Clemmensen and R. B. Andersen, "The fibrinolytic system and its relation to inflammatory diseases," *Seminars in Arthritis and Rheumatism*, vol. 11, no. 4, pp. 390–398, 1982.

[2] N. Kamio, H. Hashizume, S. Nakao, K. Matsushima, and H. Sugiya, "Plasmin is involved in inflammation via protease-activated receptor-1 activation in human dental pulp," *Biochemical Pharmacology*, vol. 75, no. 10, pp. 1974–1980, 2008.

[3] T. M. Quinton, S. Kim, C. K. Derian, J. Jin, and S. P. Kunapuli, "Plasmin-mediated activation of platelets occurs by cleavage of protease-activated receptor 4," *The Journal of Biological Chemistry*, vol. 279, no. 18, pp. 18434–18439, 2004.

[4] V. Lukic-Panin, K. Deguchi, T. Yamashita et al., "Free radical scavenger edaravone administration protects against tissue plasminogen activator induced oxidative stress and blood brain barrier damage," *Current Neurovascular Research*, vol. 7, no. 4, pp. 319–329, 2010.

[5] S. L. Raza, L. C. Nehring, S. D. Shapiro, and L. A. Cornelius, "Proteinase-activated receptor-1 regulation of macrophage elastase (MMP-12) secretion by serine proteinases," *The Journal of Biological Chemistry*, vol. 275, no. 52, pp. 41243–41250, 2000.

[6] S. C. Even-Ram, M. Maoz, E. Pokroy et al., "Tumor cell invasion is promoted by activation of protease activated receptor-1 in cooperation with the alpha vbeta 5 integrin," *The Journal of Biological Chemistry*, vol. 276, no. 14, pp. 10952–10962, 2001.

[7] E. Sokolova and G. Reiser, "Prothrombin/thrombin and the thrombin receptors PAR-1 and PAR-4 in the brain: localization, expression and participation in neurodegenerative diseases," *Thrombosis and Haemostasis*, vol. 100, no. 4, pp. 576–581, 2008.

[8] V. J. Marder, "Historical perspective and future direction of thrombolysis research: the re-discovery of plasmin," *Journal of Thrombosis and Haemostasis*, vol. 9, no. 1, pp. 364–373, 2011.

[9] F. Olldashi, M. Kerçi, T. Zhurda et al., "The importance of early treatment with tranexamic acid in bleeding trauma patients: an exploratory analysis of the CRASH-2 randomised controlled trial," *The Lancet*, vol. 377, no. 9771, pp. 1096–1101, 1101.e1-1101.e2, 2011.

[10] D. A. Henry, A. J. Moxey, P. A. Carless et al., "Anti-fibrinolytic use for minimising perioperative allogeneic blood transfusion," *Cochrane Database of Systematic Reviews*, no. 1, Article ID CD001886, 2001.

[11] S. Fujimoto, H. Katsuki, M. Ohnishi, M. Takagi, T. Kume, and A. Akaike, "Plasminogen potentiates thrombin cytotoxicity and contributes to pathology of intracerebral hemorrhage in rats," *Journal of Cerebral Blood Flow and Metabolism*, vol. 28, no. 3, pp. 506–515, 2008.

[12] J. J. Sheehan, C. Zhou, I. Gravanis et al., "Proteolytic activation of monocyte chemoattractant protein-1 by plasmin underlies excitotoxic neurodegeneration in mice," *Journal of Neuroscience*, vol. 27, no. 7, pp. 1738–1745, 2007.

[13] S. E. Tsirka, T. H. Bugge, J. L. Degen, and S. Strickland, "Neuronal death in the central nervous system demonstrates a non-fibrin substrate for plasmin," *Proceedings of the National Academy of Sciences of the United States of America*, vol. 94, no. 18, pp. 9779–9781, 1997.

[14] S. E. Tsirka, A. D. Rogove, T. H. Bugge, J. L. Degen, and S. Strickland, "An extracellular proteolytic cascade promotes neuronal degeneration in the mouse hippocampus," *Journal of Neuroscience*, vol. 17, no. 2, pp. 543–552, 1997.

[15] B. Niego, R. Freeman, T. B. Puschmann, A. M. Turnley, and R. L. Medcalf, "t-PA-specific modulation of a human blood-brain barrier model involves plasmin-mediated activation of the Rho kinase pathway in astrocytes," *Blood*, vol. 119, no. 20, pp. 4752–4761, 2012.

[16] Y. F. Wang, S. E. Tsirka, S. Strickland, P. E. Stieg, S. G. Soriano, and S. A. Lipton, "Tissue plasminogen activator (tPA) increases neuronal damage after focal cerebral ischemia in wild-type and tPA-deficient mice," *Nature Medicine*, vol. 4, no. 2, pp. 228–231, 1998.

[17] F. Adhami, D. Yu, W. Yin et al., "Deleterious effects of plasminogen activators in neonatal cerebral hypoxia-ischemia," *American Journal of Pathology*, vol. 172, no. 6, pp. 1704–1716, 2008.

[18] B. Reinsfelt, S.-E. Ricksten, H. Zetterberg, K. Blennow, J. Fredén-Lindqvist, and A. Westerlind, "Cerebrospinal fluid markers of brain injury, inflammation, and blood-brain barrier dysfunction in cardiac surgery," *Annals of Thoracic Surgery*, vol. 94, no. 2, pp. 549–555, 2012.

[19] T. K. H. Vu, V. I. Wheaton, D. T. Hung, I. Charo, and S. R. Coughlin, "Domains specifying thrombin-receptor interaction," *Nature*, vol. 353, no. 6345, pp. 674–677, 1991.

[20] T. K. H. Vu, D. T. Hung, V. I. Wheaton, and S. R. Coughlin, "Molecular cloning of a functional thrombin receptor reveals a novel proteolytic mechanism of receptor activation," *Cell*, vol. 64, no. 6, pp. 1057–1068, 1991.

[21] M. Poullis, R. Manning, M. Laffan, D. O. Haskard, K. M. Taylor, and R. C. Landis, "The antithrombotic effect of aprotinin: actions mediated via the protease-activated receptor 1," *Journal of Thoracic and Cardiovascular Surgery*, vol. 120, no. 2, pp. 370–378, 2000.

[22] C. E. Junge, T. Sugawara, G. Mannaioni et al., "The contribution of protease-activated receptor 1 to neuronal damage caused by transient focal cerebral ischemia," *Proceedings of the National Academy of Sciences of the United States of America*, vol. 100, no. 22, pp. 13019–13024, 2003.

[23] E. E. Olson, P. Lyuboslavsky, S. F. Traynelis, and R. J. McKeon, "PAR-1 deficiency protects against neuronal damage and neurologic deficits after unilateral cerebral hypoxia/ischemia," *Journal of Cerebral Blood Flow and Metabolism*, vol. 24, no. 9, pp. 964–971, 2004.

[24] Y. Wang, W. Luo, and G. Reiser, "Activation of protease-activated receptors in astrocytes evokes a novel neuroprotective pathway through release of chemokines of the growth-regulated oncogene/cytokine-induced neutrophil chemoattractant family," *European Journal of Neuroscience*, vol. 26, no. 11, pp. 3159–3168, 2007.

[25] F. M. Donovan and D. D. Cunningham, "Signaling pathways involved in thrombin-induced cell protection," *The Journal of Biological Chemistry*, vol. 273, no. 21, pp. 12746–12752, 1998.

[26] M. B. Gingrich, C. E. Junge, P. Lyuboslavsky, and S. F. Traynelis, "Potentiation of NMDA receptor function by the serine protease thrombin," *Journal of Neuroscience*, vol. 20, no. 12, pp. 4582–4595, 2000.

[27] G. Mannaioni, A. G. Orr, C. E. Hamill et al., "Plasmin potentiates synaptic N-methyl-D-aspartate receptor function in hippocampal neurons through activation of protease-activated receptor-1," *The Journal of Biological Chemistry*, vol. 283, no. 29, pp. 20600–20611, 2008.

[28] L. J. Houenou, "Thrombin perturbs neurite outgrowth and induces apoptotic cell death in enriched chick spinal motoneuron cultures through caspase activation," *Journal of Neuroscience*, vol. 18, no. 17, pp. 6882–6891, 1998.

[29] J. R. S. Day, K. M. Taylor, E. A. Lidington et al., "Aprotinin inhibits proinflammatory activation of endothelial cells by thrombin through the protease-activated receptor 1," *Journal of Thoracic and Cardiovascular Surgery*, vol. 131, no. 1, pp. 21–27, 2006.

[30] L. F. Brass, S. Pizarro, M. Ahuja et al., "Changes in the structure and function of the human thrombin receptor during receptor activation, internalization, and recycling," *The Journal of Biological Chemistry*, vol. 269, no. 4, pp. 2943–2952, 1994.

[31] A. Maglott, P. Bartik, S. Cosgun et al., "The small $\alpha5\beta1$ integrin antagonist, SJ749, reduces proliferation and clonogenicity of human astrocytoma cells," *Cancer Research*, vol. 66, no. 12, pp. 6002–6007, 2006.

[32] Y. Fukushima, M. Tamura, H. Nakagawa, and K. Itoh, "Induction of glioma cell migration by vitronectin in human serum and cerebrospinal fluid," *Journal of Neurosurgery*, vol. 107, no. 3, pp. 578–585, 2007.

[33] Z. Suo, B. A. Citron, and B. W. Festoff, "Thrombin: a potential proinflammatory mediator in neurotrauma and neurodegenerative disorders," *Current Drug Targets*, vol. 3, no. 1, pp. 105–114, 2004.

[34] R. C. Landis and K. D. Hall, "Plasmin but not thrombin activates A172 glial cells via serine proteolytic cleavage of preotease-activated receptor (PAR)1," *Heart Surgery Forum*, vol. 11, no. 5, article 278, 2008.

[35] C. E. Hamill, G. Mannaioni, P. Lyuboslavsky, A. A. Sastre, and S. F. Traynelis, "Protease-activated receptor 1-dependent neuronal damage involves NMDA receptor function," *Experimental Neurology*, vol. 217, no. 1, pp. 136–146, 2009.

[36] H. S. Suidan, C. D. Nobes, A. Hall, and D. Monard, "Astrocyte spreading in response to thrombin and lysophosphatidic acid is dependent on the Rho GTPase," *GLIA*, vol. 21, no. 2, pp. 244–252, 1997.

[37] O. Nicole, A. Goldshmidt, C. E. Hamill et al., "Activation of protease-activated receptor-1 triggers astrogliosis after brain injury," *Journal of Neuroscience*, vol. 25, no. 17, pp. 4319–4329, 2005.

[38] K. P. Cavanaugh, D. Gurwitz, D. D. Cunningham, and R. A. Bradshaw, "Reciprocal modulation of astrocyte stellation by thrombin and protease nexin-1," *Journal of Neurochemistry*, vol. 54, no. 5, pp. 1735–1743, 1990.

[39] D. D. Cunningham and D. Gurwitz, "Proteolytic regulation of neurite outgrowth from neuroblastoma cells by thrombin and protease nexin-1," *Journal of Cellular Biochemistry*, vol. 39, no. 1, pp. 55–64, 1989.

[40] S. F. Traynelis and J. Trejo, "Protease-activated receptor signaling: new roles and regulatory mechanisms," *Current Opinion in Hematology*, vol. 14, no. 3, pp. 230–235, 2007.

[41] T. Okamoto, M. Nishibori, K. Sawada et al., "The effects of stimulating protease-activated receptor-1 and -2 in A172 human glioblastoma," *Journal of Neural Transmission*, vol. 108, no. 2, pp. 125–140, 2001.

[42] M. B. Gingrich and S. F. Traynelis, "Serine proteases and brain damage—is there a link?" *Trends in Neurosciences*, vol. 23, no. 9, pp. 399–407, 2000.

[43] C. Landis, "Why the inflammatory response is important to the cardiac surgical patient," *Journal of Extra-Corporeal Technology*, vol. 39, no. 4, pp. 281–284, 2007.

[44] D. A. Stump, "Deformable emboli and inflammation: temporary or permanent damage?" *Journal of Extra-Corporeal Technology*, vol. 39, no. 4, pp. 289–290, 2007.

[45] A. M. Schuller, J. Windolf, R. Blaheta et al., "Degradation of microvascular brain endothelial cell β-catenin after co-culture with activated neutrophils from patients undergoing cardiac surgery with prolonged cardiopulmonary bypass," *Biochemical and Biophysical Research Communications*, vol. 329, no. 2, pp. 616–623, 2005.

[46] M. Scholz, J. Cinatl, M. Schädel-Höpfner, and J. Windolf, "Neutrophils and the blood-brain barrier dysfunction after trauma," *Medicinal Research Reviews*, vol. 27, no. 3, pp. 401–416, 2007.

[47] P. Tricoci, Z. Huang, C. Held et al., "Thrombin-receptor antagonist vorapaxar in acute coronary syndromes," *The New England Journal of Medicine*, vol. 366, no. 1, pp. 20–33, 2012.

[48] C. E. Junge, C. J. Lee, K. B. Hubbard et al., "Protease-activated receptor-1 in human brain: localization and functional expression in astrocytes," *Experimental Neurology*, vol. 188, no. 1, pp. 94–103, 2004.

[49] O. Eser, E. Kalkan, M. Cosar et al., "The effect of aprotinin on brain ischemic-reperfusion injury after hemorrhagic shock in rats: an experimental study," *Journal of Trauma*, vol. 63, no. 2, pp. 373–378, 2007.

[50] K. Durgut, K. Hosgor, N. Gormus, U. Ozergin, and H. Solak, "The cerebroprotective effects of pentoxifylline and aprotinin during cardiopulmonary bypass in dogs," *Perfusion*, vol. 19, no. 2, pp. 101–106, 2004.

[51] V. Anttila, I. Hagino, Y. Iwata et al., "Aprotinin improves cerebral protection: evidence from a survival porcine model," *Journal of Thoracic and Cardiovascular Surgery*, vol. 132, no. 4, pp. 948–953, 2006.

[52] V. L. Turgeon and L. J. Houenou, "The role of thrombin-like (serine) proteases in the development, plasticity and pathology of the nervous system," *Brain Research Reviews*, vol. 25, no. 1, pp. 85–95, 1997.

[53] P. Rossignol, B. Ho-Tin-Noé, R. Vranckx et al., "Protease nexin-1 inhibits plasminogen activation-induced apoptosis of adherent cells," *The Journal of Biological Chemistry*, vol. 279, no. 11, pp. 10346–10356, 2004.

23

Salivary and Urinary Total Antioxidant Capacity as Biomarkers of Oxidative Stress in Humans

Ilaria Peluso and Anna Raguzzini

Center of Nutrition, Council for Agricultural Research and Economics (CREA-NUT), Via Ardeatina 546, 00178 Rome, Italy

Correspondence should be addressed to Ilaria Peluso; i.peluso@tiscali.it

Academic Editor: Runjan Chetty

Total Antioxidant Capacity (TAC) is a biomarker often used in order to investigate oxidative stress in many pathological conditions. Saliva and urine can be collected noninvasively and represent attractive diagnostic fluids for detecting biomarkers of various pathological conditions. The reviewed case-control and intervention studies that measured salivary or urinary TAC revealed that diseases, antioxidant foods, or supplements and age, gender, and lifestyle factors influenced salivary or urinary TAC. Salivary and urinary TAC were particularly affected by oral or renal status, respectively, as well as by infection; therefore these factors must be taken into account in both case-control and intervention studies. Furthermore, some considerations on sample collection and normalization strategies could be made. In particular, unstimulated saliva could be the better approach to measure salivary TAC, whereas 24 h or spontaneous urine collection should be chosen on the basis of the study outcome and of the creatinine clearance. Finally, the uric acid-independent TAC could be the better approach to evaluate red-ox status of body, in particular after nutritional interventions and in diseases associated with hyperuricaemia.

1. Introduction

Oxidative stress, defined as the imbalance between Reactive Oxygen Species (ROS) production and antioxidant defense inside human organism, is a risk factor playing a significant pathogenetic role for noncommunicable diseases [1]. A nonphysiological ROS production originates either by xenobiotics or by endogenous sources [2], such as the respiratory burst [3]. Synergistic interactions between antioxidants, in part involving antioxidant regeneration, must be taken into account in order to properly assess antioxidant status in vivo. Total Antioxidant Capacity (TAC), defined as the moles of oxidants neutralized by one litre of solution, is a biomarker measuring the antioxidant potential of body fluids [4]. Several reviews described the various assays commonly used for the measurement of TAC [5–8] and a good correlation between the results obtained with different methods was found [9, 10]. Salivary and urinary collections are simple and noninvasive and this is the reason why TAC of saliva or urine has led to increasing interest. It has been suggested that saliva could constitute a first line of defense against free radical-mediated oxidative stress [11], whereas the composition of urine reflects the continuously changing environment of the body, which is affected, among other factors, by diet and in particular by polyphenol metabolites excreted in urine [12].

We aimed to review case-control and intervention studies that measured salivary [13–138] or urinary [138–179] TAC.

2. Infection and Oral and Renal Status

Saliva and urine are particularly affected by oral or renal status, respectively, as well as by infection; therefore the relationships of salivary and urinary TAC with these conditions have been investigated in many studies (Table 1). Urinary TAC increased during urinary tract infection [148, 149], while decreased levels of salivary TAC were observed during *H. pylori* [130] and HIV [98, 112] infections and after a single consumption of enterococci containing Bryndza cheese [63]. The latter temporally affected the composition of oral microbiota [63].

On the contrary, dental caries, one of the most common infectious diseases worldwide, was associated with higher salivary TAC (Table 1). Therefore, the relationship between

TABLE 1: Infection and oral and renal status.

References	Case-control studies	Salivary TAC percentage (n°)	Urinary TAC percentage (n°)	Treatment effect percentage (n°)
[98, 112, 130, 148, 149]	Infection	↓ 100% (3/3)	↑ (100%, 2/2)	Salivary TAC ↑ HAART in HIV+
[16, 45, 47, 60, 61, 64, 72, 73, 75, 78, 84, 90, 99, 103, 104, 122, 124, 125]	Caries	↑ 81.2% (13/16) ↔ 6.3% (1/16) ↓ 12.5% (2/16)		Dental hygiene procedures ↑ 100% (3/3)
[26, 28, 34, 35, 37, 39, 40, 44, 52, 53, 66, 68, 76, 87, 89, 95, 96, 100, 101, 110, 114, 115]	Periodontitis	↓ 66.7% (14/21) ↔ 23.8% (5/21) ↑ 9.5% (2/21)		Dental hygiene procedures or scaling and root planing ↑ 50% (3/6) ↔ 50% (3/6)
[13–15, 17, 22–24, 29, 36, 49, 83, 88, 92, 113, 128]	Severe oral diseases	↓ 66.7% (10/15) ↔ 26.7% (4/15) ↑ 6.6% (1/15)		
[30, 31, 86, 142, 154, 158, 162, 179]	Renal diseases	↑ 50% (2/4) ↓ 50% (2/4)	↓ 60% (3/5) ↔ 20% (1/5) ↑ 20% (1/5)	

HAART: highly active antiretroviral therapy; TAC: total antioxidant capacity; ↑: increase; ↓: decrease; ↔: unchanged.

infection and TAC depends on the type and on the site of infection.

On the other hand, oxidative stress is implicated in the pathogenesis of many oral diseases and meta-analysis results showed that TAC levels from peripheral blood samples were significantly different between periodontitis (PD) patients and healthy subjects, suggesting that chronic periodontitis is associated with systemic oxidative stress in human bodies [180]. In agreement with this finding, lower values of salivary TAC were found in PD patients versus healthy subjects in 66.7% of the studies (Table 1). When increased salivary TAC levels were observed, it has been suggested that this increase may represent an adaptive response to oxidative stress in PD [115]. Dental hygiene procedures and scaling and root planing increased salivary TAC in 100% of the studies conducted on healthy subjects with caries and in 50% of the studies on patients with PD (Table 1). Therefore, the antioxidant status in saliva is related to both oral hygiene and periodontal status.

On the other hand, 66.7% of the studies that have investigated the salivary TAC in more serious oral diseases, including recurrent aphthous stomatitis (RAS) (the most common oral ulcerative condition) [36, 88], stem cell transplantation- (SCT-) related salivary gland injury due to graft versus host disease (GVHD) [92], oral mucositis induced by high-dose therapy of melphalan in myeloma patients treated with autologous SCT [22], cleft lip and palate [17], oral premalignant lesions (leukoplakia, lichen planus, and erythroplakia) [13–15, 23, 29, 49, 83, 113, 128], and oral cancers [14, 24], found decreased levels of salivary TAC in these patients (Table 1). Furthermore, salivary TAC was decreased also in patients with peri-implant disease [81] and in children undergoing fixed orthodontic therapy [54].

Concerning renal status, decreased levels of urinary TAC have been reported in renal diseases including secondary (induced by hypertension and diabetes) and primary renal disease, chronic and acute renal failure, and shockwave lithotripsy- (SWL-) induced acute kidney injury (Table 1).

Decreased urinary TAC has been reported 120 minutes after SWL in both patients with kidneys stone and controls [158], but others reported that SWL did not change urinary TAC measured in the 24-h urine [179]. On the contrary, urinary TAC was higher in childhood urolithiasis and was associated with hyperuricosuria [154].

Chronic renal failure is often treated with peritoneal dialysis and chronic renal failure patients undergoing dialysis are characterized by decreased urinary TAC [142]. However, both increased and decreased salivary TAC was found in these patients [30, 31, 86] (Table 1), probably due to the hyperuricaemia. Kidney transplantation is the treatment of choice for most patients with end-stage renal disease and it has been suggested that urinary biomarkers of oxidative stress could be useful in the assessment of kidney quality before transplantation, which is needed to predict recipient outcomes and to optimize management and allocation of the allograft [181]. In particular, TAC was found to be significantly lower in donor urine for kidneys from poor cadaveric donors, based on clinical impression or renal transplant outcome, compared to urinary TAC of living related donors and good cadaveric donors [173, 174]. On the other hand, increased urinary TAC was found in patients with delayed graft function, but not with early graft function [174].

3. Systemic Diseases

Oxidative stress is associated with the metabolic syndrome, a cluster of cardiovascular risk factors including dyslipidemia, abnormal glucose tolerance, hypertension, and obesity [182]. Despite the antioxidant effect of uric acid (UA), hyperuricaemia is associated with obesity and insulin resistance [183] and has been proposed as a component of the metabolic syndrome [184, 185].

TABLE 2: Systemic diseases.

References	Case-control studies	Salivary TAC percentage (n°)	Urinary TAC percentage (n°)	Treatment effect percentage (n°)
[19, 37, 46, 50, 55, 56, 91, 100, 101, 107, 119, 129, 144]	Metabolic syndrome symptoms	↑ 41.7% (5/12) ↔ 33.3% (4/12) ↓ 25% (3/12)		Salivary TAC ↔ 100% (1/1) enalapril ↓ 100% (1/1) metoprolol ↓ 100% (1/1) rasburicase Urinary TAC ↓ 100% (1/1) PCI ↔ 100% (1/1) NAC before and after PCI
[59, 74, 118, 152, 165]	Cancer	↓ 66.7% (2/3) ↑ 33.3% (1/3)	↓ 66.7% (2/3) ↔ 33.3% (1/3)	Salivary TAC ↓ chemotherapy
[42, 105, 111, 117, 150, 167]	Neuropsychiatric disorders	↓ 75% (3/4) ↑ 25% (1/4)	↓ 100% (2/2)	
[43, 82, 116, 146, 151, 156, 163, 169]	Congenital and genetic diseases	↓ 33.3% (1/3) ↔ 33.3% (1/3) ↑ 33.3% (1/3)	↓ 83.3% (5/6) ↑ 16.7% (1/6)	Urinary TAC: ↑ 100% (3/3) low-protein diet + L-carnitine in IEM patients
[33, 38, 48, 58, 65, 106, 108, 109, 123, 126, 132, 135]	Immune mediated and inflammatory diseases	↓ 60% (6/10) ↑ 40% (4/10)		Salivary TAC ↔ 100% (1/1) corticosteroid ↔ 100% (2/2) CPAP in OSAS ↔ 100% (1/1) anti-TNFα therapy

CPAP: continuous positive airway pressure; IEM: inborn errors of metabolism; NAC: N-acetylcysteine; OSAS: obstructive sleep apnea syndrome; PCI: percutaneous coronary intervention; TAC: total antioxidant capacity; TNFα: tumor necrosis factor alpha; ↑: increase; ↓: decrease; ↔: unchanged.

Contrasting results came from the studies that investigated salivary TAC in subjects with at least one of the metabolic syndrome symptoms (Table 2).

Pregnant women with diabetes were found to have increased salivary TAC, but also markedly increased indexes of caries activity [119]. Besides the authors [119] found increased *Lactobacillus* and *Streptococcus* species in saliva of pregnant women with diabetes having systemic complications as compared to healthy individuals and other patients. However, increase in salivary TAC was observed also in obese subjects with hyperuricaemia [50] and in obese children despite their good oral hygiene status [56]. While rasburicase infusion decreased salivary TAC [50], intravenous N-acetylcysteine failed to prevent renal dysfunction and oxidative stress after contrast media administration during percutaneous coronary interventions [144] (Table 2). On the other hand, only hypertensive patients in treatment with metoprolol had lower salivary TAC compared to controls [46] (Table 2).

Salivary or urinary TAC was studied also in other diseases, such as cancer, neuropsychiatric disorders, congenital and genetic diseases, and immune mediated and inflammatory diseases (Table 2).

Urinary TAC was decreased in bladder cancer [165] and in nonsmokers with lung cancer [152], but not in smokers with lung cancer. Decreased salivary TAC was observed in patients with squamous cell carcinoma of head and neck [74] and with brain tumor [118], but increased salivary TAC was reported in acute lymphoblastic leukemia (ALL) children [59] (Table 2). Only children with more than 2 weeks of chemotherapy had decreased levels of salivary TAC [59].

Increased levels of salivary TAC were found in patients with neurological disorders and tube-feeding [42], whereas decreased levels were reported in cerebral palsy [117], intractable epilepsy [111], and autistic children [105]. Also urinary TAC levels were lower in autistic compared to healthy children [150, 167].

On the other hand, case-control studies on congenital or genetic diseases such as Down syndrome [43, 116] and cystic fibrosis [82] reported conflicting results on salivary TAC (Table 2). Besides, Campos et al. [146] found increased and decreased levels of urinary TAC in children and adults with Down syndrome, respectively (Table 2). On the contrary, urinary TAC resulted in a good marker of oxidative stress in patients with inborn errors of metabolism (IEM), such as maple syrup urine disease (MSUD), propionic aciduria (PA), methylmalonic aciduria (MMA), 3-hydroxy-3-methylglutaric aciduria (HMGA), and ornithine transcarbamylase deficiency (OTC), both before and after treatment (Table 2).

On the other hand, salivary TAC was lower in asthma [58], Crohn's disease [106], multiple sclerosis [65, 135], and Sjögren's syndrome [109] patients compared to healthy individuals (Table 2), but neither corticosteroid therapy, in multiple sclerosis patients [65], nor continuous positive airway pressure (CPAP) in obstructive sleep apnea syndrome (OSAS) improved salivary TAC [38, 123]. Furthermore, increased salivary TAC levels were found in chronic obstructive pulmonary disease (COPD) [132] and in juvenile idiopathic arthritis (JIA) [33]. Children with JIA, whether treated or not treated with anti-tumor necrosis factor- (TNF-) α agents (Infliximab or Etanercept), had higher salivary TAC and the increase of the active patients was nearly two times higher than that of nonactive patients [33]. Increased salivary TAC levels were found also in pre- and postsurgical patients, where surgical procedures, involving stress such as extended general anaesthesia and a long presurgical fasting period, may cause systemic inflammation and oxidative stress [126].

TABLE 3: Nutritional and supplement interventions.

References	Intervention	Number of bolus/repeated consumptions	Salivary TAC percentage (n°)	Urinary TAC percentage (n°)
[80, 94, 120, 127, 138, 141, 147, 168]	Caffeinated or alcoholic antioxidant beverages	5/4	↑ 50% (2/4) ↔ 50% (2/4)	↑ 40% (2/5) ↔ 60% (3/5)
[160, 166, 170]	Cocoa powder and walnuts	2/1		↑ 100% (3/3)
[137, 147, 153, 155, 157, 161, 164]	Fruit, juices, and vegetables	6/3	↔ 100% (1/1)	↑ 62.5% (5/8) ↓ 12.5% (1/8) ↔ 25% (2/8)
[25, 27, 64, 127, 142, 147, 159, 161, 171, 175–178]	Supplements and supplemented foods	4/12	↑ 50% (2/4) ↔ 50% (2/4)	↑ 58.3% (7/12) ↔ 41.7% (5/12)
[32, 143, 160, 164]	Other dietary interventions	1/3	↔ 100% (1/1)	↑ 66.7% (2/3) ↔ 33.3% (1/3)

TAC: Total Antioxidant Capacity.

Increased salivary TAC was also observed in Regional Pain Syndrome type I [48], whereas decreased salivary TAC levels were reported in temporomandibular disorders [108].

4. Nutritional and Supplement Interventions

Although body possesses a sophisticated and cooperative array of endogenous antioxidant defenses, dietary consumption of antioxidant-rich foods may lower the risk of noncommunicable diseases, by increasing TAC. In fact, 70% of the interventions with plant foods or supplements conducted on subjects characterized by oxidative stress conditions such as cardiovascular risk factors (smoking, hypercholesterolemia, metabolic syndrome, hyperlipidemia, and hypertension) or with pathologies reported an increase of plasma/serum TAC [186]. In the studies that investigated the effect of dietary or supplementation interventions on salivary or urinary TAC (Table 3), volunteers were prevalently healthy; however, in some studies, overweight (OW) [164] or elderly [94, 143, 147, 153] subjects, smokers [25], or patients with PD [137] or dialyzed [142] were enrolled. A review of 41 interventions, from 29 studies, has been performed (Table 3). Of these interventions, 18 regard a single ingestion (bolus) and the other 23 were related to repeated supplementations.

Caffeinated or alcoholic antioxidant beverages increased salivary TAC in 50% and urinary TAC in 40% of the interventions. In particular, green tea (GT) consumption for 4 or 12 weeks increased salivary TAC in laboratory workers and elderly subjects [94, 120], whereas it did not affect salivary TAC of Taekwondo (TKD) athletes after training [80]. Besides, Benzie et al. [141] found a significant correlation between urinary FRAP values and urinary total phenolic concentrations after GT consumption. Red wine bolus consumption did not change salivary TAC [127] but increased urinary TAC in elderly women [147]. After a single or 2 weeks of consumption of green or black coffee urinary TAC did not change [138, 168].

On the other hand, walnuts [160, 166] increased urinary TAC both after 4 weeks and after a single consumption and cocoa increased urinary TAC at 6–12 h after intake concomitantly with the excretion of epicatechin urinary metabolites [170] (Table 3).

Concerning fruit, juices, and vegetables, only Zare Javid et al. [137] investigated the effect of fruits, vegetables, and whole grains (3 and 6 months) consumption on salivary TAC of PD patients and did not find any change in this marker. Only one study reported decreased urinary TAC levels after a single consumption of blackberry juices [157]. On the contrary, urinary TAC increased after bolus consumption of spinach [147], strawberries [147], Jerte Valley cherry [153], and a fruit based drink (86% of a mix of apple, grape, blueberry and pomegranate juices and grape skin, grape seed, and green tea extracts) ingested during a high fat meal (HFM) [164]. In the same postprandial study, a less antioxidant fruit based drink (63% of a mix of pineapple, black currant, and plum juices) during HFM did not affect urinary TAC, a well as plasma TAC [164]. Also grape juice consumption for 5 days increased urinary TAC [155], whereas tomato juice consumption for 2 weeks did not [161]. The same study found increased urinary TAC levels when tomato juice was supplemented with vitamin C (870 mg/L) fortification [161]. Vitamin C (250 mg) with vitamin E (400 i.u.) supplementation for 8 weeks increased urinary TAC in dialyzed patients [142] and vitamin C in bolus administration increased urinary TAC in elderly women (1250 mg) [147] and salivary TAC in healthy subjects (250 mg) [64]. On the contrary neither vitamin C after 3 weeks (500 mg) of consumption in smokers [25] nor 90 days of astaxanthin supplementation in trained male soccer players in preexercise conditions [27] changed salivary TAC.

TABLE 4: Life-style factors.

References	Factor	Salivary TAC percentage (n°)	Urinary TAC percentage (n°)
[21, 80, 85, 134, 140]	Exercise	↓ 75% (3/4) ↑ 25% (1/4)	↓ 100% (1/1)
[32, 35, 41, 53, 71, 77, 93, 132, 136, 138, 145]	Smoking habit	↑ 20% (2/10) ↔ 50% (5/10) ↓ 30% (3/10)	↔ 100% (1/1)
[102]	Alcohol dependence	↓ 100% (1/1)	
[51, 139]	Occupational exposure to toxicants	↓ 100% (1/1)	↑ 100% (1/1)
[18, 20, 57, 67]	Cell phone and watching TV	↑ 75% (3/4) ↓ 25% (1/4)	

TAC: Total Antioxidant Capacity.

Conversely, red wine extract administration caused a marked rise in salivary TAC, within 30 min, and the same treatment raised also salivary polyphenol concentration [127]. Helbig et al. [159] reported the same increase in urinary TAC versus baseline with both control bread and bread enriched with black currant press residue (4 weeks). Besides, urinary TAC was unchanged after 21 days consumption of a dried fruit and vegetable extracts fortified with antioxidants [176], after 2 weeks of Pycnogenol (200 mg/day) supplementation [175] and after 24 days of administration of an antioxidant mixture containing vitamin E, beta-carotene, ascorbic acid, selenium, alpha-lipoic acid, N-acetyl 1-cysteine, catechin, lutein, and lycopene [171]. On the contrary, ganoderma lucidum (Lingzhi, woody mushroom) supplements increased urinary TAC both in bolus and in repeated administration [177, 178].

Concerning other dietary interventions, a low fat diet did not affect salivary TAC compared to a high fat diet [32] and a HFM did not affect urinary TAC [164]. On the contrary, a fish diet (8 oz/week of salmon) for 4 weeks [160] and the consumption of tryptophan-enriched cereals for 1 week [143] increased urinary TAC.

5. Age, Gender, and lifestyle Factors

Age and gender differences were observed in oxidative stress markers in plasma [187]. It was found that salivary TAC increased with the age of the children with caries [60], as well as during aging [62, 69]. On the contrary, others reported that salivary TAC was higher in younger subjects [73] and negative correlations with age were found for urinary TAC [146]. Women had significantly lower salivary TAC than men [79, 110, 114]. In this context Kawamoto et al. [66] reported decreased levels of salivary TAC during the ovulatory phase compared to follicular phase in women with PD, but not in healthy women. TAC was negatively correlated with bacterial counts during the ovulatory phase, but not during the follicular phase [66]. Besides, salivary TAC was lower during uncomplicated pregnancy [70] and in osteoporotic subjects compared to age-matched healthy women [133].

Apart from age, gender, diseases, and dietary habit, also lifestyle factors could affect salivary and urinary TAC. Within lifestyle factors, many studies investigated the effect of exercise and smoking habit on salivary or urinary TAC (Table 4).

In agreement with the well-known reduction of antioxidant defenses after physical stress, strong correlation was found between the variations of salivary and plasma TAC during the training season in triathletes [134]. Both 2 hr TKD training session and 1 hr exhaustive aerobic dance exercise decreased salivary TAC [21, 80]. Besides also urinary TAC decreased after 3 hours or more of TKD training camp/d for 5–8 days [140]. Only a study found increased salivary TAC in older adults with PD who performed Tai Chi during a period of 6 months; however this increase was accompanied by a statistically significant decrease in the Periodontal Disease Index (PDI) [85].

More conflicting are results on smoking habit; higher, lower, or nonsignificant different levels of salivary TAC have been found in smokers compared to nonsmokers, whereas no significant differences were found in urinary TAC between smokers and nonsmokers (Table 4).

On the contrary, alcohol-dependent subjects showed significantly lower TAC in blood and saliva as compared to those in the controls and the alcohol withdrawal caused an increase in the TAC to near-control values [102].

Decreased levels of salivary TAC were found also in workers subjected to occupational exposure to nonferrous metal mine conditions [51], whereas exposure to trichloroethylene increased urinary TAC [139].

Although there was no statistically significant effect of cell phone talking time on the salivary TAC, the latter progressively increased with time and reached maximum at 30 min, probably due to exposure to radio frequency radiation [67]. However, both increased [57] and decreased [18] levels of salivary TAC in mobile phone users were found.

On the other hand, it has been observed that salivary TAC was affected by emotional and psychological factors [20]. In particular, watching a cheerful comical video for 30 min increased salivary TAC [20].

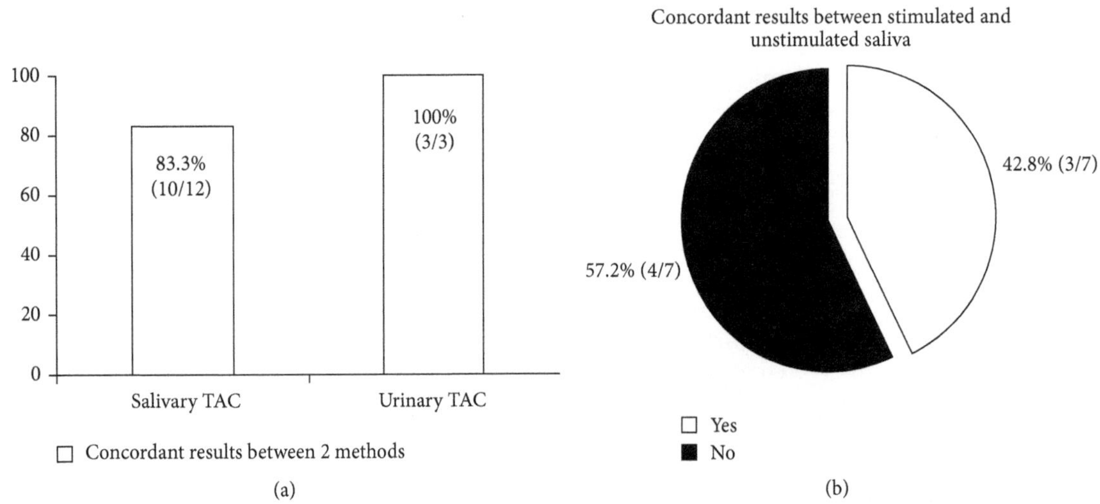

FIGURE 1: Concordat results between two different methods used in the same study to measure salivary or urinary TAC (a). Concordant results between unstimulated and stimulated saliva samples analyzed in the same study (b). References [22, 24, 34, 38, 50, 62, 64, 65, 67, 72, 78, 81, 111, 127, 135, 137, 161, 166, 175, 188–190].

6. Methodological Issues

Despite the differences between the assays [8], concordant results were found in the majority of the cases between the results obtained when two different methods (Trolox Equivalent Antioxidant Capacity (TEAC), Ferric Reducing Antioxidant Potential (FRAP), Oxygen Radical Antioxidant Capacity (ORAC), Total-radical Trapping Antioxidant Parameter (TRAP), or enzyme-linked immunosorbent assay (ELISA) colorimetric kit) were used in the same study to measure salivary or urinary TAC (Figure 1(a)).

In particular, although FRAP was significantly lower in multiple sclerosis patients, whereas no significant difference in salivary TEAC between patients and controls was observed [65], the authors pointed out that their study had some limitations, such as the low number of patients included, the variability of the clinical status, and the different treatment of patients. Therefore, method choice does not seem to be a critical point for salivary TAC measure. On the contrary, major concerns came from saliva collection (Figure 1(b)).

Saliva sampling has been improved by cotton and polypropylene Salivette collection systems, but the latter altered the determination of some markers [188]. It has been reported that in samples collected using the cotton Salivette TAC was comparable, but higher thiobarbituric acid reacting substances (TBARS) concentrations were determined compared with unstimulated saliva [188].

In healthy subjects values were higher under stimulated conditions for saliva flow and were higher under unstimulated conditions with respect to TAC and UA [189]. When TAC was examined with respect to flow rate, a significantly lower rate of antioxidant production was noted in patients with PD compared with controls for unstimulated saliva but not for stimulated saliva [34]. Besides, a significant decrease in UA and TAC was observed in unstimulated saliva as well as a significant increase in all antioxidants examined in stimulated saliva of systemic sclerosis women with normal salivary flow rate as compared to the healthy controls [135].

Nagler et al. [190] examined the correlation between the levels of various salivary antioxidant components and the TAC in whole saliva in comparison with those in saliva secreted specifically from the major salivary glands: the parotid and the submandibular/sublingual (Sm_Sl) glands. While the secretory IgA and lysozyme concentrations were similar in parotid and Sm_Sl saliva, the authors [190] found higher levels of the various antioxidant parameters (antioxidant enzymes, UA and TAC) in the parotid saliva as compared with the Sm_Sl saliva, especially under resting condition. Under resting condition parotid saliva was the major source of salivary antioxidants, especially of UA [190]. After stimulation (i.e., eating), the various parameters of antioxidants of parotid saliva were considerably reduced, in light of the well-reported "dilution effect" that follows stimulation. In addition, fluids by nonglandular sources contributed to the possible dilution of the whole saliva, after meal. Therefore, unstimulated saliva with and without flow rate normalization could be the better approaches to measure salivary TAC.

Also urine can be more or less diluted, complicating the evaluation of parameters in spontaneous urine. Particularly after physical stress [140] more concentrated urine is to be expected due to sweating. In order to obviate this problem and provided that the creatinine excretion is relatively constant over 24 h, the mean creatinine excretion can serve as a reference for the measured values of excretion. Generally, an average creatinine excretion of 1 g/24 h is assumed [140]. However, it must be taken into consideration that age, sex, muscle mass, and diet all have an influence on creatinine excretion [191]. Although analyzing 24 h urine collection would have been preferable in case-control studies, it was logistically impossible in some cases. On the other hand, 24 h urine collection could not appreciate the increase in TAC due to intervention with polyphenol-rich foods, considering

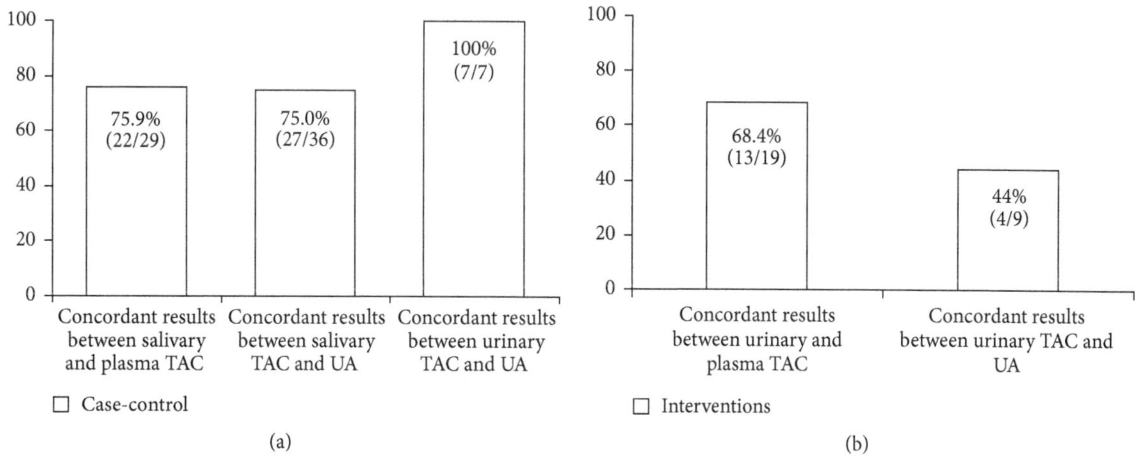

FIGURE 2: Concordant results between salivary or urinary TAC and UA levels or plasma TAC in case-control (a) or antioxidant/nutritional intervention (b) studies. References [17, 19, 21–24, 26, 28–31, 34, 37, 38, 40–44, 48–51, 55, 57, 61, 62, 65, 71, 77, 78, 81, 82, 86–89, 91, 92, 95–97, 102, 106–111, 119, 126, 132–136, 140–142, 144, 146, 147, 150, 154, 157, 159–162, 164, 166, 171, 175–178].

the rate of elimination of polyphenols [12]. Therefore, 24 h or spontaneous urine collection should be chosen on the basis of the study outcome and of the creatinine clearance.

7. Uric Acid-Independent TAC versus TAC

UA is a powerful scavenger of free radicals and provides 60–80% of TAC in plasma [192, 193]. It has been also reported that TAC of both plasma and urine is mainly related to the UA concentration of the samples [194]. Besides, UA contributes approximately 70% of the salivary TAC [89], with the antioxidant role of the ascorbic acid being secondary [89] and correlation between concentrations of UA in both saliva and plasma points to the latter as the origin of salivary UA [71, 190]. According to this hypothesis, when salivary or urinary TAC, UA, and plasma or serum TAC were measured in the same study, it turned out that there was a clear accordance between UA concentration and TAC, as well as between salivary or urinary TAC and plasma or serum TAC in case-control studies (Figure 2(a)). Furthermore, rasburicase i.v. infusion in obese subjects with hyperuricaemia caused a marked decrease in both plasma and saliva TAC values [50].

Increase in serum UA levels can be due to increased intake of dietary purines, alcohol and fructose [195], impaired renal function and renal microvascular disease, which can increase UA production and/or decrease UA clearance [196], and hyperinsulinemia, which increases renal UA reabsorption [197]. In particular, the plasma level of UA is regulated by renal function [162]. However, although urine from renal disease patients had more proteins and UA compared to controls, urinary TAC from acute renal failure patients did not correlate with UA [162]. Furthermore, contrasting results came from patients with severe chronic renal failure (CRF) (dialytic) without diabetes and severe CRF (dialytic) with diabetes [30]. In severe-CRF patients without diabetes, median TAC and UA levels decreased following dialysis, whereas in severe-CRF patients with diabetes, median TAC increased following dialysis while median UA decreased [30].

Although UA in urine samples constitutes about 75% of urinary TAC [140], the composition of urine is unpredictable, reflecting the continuously changing environment of the body, which is affected, among other factors, by diet [162]. In fact, only in 44% (4/9) of the interventions with antioxidant foods, beverages or supplements urinary TAC was related to UA (Figure 1(b)). These findings are probably due to the fact that low molecular weight antioxidants, such as polyphenols, are cleared from the blood by kidney [12]. The only study that [137] investigated the effect of fruits, vegetables, and whole grains consumption on both salivary and plasma TAC did not find any change in salivary TAC, despite the increase in plasma TAC.

In order to avoid the UA interference, methods for UA-independent TAC have been proposed, by using the uricase reaction, in both plasma and urine [198], or by using the corrected TAC, the calculated parameter that represents the fraction of circulating antioxidants after the elimination of the interference of UA [140, 199].

Similar calculated urinary TAC has been proposed by Campos et al. [146]. Authors suggested that TAC-UA/Cr could provide more reliable information about the antioxidant status, at least in Down syndrome, because children had higher TAC/Cr and UA/Cr, whereas levels of TAC-UA/Cr of adult patients were lower compared to healthy subjects.

On the contrary, uricase methods could be biased by the generation of H_2O_2 during the action of uricase [200]. Therefore, the calculated corrected TAC-UA could be the better approach.

8. Conclusion

The reviewed case-control and intervention studies that measured salivary or urinary TAC revealed that these markers can be useful in the evaluation of the antioxidant status of the body taking into account some factors. First of all, salivary and urinary TAC were particularly affected by oral or renal status, respectively, as well as by infection

(Table 1); therefore these factors could bias results in some studies [66, 85, 119]. Second, samples collection (Figure 1) and normalization strategies should be chosen on the basis of the type of biological fluid, of the study outcome, and of the creatinine clearance. Again, TAC is related to both UA (Figure 2) and nutritional antioxidant levels in biological fluids [127, 141, 147, 170]. From that, the UA-independent TAC could be the better approach to evaluate red-ox status of body both after nutritional interventions and in diseases associated with hyperuricaemia. Finally, TAC is sensitive also to the endogenous antioxidant response induced by some pathological and environmental conditions [20, 33, 48, 57, 59, 67, 115, 126, 132, 139, 142].

Conflict of Interests

The authors declare that there is no conflict of interests regarding the publication of this paper.

References

[1] K.-H. Wagner and H. Brath, "A global view on the development of non communicable diseases," *Preventive Medicine*, vol. 54, supplement, pp. S38–S41, 2012.

[2] J. Limón-Pacheco and M. E. Gonsebatt, "The role of antioxidants and antioxidant-related enzymes in protective responses to environmentally induced oxidative stress," *Mutation Research/Genetic Toxicology and Environmental Mutagenesis*, vol. 674, no. 1-2, pp. 137–147, 2009.

[3] M. Valko, D. Leibfritz, J. Moncol, M. T. D. Cronin, M. Mazur, and J. Telser, "Free radicals and antioxidants in normal physiological functions and human disease," *International Journal of Biochemistry and Cell Biology*, vol. 39, no. 1, pp. 44–84, 2007.

[4] E. Niki, "Assessment of antioxidant capacity in vitro and in vivo," *Free Radical Biology and Medicine*, vol. 49, no. 4, pp. 503–515, 2010.

[5] G. Bartosz, "Non-enzymatic antioxidant capacity assays: limitations of use in biomedicine," *Free Radical Research*, vol. 44, no. 7, pp. 711–720, 2010.

[6] S. Knasmüller, A. Nersesyan, M. Mišík et al., "Use of conventional and -omics based methods for health claims of dietary antioxidants: a critical overview," *British Journal of Nutrition*, vol. 99, supplement 1, pp. ES3–ES52, 2008.

[7] I. Pinchuk, H. Shoval, Y. Dotan, and D. Lichtenberg, "Evaluation of antioxidants: scope, limitations and relevance of assays," *Chemistry and Physics of Lipids*, vol. 165, no. 6, pp. 638–647, 2012.

[8] V. Dilis and A. Trichopoulou, "Assessment of antioxidants in foods and biological samples: a short critique," *International Journal of Food Sciences and Nutrition*, vol. 61, no. 5, pp. 441–448, 2010.

[9] G. Cao and R. L. Prior, "Comparison of different analytical methods for assessing total antioxidant capacity of human serum," *Clinical Chemistry*, vol. 44, no. 6, part 1, pp. 1309–1315, 1998.

[10] C. Campos, R. Guzmán, E. López-Fernández, and Á. Casado, "Evaluation of the copper(II) reduction assay using bathocuproinedisulfonic acid disodium salt for the total antioxidant capacity assessment: the CUPRAC-BCS assay," *Analytical Biochemistry*, vol. 392, no. 1, pp. 37–44, 2009.

[11] M. Greabu, M. Battino, M. Mohora et al., "Could constitute saliva the first line of defence against oxidative stress?" *Romanian Journal of Internal Medicine*, vol. 45, no. 2, pp. 209–213, 2007.

[12] J. Pérez-Jiménez, J. Hubert, L. Hooper et al., "Urinary metabolites as biomarkers of polyphenol intake in humans: a systematic review," *The American Journal of Clinical Nutrition*, vol. 92, no. 4, pp. 801–809, 2010.

[13] H. Abdolsamadi, N. Rafieian, M. T. Goodarzi et al., "Levels of salivary antioxidant vitamins and lipid peroxidation in patients with oral lichen planus and healthy individuals," *Chonnam Medical Journal*, vol. 50, no. 2, pp. 58–62, 2014.

[14] F. Agha-Hosseini, I. Mirzaii-Dizgah, N. Farmanbar, and M. Abdollahi, "Oxidative stress status and DNA damage in saliva of human subjects with oral lichen planus and oral squamous cell carcinoma," *Journal of Oral Pathology and Medicine*, vol. 41, no. 10, pp. 736–740, 2012.

[15] F. Agha-Hosseini, I. Mirzaii-Dizgah, S. Mikaili, and M. Abdollahi, "Increased salivary lipid peroxidation in human subjects with oral lichen planus," *International Journal of Dental Hygiene*, vol. 7, no. 4, pp. 246–250, 2009.

[16] F. Ahmadi-Motamayel, M.-T. Goodarzi, S.-S. Hendi, S. Kasraei, and A. Moghimbeigi, "Total antioxidant capacity of saliva and dental caries," *Medicina Oral, Patología Oral y Cirugía Bucal*, vol. 18, no. 4, pp. e553–e556, 2013.

[17] D. Aizenbud, Y. Peri-Front, and R. M. Nagler, "Salivary analysis and antioxidants in cleft lip and palate children," *Archives of Oral Biology*, vol. 53, no. 6, pp. 517–522, 2008.

[18] F. Arbabi-Kalati, S. Salimi, A. Vaziry-Rabiee, and M. Noraeei, "Effect of mobile phone usage time on total antioxidant capacity of saliva and salivary immunoglobulin A," *Iranian Journal of Public Health*, vol. 43, no. 4, pp. 480–484, 2014.

[19] F. Astaneie, M. Afshari, A. Mojtahedi et al., "Total antioxidant capacity and levels of epidermal growth factor and nitric oxide in blood and saliva of insulin-dependent diabetic patients," *Archives of Medical Research*, vol. 36, no. 4, pp. 376–381, 2005.

[20] T. Atsumi, S. Fujisawa, Y. Nakabayashi, T. Kawarai, T. Yasui, and K. Tonosaki, "Pleasant feeling from watching a comical video enhances free radical-scavenging capacity in human whole saliva," *Journal of Psychosomatic Research*, vol. 56, no. 3, pp. 377–379, 2004.

[21] T. Atsumi, I. Iwakura, Y. Kashiwagi, S. Fujisawa, and T. Ueha, "Free radical scavenging activity in the nonenzymatic fraction of human saliva: a simple DPPH assay showing the effect of physical exercise," *Antioxidants and Redox Signaling*, vol. 1, no. 4, pp. 537–546, 1999.

[22] I. Avivi, S. Avraham, M. Koren-Michowitz et al., "Oral integrity and salivary profile in myeloma patients undergoing high-dose therapy followed by autologous SCT," *Bone Marrow Transplantation*, vol. 43, no. 10, pp. 801–806, 2009.

[23] A. Azizi and F. Farshchi, "Comparison of salivary and plasma antioxidant levels in lichen planus patients and healthy subjects," *Journal of Oral Pathology and Medicine*, vol. 41, no. 7, pp. 524–526, 2012.

[24] G. Bahar, R. Feinmesser, T. Shpitzer, A. Popovtzer, and R. M. Nagler, "Salivary analysis in oral cancer patients: DNA and protein oxidation, reactive nitrogen species, and antioxidant profile," *Cancer*, vol. 109, no. 1, pp. 54–59, 2007.

[25] S. Bakhtiari, J. B. Taheri, M. Bakhshi et al., "Effect of vitamin C on salivary total antioxidant capacity in smokers," *Iranian Journal of Pharmaceutical Research*, vol. 11, no. 4, pp. 1045–1049, 2012.

[26] E. Baltacıoğlu, P. Yuva, G. Aydın et al., "Lipid peroxidation levels and total oxidant/antioxidant status in serum and saliva from patients with chronic and aggressive periodontitis. Oxidative stress index: a new biomarker for periodontal disease?" *Journal of Periodontology*, vol. 85, no. 10, pp. 1432–1441, 2014.

[27] I. Baralic, M. Andjelkovic, B. Djordjevic et al., "Effect of astaxanthin supplementation on salivary IgA, oxidative stress, and inflammation in young soccer players," *Evidence-Based Complementary and Alternative Medicine*, vol. 2015, Article ID 783761, 9 pages, 2015.

[28] U. Baser, H. Gamsiz-Isik, E. Cifcibasi, E. Ademoglu, and F. Yalcin, "Plasma and salivary total antioxidant capacity in healthy controls compared with aggressive and chronic periodontitis patients," *Saudi Medical Journal*, vol. 36, no. 7, pp. 856–861, 2015.

[29] M. Battino, M. Greabu, A. Totan et al., "Oxidative stress markers in oral lichen planus," *BioFactors*, vol. 33, no. 4, pp. 301–310, 2008.

[30] I. Ben-Zvi, Y. Green, F. Nakhoul, Y. Kanter, and R. M. Nagler, "Effects of diabetes mellitus, chronic renal failure and hemodialysis on serum and salivary antioxidant status," *Nephron—Clinical Practice*, vol. 105, no. 3, pp. c114–c120, 2007.

[31] G. Bibi, Y. Green, and R. M. Nagler, "Compositional and oxidative analysis in the saliva and serum of predialysis chronic kidney disease patients and end-stage renal failure patients on peritoneal dialysis," *Therapeutic Apheresis and Dialysis*, vol. 12, no. 2, pp. 164–170, 2008.

[32] M. Bogucka, J. Giebułtowicz, K. Zawada et al., "The oxidation status of ALDH3A1 in human saliva and its correlation with antioxidant capacity measured by orac method," *Acta Poloniae Pharmaceutica*, vol. 66, no. 5, pp. 477–482, 2009.

[33] R. Brik, I. Rosen, D. Savulescu, I. Borovoi, M. Gavish, and R. Nagler, "Salivary antioxidants and metalloproteinases in juvenile idiopathic arthritis," *Molecular Medicine*, vol. 16, no. 3-4, pp. 122–128, 2010.

[34] G. R. Brock, C. J. Butterworth, J. B. Matthews, and I. L. C. Chapple, "Local and systemic total antioxidant capacity in periodontitis and health," *Journal of Clinical Periodontology*, vol. 31, no. 7, pp. 515–521, 2004.

[35] N. Buduneli, L. Kardeşler, H. Işik et al., "Effects of smoking and gingival inflammation on salivary antioxidant capacity," *Journal of Clinical Periodontology*, vol. 33, no. 3, pp. 159–164, 2006.

[36] F. Çağlayan, Ö. Miloglu, O. Altun, Ö. Erel, and A. B. Yilmaz, "Oxidative stress and myeloperoxidase levels in saliva of patients with recurrent aphthous stomatitis," *Oral Diseases*, vol. 14, no. 8, pp. 700–704, 2008.

[37] V. Canakci, A. Yildirim, C. F. Canakci, A. Eltas, Y. Cicek, and H. Canakcit, "Total antioxidant capacity and antioxidant enzymes in serum, saliva, and gingival crevicular fluid of preeclamptic women with and without periodontal disease," *Journal of Periodontology*, vol. 78, no. 8, pp. 1602–1611, 2007.

[38] P. Celec, J. Hodosy, M. Behuliak et al., "Oxidative and carbonyl stress in patients with obstructive sleep apnea treated with continuous positive airway pressure," *Sleep and Breathing*, vol. 16, no. 2, pp. 393–398, 2012.

[39] V. Celecová, N. Kamodyová, L'. Tóthová, M. Kúdela, and P. Celec, "Salivary markers of oxidative stress are related to age and oral health in adult non-smokers," *Journal of Oral Pathology and Medicine*, vol. 42, no. 3, pp. 263–266, 2013.

[40] I. L. C. Chapple, G. I. Mason, I. Garner et al., "Enhanced chemiluminescent assay for measuring the total antioxidant capacity of serum, saliva and crevicular fluid," *Annals of Clinical Biochemistry*, vol. 34, part 4, pp. 412–421, 1997.

[41] K. Charalabopoulos, D. Assimakopoulos, S. Karkabounas, V. Danielidis, D. Kiortsis, and A. Evangelou, "Effects of cigarette smoking on the antioxidant defence in young healthy male volunteers," *International Journal of Clinical Practice*, vol. 59, no. 1, pp. 25–30, 2005.

[42] A. S. Cunha-Correia, A. H. Neto, A. F. Pereira, S. M. H. C. Á. Aguiar, and A. C. D. M. S. Nakamune, "Enteral nutrition feeding alters antioxidant activity in unstimulated whole saliva composition of patients with neurological disorders," *Research in Developmental Disabilities*, vol. 35, no. 6, pp. 1209–1215, 2014.

[43] M. C. de Sousa, R. B. Vieira, D. S. Dos Santos et al., "Antioxidants and biomarkers of oxidative damage in the saliva of patients with Down's syndrome," *Archives of Oral Biology*, vol. 60, no. 4, pp. 600–605, 2015.

[44] R. Diab-Ladki, B. Pellat, and R. Chahine, "Decrease in the total antioxidant activity of saliva in patients with periodontal diseases," *Clinical Oral Investigations*, vol. 7, no. 2, pp. 103–107, 2003.

[45] R. A. DiSilvestro, D. J. DiSilvestro, and D. J. DiSilvestro, "Pomegranate extract mouth rinsing effects on saliva measures relevant to gingivitis risk," *Phytotherapy Research*, vol. 23, no. 8, pp. 1123–1127, 2009.

[46] L. Djukić, J. Roganović, M. D. Brajović, D. Bokonjić, and D. Stojić, "The effects of anti-hypertensives and type 2 diabetes on salivary flow and total antioxidant capacity," *Oral Diseases*, vol. 21, no. 5, pp. 619–625, 2015.

[47] R. Dodwad, A. V. Betigeri, and B. P. Preeti, "Estimation of total antioxidant capacity levels in saliva of caries-free and caries-active children," *Contemporary Clinical Dentistry*, vol. 2, no. 1, pp. 17–20, 2011.

[48] E. Eisenberg, S. Shtahl, R. Geller et al., "Serum and salivary oxidative analysis in Complex Regional Pain Syndrome," *Pain*, vol. 138, no. 1, pp. 226–232, 2008.

[49] S. Ergun, Ş. C. Troşala, S. Warnakulasuriya et al., "Evaluation of oxidative stress and antioxidant profile in patients with oral lichen planus," *Journal of Oral Pathology and Medicine*, vol. 40, no. 4, pp. 286–293, 2011.

[50] E. Fabbrini, M. Serafini, I. Colic Baric, S. L. Hazen, and S. Klein, "Effect of plasma uric acid on antioxidant capacity, oxidative stress, and insulin sensitivity in obese subjects," *Diabetes*, vol. 63, no. 3, pp. 976–981, 2014.

[51] M. Greabu, A. Didilescu, L. Puiu, D. Miricescu, and A. Totan, "Salivary antioxidant biomarkers in non-ferrous metals mine workers—a pilot study," *Journal of Oral Pathology and Medicine*, vol. 41, no. 6, pp. 490–493, 2012.

[52] M. Greabu, M. Purice, A. Totan, T. Spînu, and C. Totan, "Salivary cortisol-marker of stress response to different dental treatment," *Romanian Journal of Internal Medicine*, vol. 44, no. 1, pp. 49–59, 2006.

[53] A. Guentsch, P. M. Preshaw, S. Bremer-Streck, G. Klinger, E. Glockmann, and B. W. Sigusch, "Lipid peroxidation and antioxidant activity in saliva of periodontitis patients: effect of smoking and periodontal treatment," *Clinical Oral Investigations*, vol. 12, no. 4, pp. 345–352, 2008.

[54] C. Guler, E. Toy, F. Ozturk, D. Gunes, A. B. Karabulut, and O. Otlu, "Evaluation of salivary total oxidant-antioxidant status and DNA damage of children undergoing fixed orthodontic therapy," *The Angle Orthodontist*, vol. 85, no. 2, pp. 239–244, 2015.

[55] P. Gümüş, N. Buduneli, Ş. Çetinkalp et al., "Salivary antioxidants in patients with type 1 or 2 diabetes and inflammatory

periodontal disease: a case-control study," *Journal of Periodontology*, vol. 80, no. 9, pp. 1440–1446, 2009.

[56] G. Gunjalli, K. N. Kumar, S. K. Jain, S. K. Reddy, G. R. Shavi, and S. L. Ajagannanavar, "Total salivary anti-oxidant levels, dental development and oral health status in childhood obesity," *Journal of International Oral Health*, vol. 6, no. 4, pp. 63–67, 2014.

[57] Y. Hamzany, R. Feinmesser, T. Shpitzer et al., "Is human saliva an indicator of the adverse health effects of using mobile phones?" *Antioxidants and Redox Signaling*, vol. 18, no. 6, pp. 622–627, 2013.

[58] A. M. Hegde, K. Raj, and S. Shetty, "Relation of caries status on the salivary total antioxidant levels in asthmatic children," *Contemporary Clinical Dentistry*, vol. 3, no. 4, pp. 402–405, 2012.

[59] A. M. Hegde, S. Joshi, K. Rai, and S. Shetty, "Evaluation of oral hygiene status, salivary characteristics and dental caries experience in Acute Lymphoblastic Leukemic (ALL) children," *Journal of Clinical Pediatric Dentistry*, vol. 35, no. 3, pp. 319–323, 2011.

[60] A. M. Hegde, K. Rai, and V. Padmanabhan, "Total antioxidant capacity of saliva and its relation with early childhood caries and rampant caries," *Journal of Clinical Pediatric Dentistry*, vol. 33, no. 3, pp. 231–234, 2009.

[61] M. N. Hegde, N. D. Hegde, A. Ashok, and S. Shetty, "Evaluation of total antioxidant capacity of saliva and serum in caries-free and caries-active adults: an in-vivo study," *Indian Journal of Dental Research*, vol. 24, no. 2, pp. 164–167, 2013.

[62] O. Hershkovich, I. Shafat, and R. M. Nagler, "Age-related changes in salivary antioxidant profile: possible implications for oral cancer," *Journals of Gerontology, Series A: Biological Sciences and Medical Sciences*, vol. 62, no. 4, pp. 361–366, 2007.

[63] N. Kamodyová, G. Minárik, J. Hodosy, and P. Celec, "Single consumption of Bryndza cheese temporarily affects oral microbiota and salivary markers of oxidative stress," *Current Microbiology*, vol. 69, no. 5, pp. 716–724, 2014.

[64] N. Kamodyová, L. Tóthová, and P. Celec, "Salivary markers of oxidative stress and antioxidant status: influence of external factors," *Disease Markers*, vol. 34, no. 5, pp. 313–321, 2013.

[65] M. Karlík, P. Valkovič, V. Hančinová, L. Krížová, Ľ. Tóthová, and P. Celec, "Markers of oxidative stress in plasma and saliva in patients with multiple sclerosis," *Clinical Biochemistry*, vol. 48, no. 1-2, pp. 24–28, 2015.

[66] A. Kawamoto, N. Sugano, M. Motohashi, S. Matsumoto, and K. Ito, "Relationship between salivary antioxidant capacity and phases of the menstrual cycle," *Journal of Periodontal Research*, vol. 47, no. 5, pp. 593–598, 2012.

[67] A. M. Khalil, K. M. Abu Khadra, A. M. Aljaberi, M. H. Gagaa, and H. S. Issa, "Assessment of oxidant/antioxidant status in saliva of cell phone users," *Electromagnetic Biology and Medicine*, vol. 33, no. 2, pp. 92–97, 2014.

[68] S.-C. Kim, O.-S. Kim, O.-J. Kim, Y.-J. Kim, and H.-J. Chung, "Antioxidant profile of whole saliva after scaling and root planing in periodontal disease," *Journal of Periodontal and Implant Science*, vol. 40, no. 4, pp. 164–171, 2010.

[69] R. Kohen, O. Tirosh, and K. Kopolovich, "The reductive capacity index of saliva obtained from donors of various ages," *Experimental Gerontology*, vol. 27, no. 2, pp. 161–168, 1992.

[70] E. Kolarzyk, A. Pietrzycka, M. Stępniewski, J. Łyszczarz, A. Mendyk, and A. Ostachowska-Gąsior, "Micronutrients and macronutrients and parameters of antioxidative ability in saliva of women: inhabitants of Krakow (Poland) in the course of uncomplicated singleton pregnancy," *Biological Trace Element Research*, vol. 114, no. 1–3, pp. 73–84, 2006.

[71] I. Kondakova, E. A. Lissi, and M. Pizarro, "Total reactive antioxidant potential in human saliva of smokers and non-smokers," *Biochemistry and Molecular Biology International*, vol. 47, no. 6, pp. 911–920, 1999.

[72] D. Krawczyk, J. Błaszczak, J. Borowicz, and M. Mielnik-Błaszczak, "Life style and risk of development of dental caries in a population of adolescents," *Annals of Agricultural and Environmental Medicine*, vol. 21, no. 3, pp. 576–580, 2014.

[73] D. Krawczyk, M. H. J. Sikorska-Jaroszyńska, M. Mielnik-Błaszczak, K. Pasternak, E. Kapeć, and M. Sztanke, "Dental caries and total antioxidant status of unstimulated mixed whole saliva in patients aged 16–23 years," *Advances in Medical Sciences*, vol. 57, no. 1, pp. 163–168, 2012.

[74] A. Kumar, M. C. Pant, H. S. Singh, and S. Khandelwal, "Determinants of oxidative stress and DNA damage (8-OhdG) in squamous cell carcinoma of head and neck," *Indian Journal of Cancer*, vol. 49, no. 3, pp. 309–315, 2012.

[75] D. Kumar, R. K. Pandey, D. Agrawal, and D. Agrawal, "An estimation and evaluation of total antioxidant capacity of saliva in children with severe early childhood caries," *International Journal of Paediatric Dentistry*, vol. 21, no. 6, pp. 459–464, 2011.

[76] A. Kurhańska-Flisykowska, W. Łojewski, and M. Wyganowska-Swiatkowska, "Effectiveness of Emdogain in the periodontal treatment," *Przegląd Lekarski*, vol. 69, no. 10, pp. 1046–1048, 2012.

[77] H. Kurku, M. Kacmaz, U. Kisa, O. Dogan, and O. Caglayan, "Acute and chronic impact of smoking on salivary and serum total antioxidant capacity," *Journal of Pakistan Medical Association*, vol. 65, no. 2, pp. 164–169, 2015.

[78] M. F. Leite, N. F. D. Ferreira, C. D. W. M. Shitsuka et al., "Effect of topical application of fluoride gel NaF 2% on enzymatic and non-enzymatic antioxidant parameters of saliva," *Archives of Oral Biology*, vol. 57, no. 6, pp. 630–635, 2012.

[79] I. Lettrichová, L. Tóthová, J. Hodosy, M. Behuliak, and P. Celec, "Variability of salivary markers of oxidative stress and antioxidant status in young healthy individuals," *Redox Report*, 2015.

[80] S.-P. Lin, C.-Y. Li, K. Suzuki, C.-K. Chang, K.-M. Chou, and S.-H. Fang, "Green tea consumption after intense taekwondo training enhances salivary defense factors and antibacterial capacity," *PLoS ONE*, vol. 9, no. 1, Article ID e87580, 2014.

[81] S. Liskmann, T. Vihalemm, O. Salum, K. Zilmer, K. Fischer, and M. Zilmer, "Characterization of the antioxidant profile of human saliva in peri-implant health and disease," *Clinical Oral Implants Research*, vol. 18, no. 1, pp. 27–33, 2007.

[82] G. Livnat, L. Bentur, E. Kuzmisnsky, and R. M. Nagler, "Salivary profile and oxidative stress in children and adolescents with cystic fibrosis," *Journal of Oral Pathology and Medicine*, vol. 39, no. 1, pp. 16–21, 2010.

[83] P. Lopez-Jornet, A. Martinez-Canovas, and A. Pons-Fuster, "Salivary biomarkers of oxidative stress and quality of life in patients with oral lichen planus," *Geriatrics and Gerontology International*, vol. 14, no. 3, pp. 654–659, 2014.

[84] S. Mahjoub, M. Ghasempour, A. Gharage, A. Bijani, and J. Masrourroudsari, "Comparison of total antioxidant capacity in saliva of children with severe early childhood caries and caries-free children," *Caries Research*, vol. 48, no. 4, pp. 271–275, 2014.

[85] V. M. Mendoza-Núñez, B. Hernández-Monjaraz, E. Santiago-Osorio, J. M. Betancourt-Rule, and M. Ruiz-Ramos, "Tai chi exercise increases SOD activity and total antioxidant status in saliva and is linked to an improvement of periodontal disease

in the elderly," *Oxidative Medicine and Cellular Longevity*, vol. 2014, Article ID 603853, 6 pages, 2014.

[86] E. Meucci, C. Littarru, G. Deli, G. Luciani, L. Tazza, and G. P. Littarru, "Antioxidant status and dialysis: plasma and saliva antioxidant activity in patients with fluctuating urate levels," *Free Radical Research*, vol. 29, no. 5, pp. 367–376, 1998.

[87] D. Miricescu, A. Totan, B. Calenic et al., "Salivary biomarkers: relationship between oxidative stress and alveolar bone loss in chronic periodontitis," *Acta Odontologica Scandinavica*, vol. 72, no. 1, pp. 42–47, 2014.

[88] J. Momen-Beitollahi, A. Mansourian, F. Momen-Heravi, M. Amanlou, S. Obradov, and M. Sahebjamee, "Assessment of salivary and serum antioxidant status in patients with recurrent aphthous stomatitis," *Medicina Oral, Patologia Oral y Cirugia Bucal*, vol. 15, no. 4, pp. e557–e561, 2010.

[89] S. Moore, K. A. C. Calder, N. J. Miller, and C. A. Rice-Evans, "Antioxidant activity of saliva and periodontal disease," *Free Radical Research*, vol. 21, no. 6, pp. 417–425, 1994.

[90] S. Muchandi, H. Walimbe, M. N. Ahmed Bijle et al., "Comparative evaluation and correlation of salivary total antioxidant capacity and salivary pH in caries-free and severe early childhood caries children," *The Journal of Contemporary Dental Practice*, vol. 16, no. 3, pp. 234–237, 2015.

[91] S. Mussavira, M. Dharmalingam, and B. O. Sukumaran, "Salivary glucose and antioxidant defense markers in type II diabetes mellitus," *Turkish Journal of Medical Sciences*, vol. 45, no. 1, pp. 141–147, 2015.

[92] R. Nagler, L. Barness-Hadar, M. Lieba, and A. Nagler, "Salivary antioxidant capacity in graft versus host disease," *Cancer Investigation*, vol. 24, no. 3, pp. 269–277, 2006.

[93] R. M. Nagler, "Altered salivary profile in heavy smokers and its possible connection to oral cancer," *International Journal of Biological Markers*, vol. 22, no. 4, pp. 274–280, 2007.

[94] B. Narotzki, A. Z. Reznick, T. Mitki, D. Aizenbud, and Y. Levy, "Green tea drinking improves erythrocytes and saliva oxidative status in the elderly," *Advances in Experimental Medicine and Biology*, vol. 832, pp. 25–33, 2014.

[95] N. Novaković, S. Cakić, T. Todorović et al., "Antioxidative status of saliva before and after non-surgical periodontal treatment," *Srpski Arhiv Za Celokupno Lekarstvo*, vol. 141, no. 3-4, pp. 163–168, 2013.

[96] N. Novakovic, T. Todorovic, M. Rakic et al., "Salivary antioxidants as periodontal biomarkers in evaluation of tissue status and treatment outcome," *Journal of Periodontal Research*, vol. 49, no. 1, pp. 129–136, 2014.

[97] L. A. S. Nunes, R. Brenzikofer, and D. V. Macedo, "Reference intervals for saliva analytes collected by a standardized method in a physically active population," *Clinical Biochemistry*, vol. 44, no. 17-18, pp. 1440–1444, 2011.

[98] V. Padmanabhan, K. Rai, A. Hegde, and S. Shetty, "Total antioxidant capacity of saliva in children with HIV," *Journal of Clinical Pediatric Dentistry*, vol. 34, no. 4, pp. 347–350, 2010.

[99] P. Pandey, N. V. Reddy, V. A. Rao, A. Saxena, and C. P. Chaudhary, "Estimation of salivary flow rate, pH, buffer capacity, calcium, total protein content and total antioxidant capacity in relation to dental caries severity, age and gender," *Contemporary Clinical Dentistry*, vol. 6, no. 5, supplement 1, pp. S65–S71, 2015.

[100] G. Pendyala, B. Thomas, and S. Joshi, "Periodontitis, diabetes mellitus, and the lopsided redox balance: a unifying axis," *Journal of Indian Society of Periodontology*, vol. 17, no. 3, pp. 338–344, 2013.

[101] G. Pendyala, B. Thomas, and S. R. Joshi, "Evaluation of total antioxidant capacity of saliva in type 2 diabetic patients with and without periodontal disease: a case-control study," *North American Journal of Medical Sciences*, vol. 5, no. 1, pp. 51–57, 2013.

[102] N. Peter, K. J. Kevin, and A. R. Shivashankara, "Effect of alcohol withdrawl on glutathione S-transferase, total antioxidant capacity and amylase in blood and saliva of alcohol-dependent males," *Journal of Clinical and Diagnostic Research*, vol. 7, no. 5, pp. 797–800, 2013.

[103] A. R. Prabhakar, R. Dodawad, and R. Os, "Evaluation of flow rate, pH, buffering capacity, calcium, total protein and total antioxidant levels of saliva in caries free and caries active children—an *in vivo* study," *International Journal of Clinical Pediatric Dentistry*, vol. 2, no. 1, pp. 9–12, 2009.

[104] B. P. Preethi, D. Reshma, and P. Anand, "Evaluation of flow rate, pH, buffering capacity, calcium, total proteins and total antioxidant capacity levels of saliva in caries free and caries active children: an in vivo study," *Indian Journal of Clinical Biochemistry*, vol. 25, no. 4, pp. 425–428, 2010.

[105] K. Rai, A. M. Hegde, and N. Jose, "Salivary antioxidants and oral health in children with autism," *Archives of Oral Biology*, vol. 57, no. 8, pp. 1116–1120, 2012.

[106] A. Rezaie, F. Ghorbani, A. Eshghtork et al., "Alterations in salivary antioxidants, nitric oxide, and transforming growth factor-beta 1 in relation to disease activity in Crohn's disease patients," *Annals of the New York Academy of Sciences*, vol. 1091, pp. 110–122, 2006.

[107] A. Z. Reznick, N. Shehadeh, Y. Shafir, and R. M. Nagler, "Free radicals related effects and antioxidants in saliva and serum of adolescents with Type 1 diabetes mellitus," *Archives of Oral Biology*, vol. 51, no. 8, pp. 640–648, 2006.

[108] D. Rodríguez de Sotillo, A. M. Velly, M. Hadley, and J. R. Fricton, "Evidence of oxidative stress in temporomandibular disorders: a pilot study," *Journal of Oral Rehabilitation*, vol. 38, no. 10, pp. 722–728, 2011.

[109] G. I. Ron', L. T. Shmeleva, A. V. Klein, and I. Elu, "Lipid peroxidation and the status of the basal membrane of the acinar cells in the minor salivary glands of patients with Sjögren's syndrome," *Stomatologiia*, no. 2, pp. 23–26, 1992.

[110] D. V. Sculley and S. C. Langley-Evans, "Periodontal disease is associated with lower antioxidant capacity in whole saliva and evidence of increased protein oxidation," *Clinical Science*, vol. 105, no. 2, pp. 167–172, 2003.

[111] E. Shahar, U. Attias, D. Savulescu, J. Genizin, M. Gavish, and R. Nagler, "Oxidative stress, metalloproteinase and LDH in children with intractable and non-intractable epilepsy as reflected in salivary analysis," *Epilepsy Research*, vol. 108, no. 1, pp. 117–124, 2014.

[112] E. Shahar, S. Pollack, E. Kedem, G. Hassoun, and R. Nagler, "Effect of HAART on salivary composition and oxidative profile in HIV-infected patients," *Current HIV Research*, vol. 6, no. 5, pp. 447–451, 2008.

[113] A. Shirzad, M. Pouramir, M. Seyedmajidi, N. Jenabian, A. Bijani, and M. Motallebnejad, "Salivary total antioxidant capacity and lipid peroxidation in patients with erosive oral lichen planus," *Journal of Dental Research, Dental Clinics, Dental Prospects*, vol. 8, no. 1, pp. 35–39, 2014.

[114] M. Shirzaiy, S. M. Ansari, J. H. Dehghan, and S. H. Ghaeni, "Total anti-oxidant capacity of saliva in chronic periodontitis patients before and after periodontal treatment," *Journal of Nepal Health Research Council*, vol. 12, no. 28, pp. 172–176, 2014.

[115] H. Su, M. Gornitsky, A. M. Velly, H. Yu, M. Benarroch, and H. M. Schipper, "Salivary DNA, lipid, and protein oxidation in nonsmokers with periodontal disease," *Free Radical Biology and Medicine*, vol. 46, no. 7, pp. 914–921, 2009.

[116] P. Subramaniam, K. Girish Babu, and L. Mohan Das, "Assessment of salivary total antioxidant levels and oral health status in children with Down syndrome," *Special Care in Dentistry*, vol. 34, no. 4, pp. 193–200, 2014.

[117] P. Subramaniam, L. Mohan Das, and K. L. Babu, "Assessment of salivary total antioxidant levels and oral health status in children with cerebral palsy," *Journal of Clinical Pediatric Dentistry*, vol. 38, no. 3, pp. 235–239, 2014.

[118] H. Suma, K. Prabhu, R. P. Shenoy, R. Annaswamy, S. Rao, and A. Rao, "Estimation of salivary protein thiols and total antioxidant power of saliva in brain tumor patients," *Journal of Cancer Research and Therapeutics*, vol. 6, no. 3, pp. 278–281, 2010.

[119] A. Surdacka, E. Ciężka, M. Pioruńska-Stolzmann et al., "Relation of salivary antioxidant status and cytokine levels to clinical parameters of oral health in pregnant women with diabetes," *Archives of Oral Biology*, vol. 56, no. 5, pp. 428–436, 2011.

[120] H. S. Tavakol, R. Akram, S. Azam, and Z. Nahid, "Protective effects of green tea on antioxidative biomarkers in chemical laboratory workers," *Toxicology and Industrial Health*, vol. 31, no. 9, pp. 862–867, 2015.

[121] A. Totan, D. Miricescu, I. Parlatescu, M. Mohora, and M. Greabu, "Possible salivary and serum biomarkers for oral lichen planus," *Biotechnic & Histochemistry*, vol. 90, no. 7, pp. 552–558, 2015.

[122] L. Tóthová, V. Celecová, and P. Celec, "Salivary markers of oxidative stress and their relation to periodontal and dental status in children," *Disease Markers*, vol. 34, no. 1, pp. 9–15, 2013.

[123] L. Tóthová, J. Hodosy, I. Mucska, and P. Celec, "Salivary markers of oxidative stress in patients with obstructive sleep apnea treated with continuous positive airway pressure," *Sleep and Breathing*, vol. 18, no. 3, pp. 563–570, 2014.

[124] Ö. Tulunoglu, S. Demirtas, and I. Tulunoglu, "Total antioxidant levels of saliva in children related to caries, age, and gender," *International Journal of Paediatric Dentistry*, vol. 16, no. 3, pp. 186–191, 2006.

[125] J. Uberos, J. A. Alarcón, M. A. Peñalver et al., "Influence of the antioxidant content of saliva on dental caries in an at-risk community," *British Dental Journal*, vol. 205, no. 2, article E5, 2008.

[126] Y. Ullmann, Y. Klein, D. Savulescu et al., "Salivary monitoring related to major surgery," *European Journal of Clinical Investigation*, vol. 40, no. 12, pp. 1074–1080, 2010.

[127] E. M. Varoni, S. Vitalini, D. Contino et al., "Effects of red wine intake on human salivary antiradical capacity and total polyphenol content," *Food and Chemical Toxicology*, vol. 58, pp. 289–294, 2013.

[128] B. Vlková, P. Stanko, G. Minárik et al., "Salivary markers of oxidative stress in patients with oral premalignant lesions," *Archives of Oral Biology*, vol. 57, no. 12, pp. 1651–1656, 2012.

[129] C. Vors, J. Drai, L. Gabert et al., "Salivary composition in obese vs normal-weight subjects: towards a role in postprandial lipid metabolism?" *International Journal of Obesity*, vol. 39, no. 9, pp. 1425–1428, 2015.

[130] M. Wnuk, A. Myszka, A. Lewinska, I. Tokarz, K. Solarska, and G. Bartosz, "*Helicobacter pylori* cagA gene polymorphism affects the total antioxidant capacity of human saliva," *Helicobacter*, vol. 15, no. 1, pp. 53–57, 2010.

[131] P. S. Yang, W. C. Huang, S. Y. Chen et al., "Scaling-stimulated salivary antioxidant changes and oral-health behavior in an evaluation of periodontal treatment outcomes," *The Scientific World Journal*, vol. 2014, Article ID 814671, 8 pages, 2014.

[132] M. Yigla, Y. Berkovich, and R. M. Nagler, "Oxidative stress indices in COPD—broncho-alveolar lavage and salivary analysis," *Archives of Oral Biology*, vol. 52, no. 1, pp. 36–43, 2007.

[133] G. Yousefzadeh, B. Larijani, A. Mohammadirad et al., "Determination of oxidative stress status and concentration of TGF-$\beta 1$ in the blood and saliva of osteoporotic subjects," *Annals of the New York Academy of Sciences*, vol. 1091, pp. 142–150, 2006.

[134] H. Youssef, C. Groussard, G. Machefer et al., "Comparison of total antioxidant capacity of salivary, capillary and venous samplings: interest of the salivary total antioxidant capacity on triathletes during training season," *Journal of Sports Medicine and Physical Fitness*, vol. 48, no. 4, pp. 522–529, 2008.

[135] A. Zalewska, M. Knaś, E. Gińdzieńska-Sieśkiewicz et al., "Salivary antioxidants in patients with systemic sclerosis," *Journal of Oral Pathology and Medicine*, vol. 43, no. 1, pp. 61–68, 2014.

[136] B. Zappacosta, S. Persichilli, P. De Sole, A. Mordente, and B. Giardina, "Effect of smoking one cigarette on antioxidant metabolites in the saliva of healthy smokers," *Archives of Oral Biology*, vol. 44, no. 6, pp. 485–488, 1999.

[137] A. Zare Javid, C. J. Seal, P. Heasman, and P. J. Moynihan, "Impact of a customised dietary intervention on antioxidant status, dietary intakes and periodontal indices in patients with adult periodontitis," *Journal of Human Nutrition and Dietetics*, vol. 27, no. 6, pp. 523–532, 2014.

[138] A. Ziobro and G. Bartosz, "A comparison of the total antioxidant capacity of some human body fluid," *Cellular and Molecular Biology Letters*, vol. 8, no. 2, pp. 415–419, 2003.

[139] S. Abusoglu, H. T. Celik, E. Tutkun et al., "8-Hydroxydeoxyguanosine as a useful marker for determining the severity of trichloroethylene exposure," *Archives of Environmental and Occupational Health*, vol. 69, no. 3, pp. 180–186, 2014.

[140] H. Benkhai, S. Lemanski, H. Below et al., "Can physical stress be measured in urine using the parameter antioxidative potential?" *GMS Krankenhaushygiene Interdisziplinär*, vol. 5, no. 2, Article ID Doc03, 2010.

[141] I. F. F. Benzie, Y. T. Szeto, J. J. Strain, and B. Tomlinson, "Consumption of green tea causes rapid increase in plasma antioxidant power in humans," *Nutrition and Cancer*, vol. 34, no. 1, pp. 83–87, 1999.

[142] G. Boudouris, I. I. Verginadis, Y. V. Simos et al., "Oxidative stress in patients treated with continuous ambulatory peritoneal dialysis (CAPD) and the significant role of vitamin C and e supplementation," *International Urology and Nephrology*, vol. 45, no. 4, pp. 1137–1144, 2013.

[143] R. Bravo, S. Matito, J. Cubero et al., "Tryptophan-enriched cereal intake improves nocturnal sleep, melatonin, serotonin, and total antioxidant capacity levels and mood in elderly humans," *Age*, vol. 35, no. 4, pp. 1277–1285, 2013.

[144] H. Buyukhatipoglu, Y. Sezen, A. Yildiz et al., "N-acetylcysteine fails to prevent renal dysfunction and oxidative stress after noniodine contrast media administration during percutaneous coronary interventions," *Polskie Archiwum Medycyny Wewnętrznej*, vol. 120, no. 10, pp. 383–389, 2010.

[145] C. Campos, R. Guzmán, E. López-Fernández, and Á. Casado, "Urinary biomarkers of oxidative/nitrosative stress in healthy smokers," *Inhalation Toxicology*, vol. 23, no. 3, pp. 148–156, 2011.

[146] C. Campos, R. Guzmán, E. López-Fernández, and Á. Casado, "Urinary uric acid and antioxidant capacity in children and

adults with Down syndrome," *Clinical Biochemistry*, vol. 43, no. 3, pp. 228–233, 2010.

[147] G. Cao, R. M. Russell, N. Lischner, and R. L. Prior, "Serum antioxidant capacity is increased by consumption of strawberries, spinach, red wine or vitamin C in elderly women," *Journal of Nutrition*, vol. 128, no. 12, pp. 2383–2390, 1998.

[148] J.-W. Chien, L.-Y. Wang, Y.-S. Cheng, Y.-G. Tsai, and C.-S. Liu, "Urinary 8-hydroxy-2′-deoxyguanosine (8-oxodG) level can predict acute renal damage in young children with urinary tract infection," *Biomarkers*, vol. 19, no. 4, pp. 326–331, 2014.

[149] H. Ciftci, A. Verit, E. Yeni, and M. Savas, "Decreased oxidative stress index of urine in patients with urinary tract infection," *Urologia Internationalis*, vol. 81, no. 3, pp. 312–315, 2008.

[150] L. P. M. Damodaran and G. Arumugam, "Urinary oxidative stress markers in children with autism," *Redox Report*, vol. 16, no. 5, pp. 216–222, 2011.

[151] M. Dos Santos Mello, G. S. Ribas, C. A. Y. Wayhs et al., "Increased oxidative stress in patients with 3-hydroxy-3-methylglutaric aciduria," *Molecular and Cellular Biochemistry*, vol. 402, no. 1-2, pp. 149–155, 2015.

[152] S.-Y. Eom, D.-H. Yim, S. I. Moon et al., "Polycyclic aromatic hydrocarbon-induced oxidative stress, antioxidant capacity, and the risk of lung cancer: a pilot nested case-control study," *Anticancer Research*, vol. 33, no. 8, pp. 3089–3097, 2013.

[153] M. Garrido, S. D. Paredes, J. Cubero et al., "Jerte valley cherry-enriched diets improve nocturnal rest and increase 6-sulfatoxymelatonin and total antioxidant capacity in the urine of middle-aged and elderly humans," *The Journals of Gerontology Series A: Biological Sciences and Medical Sciences*, vol. 65, no. 9, pp. 909–914, 2010.

[154] N. Göknar, F. Oktem, E. Ari, A. D. Demir, and E. Torun, "Is oxidative stress related to childhood urolithiasis?" *Pediatric Nephrology*, vol. 29, no. 8, pp. 1381–1386, 2014.

[155] D. González-Flores, E. Gamero, M. Garrido et al., "Urinary 6-sulfatoxymelatonin and total antioxidant capacity increase after the intake of a grape juice cv. Tempranillo stabilized with HHP," *Food and Function*, vol. 3, no. 1, pp. 34–39, 2012.

[156] G. Guerreiro, C. P. Mescka, A. Sitta et al., "Urinary biomarkers of oxidative damage in Maple syrup urine disease: the L-carnitine role," *International Journal of Developmental Neuroscience*, vol. 42, pp. 10–14, 2015.

[157] N. M. A. Hassimotto, M. D. S. Pinto, and F. M. Lajolo, "Antioxidant status in humans after consumption of blackberry (*Rubus fruticosus* L.) juices with and without defatted milk," *Journal of Agricultural and Food Chemistry*, vol. 56, no. 24, pp. 11727–11733, 2008.

[158] N. K. Hatipoğlu, O. Evliyaoğlu, B. Işik et al., "Antioxidant signal and kidney injury molecule-1 levels in shockwave lithotripsy induced kidney injury," *Journal of Endourology*, vol. 28, no. 2, pp. 224–228, 2014.

[159] D. Helbig, A. Wagner, R. Schubert, and G. Jahreis, "Tocopherol isomer pattern in serum and stool of human following consumption of black currant seed press residue administered in whole grain bread," *Clinical Nutrition*, vol. 28, no. 6, pp. 662–667, 2009.

[160] C. Hudthagosol, E. Haddad, and R. Jongsuwat, "Antioxidant activity comparison of walnuts and fatty fish," *Journal of the Medical Association of Thailand*, vol. 95, supplement 6, pp. S179–S188, 2012.

[161] K. Jacob, M. J. Periago, V. Böhm, and G. R. Berruezo, "Influence of lycopene and vitamin C from tomato juice on biomarkers of oxidative stress and inflammation," *British Journal of Nutrition*, vol. 99, no. 1, pp. 137–146, 2008.

[162] B. Kirschbaum, "Total urine antioxidant capacity," *Clinica Chimica Acta*, vol. 305, no. 1-2, pp. 167–173, 2001.

[163] P. J. Mc Guire, A. Parikh, and G. A. Diaz, "Profiling of oxidative stress in patients with inborn errors of metabolism," *Molecular Genetics and Metabolism*, vol. 98, no. 1-2, pp. 173–180, 2009.

[164] C. Miglio, I. Peluso, A. Raguzzini et al., "Fruit juice drinks prevent endogenous antioxidant response to high-fat meal ingestion," *British Journal of Nutrition*, vol. 111, no. 2, pp. 294–300, 2014.

[165] M. Patchsung, C. Boonla, P. Amnattrakul, T. Dissayabutra, A. Mutirangura, and P. Tosukhowong, "Long interspersed nuclear element-1 hypomethylation and oxidative stress: correlation and bladder cancer diagnostic potential," *PLoS ONE*, vol. 7, no. 5, Article ID e37009, 2012.

[166] B. Pfundstein, R. Haubner, G. Würtele, N. Gehres, C. M. Ulrich, and R. W. Owen, "Pilot walnut intervention study of urolithin bioavailability in human volunteers," *Journal of Agricultural and Food Chemistry*, vol. 62, no. 42, pp. 10264–10273, 2014.

[167] A. Ranjbar, V. Rashedi, and M. Rezaei, "Comparison of urinary oxidative biomarkers in Iranian children with autism," *Research in Developmental Disabilities*, vol. 35, no. 11, pp. 2751–2755, 2014.

[168] R. Revuelta-Iniesta and E. A. S. Al-Dujaili, "Consumption of green coffee reduces blood pressure and body composition by influencing 11β-HSD1 enzyme activity in healthy individuals: a pilot crossover study using green and black coffee," *BioMed Research International*, vol. 2014, Article ID 482704, 9 pages, 2014.

[169] G. S. Ribas, G. B. Biancini, C. Mescka et al., "Oxidative stress parameters in urine from patients with disorders of propionate metabolism: a beneficial effect of L:-carnitine supplementation," *Cellular and Molecular Neurobiology*, vol. 32, no. 1, pp. 77–82, 2012.

[170] E. Roura, M. P. Almajano, M. L. M. Bilbao, C. Andrés-Lacueva, R. Estruch, and R. M. Lamuela-Raventós, "Human urine: epicatechin metabolites and antioxidant activity after cocoa beverage intake," *Free Radical Research*, vol. 41, no. 8, pp. 943–949, 2007.

[171] M. C. Schmidt, E. W. Askew, D. E. Roberts, R. L. Prior, W. Y. Ensign Jr., and R. E. Hesslink Jr., "Oxidative stress in humans training in a cold, moderate altitude environment and their response to a phytochemical antioxidant supplement," *Wilderness and Environmental Medicine*, vol. 13, no. 2, pp. 94–105, 2002.

[172] K. Shermatov, D. Zeyrek, F. Yildirim, M. Kilic, N. Cebi, and A. Kocyigit, "DNA damage in children exposed to secondhand cigarette smoke and its association with oxidative stress," *Indian Pediatrics*, vol. 49, no. 12, pp. 958–962, 2012.

[173] D. A. Shoskes, A. R. Shahed, S. Kim, H. A. Gritsch, G. Danovitch, and A. Wilkinson, "Oxidant stress and antioxidant capacity in urine of renal transplant recipients predict early graft function," *Transplantation Proceedings*, vol. 33, no. 1-2, p. 984, 2001.

[174] D. A. Shoskes, R. Webster, and A. Shahed, "Oxidant stress in cadaveric and living kidney donors as markers of renal injury: utility of total antioxidant capacity and isoprostane levels in urine," *Transplantation Proceedings*, vol. 32, no. 4, pp. 804–805, 2000.

[175] K. Silliman, J. Parry, L. L. Kirk, and R. L. Prior, "Pycnogenol does not impact the antioxidant or vitamin C status of healthy

young adults," *Journal of the American Dietetic Association*, vol. 103, no. 1, pp. 67–72, 2003.

[176] R. J. Stewart, E. W. Askew, C. M. McDonald et al., "Antioxidant status of young children: response to an antioxidant supplement," *Journal of the American Dietetic Association*, vol. 102, no. 11, pp. 1652–1657, 2002.

[177] S. Wachtel-Galor, Y.-T. Szeto, B. Tomlinson, and I. F. F. Benzie, "Ganoderma lucidum ('Lingzhi'); acute and short-term biomarker response to supplementation," *International Journal of Food Sciences and Nutrition*, vol. 55, no. 1, pp. 75–83, 2004.

[178] S. Wachtel-Galor, B. Tomlinson, and I. F. F. Benzie, "Ganoderma lucidum ('Lingzhi'), a Chinese medicinal mushroom: biomarker responses in a controlled human supplementation study," *British Journal of Nutrition*, vol. 91, no. 2, pp. 263–269, 2004.

[179] E. Yilmaz, A. Haciislamoglu, U. Kisa, O. Dogan, E. Yuvanc, and E. Batislam, "Ways in which SWL affects oxidant/antioxidant balance," *Urological Research*, vol. 41, no. 2, pp. 137–141, 2013.

[180] Z. Liu, Y. Liu, Y. Song, X. Zhang, S. Wang, and Z. Wang, "Systemic oxidative stress biomarkers in chronic periodontitis: a meta-analysis," *Disease Markers*, vol. 2014, Article ID 931083, 10 pages, 2014.

[181] R. S. Bhangoo, I. E. Hall, P. P. Reese, and C. R. Parikh, "Deceased-donor kidney perfusate and urine biomarkers for kidney allograft outcomes: a systematic review," *Nephrology Dialysis Transplantation*, vol. 27, no. 8, pp. 3305–3314, 2012.

[182] F. Bonomini, L. F. Rodella, and R. Rezzani, "Metabolic syndrome, aging and involvement of oxidative stress," *Aging and Disease*, vol. 6, no. 2, pp. 109–120, 2015.

[183] W. Y. Tae, C. S. Ki, S. S. Hun et al., "Relationship between serum uric acid concentration and insulin resistance and metabolic syndrome," *Circulation Journal*, vol. 69, no. 8, pp. 928–933, 2005.

[184] B. E. K. Klein, R. Klein, and K. E. Lee, "Components of the metabolic syndrome and risk of cardiovascular disease and diabetes in Beaver Dam," *Diabetes Care*, vol. 25, no. 10, pp. 1790–1794, 2002.

[185] R. Kawamoto, H. Tomita, Y. Oka, and N. Ohtsuka, "Relationship between serum uric acid concentration, metabolic syndrome and carotid atherosclerosis," *Internal Medicine*, vol. 45, no. 9, pp. 605–614, 2006.

[186] M. Serafini, C. Miglio, I. Peluso, and T. Petrosino, "Modulation of plasma non enzimatic antioxidant capacity (NEAC) by plant foods: the role of polyphenols," *Current Topics in Medicinal Chemistry*, vol. 11, no. 14, pp. 1821–1846, 2011.

[187] F. Veglia, G. Cighetti, M. De Franceschi et al., "Age- and gender-related oxidative status determined in healthy subjects by means of OXY-SCORE, a potential new comprehensive index," *Biomarkers*, vol. 11, no. 6, pp. 562–573, 2006.

[188] N. Kamodyová and P. Celec, "Salivary markers of oxidative stress and Salivette collection systems," *Clinical Chemistry and Laboratory Medicine*, vol. 49, no. 11, pp. 1887–1890, 2011.

[189] E. Neyraud, O. Palicki, C. Schwartz, S. Nicklaus, and G. Feron, "Variability of human saliva composition: possible relationships with fat perception and liking," *Archives of Oral Biology*, vol. 57, no. 5, pp. 556–566, 2012.

[190] R. M. Nagler, I. Klein, N. Zarzhevsky, N. Drigues, and A. Z. Reznick, "Characterization of the differentiated antioxidant profile of human saliva," *Free Radical Biology and Medicine*, vol. 32, no. 3, pp. 268–277, 2002.

[191] I. R. Gunn, "Biological variation of serum and urine creatinine and creatinine clearance," *Annals of Clinical Biochemistry*, vol. 26, part 3, pp. 302–303, 1989.

[192] A. Ghiselli, M. Serafini, G. Maiani, E. Azzini, and A. Ferro-Luzzi, "A fluorescence-based method for measuring total plasma antioxidant capability," *Free Radical Biology and Medicine*, vol. 18, no. 1, pp. 29–36, 1995.

[193] I. F. F. Benzie and J. J. Strain, "The ferric reducing ability of plasma (FRAP) as a measure of 'antioxidant power': the FRAP assay," *Analytical Biochemistry*, vol. 239, no. 1, pp. 70–76, 1996.

[194] E. Lissi, M. Salim-Hanna, C. Pascual, and M. D. del Castillo, "Evaluation of total antioxidant potential (TRAP) and total antioxidant reactivity from luminol-enhanced chemiluminescence measurements," *Free Radical Biology and Medicine*, vol. 18, no. 2, pp. 153–158, 1995.

[195] B. T. Emmerson, "The management of gout," *The New England Journal of Medicine*, vol. 334, no. 7, pp. 445–451, 1996.

[196] F. H. Messerli, E. D. Frohlich, G. R. Dreslinski, D. H. Suarez, and G. G. Aristimuno, "Serum uric acid in essential hypertension: an indicator of renal vascular involvement," *Annals of Internal Medicine*, vol. 93, no. 6, pp. 817–821, 1980.

[197] A. Quiñones Galvan, A. Natali, S. Baldi et al., "Effect of insulin on uric acid excretion in humans," *American Journal of Physiology*, vol. 268, pp. E1–E5, 1995.

[198] D. Duplancic, L. Kukoc-Modun, D. Modun, and N. Radic, "Simple and rapid method for the determination of uric acid-independent antioxidant capacity," *Molecules*, vol. 16, no. 8, pp. 7058–7067, 2011.

[199] N. Malliaraki, D. Mpliamplias, M. Kampa, K. Perakis, A. N. Margioris, and E. Castanas, "Total and corrected antioxidant capacity in hemodialyzed patients," *BMC Nephrology*, vol. 4, article 4, 2003.

[200] R. Bentley and A. Neuberger, "The mechanism of the action of uricase," *The Biochemical Journal*, vol. 52, no. 4, pp. 694–699, 1952.

24

Immunoreactivity of the 14F7 Mab Raised against N-Glycolyl GM3 Ganglioside in Primary Lymphoid Tumors and Lymph Node Metastasis

Rancés Blanco,[1] Damián Blanco,[2] Yisel Quintana,[1] Xiomara Escobar,[2] Charles E. Rengifo,[3] Marta Osorio,[4] Zailí Gutiérrez,[5] Janet Lamadrid,[5] Mercedes Cedeño,[1] Milagros Frómeta,[1] Adriana Carr,[6] and Enrique Rengifo[1]

[1] *Laboratory of Recognition and Biological Activity Assays, Department of Quality Control, Center of Molecular Immunology, P.O. Box 16040, 216 Street and 15 Avenue Atabey, Playa, 11600 Havana, Cuba*
[2] *Department of Cell Biology and Tissues Banking, National Institute of Oncology and Radiobiology, 29 and F Street Vedado, Plaza de la Revolución, 10400 Havana, Cuba*
[3] *Department of Pathology, Manuel Fajardo General Hospital, Zapata and D Street Vedado, Plaza de la Revolución, 10400 Havana, Cuba*
[4] *Clinical Trials Unit, National Institute of Oncology and Radiobiology, 29 and F Street Vedado, Plaza de la Revolución, 10400 Havana, Cuba*
[5] *Department of Pathology, National Institute of Oncology and Radiobiology, 29 and F Street Vedado, Plaza de la Revolución, 10400 Havana, Cuba*
[6] *Research and Development Direction, Center of Molecular Immunology, P.O. Box 16040, 216 Street and 15 Avenue Atabey, Playa, 11600 Havana, Cuba*

Correspondence should be addressed to Rancés Blanco; rances@cim.sld.cu

Academic Editor: Shahid Pervez

The reactivity of the 14F7 Mab, a highly specific IgG1 against N-glycolyl GM3 ganglioside (NeuGcGM3) in normal tissues, lymphomas, lymph node metastasis, and other metastatic sites was assessed by immunohistochemistry. In addition, the effect of chemical fixation on the 14F7 Mab staining using monolayers of P3X63Ag.653 cells was also evaluated. Moreover, the ability of 14F7 to bind NeuGcGM3 ganglioside inducing complement-independent cytotoxicity by a flow cytometry-based assay was measured. The 14F7 Mab was reactive in unfixed, 4% paraformaldehyde, 4% formaldehyde, and acetone fixed cells. Postfixation with acetone did not alter the localization of NeuGcGM3, while the staining with 14F7 Mab was significantly eliminated in both cells fixed and postfixed with methanol but only partially reduced with ethanol. The staining with 14F7 Mab was evidenced in the 89.2%, 89.4%, and 88.9% of lymphomas, lymph node metastasis, and other metastatic sites, respectively, but not in normal tissues. The treatment with 14F7 Mab affected both morphology and membrane integrity of P3X63Ag.653 cells. This cytotoxic activity was dose-dependent and ranged from 24.0 to 84.7% (10–1000 μg/mL) as compared to the negative control. Our data could support the possible use of NeuGcGM3 as target for both active and passive immunotherapy against malignancies expressing this molecule.

1. Introduction

Lymphomas (primary malignant neoplasms of lymphoreticular origin) represent one of the major health problems worldwide [1]. Despite the availability of several options to the treatment of lymphomas [2], the identification of novel tumor-associated antigens that are universally expressed in these malignancies is necessary for the development of newer immunotherapeutic strategies [3].

On the other hand, as it is well known, the main cause of cancer-related death is due to metastasis of primary tumors to secondary sites within the body [4]. Usually, different primary tumors tend to spread to preferred metastatic sites, although both regional and distant lymph nodes are the most common metastatic targets for a variety of primary malignancies such as skin, breast, colon, stomach, and lung [5].

Gangliosides are sialic acid-containing glycosphingolipids engaged in many biological events that take place at vertebrate's cell membrane [6]. Unusual glycolylated gangliosides have been identified by immunohistochemical methods in some malignant tumors and their metastasis becoming attractive targets for immunotherapy [7–10].

The tissue reactivity of 14F7 Mab, a highly specific IgG1 against the NeuGcGM3 ganglioside, in a variety of frozen and formalin-fixed and paraffin-embedded malignant tumors have been previously published [8, 10–18]. Nevertheless, up to now, there is no evidence about the staining of 14F7 Mab in malignant lymphoma and nonmelanoma lymph node metastasis.

For these reasons, here we evaluated the reactivity of the 14F7 Mab in normal as well as in primary lymphoid tumors, lymph node, and other metastasis. Additionally, we assessed the effect of fixation in the recognition of 14F7 Mab as well as the ability of this Mab to bind NeuGcGM3 ganglioside inducing complement-independent cytotoxicity in a mouse myeloma cell line (P3X63Ag.653).

2. Materials and Methods

2.1. Cell Line and Monolayer Preparation. The mouse myeloma cell line P3X63Ag.653 (ATCC CRL-1580) was used. Cells were grown in Dulbecco's modified Eagle's media (PAA, E15-843) supplemented with 10% heat-inactivated fetal bovine serum (PAA, A15-211), respectively. Cells were maintained at 37°C in a humidified atmosphere of air containing 5% CO_2 and the media was replaced every 3 to 4 days. Afterward, cultured cells were extensively washed with PBS (PAA, H15-002) and both cell viability and concentration were calculated by trypan blue exclusion assay followed by examination with a hemacytometer under an optical microscope. Only cells suspensions with viability greater than 90% were used. Then, cells were adjusted at 0.5 $\times 10^6$ cell/mL, deposed in histological slides, and air dried. Finally, slides were stored at −20°C until they were used.

2.2. Monoclonal Antibodies. We used the 14F7 Mab (IgG1), a highly specific anti-NeuGcGM3 ganglioside antibody. This Mab was generated by immunization of Balb/c mice with NeuGcGM3 hydrophobically conjugated with human very low-density lipoproteins (VLDL) adjuvated with Complete Freud adjuvant (CFA). Afterwards, 14F7 Mab was obtained by the hybridoma resulting of the fusion of spleen cells with mouse myeloma cell line P3X63Ag.653 as described [8]. Additionally, the P3 Mab (IgM, k, anti-NeuGc-containing gangliosides and sulfated glycolipids) [7] (complement-independent cytotoxicity assays) or the 1E10 Mab (an anti-idiotypic antibody specific for P3 Mab) [19] (immunocytochemistry assays) were used as negative controls.

2.3. Fixation Protocols and Immunocytochemical Procedure. Monolayers of P3X63Ag.653 cell line were fixed according to the following fixation protocols: 4% neutral buffered formaldehyde (Spectrum, F0110) and 4% paraformaldehyde (BDH, 294474L) for 30 and 20 minutes at room temperature, respectively, and acetone (Spectrum, A1020), ethanol (Spectrum, E1028), and methanol (Spectrum, M1240) for 10 minutes at 2–8°C each one. Unfixed cells were also included. Additionally, samples were prefixed with 4% neutral buffered formaldehyde before fixation with acetone, ethanol, and methanol fixatives.

Afterwards, cells were rinsed and rehydrated in tris saline buffer, pH 7.6 (TBS) for 10 minutes at room temperature. Then, samples were incubated for 1 h with 14F7 or 1E10 (irrelevant) antibodies. After two rinses, a labelled polymer-HRP (Dako, K1494) was added and the slides were incubated for 30 minutes. Finally, the enzymatic activity was visualized with AEC (Dako, K3461) and cells were contrasted with methyl green (Dako, S1962).

2.4. Tissue Specimens. Routinely processed, formalin-fixed, and paraffin-embedded archival samples with diagnosis of normal tissue (7), human lymphoma (37), lymph node metastasis of breast carcinoma (14), cutaneous malignant melanoma (17), colonic (12) and gastric (2) adenocarcinomas, lung cancer (1), and unknown primary tumor (1) as well as, other metastasis (9) were received from the pathology departments of both the National Institute of Oncology and Radiobiology and Manuel Fajardo General Hospital. All samples were used after the approved consent by the institutional ethical committees.

2.5. Previous Processing and Immunohistochemical Staining. Five microns serial sections from each block were obtained in a Lizt 1512 micrometer and mounted on plus slides (Dako, S2024). All sections were attached to the slide by heating in a 60°C oven for 1 hour. Afterwards, the slides were kept at room temperature and they were used within 30 days.

The slides were dewaxed in xylene and rehydrated in decreasing ethanol series as usually and endogenous peroxidase activity was blocked with dual endogenous enzyme block solution (Dako, S2003) for 10 minutes. Afterwards, all sections were washed in distilled water for 10 minutes and then were rinsed with TBS (Tris/saline buffer solution) for 5 minutes. The samples were incubated with the 14F7 Mabs for 1 hour at room temperature. Negative controls were performed by substituting primary antibody for TBS and sections of colonic adenocarcinoma of known positivity for NeuGcGM3 ganglioside were taken as positive control. After two rinses in TBS, the slides were incubated with a biotinylated link universal and streptavidin-HRP (Dako, K0690) for 30 minutes in each step. Between incubations, slides were washed with TBS for 10 minutes.

Afterwards, the enzymatic activity was visualized with a DAB (Dako, K3465) solution. For lymph node metastasis of malignant melanomas, AEC (Dako, K3461) was used. Finally, all slides were counterstained with Mayer's Hematoxylin (Dako, S2020), dehydrated, and mounted.

2.6. Immunostaining Evaluation. Staining of both cell membrane and cytoplasm was considered as positive for 14F7 Mab.

TABLE 1: Effect of different fixatives in the 14F7 Mab reactivity.

Intensity of reaction	Unfixed	NBF	PFA	Acetone	Ethanol	Methanol
	+++	+++	+++	++	++	−

Legend: NBF: neutral buffered formalin; PFA: paraformaldehyde. Intensity: − negative, ++ moderate, +++ intense.

TABLE 2: Effect of postfixation in the 14F7 Mab recognition.

Intensity of reaction	NBF	NBF/acetone	NBF/ethanol	NBF/methanol
	+++	+++	++	−

Legend: NBF: neutral buffered formalin. Intensity: − negative, ++ moderate, +++ intense.

For immunocytochemical assays, the intensity of reaction of each sample was judged as negative (−), weak (+), moderate (++), and strong (+++). For immunohistochemical determinations, a semiquantitative scoring system was used to define levels of reactivity. The recognition of 14F7 Mab was evaluated for percentage of positive cells (0–100%) and the intensity of reaction (0–3+). The score was calculated for each specimen by multiplication of the intensity of reaction and the grade of positive cells, resulting in a score ranging from 0 to 300. Subsequently, these scores were grouped as follows: 0 (score 0); 1 (scores 1–100); 2 (scores 101–200), and 3 (scores 201–300).

2.7. Complement-Independent Cytotoxicity. The induction of cell death procedures as previously described [20] with minor modifications was used. Briefly, P3X63Ag.653 cells were resuspended in culture medium with 1% bovine serum albumin (BSA) (Sigma, A2153) at 0.25×10^6 cells/mL and incubated with 14F7 Mab (10–1000 μg/mL) in a 5% CO_2 atmosphere at 37°C for 2 hours. Cells were washed, resuspended in FACSFlow (Becton-Dickinson, 342003) and maintained in ice bath. Afterwards, cells were resuspended with FACSFlow and stained with propidium iodide (PI) at a final concentration of 4 μg/mL. The percentage of PI-positive cells was measured using a FACScan flow cytometer (Becton-Dickinson). Cells that were stained red with PI were considered as dead.

3. Results

3.1. The Recognition of 14F7 Mab Varies Depending on the Protocol Fixation. The effect of a variety of fixation protocols on the 14F7 Mab immunoreaction was evaluated in monolayers of P3X63Ag.653 cell line (see Section 3). A homogeneous and finely granular reactivity of 14F7 Mab was evidenced in unfixed as well as in 4% neutral-buffered formaldehyde and 4% paraformaldehyde fixed cells (Table 1, Figure 1(a)). In acetone fixed cells, both a slight diminishing in the intensity of reaction with 14F7 Mab and the appearance of cells with a grosser granular staining mainly located in the cytoplasm were observed (Figure 1(b)). On the other hand, the staining with 14F7 Mab was only partially reduced after fixation (Figure 1(c)) and postfixation with ethanol while, postfixation with acetone did not alter the localization of the ganglioside (Table 2). The reactivity with 14F7 Mab was significantly eliminated in both cells fixed and postfixed with methanol (Figures 1(d) and 1(e)). No immunoreaction, independently of the fixation protocol, was detected in cells incubated with 1E10 Mab which was used as negative control (Figure 1(f)).

3.2. No Staining with 14F7 Mab Was Evidenced in Normal Tissues. No reactivity of 14F7 Mab was evidenced in normal tonsil (0/2), lymph node (0/2), and spleen (0/3).

3.3. Higher Levels of 14F7 Mab Reactivity Were Detected in Sections of Primary Lymphoid Tumors. The 14F7 Mab reactivity was detected in 33/37 (89.2%) of all studied lymphomas not depending on the histopathological subtype (Table 3). In 21/33 (63.6%) cases, a moderate to intense reaction with 14F7 Mab in more than 40% of malignant lymphocytes was observed, while 12/33 (36.4%) sections displayed a weak staining with this Mab. In general, the recognition of 14F7 Mab was observed as a finely granular reaction mainly located in the cell membrane but also in the cytoplasm of malignant cells (Figure 2). No immunostaining was evidenced in negative controls.

3.4. The 14F7 Mab Immunostaining Was Observed in Lymph Node Metastasis. An intense reactivity of 14F7 Mab was detected in almost all tumor cells in 11/12 (91.7%) and 2/2 of lymph node metastasis of breast ductal and lobular carcinomas, respectively (Table 4). The recognition of 14F7 Mab was homogeneous and finely granular and was mainly located in the membrane of malignant cells although the cytoplasm was also decorated (Figure 3). Only one case of breast ductal carcinoma (8.3%) exhibited a weak to moderate and diffuse pattern of staining.

Concerning lymph node metastases of cutaneous melanoma, the reactivity of 14F7 Mab was detected in more than 50% of malignant cells in 15/17 (88.2%) (Table 4). The recognition of the 14F7 Mab was variable in the intensity of reaction (from weak to intense). A weak to moderate staining with 14F7 Mab was observed in 3/15 (20.0%) of samples while in 12/15 (80.0%) of them, a moderate to intense staining was evidenced. Only one case showed a moderate reaction with 14F7 Mab in less than 25% of malignant cells.

Lymph node metastasis of colonic adenocarcinomas exhibited a homogeneous and finely granular reaction with 14F7 Mab in 9/12 (75.0%) cases, not taking into account the grade of differentiation (Table 4). The intensity of this reaction varied from moderate to intense and was observed in the cell membrane and also in the cytoplasm of more than 70% of malignant glandular cells (Figure 4). Similar results were evidenced in lymph node metastasis of gastric adenocarcinoma (2/2), lung adenocarcinoma (1/1) (Figure 4), and carcinoma of unknown primary origin (1/1).

Additionally, in 3/14 (21.4%) of lymph node metastasis of breast carcinoma as well as in 2/9 (22.2%) of colon adenocarcinomas, a weak to intense reaction of 14F7 Mab was observed in lymphocytes of tumor adjacent areas (Figures 3(a), 3(b), 4(a), and 4(b)).

3.5. Other Metastatic Sites Were Also Reactive with 14F7 Mab. A moderate to intense immunoreaction with 14F7 Mab was

TABLE 3: Immunostaining of 14F7 Mab in primary lymphoid tumors.

Lymphoid tumors	Score 0	1	2	3	Total (%)
Mature B-cell neoplasms					
Small lymphocytic lymphoma	0	2	1	1	4/4
Plasma cell myeloma	0	0	1	1	2/2
Follicular lymphoma	0	3	1	0	4/4
Diffuse large B-cell lymphoma	2	4	6	6	16/18 (88.9)
Burkitt lymphoma	0	1	0	0	1/1
Classical Hodgkin lymphoma	1	1	1	0	2/3 (66.7)
Unclassified	1	0	1	3	4/5 (80.0)

Legend: 0 (score 0); 1 (scores 1–100); 2 (scores 101–200), and 3 (scores 201–300).

TABLE 4: Immunorecognition of 14F7 Mab in some lymph node metastasis.

Lymph node metastasis of	Score 0	1	2	3	Total (%)
Cutaneous melanoma	2	2	8	5	15/17 (88.2)
Breast carcinoma					
Ductal	0	0	0	12	12/12
Lobular	0	0	0	2	2/2
Peritumoral lymphocytes	11	1	1	1	3/14 (21.4)
Colonic adenocarcinoma	3	0	3	6	9/12 (75.0)
Peritumoral lymphocytes	7	1	1	0	2/9 (22.2)
Gastric adenocarcinoma	0	0	1	1	2/2
Lung carcinoma	0	0	0	1	1/1
Unknown primary origin	0	0	1	0	1/1

Legend: 0 (score 0); 1 (scores 1–100); 2 (scores 101–200), and 3 (scores 201–300).

obtained in both cutaneous (1/1) and subcutaneous (3/3) metastasis of primary malignant melanoma. The staining was homogeneous and was mainly located on the plasmatic membrane of more than 90% of malignant cells although the cytoplasm was also reactive. Other metastatic tumors such as neuroblastoma (1/1), renal cell carcinoma (1/1), and those from unknown origin (2/2) were also recognized by 14F7 Mab. No reactivity was evidenced in a metastatic thymic carcinoma (Table 5).

3.6. Treatment with 14F7 Mab Induces a Complement-Independent Cytotoxicity in a Dose-Dependent Manner. The ability of 14F7 Mab to induce a complement-independent cytotoxicity after binding to NeuGcGM3-positive cell line (P3X63Ag.653) was evaluated. This effect was tested by PI internalization and flow cytometry analysis. The treatment with 14F7 Mab affected both morphology and membrane integrity of tumor cells. After treating P3X63Ag.653 cells with 14F7 Mab, a subpopulation exhibiting both cell size (FSC-H) and internal complexity (SSC-H) alterations (Figures 5(a) and 5(b)), as well as a positive staining with PI were observed (Figures 5(c) and 5(d)). The cytotoxic activity of 14F7 Mab was dose-dependent and ranged from 24.0 to 84.7% as compared to the negative control, obtaining the maximum of cell death at 1000 μg/mL. This effect was not seen when cells were treated with P3 Mab used as negative control.

4. Discussion

The use of frozen samples is desirable for any determination of gangliosides, but it is known, this kind of samples is often difficult to obtain and, even when available, to conserve. For these reasons, the most common specimen available for immunohistochemical assays after the histopathological diagnosis is formalin-fixed, ethanol and xylene-processed, and paraffin-embedded tissues. But, gangliosides are usually damaged or extracted after the routine treatment of tissues with organic solvents, due to their glycosphingolipid chemical structure.

In this paper, we demonstrated that cells fixation plays an important role for the immunolocalization of NeuGcGM3 by mean of 14F7 Mab. As expected, both fixation and postfixation with methanol completely removed NeuGcGM3 ganglioside from P3X63Ag.653 cells, consistent with the solubility of the glycolipid antigens [21]. While fixation with acetone only lead to slight decreasing in the intensity of reaction with 14F7 Mab joint to little alterations in the localization of NeuGcGM3. These results seem to be related to a complete

TABLE 5: Immunoreactivity of 14F7 Mab in other metastasis.

Metastasis of	Score				
	0	1	2	3	Total (%)
Cutaneous melanoma					
Subcutaneous	0	0	1	2	3/3
Cutaneous	0	0	0	1	1/1
Thymic carcinoma	1	0	0	0	0/1
Neuroblastoma	0	0	0	1	1/1
Renal cell carcinoma	0	0	0	1	1/1
Unknown primary origin	0	1	0	1	2/2

Legend: 0 (score 0); 1 (scores 1–100); 2 (scores 101–200), and 3 (scores 201–300).

partial extraction and/or displacing of this ganglioside from cells, similar to previous studies [21]. Consequently, methanol and acetone should be excluded as fixatives in the detection of NeuGcGM3 because both solubilize this ganglioside to different extents.

On the other hand, paraformaldehyde is one of the most common and adequate fixatives used in the immunolocalization of gangliosides [7, 8]. It is known that paraformaldehyde is a polymerization product of formaldehyde and to prevent its formation, formalin solutions usually contain different percentages of methanol (10–15%). Here, we obtained an intense reactivity of 14F7 Mab, mainly located in the membrane of P3X63Ag.653 cells after both 4% paraformaldehyde and 4% neutral-buffered formalin (NBF) fixations. These results permit to consider that the low percentage of methanol present in the final solution of NBF is not able to be removed NeuGcGM3 from cells. In this way, our data also could support the use of NBF fixation in the immunodetection of NeuGcGM3 ganglioside.

In addition, some authors have suggested that the routine tissues processing do not extract or damage the antigenic carbohydrate determinants of gangliosides [22]. Curiously, fixation and postfixation with ethanol only induce a partial extraction and/or damage of NeuGcGM3 ganglioside from the P3X63Ag.653 myeloma cells. These results are suggestive that carbohydrate determinant recognized by 14F7 probably resists the formalin fixation and the ethanol tissues processing, permitting its detection in this kind of samples. In line with this, the expression of NeuGcGM3 and NeuGcGDla gangliosides in formalin-fixed and paraffin-embedded tissues using GMR8 Mab by immunohistochemical and TLC immunostaining methods has been recently demonstrated [23].

Aberrant and elevated expression of some gangliosides has been previously demonstrated on the surface of lymphoid derived tumors [24, 25]. In previous studies, GM3 was the predominant ganglioside found in pre-B lymphoma cells and B-cell neoplasms using over-pressured thin-layer chromatography (OPTLC) followed by scanning densitometry and high performance thin layer chromatography (HPTLC) and immune thin layer chromatography (ITLC), respectively. Nevertheless, these studies have been restricted to gangliosides containing the N-acetylated variant of sialic acid (NeuAc) [24, 25].

In the present work, we reported for the first time the tissue reactivity of the 14F7 Mab, a highly specific IgGl against the N-glycolylated variant of GM3 ganglioside, in a variety of lymphoid tumors not related with the histopathological typing, but not in normal tissues. The pattern of staining of 14F7 was finely granular, homogeneous, and mainly located in cell membrane of malignant lymphocytes, similar to that observed in preceding reports in other tumor localizations [10, 14–17].

The expression of the N-glycolylated variant of sialic acid (NeuGc) forming the structure of gangliosides and/or other glycoconjugates (Hangnutziu-Deicher antigen, HD) in humans has been considered as a tumor-associated antigen [26]. Normal cells are capable to synthetize the sialic acid N-acetylneuraminic acid but not N-glycolylneuraminic acid (as a result of a deletion in the cytidine monophospho-N-acetylneuraminic acid hydroxylase gene). The aberrant expression of NeuGc residues in humans has been related to the metabolic incorporation from red meat and dairy products in the diet due to the altered metabolism of malignant cells [27–29]. However, some authors have reported an alternative pathway to the NeuGc synthesis from other intermediates of cellular metabolism in some human tumors [27]. The expression of NeuGc also triggers the immune responses to the nonhuman sialic acid, which is the mechanism of the "serum sickness" reaction previously described as HD antibodies [30, 31]. These HD antibodies were found to react with NeuGc bound to horse serum glycoconjugates and were then discovered in the serum and tissues of patients with cancer [30] and in activated and malignant immune cells [32].

The expression of heterophile HD antigen on the cell surface of both leukemia and malignant lymphoma was evidenced by membrane immunofluorescence staining with chicken antiserum against NeuGcGM3 and fluorescein-conjugated rabbit anti-chicken IgG [26]. The aberrant expression of NeuGc forming part of human lymphoma glycosphingolipids using gas chromatography-mass spectrometry had been also demonstrated [33]. Moreover, the expression of HD antigen in both pathologic sera and extracts of cancer tissues from lymphoma and leukemia had been previously detected by means of inhibition of agglutination of bovine erythrocytes by HD antibodies [30]. However, in other studies, no serum antibodies against HD antigen were detected in patients bearing lymphomas [34].

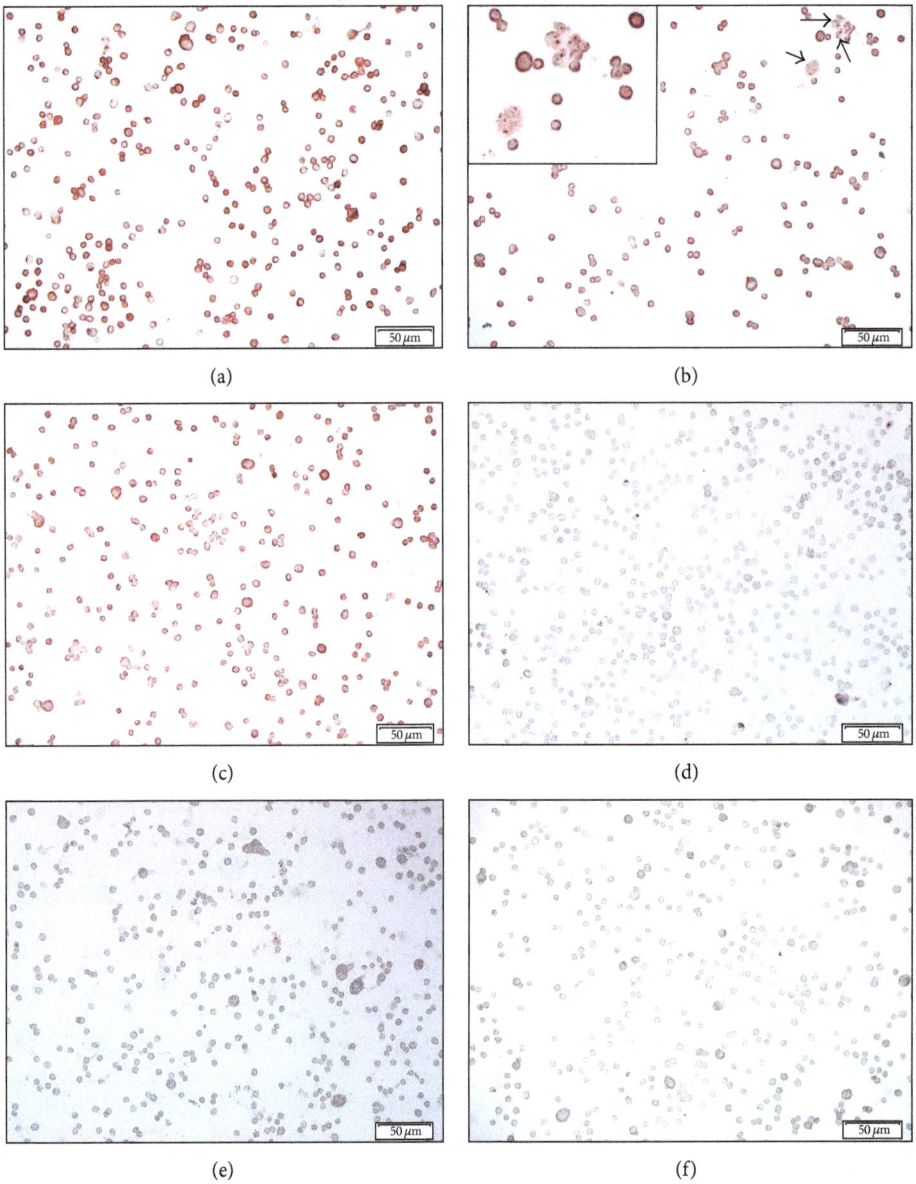

Figure 1: Microphotographs of the 14F7 Mab reactivity in P3X63Ag.653 cell line after different fixation protocols. An intense, homogeneous, and finely granular reactivity of 14F7 Mab was observed in cells fixed with 4% neutral-buffered formaldehyde (a). Observe: both the slight diminishing in the intensity of reaction and the appearance of cells with a grosser granular staining mainly located in the cytoplasm after fixation with acetone (b) (black arrows). Inset on the upper-left corner, 400x magnification. The 14F7 Mab staining was only partially diminished after fixation with ethanol (c) while, the reactivity with this Mab was significantly removed in cells fixed and postfixed with methanol (d and e, resp.). No immunoreaction was detected in cells incubated with 1E10 Mab (negative control) (d). White bar = 50 μm.

Additionally, we found the recognition of 14F7 Mab in most of lymph node metastasis of some primary tumors such as colonic and gastric adenocarcinoma, cutaneous malignant melanoma, breast tumors, and lung carcinoma. A preliminary study of the 14F7 Mab staining in cutaneous and subcutaneous metastasis of melanoma and other metastasis was also showed. Similar pattern of immunostaining and percentages of positive cells were obtained by our group in the corresponding primary malignancies [10, 14–16]. In previous reports, the 14F7 Mab was able to intensely stain cells of metastatic lymph nodes of cutaneous malignant melanoma [9, 14]. Moreover, another Mab (P3), reported by our group, binds to several NeuGc containing gangliosides and also reacts with sulfated glycolipids showed a positive staining in lymph node metastasis of breast tumors [7]. Interestingly, specific therapies anti-NeuGcGM3 ganglioside using molecular cancer vaccines have shown promising results in patients bearing lymph node metastasis of breast tumors and cutaneous malignant melanoma [35–37]. In this way, although in some cases the number of metastasis samples

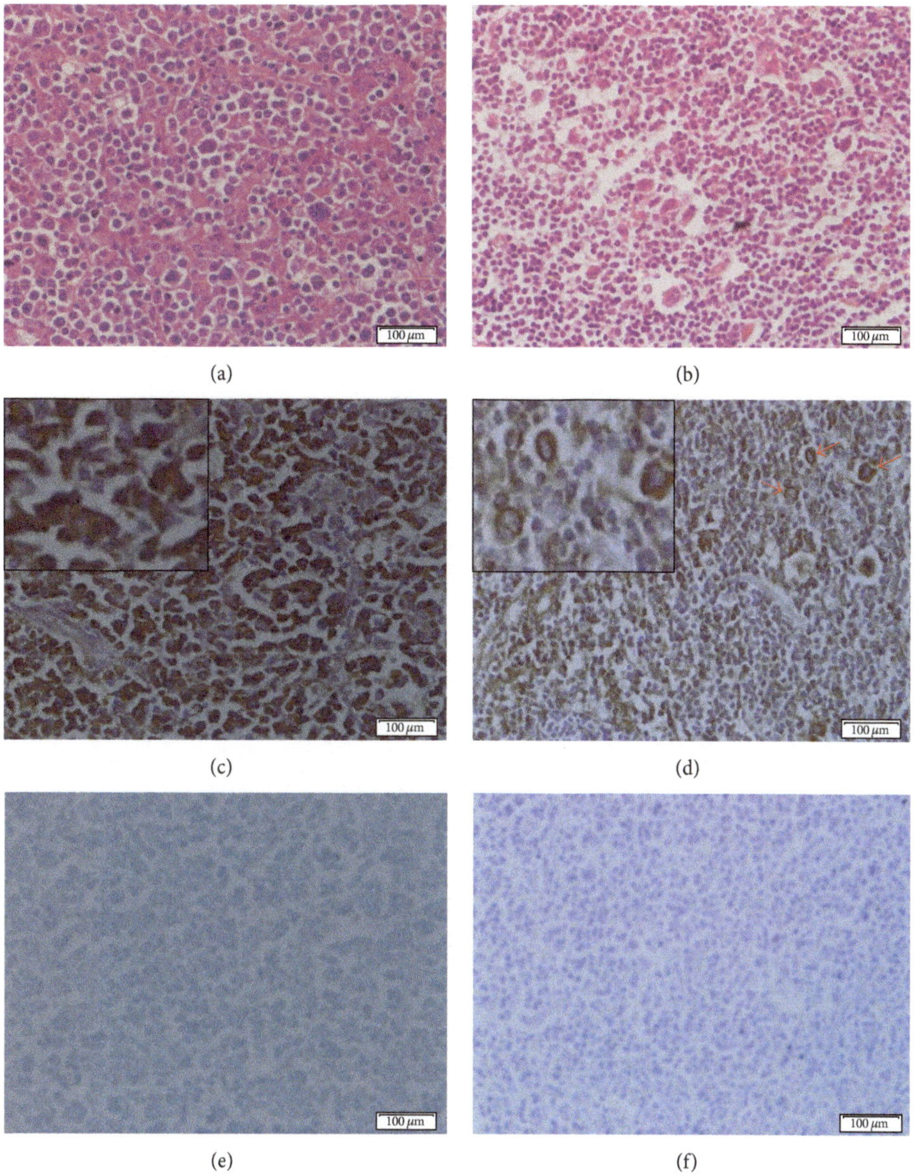

FIGURE 2: Microphotographs of the 14F7 Mab reactivity in human lymphoma. (a) and (b): Hematoxylin and eosin staining of diffuse large B-cell lymphoma and nodular sclerosis classical Hodgkin lymphoma, respectively. (c) and (d): Immunostaining with 14F7 Mab. Note: the intense reactivity of 14F7 Mab in both the cell membrane and cytoplasm of both malignant B lymphocytes (c) and Hodgkin cells (d) (red arrows). Inset on the upper-left corner, 400x magnification. (e) and (f): Negative controls. Observe: the absence of staining. White bar = 100 μm.

is small, it would be interesting to extent the evaluation of NeuGcGM3 expression in these malignancies in order to assess its potential use as target for immunotherapy.

On the other hand, gangliosides can be actively shed from the cell surface of malignant cells and taken up by other cells by insertion of their lipid anchors into the membrane [38]. In addition, shedding of immunosuppressive gangliosides to the tumor microenvironment has been reported to be an important characteristic of human malignancies [39]. These circulating gangliosides are potentially involved in tumor-host interactions contributing to cancer progression [40] and metastasis through tumor immune escape [41].

Here, it was observed a reactivity of 14F7 Mab in the cell membrane of normal lymphocytes localized around both metastatic breast carcinoma cells of axillary lymph nodes and metastatic colon adenocarcinoma cells of local lymph nodes (Figures 3(b) and 4(b), red arrows). It is known that sentinel lymph nodes are the first nodes to receive lymphatic drainage from a primary tumor and the preferential site of initial tumor metastasis. These lymph nodes are intensively exposed to the bioactive products of tumor cells and other associated cells [42]. Increased tumor-derived NeuGcGM3 ganglioside in sentinel lymph nodes have been suggested to directly influence coordinated interactions between DC

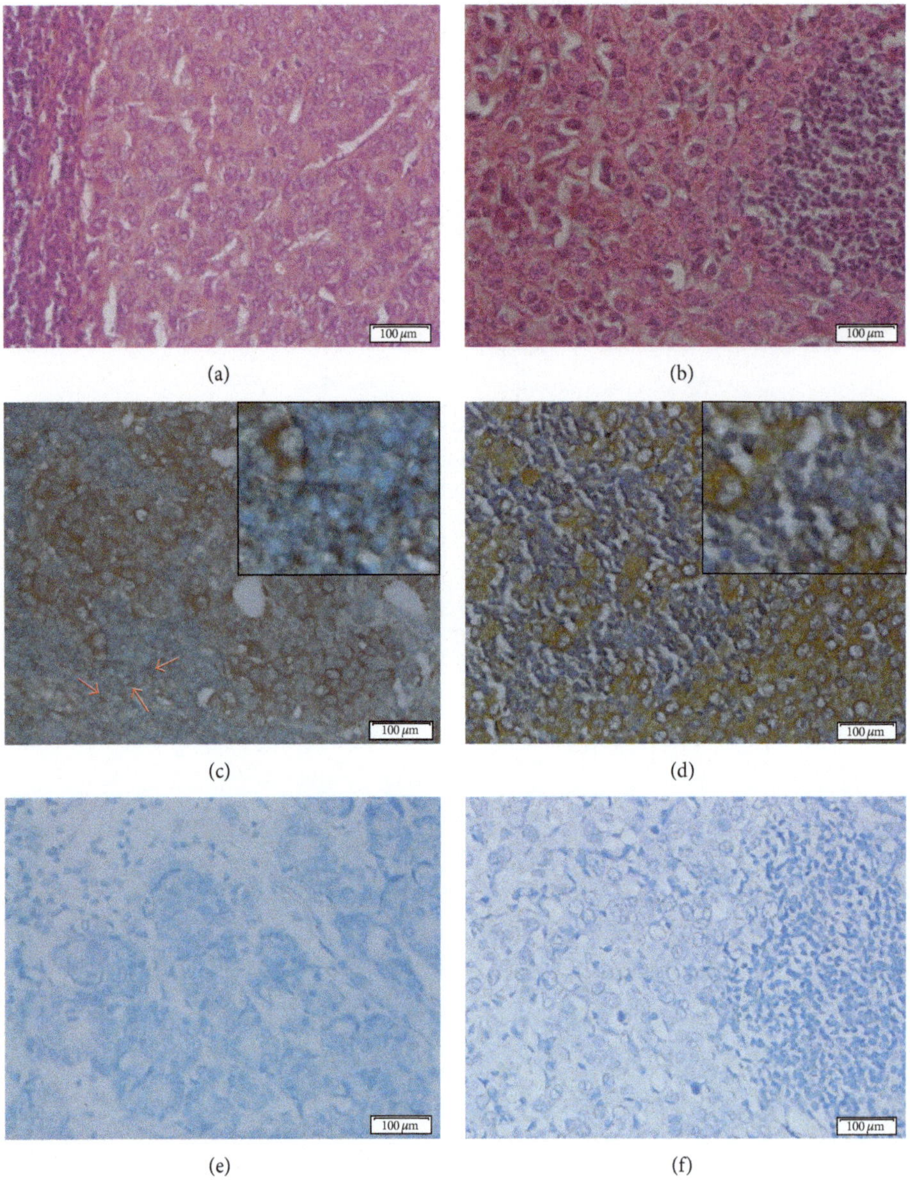

FIGURE 3: Microphotographs of the 14F7 Mab reaction in lymph node metastasis. (a) and (b): Hematoxylin and eosin staining of lymph node metastasis of breast ductal and lobular adenocarcinomas, respectively. (c) and (d): Immunostaining with 14F7 Mab. Observe: an intense reaction of 14F7 Mab located in both cell membrane and cytoplasm of malignant epithelial cells. See: an intense immunostaining in lymphocytes of tumor adjacent areas (c) (red arrows). Inset on the upper-right corner, 400x magnification. Note: the absence of reactivity in peritumoral lymphocytes (d). (e) and (f): Negative controls. Observe: the lack of staining. White bar = 100 μm.

and both helper and regulatory $CD4^+$ T cells abrogating an anti-tumor-specific immune response [41]. In this way, our results seem to be in agreement with the potential shedding of NeuGcGM3 ganglioside by metastatic epithelial cells in secondary lymphoid organs as well as with its incorporation to the cell membrane of peritumoral lymphocytes.

Finally, we showed the ability of 14F7 murine Mab to directly kill the NeuGcGM3-positive murine myeloma cells without participation of complement. This Mab, after binding to NeuGcGM3, significantly induced the appearance of a subpopulation with increased cell size and internal complexity measured by flow cytometry. In addition, a decreasing in the tumor cell viability in a dose-dependent manner using the staining with PI was also observed in this subpopulation. Similar results had been previously reported [20, 43]. Nevertheless, the selection of patients to any anti-NeuGcGM3 specific therapies has been usually based on the tissue reactivity of the 14F7 murine Mab, which is typically used only for diagnostic purposes. It is known that therapy with murine-derived Mabs is limited by their tendency to develop human anti-mouse antibodies response (HAMA), the relatively short half-life of the Mabs

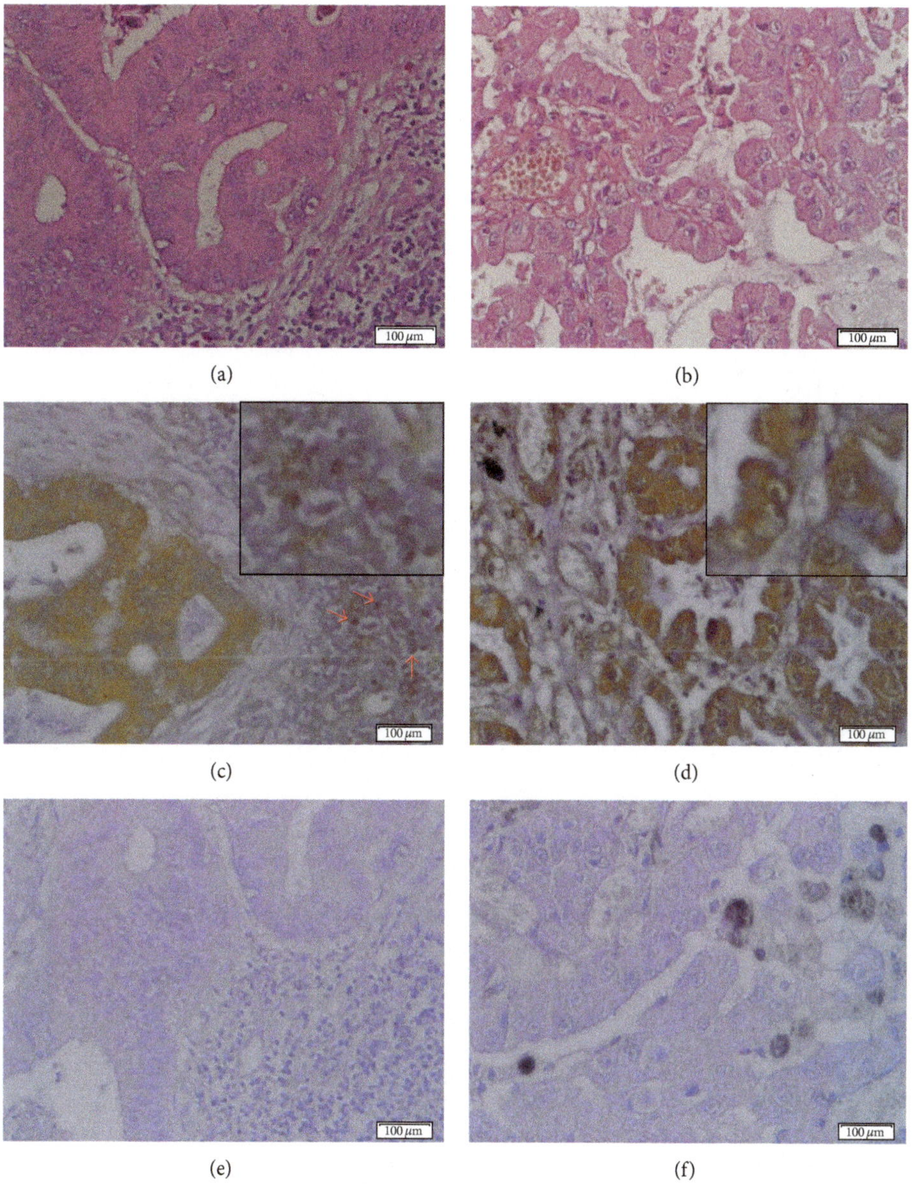

FIGURE 4: Microphotographs of the 14F7 Mab staining in lymph node metastasis. (a) and (b): Hematoxylin and eosin staining of lymph node metastasis of colonic and lung adenocarcinomas, respectively. (c) and (d): Immunoreactivity of the 14F7 Mab. Observe: an intense reaction of 14F7 Mab located in both cell membrane and cytoplasm of malignant epithelial cells. See: a moderate immunostaining in lymphocytes of tumor adjacent areas (red arrows). Inset on the upper-right corner, 400x magnification. (e) and (f): Negative controls. Observe: the lack of staining. White bar = 100 μm.

and the limited ability of murine Fc to activate human immune mechanisms [44]. For that reason, in the last few years, a chimeric and humanized variant of 14F7 Mab were developed in our center. The resulting recombinant Mabs exhibited a similar ability to bind NeuGcGM3 and to induce complement- independent cytotoxicity as compared with the murine counterpart [20, 45]. In this sense, 14F7 Mab becomes a useful tool to identify tumors that could be sensitive to anti-NeuGcGM3 specific therapies, including passive immunotherapy using a chimeric and/or the humanized version of this Mab.

5. Conclusions

In summary, we reported the tissue reactivity of 14F7 Mab in both primary and secondary malignancies of lymphoid system. Evidence that probably support the potential resistance of the antigenic determinant recognized by 14F7 to formalin fixation and tissues processing were also showed. In addition, the capacity of 14F7 Mab to induce complement-independent cytotoxicity in a myeloma-derived cell line after binding NeuGcGM3 was demonstrated. Our data could support the possible use of NeuGcGM3 as target for both active

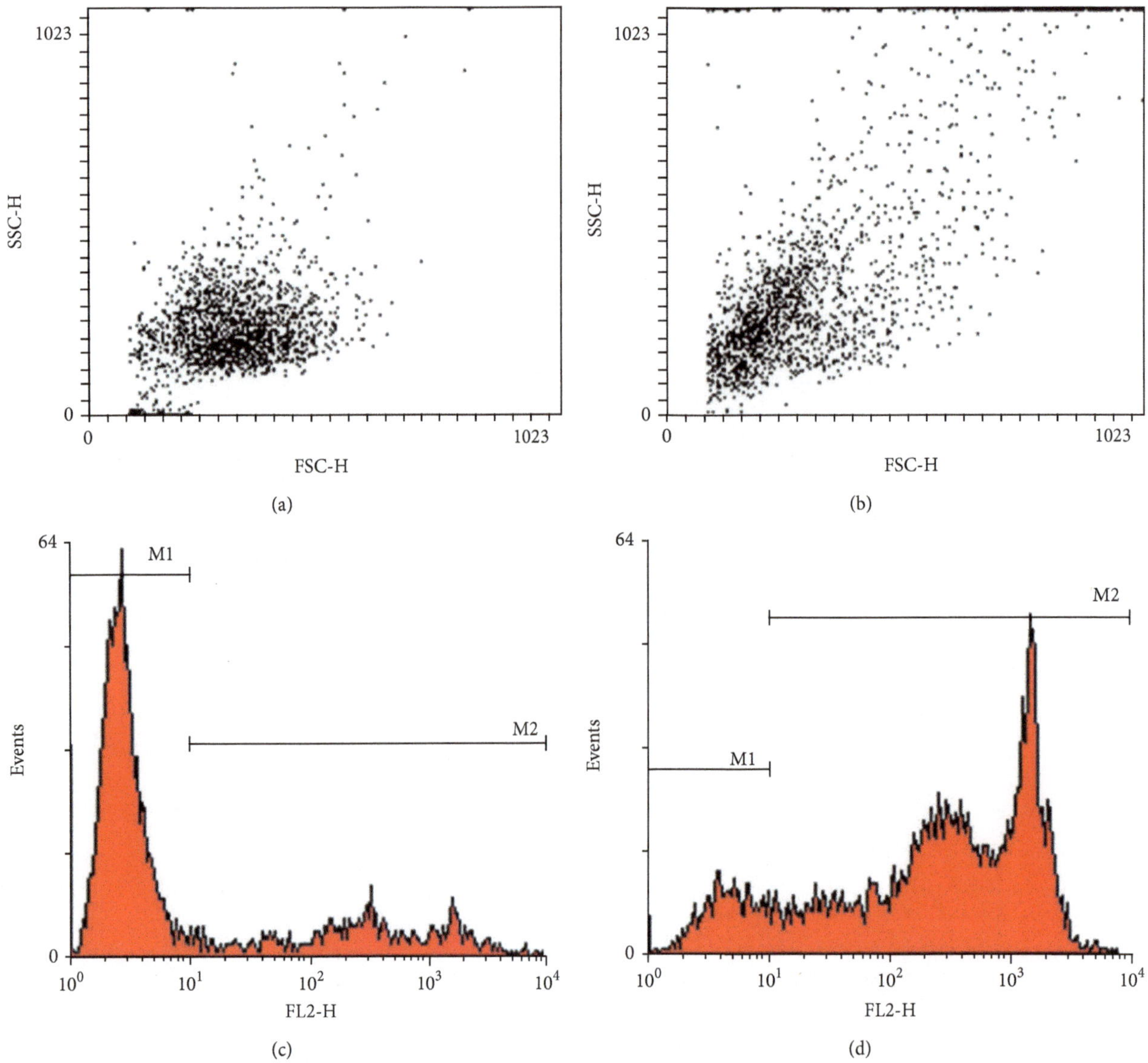

FIGURE 5: Representative flow cytometric profiles of complement-independent cytotoxicity of 14F7 Mab in the murine myeloma derived cell line, P3X63Ag.653. (a) and (b): Dot plots graphs. Correlated measurements of FSC-H (cell-surface area or size) and SSC-H (cell granularity or internal complexity) permit to detect changes in the light scattering properties of cells. Observe: a homogeneous population of cells treated with P3 Mab (irrelevant control) (a). The treatment with 14F7 Mab altered the morphology of P3X63Ag.653 cells, characterized by changes in cell size and granularity based on both FSC-H and SSC-H parameters analysis (b). (c) and (d): Histogram graphs showing the discrimination of viable (M1) and nonviable (M2) cells using the propidium iodide (PI) staining. These graphs correspond to (a) and (b), respectively. Nonviable cells uptake this dye fluorescing brightly in the red range of the visible color spectrum (FL2-H). A limited fraction of P3X63Ag.653 cells showed a positive staining with PI after incubation with P3 Mab (M2 region). Note: the dramatic decreasing in the cell viability after treatment with 14F7 Mab.

and passive immunotherapy of malignancies expressing this molecule. Moreover, our results permit to consider the use of 14F7 murine Mab to identify lymphoid tumors that could be sensitive to anti-NeuGcGM3 specific therapies. Experiments in order to evaluate the recognition of 14F7 Mab in human leukemia are ongoing by our group.

Conflict of Interests

The authors declare that there is no conflict of interests.

Authors' Contribution

Rancés Blanco and Damián Blanco equally contributed to this work.

Acknowledgment

Financial support was provided by the Center of Molecular Immunology.

References

[1] A. M. El-Sayed, M. H. El-Borai, A. A. Bahnassy, and S. M. S. El-Gerzawi, "Flow cytometric immunophenotyping (FCI) of lymphoma: correlation with histopathology and immunohistochemistry," *Diagnostic Pathology*, vol. 3, no. 1, article 43, 2008.

[2] D. Berthold and M. Ghielmini, "Treatment of malignant lymphoma," *Swiss Medical Weekly*, vol. 134, no. 33-34, pp. 472–480, 2004.

[3] J. Weng, S. Rawal, F. Chu et al., "TCL1: a shared tumor-associated antigen for immunotherapy against B-cell lymphomas," *Blood*, vol. 120, no. 8, pp. 1613–1623, 2012.

[4] E. L. Walk and S. A. Weed, "Recently identified biomarkers that promote lymph node metastasis in head and neck squamous cell carcinoma," *Cancers*, vol. 3, no. 1, pp. 747–772, 2011.

[5] G. DiSibio and S. W. French, "Metastatic patterns of cancers: results from a large autopsy study," *Archives of Pathology and Laboratory Medicine*, vol. 132, no. 6, pp. 931–939, 2008.

[6] T. Yamashita, R. Wada, T. Sasaki et al., "A vital role for glycosphingolipid synthesis during development and differentiation," *Proceedings of the National Academy of Sciences of the United States of America*, vol. 96, no. 16, pp. 9142–9147, 1999.

[7] A. M. Vazquez, M. Alfonso, B. Lanne et al., "Generation of a murine monoclonal antibody specific for N-glycolylneuraminic acid-containing gangliosides that also recognizes sulfated glycolipids," *Hybridoma*, vol. 14, no. 6, pp. 551–556, 1995.

[8] A. Carr, A. Mullet, Z. Mazorra et al., "A mouse IgG1 monoclonal antibody specific for N-glycolyl GM3 ganglioside recognized breast and melanoma tumors," *Hybridoma*, vol. 19, no. 3, pp. 241–247, 2000.

[9] M. Osorio, E. Gracia, E. Rodríguez et al., "Heterophilic NeuGcGM3 ganglioside cancer vaccine in advanced melanoma patients: results of a phase Ib/IIa study," *Cancer Biology and Therapy*, vol. 7, no. 4, pp. 488–495, 2008.

[10] R. Blanco, E. Rengifo, M. Cedeño, C. E. Rengifo, D. F. Alonso, and A. Carr, "Immunoreactivity of the 14F7 Mab raised against N-Glycolyl GM3 ganglioside in epithelial malignant tumors from digestive system," *ISRN Gastroenterology*, vol. 2011, Article ID 645641, 8 pages, 2011.

[11] H. van Cruijsen, M. Ruiz, P. van der Valk, T. D. de Gruijl, and G. Giaccone, "Tissue micro array analysis of ganglioside N-glycolyl GM3 expression and signal transducer and activator of transcription (STAT)-3 activation in relation to dendritic cell infiltration and microvessel density in non-small cell lung cancer," *BMC Cancer*, vol. 9, article 180, 2009.

[12] A. M. Scursoni, L. Galluzzo, S. Camarero et al., "Detection of N-glycolyl GM3 ganglioside in neuroectodermal tumors by immunohistochemistry: an attractive vaccine target for aggressive pediatric cancer," *Clinical and Developmental Immunology*, vol. 2011, Article ID 245181, 6 pages, 2011.

[13] A. M. Scursoni, L. Galluzzo, S. Camarero et al., "Detection and characterization of N-glycolyated gangliosides in Wilms tumor by immunohistochemistry," *Pediatric and Developmental Pathology*, vol. 13, no. 1, pp. 18–23, 2010.

[14] R. Blanco, E. Rengifo, C. E. Rengifo, M. Cedeño, M. Frómeta, and A. Carr, "Immunohistochemical reactivity of the 14F7 monoclonal antibody raised against N-glycolyl GM3 ganglioside in some benign and malignant skin neoplasms," *ISRN Dermatology*, vol. 2011, Article ID 848909, 8 pages, 2011.

[15] R. Blanco, M. Cedeño, X. Escobar et al., "Immunorecognition of the 14F7 Mab raised against N-Glycolyl GM3 ganglioside in some normal and malignant tissues from genitourinary system," *ISRN Pathology*, vol. 2011, Article ID 953803, 10 pages, 2011.

[16] R. Blanco, C. E. Rengifo, M. Cedeño, M. Frómeta, E. Rengifo, and A. Carr, "Immunoreactivity of the 14F7 MAb (raised against N-glycolyl GM3 ganglioside) as a positive prognostic factor in non-small cell lung cancer," *Pathology Research International*, vol. 2012, Article ID 235418, 12 pages, 2012.

[17] R. Blanco, Y. Quintana, D. Blanco et al., "Tissue reactivity of the 14F7 MAb raised against N-glycolyl GM3 ganglioside in tumors of neuroectodermal, mesodermal and epithelial origin," *Journal of Biomarkers Journal of Biomarkers*, vol. 2013, Article ID 602417, 9 pages, 2013.

[18] Y. Zhong, Y. Wu, C. Li et al., "N-Glycolyl GM3 ganglioside immunoexpression in oral mucosal melanomas of Chinese," *Oral Diseases*, vol. 18, no. 8, pp. 741–747, 2012.

[19] A. M. Vázquez, A. Pérez, A. M. Hernández et al., "Syngeneic anti-idiotypic monoclonal antibodies to an anti-NeuGc-containing ganglioside monoclonal antibody," *Hybridoma*, vol. 17, no. 6, pp. 527–534, 1998.

[20] L. Roque-Navarro, K. Chakrabandhu, J. de León et al., "Anti-ganglioside antibody-induced tumor cell death by loss of membrane integrity," *Molecular Cancer Therapeutics*, vol. 7, no. 7, pp. 2033–2041, 2008.

[21] A. Schwarz and A. H. Futerman, "Determination of the localization of gangliosides using anti-ganglioside antibodies: comparison of fixation methods," *Journal of Histochemistry and Cytochemistry*, vol. 45, no. 4, pp. 611–618, 1997.

[22] D. F. Alonso, "A novel hydrophobized GM3 ganglioside/Neisseria meningitidis outer-membrane-protein complex vaccine induces tumor protection in B16 murine melanoma," *International Journal of Oncology*, vol. 15, no. 1, pp. 59–66, 1999.

[23] N. Hayashi, H. Chiba, K. Kuronuma et al., "Detection of N-glycolyated gangliosides in non-small-cell lung cancer using GMR8 monoclonal antibody," *Cancer Science*, vol. 104, no. 1, pp. 43–47, 2013.

[24] N. Anh-Tuan, J. Pick, A. Mod, and S. R. Hollan, "Gangliosides in acute myeloid leukaemia (AML) and non-Hodgkin's lymphoma (NHL)," *European Journal of Cancer and Clinical Oncology*, vol. 22, no. 8, pp. 1003–1007, 1986.

[25] K. P. O'Boyle, K. Freeman, A. Kalisiak, A. Agregado, and D. A. Scheinberg, "Patterns of ganglioside expression in B cell neoplasms," *Leukemia and Lymphoma*, vol. 21, no. 3-4, pp. 255–266, 1996.

[26] H. Higashi, Y. Nishi, Y. Fukui et al., "Tumor-associated expression of glycosphingolipid Hanganutziu-Deicher antigen in human cancers," *Gann*, vol. 75, no. 11, pp. 1025–1029, 1984.

[27] Y. N. Malykh, R. Schauer, and L. Shaw, "N-glycolylneuraminic acid in human tumours," *Biochimie*, vol. 83, no. 7, pp. 623–634, 2001.

[28] P. Tangvoranuntakul, P. Gagneux, S. Diaz et al., "Human uptake and incorporation of an immunogenic nonhuman dietary sialic acid," *Proceedings of the National Academy of Sciences of the United States of America*, vol. 100, no. 21, pp. 12045–12050, 2003.

[29] M. Bardor, D. H. Nguyen, S. Diaz, and A. Varki, "Mechanism of uptake and incorporation of the non-human sialic acid N-glycolylneuraminic acid into human cells," *The Journal of Biological Chemistry*, vol. 280, no. 6, pp. 4228–4237, 2005.

[30] T. Nishimaki, K. Kano, and F. Milgrom, "Hanganutziu-Deicher antigen and antibody in pathologic sera and tissues," *Journal of Immunology*, vol. 122, no. 6, pp. 2314–2318, 1979.

[31] H. Higashi, M. Naiki, S. Matuo, and K. Okouchi, "Antigen of "serum sickness" type of heterophile antibodies in human sera: identification as gangliosides with N-glycolylneuraminic acid," *Biochemical and Biophysical Research Communications*, vol. 79, no. 2, pp. 388–395, 1977.

[32] D. H. Nguyen, P. Tangvoranuntakul, and A. Varki, "Effects of natural human antibodies against a nonhuman sialic acid that metabolically incorporates into activated and malignant immune cells," *Journal of Immunology*, vol. 175, no. 1, pp. 228–236, 2005.

[33] T. Kawai, A. Kato, H. Higashi, S. Kato, and M. Naiki, "Quantitative determination of N-glycolylneuraminic acid expression in human cancerous tissues and avian lymphoma cell lines as a tumor-associated sialic acid by gas chromatography-mass spectrometry," *Cancer Research*, vol. 51, no. 4, pp. 1242–1246, 1991.

[34] E. G. Kanduma, J. C. Mukuria, and O. W. Mwanda, "Serum total sialic acid and Hanganutziu-Deicher antibody in normals and in cancer patients," *East African Medical Journal*, vol. 84, no. 5, pp. 207–214, 2007.

[35] A. Carr, E. Rodríguez, M. D. C. Arango et al., "Immunotherapy of advanced breast cancer with a heterophilic ganglioside (NeuGcGM3) cancer vaccine," *Journal of Clinical Oncology*, vol. 21, no. 6, pp. 1015–1021, 2003.

[36] M. Osorio, E. Gracia, E. Reigosa et al., "Effect of vaccination with N-glycolyl GM3/VSSP vaccine by subcutaneous injection in patients with advanced cutaneous melanoma," *Cancer Management and Research*, vol. 4, pp. 341–345, 2012.

[37] K. Pérez, M. Osorio, J. Hernández, A. Carr, and L. E. Fernández, "NGcGM3/VSSP vaccine as treatment for melanoma patients," *Human vaccines and immunotherapeutics*, vol. 9, no. 6, pp. 1237–1240, 2013.

[38] G. Lauc and M. Heffer-Lauc, "Shedding and uptake of gangliosides and glycosylphosphatidylinositol-anchored proteins," *Biochimica et Biophysica Acta*, vol. 1760, no. 4, pp. 584–602, 2006.

[39] R. McKallip, R. Li, and S. Ladisch, "Tumor gangliosides inhibit the tumor-specific immune response," *Journal of Immunology*, vol. 163, no. 7, pp. 3718–3726, 1999.

[40] S. Birklé, G. Zeng, L. Gao, R. K. Yu, and J. Aubry, "Role of tumor-associated gangliosides in cancer progression," *Biochimie*, vol. 85, no. 3-4, pp. 455–463, 2003.

[41] J. de León, A. Fernández, M. Clavell et al., "Differential influence of the tumour-specific non-human sialic acid containing GM3 ganglioside on $CD4^{+}CD25^{-}$ effector and naturally occurring $CD4^{+}CD25^{+}$ regulatory T cells function," *International Immunology*, vol. 20, no. 4, pp. 591–600, 2008.

[42] A. J. Cochran, R. Huang, J. Lee, E. Itakura, S. P. L. Leong, and R. Essner, "Tumour-induced immune modulation of sentinel lymph nodes," *Nature Reviews Immunology*, vol. 6, no. 9, pp. 659–670, 2006.

[43] A. Carr, C. Mesa, M. D. C. Arango, A. M. Vázquez, and L. E. Fernández, "In vivo and in vitro anti-tumor effect of 14F7 monoclonal antibody," *Hybridoma and Hybridomics*, vol. 21, no. 6, pp. 463–468, 2002.

[44] A. Zhiqiang, "Antibody Therapeutics—a mini review," *Trends in Bio/Pharmaceutical Industry*, vol. 2, pp. 24–29, 2008.

[45] Y. Fernández-Marrero, L. Roque-Navarro, T. Hernández et al., "A cytotoxic humanized anti-ganglioside antibody produced in a murine cell line defective of N-glycolylated-glycoconjugates," *Immunobiology*, vol. 16, no. 12, pp. 1239–12347, 2001.

25

Histopathological Audit of 373 Nononcological Hysterectomies in a Teaching Hospital

Kanwardeep Kaur Tiwana, Sarita Nibhoria, Tanvi Monga, and Richa Phutela

Department of Pathology, GGS Medical College Faridkot, BFHUS, Punjab 151203, India

Correspondence should be addressed to Kanwardeep Kaur Tiwana; kanwardeepjhajj@gmail.com

Academic Editor: Phillip Ruiz

Hysterectomy, the most common gynecological surgery, provides a definitive cure to various diseases like DUB (dysfunctional uterine bleeding), leiomyoma, adenomyosis, chronic pelvic pain, prolapse, and malignancy. However, with advent of effective medical and conservative treatment modalities for nononcological causes it is now posing question mark on justification of hysterectomy. Therefore, an audit is required to assess the correlation between preoperative diagnosis and histopathological examination of specimen for justification of the procedure. In this study over period of one year (April 2013 to March 2014) 373 hysterectomies specimens were received in the department of pathology for nononcological causes. The age of patients ranged from 22 to 85 years with mean 45 ± 9.2 years. All cases were divided into five categories on the basis of age and audit was done. In this study the most common finding was leiomyoma (43.7%) followed by adenomyosis (19.3%). Almost 50% of hysterectomies causes were justified as preoperative diagnosis matched with histopathology. Cohen kappa statistics were used to measure agreement between preoperative and postoperative histopathological diagnosis which was found to be fair with κ value being 0.36. This study highlights that regular audit of surgeries can help improve quality of health care services and provide safe conservative option to patients.

1. Introduction

Hysterectomy means removal of uterus. Since early twentieth century it is considered definite treatment of various pelvic pathologies like leiomyoma, dysfunctional uterine bleeding (DUB), chronic pelvic pain, endometriosis, adenomyosis, prolapse, and malignancies [1]. In fact it is the second most frequently performed major surgical procedure in females all over the world next to cesarean section [2].

However, with emergence of effective medical and conservative treatment for benign conditions it is now posing a question mark regarding the justification of hysterectomy [3]. An audit is required as hysterectomy is associated with life time risk of 20–35% and this procedure would be unwarranted if not originally indicated [4–6]. According to Magon et al. hysterectomy is a surgery which has been used and misused, underused, and abused at different times in gynecology [7]. This study highlights correlation between indications of hysterectomy and histopathological evaluation of hysterectomy specimens. We want to stress on fact that uterus should not be considered for child bearing purposes only, as after hysterectomy females suffer from various psychosexual dysfunctions.

The aim of audit is to evaluate criteria based justification of hysterectomy and to analyze correlation of preoperative diagnosis with final histopathology report of all hysterectomies done in a teaching hospital. In India, very few hysterectomy audits have been published recently and this audit may provide baseline comparison with future studies.

2. Materials and Methods

This study involved all the patients who underwent hysterectomy for nononcological reasons in teaching hospital over a span of one year during period of April, 2013, to March 31, 2014. All elective as well as emergency hysterectomies (including obstetric hysterectomies) were analyzed excluding oncological hysterectomies.

Abdominal hysterectomies included subtotal hysterectomies, total abdominal hysterectomies (TAH), TAH with unilateral salpingoopherectomy, or TAH with bilateral salpingoopherectomy along with vaginal hysterectomies. In this study all indications were reviewed with special attention given to cases with age less than 30 years and in those cases where there was more than one indication. Preoperative indications were compared with histopathological report. Preoperative indications were recorded from the histopathological requisition form; however, if indication was not mentioned then direct communication was done with the concerned clinician. Hysterectomy was considered justified if pathology report verified the indication for surgery or had significant pathology. Statistical analyses were done using Cohen Kappa scale for calculation of agreement between preoperative and postoperative diagnosis and kappa value was calculated.

Gross evaluation of all specimens received in the department of pathology was done. Following parameters were recorded, that is, weight, measurements from fundus to ectocervix, cornu to cornu, and anterior to posterior. Length and diameter of cervix were measured from side to side and from anterior to posterior lip. Systematic evaluation of each component of uterus was done. Serosa was examined to see any powder burn spots for endometriosis mainly on posterior aspect. Next cervix was evaluated for any lacerations, scars, ulcers, cysts, or any mass. Using probe the uterus was incised into two halves and longitudinal sections were done on cervix at an interval of 0.2-0.3 cm and were fixed in 10% formalin. After which evaluation of transformation zone and stroma was done. Thickness of endometrium was measured, considering the age of patient if it was found to be >2 mm in postmenopausal female then whole slice was processed to rule out hyperplasia and any focus of malignant transformation. Lastly myometrium was examined with serial sections of 0.5 cm then corpus and lower uterine segment, recording maximum myometrial thickness, intramural leiomyomas, and adenomyosis. Posterior wall was specifically examined for adenomyosis as it is the common site for this pathology appearing as trabeculations or small hemorrhagic cysts. Leiomyomatous uterus was the most frequently encountered pathology. Number and size of leiomyomas were recorded with their locations. Representative sampling was done; however, if size of leiomyoma >5 cm then they were extensively sampled, that is, one section each for centimeter of tumour particularly from areas of hemorrhage and necrosis. Adnexa was examined separately particularly for foci of endometriosis or any other lesions. If no lesions were grossly identified then standard sections of uterus from endometrium, myometrium, cervix, serosa, lower uterine segment, and adnexa were examined.

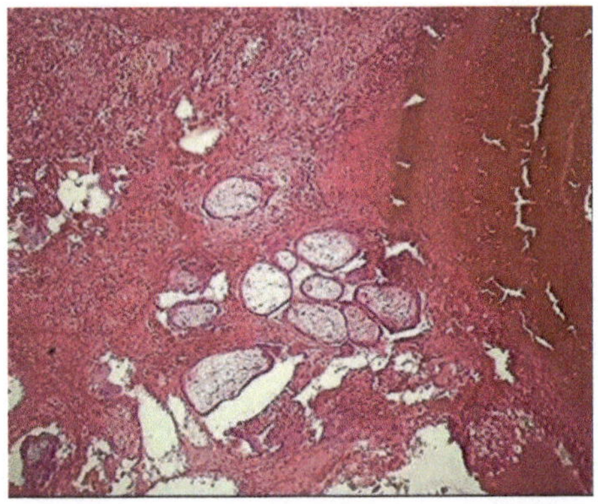

Figure 1: Sections show chorionic villi embedded in myometrium (H&E ×100).

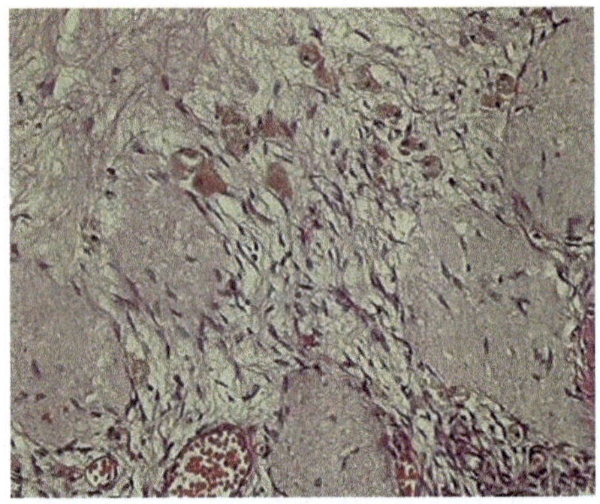

Figure 2: Sections from ovary shows collections of hemosiderin laden macrophages—endometriosis (H&E ×450).

3. Results

In this study a total number of cases were 373 over the span of one year (during April, 2013, to March 31, 2014). The patient age ranged from 22 to 85 years with mean 45 ± 9.2 years (median 45.2 years). An audit of hysterectomies was done with correlation of histopathological examination and preoperative clinical diagnosis. Of all 373 cases received leiomyoma (43.7%) was the most common pathology followed by adenomyosis (19.3%). But significant finding was absence of any pathology in 20.1% of all cases (Table 1). Age wise audit was done by dividing into five categories: 1st ≤ 30 years, 2nd 31–40 years, 3rd 41–50 years, 4th 51–60 years, and 5th ≥ 60 years (Table 2).

In the first category of age ≤30 years, a total number of hysterectomies were 18 (4.8%). All were TAH (total abdominal hysterectomies) without removal of adnexa. The preoperative indications in 11/18 (61.1%) were emergency obstetrical causes like placenta previa, placenta increta and placenta accreta (Figure 1), thus justifying all cases. However, in 7/18 (38.9%) the clinical diagnosis did not correlate with histopathological examination report as six had clinical diagnosis of chronic pelvic pain and one had unhealthy cervix. On histopathological examination 4/7 had leiomyoma but it was not clinically suspected and it is of no indication for hysterectomy in this particular age group.

In second category of age group 31–40 years, a total number of hysterectomies were 116 out of which 25/116 (21.6%) were TAH and 91/116 (78.4%) were TAH with bilateral salpingoopherectomy. In 91 cases of TAH with BSO only 2/91 (2.2%) had endometriosis (Figure 2) whereas the rest, that is, 97.8% ovaries, had no pathology; thus, their removal was not justified. In this category 1/116 was due to obstetrical reason

TABLE 1: Distribution of various pathologies on hysterectomies.

S. number	Histopathological diagnosis	Number and percentage
1	Leiomyoma	163 (43.7%)
2	Adenomyosis	72 (19.3%)
3	Prolapse	31 (8.3%)
	Simple endometrial hyperplasia	15 (4%)
4	Obstetrical causes	12 (3.2%)
5	Endometriosis	2 (0.5%)
6	CIN 1	2 (0.5%)
7	Endometritis	1 (0.26%)
8	No pathology	75 (20.1%)

TABLE 2: Distribution of hysterectomies.

Age group	Type of hysterectomy	Indications with percent distributions
≤30 years	TAH (18)	11/18 (61.1%) obstetrical causes 7/18 (38.9%) no pathology
31–40 years	TAH (25) TAH with salpingoopherectomy (91)	63/116 (54.3%) leiomyoma 45/116 (38.7%) adenomyosis 3/116 (2.6%) simple endometrial hyperplasia 2/116 (1.7%) endometriosis 2/116 (1.7%) no pathology 1/116 (0.8%) obstetrical cause
41–50 years	TAH (17) TAH with salpingoopherectomy (156)	100/173 (57.8%) leiomyoma 10/173 (6%) simple endometrial hyperplasia 2/173 (1.1%) CIN-1 61/173 (35.1%) no pathology
51–60 years	Vaginal hysterectomy (15) TAH with salpingoopherectomy (35)	15/50 (30%) prolapse 27/50 (54%) adenomyosis 2/50 (4%) simple endometrial hyperplasia 1/50 (2%) endometritis 5/50 (10%) no pathology
>60 years	Vaginal hysterectomy (3) TAH with salpingoopherectomy (13)	3/16 (18.7%) prolapse 13/16 (81.3%) prolapse

and 3/116 (2.6%) had simple endometrial hyperplasia which was an incidental histopathological diagnosis as there was no clinical suspicion. Two main pathologies in this group were leiomyoma (54.3%) followed by adenomyosis (38.7%).

In third category of age group 41–50 years had maximum cases, that is, 173 out of which 17 were TAH and rest TAH with bilateral salpingoopherectomy. The most common histopathological diagnosis was leiomyoma 100/173 (57.8%) (Figure 3). It was noted that in 51% of these 100 cases clinicians suspected leiomyoma whereas the rest made preoperative diagnosis of prolapse, DUB, unhealthy cervix and chronic pelvic pain. 10/173 (0.6%) cases had histopathological diagnosis of simple endometrial hyperplasia but the important thing is that in none of the cases clinical diagnosis was made.

Also in 2/173 cases CIN 1 (cervical intraepithelial neoplasia) was seen and it is known that hysterectomy is not the first treatment modality for it and various alternative options as there.

Fourth category of age group 51–60 years had total 50 cases out of which 15/50 (30%) were vaginal hysterectomies and rest TAH with bilateral salpingoopherectomy. All vaginal hysterectomies were done for prolapse which was justified. In three cases of clinical preoperative diagnosis of pyometra turned out to be endometrial hyperplasia (4%) (Figure 4) and endometritis (2%) (Figure 5). In this category adenomyosis was the most common diagnosis (54%) and it was incidental finding on histopathology.

In the last category >60 years total number of cases were 16 and 13/16 were TAH with bilateral salpingoopherectomy. All hysterectomies (vaginal and TAH with bilateral salpingoopherectomy) were for prolapse. But in this category almost all hysterectomies were justified and preoperative diagnosis matched with histopathological report.

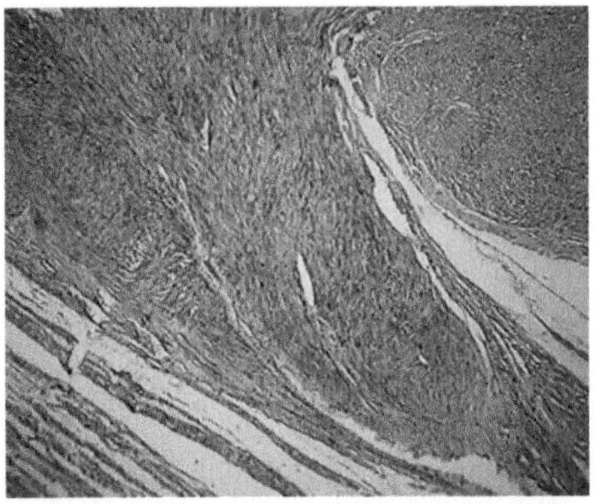

FIGURE 3: Section shows leiomyoma (H&E ×100).

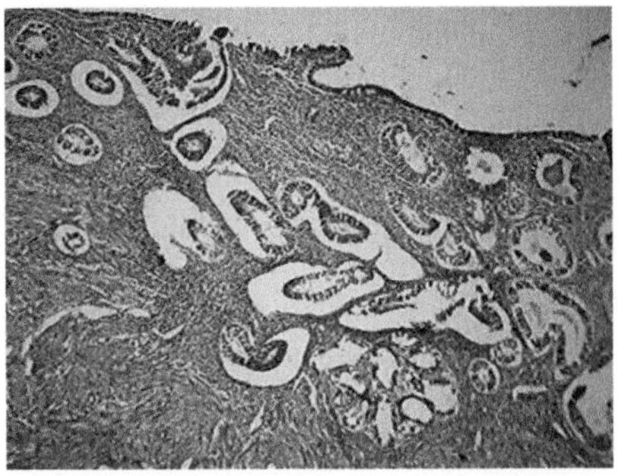

FIGURE 4: Sections show simple endometrial hyperplasia (H&E ×100).

Cohen kappa statistics were used to measure agreement between preoperative and postoperative histopathological diagnosis which was found to be fair with κ value being 0.36.

4. Discussion

Hysterectomy is the most common gynecological surgery in the world [8]. It provides definitive cure to many diseases like DUB, leiomyoma, adenomyosis, endometriosis, pelvic inflammatory disease, prolapse, and malignancy [8]. It remains a matter of debate owing to physical, emotional, economics, sexual, and medical significance to women [9]. In a study conducted in USA by Broder et al. indications for nononcological and nonemergency hysterectomy were found to be inappropriate [10]. Several questions about the indications, probable overuse, and justification of hysterectomy have been raised. Thus evaluation of appropriateness of hysterectomy should be integral part of audit. The system of reviewing preoperative diagnosis and histopathological report provide an efficient means of quality assurance and the appropriateness of surgery. This study emphasizes the need for regular audit of indications of hysterectomy with pathological findings which can help recognize malpractice and lacunae in the knowledge of health care provider.

In the present study over the period of one year 373 hysterectomies were done for nononcological causes. All different types of hysterectomy procedures were followed with

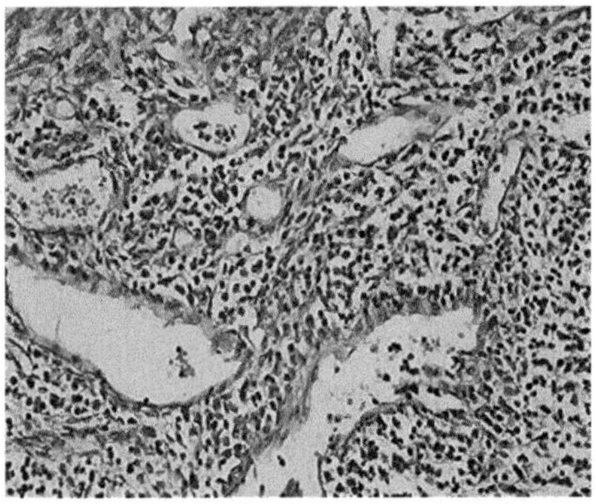

FIGURE 5: Section shows endometritis (H&E ×450).

most common being TAH with bilateral salpingoopherectomy 295/373 (79%) followed by TAH 60/373 (16%) and vaginal hysterectomy 18/373 (5%). This was in concordance with various studies which had almost same percentages [3, 11].

The patient age ranged from 22 to 85 years with mean 45 ± 9.2 years and median being 45.2 years. This is similar to study done by Gupta et al. where mean age was 45.6 years [8]. Age wise distribution of all 373 cases showed that ≤30 years age group had 18 hysterectomies out of which 11/18 were due to obstetrical reasons but 7/18 were totally unjustified. Similar findings were seen in a study done by Pandey et al. [3]. But they stressed upon the fact that hysterectomies could have been avoided by disseminating awareness among peripheral centers for early referral of high risk obstetric cause and with conservative approach.

The most common indication in all four categories, that is, 31–85 years, was leiomyomas which is in agreement with various other studies [12, 13]. But in more than 50% cases the provisional preoperative diagnosis was DUB. In this study, there were many findings which were missed preoperatively like adenomyosis and endometrial (simple and atypical). This is in concordance with findings of study done by Siwatch et al. [14].

Only few studies have done an audit by comparison of preoperative diagnosis with histopathological examination of specimens. In India no national statistics are available except for few studies where they pointed out 7-8% of rural women and 5% of urban women had undergone hysterectomy at an age of 37 years [15].

There is a concern regarding misuse of hysterectomy which is highlighted in this study where the most common diagnosis was leiomyoma (43.7%), followed by adenomyosis (19.3%), but only half the cases of leiomyoma were made preoperatively whereas adenomyosis was totally missed out. This is in concordance with study done by Miller where only 50% of preoperative diagnosis was confirmed on histopathology [16]. Also authors want to stress upon the fact of unnecessary removal of ovaries when no pathology is suspected, as it hastens up menopause and affects psychosexual health of female. Significant number of cases 75/373 (20%) with no histopathological finding was found thus questioning the preoperative indication of procedure.

This study wants to highlight the fact that reporting of all hysterectomies should be made mandatory and audit results should be used for improvement in quality of health services. As any surgical procedure hysterectomy is also associated with risk factors, thus indications should be carefully evaluated. Thus implementing targeted actions and conservative therapy for benign gynecological conditions should be effective alternatives to hysterectomies.

5. Conclusion

Hysterectomy is one of the most common gynecological surgeries. In one-year analysis of all cases it was found that preoperative diagnosis and histopathological correlation could reduce the number of hysterectomies as in many cases conservative approach could have been followed. Thus we conclude by saying that regular audit can help improve quality of health care services and provide safe conservative option to patients.

Conflict of Interests

The authors declare that there is no conflict of interests regarding the publication of this paper.

References

[1] F. Nausheen, J. Iqbal, F. A. Bhatti, A. T. Khan, and S. Sheikh, "Hysterectomy: the patient's perspective," *Annals of Gynecology*, vol. 10, pp. 339–341, 2004.

[2] J. M. Wu, M. E. Wechter, E. J. Geller, T. V. Nguyen, and A. G. Visco, "Hysterectomy rates in the United States, 2003," *Obstetrics and Gynecology*, vol. 110, no. 5, pp. 1091–1095, 2007.

[3] D. Pandey, K. Sehgal, A. Saxena, S. Hebber, J. Nambiar, and R. Bhat, "An audit of indications, complications and justification of hysterectomy at a tertiary hospital in India," *International Journal of Reproductive Medicine*, vol. 2014, Article ID 279273, 6 pages, 2014.

[4] K. Sait, M. Alkhattabi, A. Boker, and J. Alhashemi, "Hysterectomy for benign conditions in a university hospital in Saudi Arabia," *Annals of Saudi Medicine*, vol. 28, no. 4, pp. 282–286, 2008.

[5] K. Spilsbury, J. B. Semmens, I. Hammond, and A. Bolck, "Persistent high rates of hysterectomy in Western Australia: a population-based study of 83 000 procedures over 23 years," *BJOG*, vol. 113, no. 7, pp. 804–809, 2006.

[6] I. Z. MacKenzie, C. Naish, M. Rees, and S. Manek, "1170 consecutive hysterectomies: indications and pathology," *Journal of the British Menopause Society*, vol. 10, no. 3, pp. 108–112, 2004.

[7] N. Magon, H. Divakar, and A. Kirpalni, "The use, misuse, and abuse of hysterectomy," *Journal of Mid-Life Health*, vol. 4, no. 1, p. 1, 2013.

[8] G. Gupta, D. S. Kotasthane, and V. D. Kotasthane, "Hysterectomy: a clinico-pathological correlation of 500 cases," *Internet Journal of Gynecology and Obstetrics*, vol. 14, no. 1, 2009.

[9] N. Magon and M. Chahuan, "Editorial. Subtotal Hysterectomy: has it come a full circle?" *International Journal of Clinical Cases and Investigations*, vol. 4, pp. 1–4, 2012.

[10] M. S. Broder, D. E. Kanouse, B. S. Mittman, and S. J. Bernstein, "The appropriateness of recommendations for hysterectomy," *Obstetrics & Gynecology*, vol. 95, no. 2, pp. 199–205, 2000.

[11] A. Toma, W. M. Hopman, and R. H. Gorwill, "Hysterectomy at a Canadian tertiary care facility: results of a one year retrospective review," *BMC Women's Health*, vol. 4, article 10, 2004.

[12] E. Abe and L. O. Omo-Aghoja, "A decade of hysterectomy in a tertiary hospital in urban Niger-delta region of Nigeria," *Nigerian Journal of Clinical Practice*, vol. 11, no. 4, pp. 359–363, 2008.

[13] P. L. Leung, S. W. Tsang, and P. M. Yuen, "An audit on hysterectomy for benign diseases in public hospitals in Hong Kong," *Hong Kong Medical Journal*, vol. 13, no. 3, pp. 187–193, 2007.

[14] S. Siwatch, R. Kundu, H. Mohan, and A. Huria, "Histopathological audit of hysterectomy specimen in a tertiary care hospital," *Sri Lanka Journal of Obstetrics and Gynaecology*, vol. 34, pp. 155–158, 2012.

[15] S. Desai, T. Sinha, and A. Mahal, "Prevalence of hysterectomy among rural and urban women with and without health insurance in Gujarat, India," *Reproductive Health Matters*, vol. 19, no. 37, pp. 42–51, 2011.

[16] N. F. Miller, "Hysterectomy; therapeutic necessity or surgical racket?" *The American Journal of Obstetrics and Gynecology*, vol. 51, pp. 804–810, 1946.

Permissions

All chapters in this book were first published in PRI, by Hindawi Publishing Corporation; hereby published with permission under the Creative Commons Attribution License or equivalent. Every chapter published in this book has been scrutinized by our experts. Their significance has been extensively debated. The topics covered herein carry significant findings which will fuel the growth of the discipline. They may even be implemented as practical applications or may be referred to as a beginning point for another development.

The contributors of this book come from diverse backgrounds, making this book a truly international effort. This book will bring forth new frontiers with its revolutionizing research information and detailed analysis of the nascent developments around the world.

We would like to thank all the contributing authors for lending their expertise to make the book truly unique. They have played a crucial role in the development of this book. Without their invaluable contributions this book wouldn't have been possible. They have made vital efforts to compile up to date information on the varied aspects of this subject to make this book a valuable addition to the collection of many professionals and students.

This book was conceptualized with the vision of imparting up-to-date information and advanced data in this field. To ensure the same, a matchless editorial board was set up. Every individual on the board went through rigorous rounds of assessment to prove their worth. After which they invested a large part of their time researching and compiling the most relevant data for our readers.

The editorial board has been involved in producing this book since its inception. They have spent rigorous hours researching and exploring the diverse topics which have resulted in the successful publishing of this book. They have passed on their knowledge of decades through this book. To expedite this challenging task, the publisher supported the team at every step. A small team of assistant editors was also appointed to further simplify the editing procedure and attain best results for the readers.

Apart from the editorial board, the designing team has also invested a significant amount of their time in understanding the subject and creating the most relevant covers. They scrutinized every image to scout for the most suitable representation of the subject and create an appropriate cover for the book.

The publishing team has been an ardent support to the editorial, designing and production team. Their endless efforts to recruit the best for this project, has resulted in the accomplishment of this book. They are a veteran in the field of academics and their pool of knowledge is as vast as their experience in printing. Their expertise and guidance has proved useful at every step. Their uncompromising quality standards have made this book an exceptional effort. Their encouragement from time to time has been an inspiration for everyone.

The publisher and the editorial board hope that this book will prove to be a valuable piece of knowledge for researchers, students, practitioners and scholars across the globe.

List of Contributors

Neelam Sood
Department of Pathology, Deen Dayal Upadhyay Hospital, Hari Nagar, New Delhi 110066, India

Jitendra Singh Nigam
Department of Pathology, Saraswathi Institute of Medical Sciences, Anwarpur, Hapur, Uttar Pradesh 245304, India

Priyanka Bhatia Soni
Department of Pathology, Deen Dayal Upadhyay Hospital, Hari Nagar, New Delhi 110066, India

Anand Kumar Verma and Raj Kumar Chandoke
Department of Pathology, Employees' State Insurance Scheme of India (ESI) Hospital, Basaidarapur, New Delhi 110015, India

Jitendra Singh Nigam
Department of Pathology, Saraswathi Institute of Medical Sciences, Hapur, Uttar Pradesh 245304, India

Ganiyu Oboh, Ayokunle O. Ademosun, Adedayo O. Ademiluyi, Olasunkanmi S. Omojokun, Esther E. Nwanna and Kuburat O. Longe
Functional Foods and Nutraceuticals Unit, Biochemistry Department, Federal University of Technology, PMB 704, Akure 340252, Nigeria

SadiaMinhas
Department of Oral Pathology, Akhtar Saeed Medical and Dental College, Bahria Town, Lahore 54000, Pakistan

Muhammad Kashif
Department of Immunology, University of Health Sciences, Lahore, Pakistan

A. H. Nagi
Department of Morbid Anatomy and Histopathology, University of Health Sciences, Lahore, Pakistan

Bandana Sharma, Neetu Singh, Neena Gupta, Pavika Lal, Shefali Pande and Shashi Chauhan
Department of Obstetrics & Gynaecology, GSVMMedical College, Kanpur 208002, India

Joerg Schwock and William R. Geddie
Division of Anatomical Pathology, Department of Laboratory Medicine and Pathobiology, University of Toronto, Toronto General Hospital, Room E11-219, Toronto, ON, Canada M5G 2C4

Azadeh Andisheh Tadbir
Department of Oral and Maxillofacial Pathology, School of Dentistry, Shiraz University of Medical Sciences, Ghom Abad, Ghasrodasht Avenue, Shiraz 71956-15878, Iran

Bijan Khademi
Department of Otolaryngology, Khalili Hospital, Shiraz Institute for Cancer Research, Shiraz University of Medical Sciences, Shiraz 71348-45794, Iran

Mahyar Malekzadeh
Shiraz Institute for Cancer Research, Shiraz University of Medical Sciences, Shiraz 71348-45794, Iran

Maryam Mardani
Department ofOralMedicine, School of Dentistry, Shiraz University of Medical Sciences, GhomAbad, Ghasrodasht Avenue, Shiraz 71956-15878, Iran

Bahar Khademi
School of Dentistry, Shiraz University of Medical Sciences (International Branch), Azadi Square, Jahad Sazandegi Street, Shiraz 71447-16699, Iran

Payal Mehra and Anand Kumar Verma
Department Of Pathology, Employees State Insurance (ESI) Postgraduate Institute of Medical Sciences and Research and ESI Model Hospital, Basai Darapur, New Delhi 110015, India

Miroslav Sekulic
Department of Laboratory Medicine and Pathology, University of Minnesota, 420 Delaware Street SE, MMC 609 Mayo D185, Minneapolis, MN 55455, USA
Division of Nephrology, Department of Medicine, Harvard Medical School, Massachusetts General Hospital, 149 13th Street, Boston, MA 02129, USA

Simona Pichler Sekulic
University of Belgrade School of Medicine, Dr. Subotica 8, 11000 Belgrade, Serbia

Muhammad Kashif and A. H. Nagi
Department of Morbid Anatomy and Histopathology, University of Health Sciences, Lahore 54000, Pakistan

Muhammad Ishfaq
Oral & Maxillofacial Surgery Department, Nishtar Institute of Dentistry, Multan 60000, Pakistan

Neelam Sood, Jitendra Singh Nigam, Poonam Yadav, Shivani Rewri, Ankit Sharma, Anita Omhare and Jaya Malhotra
Department of Pathology, D.D.U. Hospital, Harinagar, New Delhi 110066, India

Anita Omhare
Department of Pathology, GSVM Medical College, Kanpur, Uttar pradesh 208012, India

Sanjeev Kumar Singh
Department of Pathology, M.L.B. Medical College, Jhansi, Uttar Pradesh 284128, India

Jitendra Singh Nigam
Department of Pathology, Saraswathi Institute of Medical Sciences, Anwarpur, Pilkhuwa, Hapur, Uttar Pradesh 245304, India

Ankit Sharma
Department of Pathology, D.D.U. Hospital, Harinagar, New Delhi 110066, India

Okechukwu A. Ibeanu and Teresa P. Díaz-Montes
Division of Gynecologic Oncology, Department of Gynecology and Obstetrics, The Kelly Gynecologic Oncology Service, The Johns Hopkins Medical Institutions, Baltimore, MD 21287, USA

Hayato Nakagawa
Department of Gastroenterology, University of Tokyo, 7-3-1 Hongo, Bunkyo-ku, Tokyo 113-8655, Japan
Laboratory of Gene Regulation and Signal Transduction, Departments of Pharmacology and Pathology, School of Medicine, University of California, La Jolla, CA 92093, USA

Shin Maeda
Department of Gastroenterology, Yokohama City University, 3-9 Fukuura, Kanazawa-ku, Yokohama 236-0004, Japan

Chitra Anandani and Rashmi Metgud
Department ofOral andMaxillofacial Pathology, Pacific Dental College and Hospital, PAHER University,Udaipur, Rajasthan 313024, India

Karanprakash Singh
Department of Public Health Dentistry, Genesis Institute of Dental Sciences and Research, Ferozepur, Punjab 152001, India

Jackie M. Wypij
Department of Veterinary Clinical Medicine, University of Illinois at Urbana-Champaign, HazelwoodDrive,Urbana, IL 61802, USA

Francesco Cetta
IRCCS MultiMedica, Viale Fantoli 16/15, 20138 Milan, Italy

Alpidio A. Boada-Sucre
Laboratorio deMicroscopía Electrónica, Centro de Estudios Biomédicos y Veterinarios, Instituto de EstudiosCientíficos y Tecnológicos, Universidad Nacional Experimental Simón Rodríguez, Caracas, Venezuela

Marcello Salvatore Rossi Spadafora
Unidad de Toxoplasmosis y Protozoosis, Departamento de Parasitología, Centro Nacional de Microbiología, Instituto de Salud Carlos III, Calle Alejandro Casona 7, Piso 6D, 28035 Madrid, Spain
Sección de Inmunohistoquímica y Microscopía Electrónica, Instituto Anatomopatológico "José A. O'Daly", Facultad de Medicina, Universidad Central de Venezuela, Caracas, Venezuela

LucindaM. Tavares-Marques
Grupo de Inmunobiología, Centro de Estudios Biomédicos y Veterinarios, Instituto de Estudios Científicos y Tecnológicos, Universidad Nacional Experimental Simón Rodríguez, Caracas, Venezuela

Héctor J. Finol
Centro de Microscopía Electrónica "Mitsuo Ogura", Facultad de Ciencias, Universidad Central de Venezuela, Caracas, Venezuela

Armando Reyna-Bello
Grupo de Inmunobiología, Centro de Estudios Biomédicos y Veterinarios, Instituto de Estudios Científicos y Tecnológicos, Universidad Nacional Experimental Simón Rodríguez, Caracas, Venezuela
Investigador Prometeo, Universidad de Las Fuerzas Armadas ESPE, Departamento de Ciencias de la Vida, Grupo de Investigación de Sanidad Animal y Humana (GISAH), Sangolquí, Ecuador

Valentina Cottignoli and Adriana Maras
Department of Earth Sciences, Sapienza University of Rome, Piazzale Aldo Moro 5, 00185 Rome, Italy

Elena Cavarretta
Department of Medical-Surgical Sciences and Biotechnologies, Sapienza University of Rome, Corso della Repubblica 79, 04100 Latina, Italy

Loris Salvador and Carlo Valfré
Division of Cardiac Surgery, San Bortolo Hospital, Viale Rodolfi 37, 36100 Vicenza, Italy

M. Santos and M. Gobernado
Arevalo Baca Street 3, 46010 Valencia, Spain

A. Gil-Brusola
Department of Microbiology, University Hospital La Fe, Avenida Campanar 21, 46009 Valencia, Spain

A. Escandell and M. Blanes
Infectious Diseases Unit, University Hospital La Fe, 46009 Valencia, Spain

Prajwal Boddu
Department of Internal Medicine, Advocate Illinois Masonic Medical Center, 836WestWellington Avenue, Chicago, IL 60657, USA

Vamsi Parimi
Department of Pathology, Loyola University Medical Center, 2160 S. 1st Avenue, Maywood, IL 60153, USA

Michale Taddonio
Department of Radiology, UC San Diego, 200West Arbor Drive, San Diego, CA 92103, USA

Joshua Robert Kane
Department of Anatomic Pathology, Feinberg School of Medicine, Northwestern University, 303 E. Chicago Ave., Chicago, IL 60611, USA

Anjana Yeldandi
Northwestern University, Chicago, IL, USA

André R. Greenidge, Kiana R. Hall, Ian R. Hambleton, Richelle Thomas, and R. Clive Landis
Edmund Cohen Laboratory For Vascular Research, Chronic Disease Research Centre, University of the West Indies, Cave Hill, Barbados

Dougald M. Monroe
Division of Hematology/Oncology, School of Medicine, University of North Carolina, Chapel Hill, NC, USA

Ilaria Peluso and Anna Raguzzini
Center of Nutrition, Council for Agricultural Research and Economics (CREA-NUT), Via Ardeatina 546, 00178 Rome, Italy

Rancés Blanco, Yisel Quintana, Mercedes Cedeño, Milagros Frómeta and Enrique Rengifo
Laboratory of Recognition and Biological Activity Assays, Department of Quality Control, Center of Molecular Immunology, P.O. Box 16040, 216 Street and 15 Avenue Atabey, Playa, 11600 Havana, Cuba

Damián Blanco and Xiomara Escobar
Department of Cell Biology and Tissues Banking, National Institute of Oncology and Radiobiology, 29 and F Street Vedado, Plaza de la Revoluci´on, 10400 Havana, Cuba

Charles E. Rengifo
Department of Pathology, Manuel Fajardo General Hospital, Zapata and D Street Vedado, Plaza de la Revolución, 10400 Havana, Cuba

Marta Osorio
Clinical Trials Unit, National Institute of Oncology and Radiobiology, 29 and F Street Vedado, Plaza de la Revolución, 10400 Havana, Cuba

Zailí Gutiérrez and Janet Lamadrid
Department of Pathology, National Institute of Oncology and Radiobiology, 29 and F Street Vedado, Plaza de la Revolución, 10400 Havana, Cuba

Adriana Carr
Research and Development Direction, Center of Molecular Immunology, P.O. Box 16040, 216 Street and 15 Avenue Atabey, Playa, 11600 Havana, Cuba

Kanwardeep Kaur Tiwana, Sarita Nibhoria, Tanvi Monga and Richa Phutela
Department of Pathology, GGSMedical College Faridkot, BFHUS, Punjab 151203, India

Index